Scientific Foundations of Sports Medicine

Scientific Foundations of Sports Medicine

CAROL C. TEITZ, M.D.

Associate Professor
Department of Orthopaedics
Acting Director
Division of Sports Medicine
University of Washington
Seattle, Washington

1989
B.C. Decker Inc • Toronto • Philadelphia

Contributors

GIDEON B. ARIEL, Ph.D.
President, Ariel Dynamics, Inc.,
Trabuco Canyon, California
Biomechanics

JACQUELINE R. BERNING, M.S., R.D.
Sports Nutritionist, Western Dairy Council,
Thornton, Colorado
Osteoporosis, Diet, and Exercise

GEORGE L. BRENGELMANN, Ph.D.
Professor, Physiology Department, University of Washington School of Medicine,
Seattle, Washington
Temperature Regulation

BARBARA J. DE LATEUR, M.D., M.S.
Professor, Department of Rehabilitation Medicine, University of Washington School of Medicine; Chief of Service, Department of Rehabilitation Medicine, Harborview Medical Center, Seattle, Washington
Muscle Strength and Local Endurance Training

JOHN P. FULKERSON, M.D.
Professor of Orthopaedic Surgery,
University of Connecticut School of Medicine; Director, Sport Injury and Knee Clinic, University of Connecticut Health Center,
Farmington, Connecticut
Structure and Function of Joints

PHILIP D. GOLLNICK, Ph.D.
Professor of Physiology, Department of Veterinary and Comparative Anatomy, Pharmacology, and Physiology, College of Veterinary Medicine, Washington State University, Pullman, Washington
Skeletal Muscle Physiology

GLEN A. HALVORSON, M.D.
Medical Director, Physical Medicine Clinic, Sport Training and Rehabilitation, Consultant, University of Arizona Department of Athletics, Team Physician, Santa Rita High School, and Past Chairman, Sports Medicine Special Interest Group AAPMR, Tucson, Arizona
Principles of Rehabilitating Sports Injuries

BRUCE J. MARTIN, Ph.D.
Associate Professor of Physiology, Medical Sciences Program, Indiana University School of Medicine, Bloomington, Indiana
Effect of Exercise on the Digestive System

LYLE J. MICHELI, M.D., F.A.C.S.M.
Associate Clinical Professor, Harvard Medical School; Director, Division of Sports Medicine, The Children's Hospital, Boston, Massachusetts
Pediatric and Adolescent Musculoskeletal Sports Injuries

STEPHEN G. RICE, M.D., Ph.D., M.P.H.
Lecturer, Division of Sports Medicine, Departments of Pediatrics and Orthopaedics, University of Washington School of Medicine; Clinic Director, Harborview Medical Center Sports Medicine Clinic, Seattle, Washington
Epidemiology and Mechanisms of Sports Injuries

BENGT SALTIN, M.D.
Professor of Physiology, August Krogh Institute, University of Copenhagen,
Copenhagen, Denmark
Skeletal Muscle Physiology

CHARLOTTE FEICHT SANBORN, Ph.D.
Assistant Professor of Exercise Physiology, Department of Sport Sciences, University of Denver, Denver, Colorado
Menstrual Dysfunction in the Female Athlete
Osteoporosis, Diet, and Exercise

ROBERT S. SCHWARTZ, M.D.

Associate Professor of Internal Medicine, University of Washington School of Medicine; Chief of Geriatric Medicine Section, Seattle Veterans Administration Medical Center, Seattle, Washington
Exercise and Energy Expenditure in the Treatment of Obesity

ROY J. SHEPHARD, M.D.(LOND), Ph.D., F.A.C.S.M.

Professor of Applied Physiology and Director, School of Physical and Health Education, University of Toronto; Consultant, Toronto Rehabilitation Center, Toronto, Ontario, Canada
Cardiovascular Aspects of Sports Medicine

RONALD E. SMITH, Ph.D.

Professor, Department of Psychology, University of Washington, Seattle, Washington
Competitive Stress and Young Athletes
The Psychology of "Mental Toughness": Theoretical Models and Training Approaches to Anxiety Reduction in Athletes

FRANK L. SMOLL, Ph.D.

Associate Professor, Department of Psychology, University of Washington, Seattle, Washington
Competitive Stress and Young Athletes
The Psychology of "Mental Toughness": Theoretical Models and Training Approaches to Anxiety Reduction in Athletes

CAROL C. TEITZ, M.D.

Associate Professor, Department of Orthopaedics, and Acting Director, Division of Sports Medicine, University of Washington School of Medicine, Seattle, Washington
Overuse Injuries

WILTZ W. WAGNER, Ph.D.

Associate Professor of Physiology and Anesthesiology, Indiana University School of Medicine, Indianapolis, Indiana
Osteoporosis, Diet, and Exercise

TONY G. WALDROP, Ph.D.

Assistant Professor, Department of Physiology and Biophysics, University of Illinois College of Medicine; Established Investigator, American Heart Association, Urbana, Illinois
Respiratory Responses and Adaptations to Exercise

Preface

How did I get this stress fracture? Why do I get diarrhea when I run? Is it better to train with high weights and low reps, or low weights and high reps? Should I use ice or heat? How can I improve my distance in the shot put? As we strive to improve athletic performance and medical care of athletes, we must take care not to base our recommendations on anecdote. This book provides current scientific knowledge in the disciplines that are an integral part of the practice of sports medicine. With this knowledge we can try to provide answers to these inquiries as well as recognize the missing pieces for which answers must be sought.

We must be forever vigilant and inquisitive, seeking clues to physiologic, biomechanical, and psychological aspects of performance and injury, seeking to understand nature's ways of responding to physical and psychological stress and injury. Only by so doing can we hope to discover better ways of improving performance without compromising the athlete's health, and better ways of treating our patients, ways based on firm scientific foundations.

Carol C. Teitz
Seattle, Washington

Contents

Section I
Introduction

Chapter 1
Epidemiology and Mechanisms of
Sports Injuries 3
   Stephen G. Rice

Section II
Systemic Components

Chapter 2
Cardiovascular Aspects of Sports
Medicine 27
   Roy J. Shephard

Chapter 3
Respiratory Responses and
Adaptations to Exercise 59
   Tony G. Waldrop

Chapter 4
Temperature Regulation 77
   George I. Brengelmann

Chapter 5
Menstrual Dysfunction in the
Female Athlete 117
   Charlotte F. Sanborn

Chapter 6
Osteoporosis, Diet, and Exercise 135
   Jacqueline R. Berning
   Charlotte F. Sanborn
   Wiltz W. Wagner

Chapter 7
Effect of Exercise on the
Digestive System 153
   Bruce J. Martin

Chapter 8
Exercise and Energy Expenditure in
the Treatment of Obesity 167
   Robert S. Schwartz

Section III
Musculoskeletal Components

Chapter 9
Skeletal Muscle Physiology 185
   Philip D. Gollnick
   Bengt Saltin

Chapter 10
Muscle Strength and Local
Endurance Training 243
   Barbara J. de Lateur

Chapter 11
Structure and Function of Joints 261
   John P. Fulkerson

Chapter 12
Biomechanics 271
   Gideon B. Ariel

Chapter 13
Overuse Injuries 299
   Carol C. Teitz

Chapter 14
Pediatric and Adolescent
Musculoskeletal Sports Injuries 329
  Lyle J. Micheli

Chapter 15
Principles of Rehabilitating
Sports Injuries 345
  Glen A. Halvorson

Section IV
Psychological Components

Chapter 16
Competitive Stress and
Young Athletes 375
  Frank L. Smoll
  Ronald E. Smith

Chapter 17
The Psychology of "Mental
Toughness": Theoretical Models
and Training Approaches to
Anxiety Reduction in Athletes 391
  Ronald E. Smith
  Frank L. Smoll

Index 403

Section I
Introduction

Chapter 1
Epidemiology and Mechanisms of Sports Injuries

STEPHEN G. RICE

EPIDEMIOLOGY

An *athletic injury* is a medical condition, resulting from athletic activity, that causes a limitation or restriction on participation in that activity, or for which medical treatment was received. Athletic injuries may stem from a single traumatic episode or from repeated overuse of a body part. For epidemiologic purposes, the inability to participate in a free, unrestricted manner defines athletic injury. The criteria for safe participation (and return to play following injury) include the ability to protect oneself during the sports activity.

The definition of injury thus hinges primarily on missed practices and games or participation in a limited fashion (no contact, no jumping, no cutting, etc.). A quarterback with laryngitis would be unable to participate, but no other team member would be affected by having this ailment. Likewise, by this narrow definition, a sprinter who falls and fractures his wrist after crossing the finish line during the last race of the day and who is able to participate without restriction the next day after his arm is x-rayed and casted would not be listed as "injured." For this reason, another aspect considered in defining an athletic injury is when a "sentinel event" occurs, i.e., an injury that is significant regardless of its impact on one's participation status.

When athletic injuries are studied for epidemiologic purposes, the sensitivity of the definition of injury is an important consideration. Some studies consider the status of the athlete at the end of the practice or game to determine whether a reportable injury has occurred.[1] They do not include the time loss resulting from the initial sideline examination and management. Any athlete who is able to return to play without restrictions prior to the end of the practice or game is *not* considered to have experienced a reportable injury. Some athletes may be taped or may use additional protective equipment, thus allowing unrestricted participation. In these cases, the need for ongoing medical evaluation or treatment may later qualify this episode as a reportable injury.

Other studies seek to eliminate minor or nuisance injuries from consideration.[2] Their less sensitive definition counts only those injuries that result in restriction or limitation the next time there is a game or practice. This usually means the next day, but such is not always the case. Athletes injured on Friday evenings in high school sports, for example, do not practice again until Monday. Similarly, athletes injured just prior to a holiday or vacation may not have their injuries counted.

The National Athletic Injury/Illness Reporting System (NAIRS), established during the 1970s, defined a *reportable injury* or illness as any condition causing cessation of an athlete's customary participation throughout the participation day following the day of onset.[3] NAIRS also created three categories to denote the severity of injury. Injuries causing less than 7 days of restriction are considered *minor*, those resulting in 7 to 21 days of time loss are considered *moderate*, and those injuries lasting longer than 21 days are termed *major*. Separate categories are maintained for death, quadriplegia or paralysis, and amputation.[2]

Many athletes participate despite injuries, because they are willing to accept a less than optimal physical condition as a criterion for return to play. In his long and glorious professional football career, Walter Payton missed only one game of almost 200, and he claims he could have played in that one, too. It is hardly conceivable that he played professional football for over a decade and never experienced an injury. Similarly, athletes with chronic overuse conditions try to continue playing rather than succumb to the need for treatment and rehabilitation. In order to be able to study the epidemiology of injury, it is imperative that a clear definition of injury be established and that standards for safe participation be determined.

Risk of Sports Participation

Virtually all physical activities and sports carry some risk of injury. Indeed, if total prevention of athletic injuries were the goal, elimination of sports would be the only appropriate solution. Injuries are an inevitable outcome of challenging competition; striving to push one's body to its limit entails the risk of exceeding that limit. Loss of control or facing forces greater than the body or body part can withstand frequently causes traumatic injury. Similarly, excessive training in hopes of maximizing performance may result in an overuse injury rather than in superior conditioning. Recognition that risk is always with us during physical activity and acceptance of that risk by the participants and organizers of the activities are key steps toward the prevention and management of injuries.

The goal in managing or controlling the risks associated with sports activity is to identify and quantify these risks and then to employ methods and techniques to minimize them. Risk may be assessed, predicted, or measured through careful epidemiologic studies that note the incidence or prevalence of injury in a given sport as well as the factors leading to or associated with such injury. By studying the occurrence of injuries, trends can be identified that may help in developing strategies to reduce the number of future injuries. In this light, reporting of near injuries or accidents may also be helpful.

The decision regarding the appropriateness of particular sports activities comes from balancing the risks against the benefits. If the benefits clearly outweigh the risks, then the activity is worthwhile; if the risks exceed the benefits, we may conclude that the activity is too dangerous to justify undertaking it.

Boxing has come under challenge by many organizations, including the American Medical Association, because of the object of the sport and the high risk of permanent brain damage.[4] At the high school level, this sport is not deemed to have adequate benefits to justify the risks. At the community (Golden Gloves), Olympic, and professional levels, boxing still enjoys great popularity among its advocates. The debate to ban boxing focuses directly on the benefits versus the risks.

Injury Reporting

Recognition

In order to gain knowledge about athletic injuries, it is necessary to record and report injuries. It is essential that those who report injuries be properly educated about terms and definitions of injury, what information to gather, and how to record this information on the appropriate forms. There must be completeness, uniformity, accuracy, and standardization of methodology to be able to make meaningful comparisons among different reporters of injuries. The reports must be submitted in a timely fashion to allow for collection, summarization, and analysis of the data.

Recognition of injuries is the critical first step in the process of reporting. Failure to recognize injuries, especially minor injuries, frequently accounts for wide differences in apparent injury rates among various studies. Those with the least amount of training in sports medicine usually miss minor injuries and report low rates of injury; those with the greatest experience and expertise generally report higher rates of injury (despite their superior knowledge and skills in the areas of prevention and management of injuries). This phenomenon often confuses the lay public, who are shocked to discover that an improvement of the athletic health care available to their athletes seems to result in more injuries than ever before!

Recognition of injuries is also a function of the attitude and sensitivity of the coach toward injuries. Many athletes are afraid to report injuries to their coach because of the anticipated negative response: anger, disappointment, or lack of concern. An athlete in pain who gets yelled at by a coach is unlikely to present future injuries to this person. This is especially true among "oldtime" coaches who are not aware of the many techniques available today to treat and rehabilitate injuries. They remember the "good old days" when "athletes were athletes"; they regale their players with stories about playing while hurt or how tough they were. These coaches view today's athletes who refuse to "play hurt" as weaklings. Another reason for a negative attitude toward injury among unknowledgeable coaches may be their inability to deal with the injuries properly or the lack of appropriate assistance of athletic trainers and team doctors. When the coach is the single individual responsible for the athletes playing the sport, he or she does not relish having the additional responsibility of recognizing, assessing, and providing first aid treatment for athletic injuries; to this person, it may be better never to know about an injury than to have to deal with it.

Other athletes refuse to accept the reality of being hurt and turn to denial. Unless a coach or trainer is perceptive in recognizing injuries, these injuries may go unnoticed until they inflict significant disability on the athlete's performance. Minor injuries, especially overuse injuries, when recognized early and treated effectively, may cause little or no time loss. When recognition is delayed, complete treatment and rehabilitation often take weeks.

The presence of an athletic trainer or a knowledgeable coach usually leads to a policy that all injuries, regardless of how minor they seem, must be reported. Although never happy to know that an athlete has been injured, the coach or trainer should thank the athlete for bringing this injury to his or her attention so that it can be handled promptly and properly. Because these individuals are aware and presumably equipped to deal with the management of injuries, early recognition and treatment lead to less overall "down time" and a healthier team performance. The knowledgeable coach and athletic trainer are willing to accept the fact that many insignificant "injuries" may pass before them for evaluation (perhaps from athletes simply seeking attention). These coaches and athletic trainers save their anger and disappointment for the athlete who fails to disclose an injury at the time of occurrence. Athletes who wait days or weeks before informing the coach or trainer of their injuries learn quickly that such behavior is unacceptable; the selfishness displayed by continuing to play when it may not be safe to do so and by denying valuable practice or game experience to those athletes who are fit for play is clearly not appreciated.

Data Collection

A data collection system must consider exactly what information is to be gathered and who will record the data. The forms utilized must be appropriate for the task. All reporters should be carefully educated, clearly understanding all terms and definitions. Completeness, accuracy, and uniformity are essential in conducting any injury study.

The research investigator must appreciate the motivation and willingness of the reporters when devising the study. A researcher or athletic trainer is far more likely to compile detailed information than a coach or even a physician (both of whom have other agendas). Many universities that participated in the NAIRS study assigned one student trainer for the entire year to complete the detailed injury form on each injury for that sport. The ease of data collection is a key determinant in conducting injury studies. In many studies, the initial recording of injuries by a coach, athlete, or doctor may trigger a second level of investigation by the research team, such as a follow-up of specific diagnoses or severe injuries.

The injury information generally desired includes the following: identification of time, place, and activity; participant identification; participant complaint; description of the accident or injury; mechanism of injury; medical diagnosis and disposition—treatment or rehabilitation program; nature of medical clearance and day of return to a conditioning program; and day of medical clearance for return to complete participation. These items provide data regarding the details of the injury.[2]

Study Design

The study design is critical in determining whether any meaningful information can be gathered and inferences drawn from the study. Is the protocol adequate to study the problem? How are athletes selected for inclusion in the study? Are these athletes a representative sample of the entire population? Did the athletes volunteer for the study or were they selected by others? Are there sufficient numbers of subjects or injuries to draw meaningful conclusions?

The two best techniques for ensuring quality studies are controlled studies and random allocation of eligible participants, preferably using a double-blind technique in which the researchers do not know which participants are in the treatment group and which are serving as controls.

Controlling for confounding variables is another hurdle to overcome when designing studies. The use of multivariate analysis has greatly improved the ability to reduce the impact of such variables and to yield meaningful research studies.[5]

Data Analysis and Display

Analysis and display of the data allow one to determine injury trends and to make comparisons among sports, schools, or regions of the country. Raw data, such as the number of injuries, may be misleading unless they are comparable to prior data or other current data. As an analogy, if one were to report 10 deaths in automobile highway accidents over a holiday weekend in each of two states, can it be concluded that the risk of death in the two states is identical? If the two states are California and Delaware, it cannot be. But if comparisons were made to the same holiday weekend in the same two states the previous year, then the data may be meaningful (as long as one assumes similar conditions and risks existed).

To establish injury rates, information regarding the total number of participants or the total amount of athletic exposures is also required. Risk is usually expressed in terms of athletic exposures (days or hours) or in terms of the number of participants involved in the activity. An athletic exposure, a unit of risk, is defined as "one athlete participating in one practice or contest, where he or she is exposed to the possibility of an athletic injury" (an opportunity to become injured through participation).[6] Data about the number of injuries give numerator information; data about the population at risk give denominator information. Rate data are expressed as the fraction of injuries per unit of participation or risk. The quality of the denominator often determines the accuracy and power of the data. However, some methods of analysis and display are much more accurate than others:

1. Injuries per 100 athletes per season are the most common units used to express injury rate data. Data collection problems are minimal. Count the number of injuries and participants participating during the season. Divide the injuries by the participants and multiply by 100. This method assumes that participants are counted in a standard way and that seasons are of the same length. It can produce misleading data unless all definitions are standardized.
2. Counting injuries per 1,000 athletic exposures is a more accurate method, but it requires checking attendance every day to record all absences. The data are more meaningful because the number of participants and the length of the season are no longer confounding factors. Count the num-

ber of injuries and sum the number of participants each day of the season. Divide the number of injuries by the total athletic exposures and multiply by 1,000. The assumption here is that each athletic exposure (practice or game) is comparable in length and risk of injury.
3. Injuries per 100,000 participants are usually reported from large studies in which the type of injury studied is well reported, but estimates of participants at risk must be made. What is the time span studied—a year, a lifetime?[2]

To appreciate the significance of these reporting techniques, consider the following example.

In a high school basketball tryout, 100 athletes turn out for basketball practice daily for 1 week (five turnouts). The coach selects 50 athletes to continue practicing. After a second week of five turnouts, 15 athletes are selected to the varsity roster and 15 to the junior varsity roster. The teams then compete for 12 weeks during the regular season, having five games or practices per week. The varsity team qualifies for playoffs, extending their season an additional 3 weeks (a total of 15 more games and practices). The athletes suffered 12 injuries during the preseason and regular season plus an additional three injuries during the playoffs. What is the injury rate for this basketball team?

According to the first method described above (injuries per 100 athletes per season), the number of injuries would be 15, but should the denominator be 30, 50, or 100 athletes? In fact, 100 athletes had an opportunity to be injured during the 17-week season but only 30 of those 100 participated for more than 2 weeks. Rational and reasonable arguments can be made for either choice. However, in order to compare injury experiences among different schools, it is necessary to be sure that everyone is reporting information on the same basis.

The rate, if the squad size is 30, would be 50 injuries per 100 athletes per season. If the squad size is 100, the rate would be 15 injuries per 100 athletes per season.

Is it appropriate to compare the injury rates of those schools that participated in postseason playoffs with those that did not? If the team had not qualified for the playoffs, the number of in-

TABLE 1–1 Data for Calculating Injuries per 1,000 Athletic Exposures

Week number	Athletes	Weekly exposures	Total exposures
1	100	500	500
2	50	250	250
3–14	30	150	1,800
			2,550 (subtotal)
15–17	15	75	225
			2,775 (total)

juries would have been only 12, yielding rates of 40 injuries per 100 athletes per season if the squad size was 30, and 12 injuries per 100 athletes per season if the squad size was 100.

With the second method listed above (injuries per 1,000 athletic exposures), the two confounding factors of number of participants and length of the season are eliminated by expressing the injury rate in terms of athletic exposures. The season can be presented as shown in Table 1–1 (assuming perfect attendance throughout the season).

The composition of the 2,775 athletic exposures is as follows:

1. 15 varsity athletes: 15 athletes × 17 weeks × 5 per week = 1,275
2. 15 junior varsity athletes: 15 athletes × 14 weeks × 5 per week = 1,050
3. 50 athletes cut first week: 50 athletes × 1 week × 5 per week = 250
4. 20 athletes cut second week: 20 athletes × 2 weeks × 5 per week = 200

The 450 athletic exposures accumulated by the 70 athletes who did not make the basketball team accounted for only 16.2 percent of the total of all athletic exposures for the sport. Thus, the following rates result:

1. Rate: 15/2,775 = 5.4 injuries per 1,000 athletic exposures (full season)
2. Rate: 12/2,550 = 4.7 injuries per 1,000 athletic exposures (regular season)
3. Rate: 3/225 = 13.3 injuries per 1,000 athletic exposures (postseason)

In the mid-1970s, football injury data from several studies were combined into a single table (Table 1–2). The conclusion from these

TABLE 1-2 Football Injuries/100 Athletes/Season

Level	Ages	Injury Rate
Youth[7-8]	8–10	1
	10–12	8
Jr. high school[8]	12–14	15
Sr. high school[9-14]	15–18	30–80
College[10-11]	19–23	100
Professional[15]	23+	133

data expressed as injuries per 100 athletes per season, was that injuries increased as the athletes became older and increased in maturity, size, and speed.

At first glance, the hypothesis appears to be supported by the numbers. At puberty, there is a sharp increase from less than 10 injuries per 100 athletes per season to 15 in junior high school and as high as 80 in high school. But if the length of the season is considered, the conclusions become less clear. Professional football has 16 regular season games and four preseason games plus the playoffs. College football has an 11-game season, a bowl game, and spring practice (with several scrimmages). High school football has eight or nine games plus playoffs. Junior high school football usually involves five or six games in a season. And how many days per week do the youth football teams meet to practice and play?

Injury reporting that provides a profile of information often makes it possible to compare the injury experiences of different teams and sports. Through the maintenance of a "daily injury report," which combines an attendance list with a record of those athletes unable to participate in an unrestricted manner, one can obtain sophisticated injury statistics (Fig. 1-1).

This author has developed an injury reporting system incorporating such a "daily injury report." Data from this report can be presented in a number of formats. Month-to-month statistics (Fig. 1-2), year-to-year comparisons of the same team (Fig. 1-3) and same-season comparisons with other teams (Fig. 1-4) help create perspective on the interpretation of the statistical information. By measuring the number of injuries and the time loss associated with each injury, injury rate and severity data can be calculated to provide an overview of the injury experience. Table 1-3 shows data from nearly 26,000 athletes from the 20 high schools that have been providing injury data during the past decade.

As the number of schools and teams providing injury data grows over the years, some frequent questions can be answered: Do boys' sports or girls' sports report more injuries? Are the alleged high-risk sports of football, wrestling, and gymnastics the sports with the highest number of injuries (frequency) and with the most significant injuries (severity)? Is the sport of soccer, heralded for its fitness and competitive aspects and offered as an alternative to football, a significantly safer sport than football? Is the lifetime activity of aerobic running (cross-country) relatively free of injuries?

Girls' sports report more injuries than boys' sports (see Table 1-3). In every sport in which boys and girls do the same activities (cross-country running, soccer, basketball, track, and swimming), the injury rates for girls are higher. The reasons for this difference are still under investigation.

The sport reporting the highest injury frequency and severity was girls' cross-country running. The fact that this noncontact endurance activity has more injuries than wrestling and football demonstrates that "overuse" injuries can be considerable in poorly conditioned, intensely training athletes. The injury rates in girls' soccer have risen steadily over the years while all other sports have shown decreasing rates in recent years. Both girls' and boys' soccer have relatively high rates of injury compared to basketball, baseball, and track.

MECHANISMS OF INJURY

When assessing factors leading to injury, one must consider a broad spectrum of possibilities, including equipment, the environment, biomechanical factors, coaching, and the skill and personality of the athlete.

Equipment

Athletic equipment serves one or more of the following purposes: to provide protection and safety from major significant injuries, to increase the comfort and pleasure of participa-

SAMPLE

ATHLETIC HEALTH CARE SYSTEM

DAILY INJURY REPORT

SCHOOL: WILSON HIGH MONTH: DECEMBER YEAR: 1986

SPORT: WRESTLING, V. COACH: JOHN JAMES ROSTER NUMBER: ______

DAY OF WEEK	T	W	Th	F	Sa	Su	M	T	W	Th	F	Sa	Su	M	T	W	Th	F	Sa	Su	M	T	W	Th	F	Sa	Su	M	T	W	Th	INJURY TYPE AND PART OF BODY INJURED
DATE	1	2	3	4	5	6	7	8	9	10	11	12	13	14	15	16	17	18	19	20	21	22	23	24	25	26	27	28	29	30	31	
PRACTICE = P; GAME = G / ROSTER	P	P	P	G	–	–	P	G	P	P	G	–	–	P	G	P	P	P	G	–	P	G	P	P	G	–	–	P	P	P	P	
Bob Arnold																																
Jerry Brooks			S	S			S																									
Hal Cannon										X	X																					
Jeff Davidson																																
Al East									N	I	I			I	I	L	L															SPRAIN (R) ANKLE
Mike Fredrich																					X	X	X									
George Gillespie																																
Steve Harris			I*	I*			L*																									STRAIN (L) HAMSTRING
Wayne Jones																																
Charlie King																							NS	S	S							FLU
Pat Long	N	I	I	I																												CONTUSION (L) FOREARM
Jim Murray																	X	X	X			T										
Bill Newton								NL	L																							SPRAIN (R) WRIST
Larry Post																																
Dick Ross															N		R	I	I			R	I	L				L				STRAIN (L) GASTROC
Bruce Storey																																
Mark Tunney																					N	I	O									FRACTURE (R) ELBOW
Dave Vinson																																
Barry Watkins				N			I	I	L	L												R	I	I	I			I	I	I	I	CONCUSSION
Max Young																																

LEGEND:

- I = Injured (prior to practice)—did not practice at all.
- S = Sick or ill, did not practice at all.
- X = Did not practice for other reasons (personal, disciplinary, cut practice, etc.).
- L = Limited practice (no cutting, no contact, etc.).
- N = New injury; began practice full go, got hurt, had to stop.
- R = Reinjury to same body part; began full go, got hurt, stopped.
- NL = New Injury; began practice full go, got hurt, returned on limited basis.
- RL = Reinjury; began practice full go, got hurt, returned on limited basis.
- NS = New Sickness; began full go, got sick, had to stop.
- * = Any injury that occurred unrelated to game or practice should be noted by adding a * after N, NL, I, R, or L.
- T = Terminated or quit for non-injury related reason; enter T in the box for the day *after* the last participation.
- O = Out-for-season for injury-related reason.

Figure 1–1 Daily injury report.

Monthly Injury Summary

Wilson High School Wrestling; Winter 1985–86

	Nov.	Dec.	Jan.	Feb.	Season total or average
Squad size	22	21	20	14	22
Total games and practices	11	24	25	20	80
Athletic exposures (risk days)	237	448	375	154	1,214
Number of injuries	4	1	1	0	6
Total injury time loss—practices and games	12	37	26	20	95
Injury rate/100 athletes/season	18.2	4.8	5.0	0	27.3
Injury rate/1,000 athletic exposures	16.9	2.2	2.7	0	4.9
Median injury time loss—practices and games	—	—	—	0	4.5
Mean injury time loss—practices and games	3.0	37.0	26.0	0	15.8
Number of *significant* injuries	2	1	0	0	3
Significant injuries/total injuries (%)	50	100	0	0	50
Significant injury rate/100 athletes/season	9.1	4.8	0	0	13.6
Significant injury rate/1,000 athletic exposures	8.4	2.2	0	0	2.5
Number of *major* injuries	1	0	0	0	1
Major injuries/total injuries (%)	25	0	0	0	16.7
Major injury rate/100 athletes/season	4.5	0	0	0	4.5
Major injury rate/1,000 athletic exposures	4.2	0	0	0	0.8
Out-for-season injuries	1	0	0	0	1
Number of different athletes with an injury	4	1	1	0	6
Percent of different athletes with injury	18.2	4.8	5.0	0	27.3
Percent of injury days athletic exposures	5.1	8.3	6.9	13.0	7.8

Figure 1–2 Monthly injury summary. *Total injury time loss* is the total number of practices and games in which an athlete either (a) did not practice or (b) practiced on a limited basis because of an injury incurred during a practice or game. *Median injury time loss* is determined by arranging all injuries according to the length of time lost and dividing the number of injuries by 2. The number of days lost for that nth/2 injury is the median injury time loss. *Mean injury time loss* is the injury days divided by the number of injuries (average). *Significant injury* is injury that results in time loss of five or more practices and games. A *major injury* is an injury that results in time loss of 15 or more practices and games. The *percent of different athletes injured* is the percent of the team that sustained an injury. The *percent of days lost to injury* is the injury days divided by athletic exposures.

tion (often through decreasing the risk of minor "nuisance" injuries), and to increase the performance potential of the athlete.

Bicycle equipment provides an excellent illustration of these purposes. Helmets for biking, which serve as protective devices to avoid catastrophic head injury, not only have to absorb and disperse the shock of hitting the ground but also must not come off after the first collision, because bikers often bounce on the ground several times before coming to a halt.[16] The helmet also must be able to be applied and removed with relative ease. The buckle must be easily attached yet stay together during a collision. Helmets should be vented to provide cooling of the head through the flow of air. (This feature allows the rider to avoid excessive sweating in a confined helmet.) Two organizations, the American National Standards Institute (ANSI) and the Snell Memorial Foundation, have set standards for construction and functional performance of bicycle helmets.

Gloves for biking serve several purposes. The biker who falls usually puts his hands out in front of him to cushion the fall. Scraping of the palms on the road surface while falling at a high speed can devastate the tendons, nerves, and blood vessels. The thickened, padded palm of the glove is designed to protect this delicate area during a fall. The palm pad and the part

Yearly Injury Summary

	Wilson High School Wrestling		
	1983–84	1984–85	1985–86
Squad size	34	38	22
Total games and practices	81	70	80
Athletic exposures (risk days)	1,833	1,723	1,214
Number of injuries	50	15	6
Total injury time loss—practices and games	156	42	95
Injury rate 100 athletes/season	147.1	39.5	27.3
Injury rate/1,000 athletic exposures	27.3	8.7	4.9
Median injury time loss—practices and games	2	3	4.5
Mean injury time loss—practices and games	2	2.8	15.8
Number of *significant* injuries	9	2	3
Significant injuries/total injuries (%)	18.0	13.3	50
Significant injury rate/100 athletes/season	26.5	5.3	13.6
Significant injury rate/1,000 athletic exposures	4.9	1.2	2.5
Number of *major* injuries	0	0	1
Major injuries/total injuries (%)	0	0	16.7
Major injury rate/100 athletes/season	0	0	4.5
Major injury rate/1,000 athletic exposures	0	0	0.8
Out-for-season injuries	0	0	1
Number of different athletes with an injury	21	11	6
Percent of different athletes with injury	61.8	28.9	27.3
Percent of injury days/athletic exposures	8.5	2.4	7.8

Figure 1–3 Yearly injury summary (see Fig. 1–2 for explanation of terms).

covering the proximal portions of the fingers help reduce the pressure that comes from gripping the handlebars tightly. This also lessens the chance of blisters and ulnar nerve compression.[17] The backs of the gloves are frequently made of a meshed material that allows the hands to "breathe" and remain cool.

Shoes for biking have an entirely different construction from all other athletic shoes. Because pedaling is done with the midfoot and metatarsal heads, bicycle shoes are rigid in the midsole. All other athletic shoes are flexible in this area. Shoes designed for biking permit greater efficiency when riding, thus increasing performance potential in competitive riders. Coupled with toe clips, which ensure proper foot placement on the pedals and allow effective rotation of the pedals by the hamstrings as well as the quadriceps muscles, the specialized shoe enhances the pleasure and efficiency of bicycle riding.

Polypropylene fabrics permit the sweat generated during bicycling to pass through the fabric. Because of sweat evaporation and air convection caused by riding, the bicyclist is able to remain cool and dry. During long rides on cold days, hypothermia can become a concern. The familiar skintight, black Lycra bicycle pants with the inner chamois cloth lining pad increase the comfort and pleasure of the rider. Some bicycle riders experience chafing of the thighs as they ride. The smooth Lycra surface that extends down the thigh greatly diminishes the friction. Other bicycle riders get "saddle sores" from the pressure of sitting on the seat. The chamois cloth liner (and a padded bicycle seat) minimize this pressure.

To be considered "acceptable," a piece of athletic equipment must meet four requirements. First, the equipment must function as designed or intended, demonstrating its efficacy. Second, the equipment must fit properly and maintain its position during participation. Third, the equipment must not predispose the athlete to another injury. Fourth, the equipment, when used correctly, must not be harmful to others.

Much athletic equipment is designed to

Interscholastic Injury Summary; Girls' Soccer, Fall 1986

School	A	B	C	D	E	Mean for 16 teams (A thru P)	Mean for all seasons to date
Squad size	32	31	54	21	25	25.4	24.5
Total games and practices	50	48	45	54	48	48.9	46.9
Athletic exposures—total risk days	1,404	1,188	1,711	648	1,130	971.1	883.4
Number of injuries	16	18	21	12	21	12.3	11.1
Total injury time loss—practices and games	62	77	80	80	69	51.7	47.0
Injury rate/100 athletes/season	50	58	38.9	57.1	84	48.4	45.3
Injury rate/1,000 athletic exposures	11.4	15.2	12.3	18.5	18.6	12.7	12.6
Median injury time loss—practices and games	3	2	2	5	2	—	—
Mean injury time loss—practices and games	3.9	4.3	3.8	6.7	3.3	4.2	4.2
Number of *significant* injuries	5	5	6	7	2	3.4	2.8
Significant injuries/total injuries (%)	31.3	27.8	28.6	58.3	9.5	27.6	25.2
Significant injury rate/100 athletes/season	15.6	16.1	11.1	33.3	8	13.4	11.4
Significant injury rate/1,000 athletic exposures	3.6	4.2	3.5	10.8	1.8	3.5	3.2
Number of *major* injuries	0	2	0	1	0	0.4	0.5
Major injuries/total injuries (%)	0	11.1	0	8.3	0	3.3	4.5
Major injury rate/100 athletes/season	0	6.5	0	4.8	0	1.6	2.0
Major injury rate/1,000 athletic exposures	0	1.7	0	1.5	0	0.4	0.6
Out-for-season injuries	0	1	1	1	1	0.4	0.6
Number of different athletes with an injury	12	11	14	8	15	9.3	8.1
Percent of different athletes with an injury	37.5	35.5	25.9	38.1	60	36.6	33.1
Percent of injury days/athletic exposures	4.4	6.5	4.5	12.3	6.1	5.3	5.3

Figure 1–4 Interscholastic injury summary (see Fig. 1–2 for explanation of terms).

serve a protective function. The status of the body part and the degree of protection desired dictate the type of protective equipment needed, as noted in Table 1–4.

The most basic form of protective athletic equipment is padding. Sponge rubber or foam rubber acts well as a resilient, nonabsorbent protective padding. This material comes in thicknesses ranging from 1/8 inch to 3/4 inch and may have an adhesive coating on one side to prevent slippage of the protective pad. Also, the sponge or foam rubber is often contained in circumferential elastic casings to fit snugly around body parts. Felt padding is composed of pressed and matted wool or synthetic fibers. The material gives a comfortable semiresilient protection that has less tendency to slip from the area than does foam rubber.

Many newer materials possess considerable shock-absorbent properties. The polyurethane liners in bicycle helmets absorb much of the force resulting from a fall.[16] Sorbothane, commonly used in runners' shoes, also reduces the jarring shock the feet receive during running.

TABLE 1-3 Injury Data Analysis 1979-1987

Rank and Sport	Number of Seasons	Total Athletes	Injury Rate/100 Athletes/Season	Injury Rate/1,000 Athletic Exposures	Significant Injury Rate/1,000 Athletic Exposures	Major Injury Rate/1,000 Athletic Exposures	Percent of Different Athletes Injured
1 Cross-country:girls	57	604	56.3	15.9	3.2	1.0	34.3
2 Wrestling	46	1,494	50.9	12.8	2.6	0.9	31.4
3 Soccer:girls	52	1,272	45.5	12.6	3.2	0.6	33.1
4 Football	61	3,695	54.8	12.2	2.9	0.7	33.6
5 Gymnastics:girls	30	526	37.5	10.2	3.0	0.9	27.2
6 Soccer:boys	64	1,807	38.2	10.0	2.0	0.2	27.2
7 Cross-country:boys	58	1,180	34.2	9.6	2.2	0.5	23.4
8 Basketball:girls	86	1,501	31.4	6.6	1.7	0.5	22.9
9 Track:girls	56	1,764	22.3	6.1	1.4	0.3	16.7
10 Volleyball:girls	62	1,410	21.5	6.0	1.1	0.3	17.1
11 Basketball:boys	102	1,584	31.3	5.8	1.4	0.3	25.4
12 Baseball	69	1,503	22.4	5.5	1.2	0.3	18.0
13 Softball:girls	66	1,293	18.7	4.9	1.2	0.3	15.3
14 Track:boys	57	2,140	16.5	4.5	1.1	0.2	13.4
15 Swimming:girls	19	520	14.2	3.9	1.0	0.3	10.8
16 Tennis:co-ed	48	1,552	6.8	1.9	0.4	0.1	5.6
17 Swimming:boys	31	1,017	5.0	1.3	0.5	0.2	4.7
18 Golf:co-ed	41	737	1.4	0.7	0.0	0.0	1.4
TOTALS	1,005	25,599					

Ranking based on injury rate/1,000 athletic exposures.
Significant injury, injury that results in time loss of five or more practices and games.
Major injury, injury that results in time loss of 15 or more practices and games.
Percent of different athletes injured, percent of the team that sustained an injury.

14 / Scientific Foundations of Sports Medicine

TABLE 1-4 Choosing Protective Equipment

Status of body part	Degree of protection	Type of protection
Uninjured	Ordinary	Absorbency/padding: foam, felt, sorbothane
Uninjured	Additional	Dispersion: thermoplastic, metal
Uninjured	Maximal	"Donut," dispersion, and absorbency/padding
Injured	Maximal	"Donut," dispersion, and absorbency/padding

When additional protection is indicated to safeguard a body part, such as the shins in soccer players, dispersion of the force of the blow is necessary. Plastic or metal is most commonly used for this purpose, spreading the force from the small area of contact over the entire surface of the protective pad. Thermoplastic forms to nearly any shape in warm water and, once cooled, retains that shape as a firm shell. Use of soft shock-absorbing padding over these "splints" helps to protect other participants from injury. In contact sports such as football, thermoplastic padding worn on the arms or lower legs is closely regulated by the officials to protect opponents and teammates from injury.[18,19]

When maximal protection of a body part is necessary (for example, the quadriceps muscle of the thigh in football players), use of the "donut principle" is mandatory. The same maximal protection is required for any body part that is injured. The donut principle distributes the padding around the perimeter of, but not directly over, the part requiring protection. By distributing the impact or friction stress to the peripheral areas, the protected area does not experience pressures and trauma associated with contact applied directly over it. Donut padding also incorporates the principles of force dispersion through the use of plastic or metal, and absorbency or padding through the use of felt, foam, or other absorbent material.

Wrestlers' headgear provides a good example of protective equipment design. Shear stresses between the ear lobe and the wrestling mat can produce hemorrhage in the ear cartilage, causing cauliflower ear—a painful and potentially disfiguring condition.[20] With proper headgear, the risk of this potential injury can be completely eliminated. An oval piece of thin metal that extends about 3/4 inch beyond the ear lobe is used (Fig. 1–5). The metal is domed over the ear lobe. When placed over the ear, the metal contacts the skull around the periphery of the ear but does not touch the lobe. Thus, when the metal piece is properly secured, there is no possible way in which the ear lobe can make contact with the metal or the mat. The metal piece is padded with foam where it touches the skin, as well as over the entire exposed outer side. Straps to secure the ear guards pass through the foam padding around the head and under the chin. The straps are adjustable and have snap attachments to secure the headgear in place. A similar ear guard was made using all plastic rather than metal for the dome. The plastic was semiflexible. After reports of cauliflower ear despite use of these ear guards, their efficacy is being reevaluated, and these will probably be withdrawn from the marketplace.

Protective equipment also plays a vital role in permitting athletic participation for individuals with certain medical conditions or disabilities. For many years, the absence of a paired organ was a contraindication to participation in contact sports. Loss of vision in one eye or having only one working kidney was sufficient ground to preclude play in football and perhaps basketball and baseball. The development of eye guards has virtually eliminated any risk

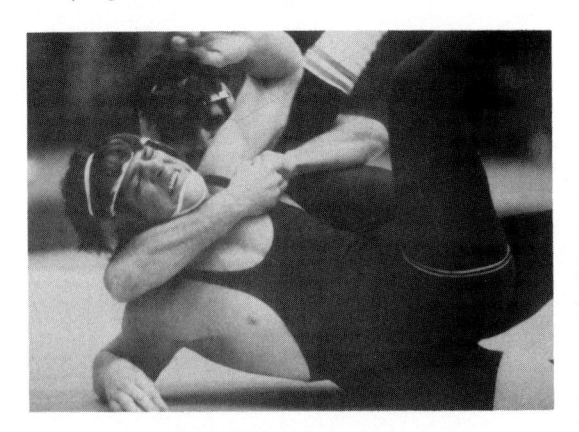

Figure 1–5 Headgear designed to protect wrestlers' ears.

of eye damage; the development of high-quality rib and kidney protector pads has substantially reduced this risk of injury.

Equipment is now available to assist athletes with joint instabilities to participate. Several types of knee braces can help stabilize the knees of athletes with anterior cruciate ligament deficiencies, and other braces can help reduce the risk of recurrent shoulder dislocations.[21,22]

Development of new athletic equipment requires knowledge not only of the demands of the sport and of biomechanics, but also of material properties such as durability, shock absorption and ease of cleaning. Other considerations include the number of sizes available, the ability to adjust equipment for persons of various shapes and sizes, the routine maintenance required, and daily and off-season storage capabilities. The process of creating new products entails going from an idea in the inventor's mind to a prototype, to testing, to test marketing, to the marketplace. Each step can be timeconsuming and expensive. In some cases, promising products reach the marketplace before they have unequivocally demonstrated their efficacy. A case in point is the "preventive" knee brace worn by football players to reduce injuries to the medial collateral ligament of the knee. In theory, these devices could save many thousands of football players from knee surgery each year. The braces usually contain a firm, hinged metal piece that is placed over the lateral aspect of the knee. The brace is attached by straps to the thigh and calf. When the knee is struck from the outside, the hinge of the brace is supposed to absorb the shock of the blow, protecting the leg from these forces. Such devices are widely manufactured and cost about $35 to $60 each. Recent studies question the effectiveness of the braces; some studies indicate a greater chance of injury rather than a reduced chance when the "preventive" knee braces are used.[23,24] The fundamental issues raised when knee brace efficacy is challenged are whether the brace functions as designed or intended, whether the brace is fitted properly, and whether the brace maintains its position during play.

Sizing is not a critical issue in athletics shoes, because they are not "reissued." However, the athlete's function during a particular activity, and the structure and biomechanics of the foot and ankle, are taken into account as shoe manufacturers become increasingly sophisticated in the production of shoes for use during sports. Shoe companies have entire lines of shoes designed to address major problems in runners: ankle stability, shock absorption, and pronation. There are shoes for training, others for racing, shoes for those who weigh less than 150 pounds, and others for heavier runners. In fact, if you look in your own closet, you may find several pairs of athletic shoes. Once, a single pair of "sneakers" sufficed, but today there are running shoes, court shoes, soccer shoes, and walking shoes. If you are a "serious" athlete in a given sport, this specificity cannot go too far. It is most helpful to have equipment and shoes designed to meet the precise demands of your sport. (The one sport still waiting for its special shoe is volleyball.)

One manufacturer is now developing athletics shoes for young children, on the premise that their ability to handle the shocks of activity may not be as good as that of adults. However, most children have the good sense to keep their activities within the limits of pain, stopping participation before the body reaches the point of fatigue. Therefore, whether risk exists in this population has not been determined.

Obviously, designing and mandating use of athletic equipment may often require weighing risks against benefits and costs against benefits to determine whether such equipment is justified for widespread marketing or mandatory use. During the 1970s, the Consumer Product Safety Commission followed injuries and deaths in youth sports. Over an 8-year period, 20 children between the ages of 5 and 14 years died from being hit in the chest with a batted or thrown baseball.[25] Death was caused by damaging the heart muscle through cardiac compression, created when the ball depressed the soft chest wall and sternum and squeezed the heart against the spinal column. Older children do not face this risk, because their bones become firmer with age, the space between the sternum and heart and the heart and spinal column enlarges with growth, and the athletes are able to get their gloves up in time to catch or block the ball. The commission recognized that a chest protector could be developed to absorb sufficient shock to protect these children from this potential cause of death. The agency is currently proceeding with plans to develop such chest protection.

Is this safety device a good idea? What is the death rate from this type of injury? On average, 2.5 children per year die from this mechanism of injury. More than 2 million children between 5 and 11 years of age play baseball annually. The anticipated cost of these protectors is between $20 and $35. Each year, about $40 to $70 million would be spent to save two or three lives. Is it worth it?

To compare this situation in children with that of using helmets to prevent head injuries in children riding bicycles, we must compare the relative risks between bicycling and baseball and consider the number of children between 5 and 11 years who ride bicycles and play baseball, as well as the number of hours per year spent doing each activity. Bicycle injuries are the most common cause of all injuries involving athletic equipment in all age groups.[26] Significant morbidity and mortality are incurred by our youth through head injuries resulting from bicycle accidents. Encouraging the use of bicycle helmets in children (as well as adults) can substantially reduce the enormous hospital costs and mortality or morbidity of head injuries.[16] The cost of children's bicycle helmets generally range from $25 to $50.

Because of the very high collision forces experienced among professional football players (who combine large, heavy muscular bodies and remarkable speed), better ways to protect certain vulnerable areas, such as the ribs, were sought. The result was a new line of high-quality, very expensive protective padding. For those athletes who make an excellent living playing professional football, such expenditures are clearly justified. Does the same hold true for the average youthful football player or high school varsity athlete?

Occasionally, the introduction of athletic equipment reduces the risk of one type of injury and increases the frequency of other injuries. One need only study the history of the football helmet to appreciate this point. Originally, the football helmet was made of leather and afforded little protection against concussions and injuries to the mouth, teeth, nose, and eyes. The introduction of the plastic hard-shelled helmet led to dispersal of the collision force to the entire skull and greatly reduced the frequency and severity of concussions.[20] But, only with the introduction of the face mask bar in the 1950s was there any significant protection of the face. From the single face bar to the current cage structure, the equipment sophistication has essentially led to the elimination of facial injuries in football. However, these were replaced during the 1970s by an alarming increase in the number of spinal cord and neck injuries for two reasons: use of the head as the initial point of contact during tackling, and grasping the face mask during tackling, resulting in twisting or bending of the neck.[2,27,28] Those who played football during the leather helmet days would be surprised by the false sense of security that today's football players feel when they don the hard-shelled plastic helmet. This sense of invulnerability has led to an increase in high-risk behaviors, such as "spearing" (flexing the neck and using the crown as the point of contact). Spearing is outlawed in football, but many players continue to use this technique. The face mask is an easy handle for tacklers to grasp. This, too, is illegal, and officials closely enforce this rule. The education of athletes to the dangers of spearing and grabbing the face mask, coupled with strict enforcement of these rules by the officials, has led to a decline in catastrophic neck injuries in recent years.

In hockey, the introduction of helmets and face masks has greatly decreased the number of concussions, lacerations, broken teeth, broken noses, and eye injuries.[29] But the hockey players, now less fearful of head injuries in the corners of the rink, have been suffering an increasing rate of neck injuries. It is speculated that more vigorous body checking is taking place in the corners now that athletes are no longer worried about damage to their heads (or retaliation by their opponent with the stick.)[30]

Product liability law is another important factor in developing and manufacturing athletic equipment. Today, lawsuits are commonly brought against manufacturers of football helmets and other athletic equipment when permanent major injuries such as death or paralysis occur.[31] A product coming under such scrutiny is the protective eye guard. With the increased popularity of racquetball and squash, the number of eye injuries during athletic activity skyrocketed in the late 1970s. Eye guards were able to reduce the risk of injury significantly. One type of eye guard was a pair of "glasses" with a plastic frame and no lens; protection was afforded because of the narrowed shape of the eye opening, which was smaller than the racquetball and squash ball (Figure 1–6). However, it appears now that injuries to the eye can occur using these protective devices; if the ball strikes that guard in a certain way, the rubber ball can distort and slip into the narrow eye opening.[32] Litigation is underway to determine whether the manufacturer is liable for these injuries.

Manufacturers' liability may decrease when equipment safety standards are developed and accepted by all participants and equipment is then designed to meet those standards. Because of the need for standards in the construction of athletic equipment, the National Operating Committee on Standards for Athletic Equipment (NOCSAE) was formed in 1969 and initially concentrated its efforts on developing safety standards to be met by football helmet manufacturers.[2] Both the National Federation of State High School Associations and the National Collegiate Athletic Association adopted rules mandating that all football helmets meet such standards. Part of those standards included the recommendation that all helmets undergo periodic testing and reconditioning as needed. Construction of baseball helmets is now governed by similar standards.

Area Safety

An important factor in injury reduction and prevention is to maintain area safety on the playing surface itself and in the immediately surrounding area. Hazards within the playing area include goal posts, volleyball net standards, basketball stanchions, the undersurface of the basketball backboard, backstops, gymnastics apparatus, and wrestling and gymnastics mats. These fixed hazards should be padded to protect the athlete from injury during participation. There are other fixed hazards around playing areas, such as indoor walls, doors, water fountains, fire extinguishers, electrical switches, as well as outdoor light poles, fences, ditches, water fountains, and benches. Many portable items regularly brought to the sidelines may become hazards as well, including the first aid kit, water supply, personal equipment, and emergency stretchers, splints, and crutches.

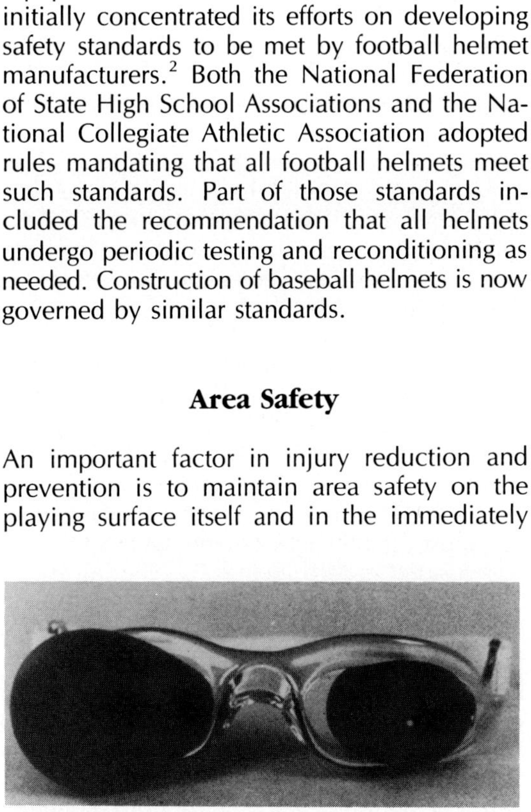

The playing surface should be inspected on a predetermined, regular schedule. At the end of the season and prior to the beginning of a new season, formal inspections should be conducted and arrangements should be made to correct hazards or to do maintenance or repair. On a monthly basis during the season, another careful inspection should be made. Each day, the coaching staff, athletic training staff, managers, and athletes should check the playing surface and perimeter for any problems. In some inner city high schools, track and field coaches report finding glass in the long jump pit every day, so daily raking is imperative to ensure that such hazards are not present. Gymnastics coaches are trained to check all the apparati each day before permitting athletes to participate. Wrestling coaches should make sure there are no gaps between mats. One effective technique for checking the playing surface of outdoor playing fields is to have the players line up along one sideline at arms distance and walk across the field picking up rocks, glass, and other hazards. The team manager then can walk past all the players with a plastic garbage bag and collect the items.

The nature of the playing surface itself may be a factor in causing or preventing injuries. The use of artificial turf has produced great controversy in the nearly 25 years since its introduction in the Houston Astrodome.[20,33,34] The artificial surfaces generally are harder than grass, predisposing athletes to contusions and overuse injuries. These surfaces also tend to become sticky in warm weather, causing the ath-

Figure 1–6 Eyeguard without lens. (From Easterbrook M. Phys Sportsmed 1982; 10:47–56.)

lete's shoes to remain in contact with the ground during key periods of acceleration and deceleration. Turf toe (hyperextension of the big toe) is an example of an injury common to artificial turf. Rug burns or turf burns (abrasions) associated with artificial turf are common and very prone to infection. For these reasons, many artificial surfaces are watered down prior to use. The even, predictable playing surface of artificial turf is believed to encourage athletes to play at higher rates of speed, thus increasing the forces associated with collisions.

Grass fields are not without their own problems. In many areas, it is difficult to maintain the grass. Patches of dirt are exposed in heavily used areas, such as the center of a football field, in front of soccer goals, and where outfielders and infielders stand. Sometimes entire fields of dirt (and rocks) soon appear where a beautiful grass field once existed. In order to maintain the fields, a sprinkler system is usually installed, but then the sprinkler heads become potential hazards for injuries such as ankle sprains. Occasionally, the sprinkler heads malfunction and produce large holes around them, creating the infamous "ankle buster" holes. Because of rainy weather and extensive use, athletic fields may become muddy and the surface, irregular. The uneven surface becomes both a potential source of injury and a detractor from play in a game like soccer or baseball, in which the athletes expect to have true bounces. A gopher-infested field can create major havoc for athletes and coaches trying to maintain a safe playing area.

Studies have been done to determine the appropriate size of the clear zone around the perimeter of playing fields.[35] Unfortunately, such distances are rarely respected because of the many coaches, athletes, officials, photographers, journalists, cheerleaders, and others who "need" to be as close to the sidelines as possible. In football, it is recognized that in the area near the goal lines (where athletes run at maximum speed to try to score or prevent a touchdown), a clear zone of 18 feet (6 yards) is sufficient to handle 95 percent of the out-of-bounds excursions. Nearer the middle of the field, a smaller zone is adequate (about 12 feet or 4 yards). One need only watch a single football game to see how many times an athlete goes careening into photographers, cheerleaders, and team members to recognize how little these zones are enforced. In basketball, because of the desire to have seats close to the court, athletes must regularly dive over the scorer's table or into the stands for loose balls. Inadequate space at the ends of the court causes rapidly moving players to mingle with the cheerleaders and fans if they are fortunate enough to avoid the backboard stanchion.

In many communities, space for athletic facilities is limited. Collisions may occur with members of other sports teams playing in adjacent areas, with projectiles from other sports teams playing in adjacent areas, with spectators or those walking through participation areas, and with vehicles for those "playing" near motor traffic, such as cross-country runners. Tracks are frequently built around football fields. This arrangement allows the football team to use the field in the fall and the track and field team to use the track and perimeter of the football field for the field events in the spring. With the increased popularity of soccer, it is common to have soccer athletes on the field and track athletes running on the track simultaneously. Errant soccer balls or footballs can stray onto the track and cause injuries to unsuspecting runners. One track layout placed the long jump runway and pit behind the endzone in the turn of the track oval. The layout was such that excellent long jumpers would land toward the back of the pit, and their momentum would cause them to fall onto the track, where they were at risk for colliding with track runners. At another high school, the long jump and pole vault runways and pits were located along the 300-foot left field foul line of the baseball field. Although these runways were about 30 feet into foul territory and behind a fence, the field athletes found it hard to concentrate on their sport, not knowing if the crack of the bat meant a ball was headed toward them.

Because teams practice on a year-round basis, indoor training space may also be at a premium. At one university during the winter months, the women's tennis team had to dodge javelins thrown by the men's track and field team. There have been several grisly stories of athletes and officials being hit by javelins, shots, and disci during major field sports competitions. Surprisingly, few accidents or injuries occur from errant tennis balls. Traffic patterns for spectators during practices and games are important, to minimize the risk of collisions with athletes or projectiles.

Those who participate in aerobic dance classes know that the characteristics of the floor make a difference in the incidence of injury.[36] Firm, unyielding floors of concrete predispose to many more overuse injuries than does a "sprung" wooden floor that is able to absorb some of the shock of a bouncing body.

Other hazards worthy of brief mention are slippery deck surfaces around swimming pools, the unevenness of many cross-country running trails, the absence of warning tracks on some baseball fields, and curling chain link fences that cause hand lacerations when baseball athletes try to retrieve overthrown or batted balls by the fence.

Environment

The environment also may pose some special risks of injury. With indoor facilities, concerns about lighting, heating, and ventilation come to mind. With outdoor facilities, weather and wind, as well as lighting for night play, are factors to consider.

Poor lighting may put athletes at risk for injury, because they cannot see rapidly moving balls. Poor indoor heating may predispose to illness. Excessive heating and inadequate ventilation may create an environment in which heat problems such as heat fatigue, heat exhaustion, or heat stroke may arise. Wrestlers are subject to such conditions, because many athletes compete intensively in a small room with little ventilation. With outdoor facilities, the temperature, humidity, and precipitation can affect play. Each year, professional football offers insights into the importance of the weather, from the sweltering, humid preseason football games in Miami or Atlanta to the winter wonderland December games in Green Bay or Chicago.

Biomechanical Factors: Mass and Speed

A critical factor in athletic injury is the force that produces the injury. Most injuries occur as a result of a collision or from rapid acceleration or deceleration. Two formulas from basic physics are useful: $F = ma$ and $KE = (1/2)mv^2$.

The first equation, *force equals mass times acceleration,* is important for understanding the collisions that result when two football linemen make contact at the line of scrimmage after the ball is snapped. Sudden acceleration or deceleration, often mentioned in terms of explosive power of an athlete, is directly proportional to the force generated; thus the action of rapid initiation or termination of movement places considerable stress on the body. Acceleration also is important when considering airborne objects, such as footballs or javelins, contacting players or spectators. The acceleration caused by gravity increases the velocity of the falling object with time; the farther the object falls, the greater the velocity and kinetic energy at the time of collision.

The second equation, *kinetic energy equals one-half of the mass times the velocity squared,* again demonstrates the significance of speed in determining the amount of energy created during a collision. The most severe injuries in sports usually are associated with high velocity, often involving a moving vehicle, animal, or conveyance. An automobile, bicycle, skateboard, motorcycle, horse, sled, or pair of skis are likely to be part of the injury scene. The recent controversy and publicity about three-wheel, all-terrain vehicles (ATVs) and the astonishingly high number of deaths in children under 16 underscore the effect of speed on injury severity.[37] By comparison, injuries from the usual team sport activities, such as football, basketball, soccer, and volleyball, do not involve such high velocity and kinetic energy as those noted above. The rehabilitation medicine section of most hospitals has few patients whose catastrophic injuries arose from standard team sports; usually, a high-velocity collision was involved. To dramatize this point, it has been noted that the risk of a teenage athlete's dying is nearly 20 times greater when he drives to and from a football game than when he plays the game itself![38,39]

The kinetic energy is directly proportional to the mass or weight involved. The larger the objects colliding, the more force or energy created. This should come as no surprise to anyone who has ever done battle with an older or younger sibling. As athletes grow larger in sports like football or basketball, injuries tend to become more severe. It is common today to have a 290-pound offensive lineman who can run a 40-yard dash in 5.4 seconds. When two of these large, fast athletes collide, the force is far greater than when the smaller, slower men of prior generations knocked heads on the gridiron.

These mathematical formulas help explain why injury rates increase as athletes grow. Table 1–5 compares two imaginary 11-year-old football players, two high school athletes, two college athletes, and two professional athletes.

If the estimated relative velocity of two 11-year-old athletes making contact on the football field is given an arbitrary value of 1, two high school athletes, 1.5, two college athletes, 2 and two professional football players, 2.5, Table 1–5 shows that the kinetic energy of the collisions of college and professional athletes is between nine and 18 times greater than the kinetic energy of collision involving two 11-year-olds. It should then come as no surprise that football injury studies reveal that prepubertal athletes suffer an injury rate of less than 10 injuries per 100 athletes per season, but that major college football players are hurt at a rate of 100 injuries per 100 athletes per season and professional athletes, at a rate of 133 injuries per 100 athletes per season.[15] (See Table 1–2.) Although football is a violent game, the injury rates among prepubertal football athletes are relatively low when compared to those among 11-year-olds falling from trees, bicycles, or skateboards.[26]

Skill Level and Personality Characteristics

The ability and skill of the athlete are significant factors influencing injury. A lack of ability and skill can place the novice at risk for virtually every kind of injury. However, possession of great skill and ability do not guarantee a safe athletic experience, because elite athletes seek competition that maximally challenges those assets. The safest athletic experiences come from being "in control." The benefits of coaching, training, and practice include adequate neuromuscular training, practical experience, and personal confidence. The

TABLE 1–5 Theoretical Kinetic Energy of Collision of Two Football Players

Age	Weight (kg)	Estimated relative velocity	Kinetic energy ($KE = 1/2mv^2$)
11	40	1x	$20x^2$
16	75	1.5x	$84x^2$
21	90	2x	$180x^2$
26	110	2.5x	$344x^2$

x = velocity

"natural" athlete is also able to take advantage of instinct, an innate sense of what one's body should be doing at any given moment.

Beginners are at risk because of inexperience, lack of awareness of potential risks, lack of confidence, lack of skills, and subsequent inability to relax during activity. They require coaching and close supervision while learning the basics of any new sports activity. Individual attention is usually required to gain confidence. Consider your own experiences as you learned to catch a ball, ride a bike, swim, or ride a horse. Among the most important items to learn is what to do when the unexpected occurs. Instilling the correct instinctive maneuvers is vital for the beginner. However, naivete and denial may place the partly trained beginner at even greater risk; overestimating one's skills and having a cocky attitude that "nothing can happen to me" can spell disaster. The ski patrol has had to assist many a beginning skier who attempted to challenge the intermediate or advanced slope.

The process of gaining confidence can be subdivided into three areas: commitment, control, and concentration. An athlete who makes the commitment and required investment in training for his sport, practicing and mastering the necessary skills, can feel comfortable with his preparation. Having control over numerous personal and environmental factors allows the athlete to relax in the familiar setting and draw on the fact that these conditions are essentially the same as those that have prevailed during the prior training sessions. Having made the commitment to prepare and having control over possible extraneous distractions, the athlete can concentrate on the task at hand, athletic performance. This foundation of commitment, control, and concentration allows the athlete to perform with confidence. When a confident athlete stays within his level of ability, the chances for injury are low.

Intermediate and advanced athletes thus can experience great enjoyment and relatively low risk of injury by proper preparation and by being in control. However, for many athletes, such as skiers, being in control diminishes the fun of the sport. Being on the edge of control is where the thrills are. Very few skiers enjoy going down the mountain slowly in total control. The excitement comes from having to make difficult maneuvers under pressure.

The motives for athletic participation are also a factor. Recreation is an essential part of any person's life, and pleasure is the driving force behind recreation. Some seek exhilaration, others challenge, competition, or the acquisition of new skills. Other considerations include the social benefits of playing with others or gaining recognition for achievement. Many today are driven by concerns of health, weight control, cessation of smoking, or improvement of their self-image. When selecting a sport, one must weigh the inherent risks of that sport against the reasons for participating. Realistic goals are most compatible with safe athletic performance.

Colleges are training grounds for professional sports—their minor leagues. It is from this showcase that the athlete's economic worth to professional teams is determined. At best, only a small fraction of those who begin as freshman scholarship recipients rise to success in professional sports. For most athletes, college may represent the last chance to play the sport. Professional and Olympic athletes serve as the role models for the masses, permitting us to fantasize that we are out there playing for the championship or a medal. Today we can play for the Boston Celtics or the Dallas Cowboys, the St. Louis Cardinals or the Edmonton Oilers. Maybe our dream is to win the gold medal in gymnastics, heavyweight boxing, or the marathon.

The Olympic games are indeed special and unique. Anyone who is a medal winner not only gains lifetime recognition for that achievement but also has many economic doors opened to him or her. Though not professionals, Olympic athletes who win a gold medal may obtain more product endorsement contracts than those received by many professional athletes. For professional ice skaters, the Olympic games are where name recognition and fame are established. Corporate sponsorship of the United States teams' efforts is staggering; hundreds of millions of dollars are donated in exchange for the right to be declared an official sponsor.

For the excellent, world class athlete, sport moves beyond recreation (and pleasure) into the realm of competition. Taking risks to gain the benefits of fame and accomplishment, and striving for a personal and world record are reasons these athletes participate. The introductory film clip on ABC's "Wide World of Sports" in which the ski jumper symbolizes the thrill of victory and the agony of defeat is etched in the minds of competitors and viewers the world over. When one is seeking to be the best, to do what no one has ever done before, risk taking and pushing to the limit are inherent elements of the sport.

Acceptance of the risks associated with athletic activity implies being prepared for injury rather than denying the possibility of getting hurt. The "macho" approach of ignoring injuries, a "no pain, no gain" philosophy, runs counter to common sense. One must make an effort to recognize, assess, and manage all athletic injuries. There can be great comfort in knowing that early recognition and treatment minimize time loss and keep many injuries from developing into chronic or more serious problems.

Coaching

Coaching is a primary factor influencing injury. The coach is entrusted with great responsibility and is expected to produce "results" for his or her efforts. Does this mentor have the appropriate sensitivity toward the athletes and reasonable goals in mind? What is the ultimate purpose for this coach/team/athlete relationship? Is a proper perspective established?

The professional athlete and the highly visible amateur athletes in the Olympic games and major colleges should possess far different expectations than a high school athlete, a youth athlete, or a recreational adult athlete. Professional sports are businesses, dependent on having customers pay to watch or sponsors pay to advertise their products. Individual players come

intensity.[5,6] In tests of the general population, the best results are obtained by uphill treadmill running, but in the case of a competitive athlete, performance depends critically upon the ability to develop a matching oxygen transport while simulating the specific sport. Thus, swimmers have been tested in a millrace like the Swedish flume or a circular tank, and paddlers have been evaluated either in their boats or using some form of rowing or kayak ergometer.[7–10]

Oxygen transport has traditionally been expressed in units of milliliters per kilogram per minute standard temperature and pressure, dry gas (STPD). Such units are appropriate for a sport such as running, in which the energy cost varies almost directly with body mass. However, in endurance sports such as swimming or rowing, in which the body mass is largely supported, it is more useful to consider absolute values (liters per minute STPD).

Oxygen transport may be conceived as proceeding from the atmosphere to the active tissues by a chain of resistances (or more precisely, conductances, the reciprocal of resistance).[5] These include ventilation (making due allowance for respiratory effort "wasted" in both ventilation of the dead space of the airways and the oxygen cost of respiration), the interaction between the diffusing capacity of the lungs and blood transport, blood transport itself, and the interaction between blood transport and the diffusing capacity of the tissues (Fig. 2–1). In disease states, any one of these links can limit oxygen transport. Attention has recently been directed to the respiratory system as a potentially weak link, particularly in prolonged bouts of exercise (30 to 60 minutes).[11,12] However, when the average, healthy young competitor performs an event of 5 to 10 minutes' duration, by far the smallest conductance (25 to 35 L per minute), and thus the largest resistance, is presented by the blood transport term.

Carbon Dioxide Homeostasis

Normal tissue function may be disturbed by excessively high or low partial pressures of carbon dioxide. Problems are particularly likely during scuba diving. The form of the respective dissociation curves is such that carbon dioxide has four to five times the effective blood solubility of oxygen.[5] This advantage is somewhat offset by a smaller acceptable partial pressure gradient from the tissues to ambient air (70 to 80 rather than 150 torr); nevertheless, problems of CO_2 transport are more likely to arise in the respiratory than in the cardiovascular system. While underwater, respiration is hampered by a decrease of maximum exercise ventilation (because of the pressure of the water on thorax and abdomen, the increased density of respired gas, expiratory collapse of the airway, and external resistance imposed by the valves of the scuba set), the dead space of the breathing equipment, and rapidly exhausted CO_2-absorbing cannisters.[3]

The climber may face the opposite problem: hyperventilation to compensate for the low oxygen pressure, causing excessive carbon dioxide elimination and leading to an intermittent pattern of ventilation with mountain sickness. Initially, the problem is respiratory, although secondary changes of mineral and fluid balance may reduce blood volume, with a reduction of cardiac stroke volume and maximum cardiac output.[13]

Thermal Homeostasis

The mechanical efficiency of exercise is poor, even in an athlete. During a typical aerobic activity such as cycling, the best that can be accomplished is a net mechanical efficiency of about 23 percent. At least three-quarters of the chemical energy consumed by the athlete thus appears as heat. Intramuscular temperature increases rapidly during the first 5 minutes of exercise (the "warm-up"). The general body temperature continues to rise for at least the first 15 minutes of work, as surplus heat is transferred from the limbs to the body core, but if effort is further prolonged, a new thermal plateau is established.[14] This reflects the increased thermal gradient from the body to its immediate environment, the onset of copious sweating, and an increase of subcutaneous blood flow.

With very prolonged bouts of exercise such as a marathon race, a sequence of circulatory changes makes it progressively more difficult for the runner to sustain thermal equilibrium. In the first few minutes of the event, there is an

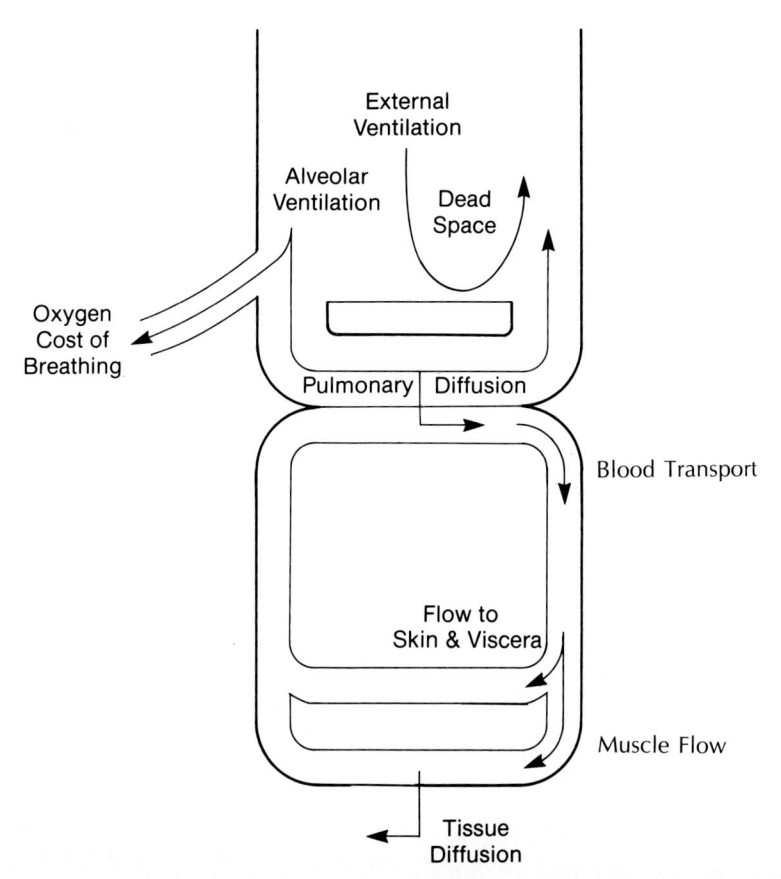

Figure 2–1 The transport of gases between the atmosphere and the working muscles can be conceived as occurring through a closely linked series of conductances. (From Shephard RJ. Exercise physiology. Toronto: BC Decker, 1987: 73.)

enhanced formation of tissue fluid, and the capacity of the peripheral veins also rises at an equal pace with the increase of core temperature.[15] In a hot, dry climate, there may also be a substantial continuing water loss in respired gas. As sweating develops, this contributes heavily to the overall decrease of blood volume; in adverse weather, sweat secretion may amount to 2 or more liters per hour.

The immediate effect of the rise in limb temperature is to improve physical performance. The viscosity of the limb muscles is reduced, the antagonists are relaxed, and intramuscular blood vessels are widely dilated.[16] However, the rising core temperature also increases oxygen consumption in regions other than muscle (the Q_{10} effect—a doubling of metabolism for a 10° C rise of temperature), and a substantial proportion of the total cardiac output is directed to the skin. At first, dilatation of the subcutaneous vessels may reduce peripheral vascular resistance, allowing a higher peak cardiac output than was possible while vessels were vasoconstricted, but as fluid is lost from the circulation, blood flow to the active muscles drops, with a decrease in physical work capacity.[17] There is also progressive difficulty in sustaining circulation to the brain (heat collapse), the kidneys (renal failure), the adrenals (thermal shock), and the skin (fatal hyperpyrexia).[3,18]

If there is repeated exposure to heat with prolonged and heavy sweating, a salt deficit may develop. Not only does this cause muscle weakness and cramps, but there is an associated reduction of blood volume. The latter impairs performance, leaving the affected individual more vulnerable to heat collapse. This problem can usually be averted by extra salting of food, without recourse to salt tablets.

DETERMINANTS OF CARDIOVASCULAR OXYGEN TRANSPORT

The Fick Equation

The basic relationship between oxygen transport and cardiovascular function was enunciated many years ago by Fick.[3] The Fick equation, originally used to determine cardiac output, can be rearranged in the following form:

$$\dot{V}_{O_2} = \dot{Q}(Ca, O_2 - C\bar{v}, O_2)$$

where $\dot{V}_{O_2}$ is the oxygen consumption, $\dot{Q}$ is the cardiac output, Ca, O_2 is the oxygen content of arterial blood, and $C\bar{v}, O_2$ is the oxygen content of mixed venous blood. In maximal effort, a $\dot{V}_{O_2}$ of 3 L per minute STPD might reflect a cardiac output of 20 L per minute and an arteriovenous oxygen difference of 0.15 L per liter.

Notice that cardiac output depends upon the product of heart rate and stroke volume, whereas the arterial blood oxygen content depends upon both oxygenation in the lungs and hemoglobin concentration. In this section, I discuss typical data for young women and men. The question of variations with age is addressed below.

Cardiac Output

Under resting conditions, the cardiac output is 5 to 6 L per minute, depending on body size. As with basal metabolism, resting cardiac output is commonly standardized per square meter of body surface area, the anticipated normal value of this "cardiac index" being 3.0 to 3.5 L per minute per square meter.[3]

During maximum effort, the cardiac output rises to 20 to 35 L per minute, depending on body size and the degree of endurance training that has been undertaken. The peak value reflects a heart rate of almost 200 beats per minute and a stroke volume of 100 to 175 mL.

Heart Rate

Because the resting cardiac index is relatively constant from one subject to another, the resting heart rate provides a useful rough estimate of resting stroke volume and thus of cardiac condition. Although the resting heart rate of a sedentary person may be 70 or even 80 beats per minute, there have been instances in which the resting heart rate of an endurance athlete was less than 30 beats per minute.[3]

In practice, the resting heart rate is influenced by recent meals or exercise and by interaction with the observer. Nevertheless, useful information can be obtained if the pulse is counted immediately on waking, while the athlete is still lying in her or his sleeping quarters.

The maximum heart rate has been estimated at an average of 198 beats per minute in young women and 195 beats per minute in young men, although there is an appreciable (5 to 10 beats per minute) variation among individuals.[5,19] The peak rate observed also varies with the type of activity performed, being a little lower with cycling or stepping and much lower with arm than with treadmill exercise.[20] Finally, there have been suggestions that the peak heart rate of an endurance competitor is somewhat lower than that of a sedentary person, although only if tested during the type of exercise for which training has been undertaken.[3,21,22]

Stroke Volume

The resting stroke volume depends on posture; if sitting, it is only 70 to 80 mL, but if lying, it is at least 100 to 120 mL, depending on body size and physical condition.[23-25]

If the subject is sitting or standing, the stroke volume rises briskly with moderate exercise, tending to a plateau at 60 to 70 percent of maximum oxygen intake.[26,27] The peak value of 100 to 175 mL depends on posture, body size, physical condition, and the type of exercise being performed (for example, Simmons and Shephard found that the stroke volume was

15 mL greater during uphill treadmill running than during cycle ergometry).[28] In the lying position, the animal experiments of Rushmer in 1959 suggest that the cardiac output during exercise is increased relatively little over the resting figure.[29]

During upright exercise, the increase of stroke volume with moderate activity reflects a combination of greater preloading and reduced after-loading of the left ventricle.[30,31] The venous return of an active person is encouraged by an increase of venous tone and operation of the muscle pump. The end-diastolic volume thus shows some rise, and a more forceful contraction is initiated through the Frank-Starling mechanism.[27,32-37] In contrast, most studies of supine exercise, whether on land or in water, have shown little increase of end-diastolic volume.[38-45] However, Bar-Shlomo and co-workers and Steingart and associates did observe some increase of end-diastolic volume in untrained subjects.[46,47] Wide dilatation of blood vessels in the active muscles reduces peripheral vascular resistance, allowing a more complete expulsion of the ventricular contents.[48-50] There is thus an increase of ejection fraction, sometimes from the resting figure of about 50 percent to as much as 75 percent, with a corresponding decrease in the end-systolic volume.[51-53]

If exercise is continued to work rates above the anaerobic threshold, at least two additional factors become operative. The active muscles are now contracting at a substantial fraction of their maximum voluntary force (for instance, 25 to 35 percent in cycle ergometry). This creates an extravascular impedance to blood flow.[54-56] There is also a progressively greater secretion of catecholamines;[57] these exert both a chronotropic and an inotropic effect on the left ventricle, increasing both heart rate and the force of contraction for a given end-diastolic volume. Although the end-diastolic volume remains greater than at rest, there is little further increase of relaxed dimensions, at least in the healthy heart.[40,47,49,58-62] Depending on the relationship of the increase in myocardial contractility to the rising intravascular and extravascular impedance, the stroke volume may be maintained or may even show a small further increase as maximum oxygen intake is approached.

Cardiac Volume

Early literature contained much discussion of the "athlete's heart."[63,64] The volume of the cardiac shadow, as estimated from posteroanterior and lateral radiographs, is increased from the sedentary value of 10 to 11 mL per kilogram to 13 to 15 mL per kilogram in an endurance athlete.[65] At first, the enlargement of the heart was confounded with the pathologic dilatation seen in various forms of cardiac disease. Subsequently, it was recognized that a large heart shadow was a normal response to endurance training, although it remained unclear to what extent the enlargement was caused by ventricular hypertrophy, and to what extent it reflected an increase of the end-diastolic volume. Echocardiography has clarified that both processes are involved.[64]

Arterial Oxygenation

The traditional view has been that the lungs function as a perfect tonometer, allowing a complete equilibration of alveolar gas and pulmonary capillary blood, both at rest and in exercise. According to this hypothesis, the oxygen saturation of blood leaving the lungs through the pulmonary veins is thus close to 100 percent; any small unsaturation of peripheral arterial blood is due to either a poor matching of ventilation and perfusion in some parts of the lungs, or vascular pathways that bypass the lungs completely. Dempsey and co-workers have recently queried this concept.[11] They noted that the average transit time for the passage of red cells through the pulmonary capillaries dropped from 0.75 seconds at rest to about 0.33 seconds during vigorous exercise. Moreover, in some vascular pathways the transit time was inevitably much less than the average figure. Thus, in athletes with a large maximum oxygen intake and a large maximum cardiac output, equilibration was incomplete in the shorter capillaries. In short, it seems that appreciable arterial oxygen unsaturation can develop during vigorous exercise.

Venous Oxygenation

The mixed venous oxygen content is no lower than 40 to 60 mL per liter, even during maximum exercise. This has led some authors to speculate that the activity of aerobic enzymes within the working muscles is inadequate to extract available oxygen from the circulation during maximum effort.

In fact, there is little evidence to substantiate this hypothesis. The classic studies of Millikan in 1937 showed that the partial pressure of oxygen in myoglobin dropped to 3 to 4 torr during a tetanic contraction of the gastrocnemius muscle, and the oxygen pressure in the vicinity of the aerobic enzymes is often as low as 0.01 torr.[66,67] Even in femoral venous blood, an oxygen content of only 6 mL per liter has been reported during maximal effort.[17]

The substantial residual oxygen content of mixed venous blood thus reflects the contribution of well-oxygenated blood from circuits other than the muscle—particularly the subcutaneous vessels, where the function of the circulation is thermal homeostasis rather than the delivery of oxygen.

Hemoglobin Concentration

When fully saturated, each gram of hemoglobin carries 1.34 mL of oxygen. Maximization of the blood hemoglobin concentration is thus important to physical performance. The average hemoglobin level is less in women (13.8 g per 100 mL) than in men (15.6 g per 100 mL), partly because of blood loss in menstruation, and partly because women secrete smaller amounts of androgens. Taking account also of oxygen dissolved in physical solution in the plasma (2 mL per liter in both sexes), women necessarily have a smaller potential arterial oxygen content than men (maximum 187 versus 211 mL per liter).

Several studies of international athletes have shown some tendency to anemia, more often expressed as a latent iron deficit than as an overt decrease of blood hemoglobin concentrations. Thus, the Dutch Olympic team had approximately the same hemoglobin concentration as track officials, but a higher proportion of competitors showed iron depletion or a low iron saturation of serum carrier proteins.[68]

A variety of factors predispose to iron deficiency in top-level athletes, even though the diet usually provides a fair quantity of iron. One survey of Italian athletic teams showed an average intake of 14 to 17 mg per day, and we found an ultra-long distance runner to be consuming 23 to 33 mg of iron per day.[69,70] On the other hand, the athlete's demand for iron is enhanced by an increased formation of red cells in iron-containing tissues such as muscle during training. In some sports such as running, the vigorous circulation of the red cells and the repeated mechanical trauma in the feet lead to an unusually rapid rate of red cell destruction.[71] At the same time, a high total energy intake is commonly achieved by the undesirable practice of boosting the proportion of fat in the diet, a nutritional technique that reduces the 10 percent or so of dietary iron that is normally absorbed from the intestines. Such problems are compounded by an appreciable iron loss in sweat. Our data for marathon runners show a total excretion of 1.8 mg of iron in the course of a marathon race (Verde 1984), at least the equal of the usual alimentary absorption.[72] Finally, endurance training may boost plasma volume, creating a "pseudo-anemia."

Maximum oxygen intake and endurance performance are unaffected by a latent iron deficiency, but oxygen transport drops almost proportionally if there is severe anemia (as may occur in people from developing countries who have had an inadequate diet or have suffered parasitic infections). In such individuals, oxygen transport is restored as the anemia is corrected.[73]

CHANGES ASSOCIATED WITH AGE

Cardiac Output

In the young competitor, cardiac function has been described as "hypokinetic," implying that the cardiac output at any given oxygen consumption is less than in an adult.[74] Among possible explanations for this phenomenon are, first, a smaller relative blood flow to parts of the body other than muscle, and second, a more ready heat dissipation (a larger relative body surface and a lesser thickness of subcutaneous fat in the growing child).

In the older adult, the relationship between cardiac output and oxygen consumption remains essentially unaltered, but most studies show a progressive decrease of maximum cardiac output and thus maximum oxygen intake with age. However, Rodeheffer and associates have argued that if individuals with undetected myocardial ischemia are excluded by a combination of exercise electrocardiography and scintigraphy, the maximum cardiac output is well sustained to a relatively advanced age.[27]

Heart Rate

Most authors have set the maximum heart rate of children in the range of 195 to 200 beats per minute, although somewhat higher figures (210 to 215 beats per minute) seem possible in well-motivated samples.[19,75,75a]

The maximum heart rate of the adult declines progressively with age (Fig. 2–2).[65,76] The commonly stated equation

Maximum rate = 220 − age (years)

probably exaggerates the rate of decline, and average values as high as 170 beats per minute or even 177 beats per minute have been described in sedentary North Americans.[76,77] There are several explanations for the decline in maximum heart rate with age: a slowing of myocardial relaxation and thus diastolic filling, a decreased sensitivity of catecholamine receptors, and possibly a reduced local secretion of noradrenaline.[65] In occasional patients (those with the "sick sinus syndrome"), the problem of a low maximum rate can be traced to ischemia of the sinus pacemaker; however, this does not seem a generalizable explanation, because the youthful maximum cannot be restored in the average old person simply by the administration of oxygen. In other instances, effort may be limited by chronic chest disease or weak peripheral muscles, before the heart has been fully stressed.

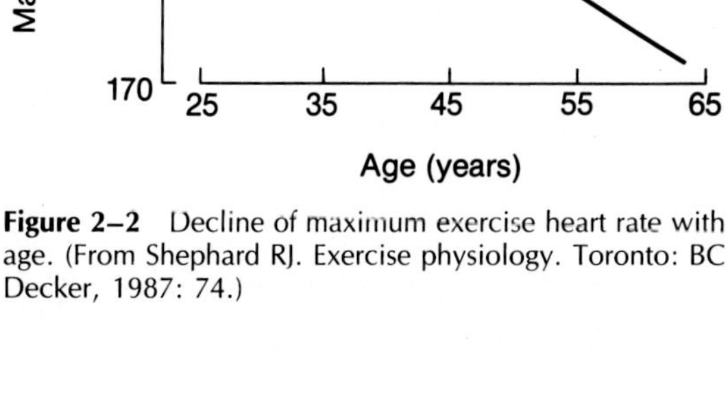

Stroke Volume

Given a high maximum heart rate and the tendency to a hypokinetic circulation, the maximum stroke volume tends to be relatively smaller in a child than in an adult.[75a]

At moderate work rates, the older adult tends to compensate for a lesser exercise-induced increase of heart rate by invoking the Frank-Starling mechanism (an increase of end-diastolic volume increasing stroke volume).[78] However, there is difficulty in sustaining ventricular ejection as maximum effort is approached, and the stroke volume may show a 3 to 6 percent decline at this stage (Fig. 2–3).[26] Rodeheffer and co-workers suggested that any decrease of ejection fraction in vigorous effort was a reflection of myocardial ischemia.[27] After screening longitudinal study volunteers by a combination of exercise electrocardiography and scintigraphy, the residual ischemia-free sample showed a large increase of end-diastolic volume and little decrease of maximal cardiac output relative to younger adults.[78] However, critics of the Rodeheffer study have questioned the realism of a population sample in which all 65-year-olds with laboratory evidence of ischemia are excluded.

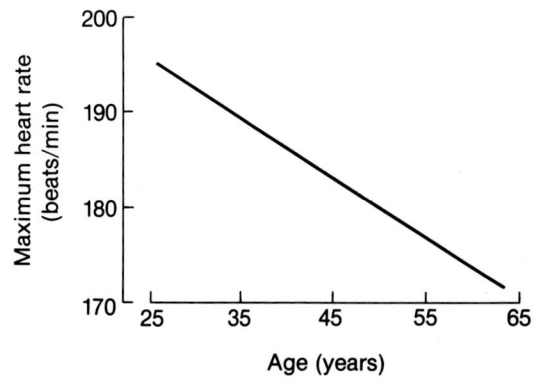

Figure 2–2 Decline of maximum exercise heart rate with age. (From Shephard RJ. Exercise physiology. Toronto: BC Decker, 1987: 74.)

Heart Volume

It has generally been assumed that ventricular mass decreases at the same time as the overall age-related decrease of lean tissue. Such a trend was indeed suggested by early analyses of chest radiographs, but more recent data for continuing athletes have shown a stable or even an increasing heart shadow in older competitors.[79] Echocardiography has further confirmed that there is some increase of left ventricular wall thickness with age.[78]

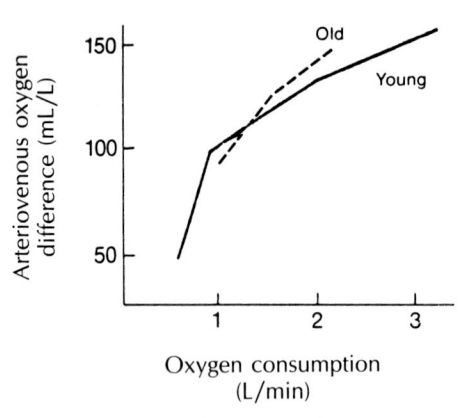

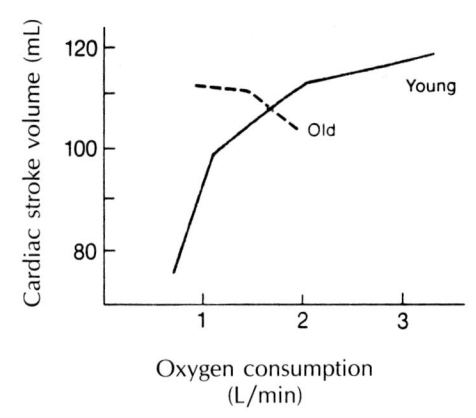

Figure 2–3 A comparison of cardiovascular responses to exercise in 25- and 65-year-old subjects. (From Shephard RJ. Exercise physiology. Toronto: BC Decker, 1987: 152.)

Arterial Oxygenation

The completeness of arterial oxygen saturation in the lungs depends on the ratio of diffusing capacity to perfusion.[5] Considering the effects of aging upon the lungs as a whole, maximum diffusing capacity decreases at about the same rate as maximum perfusion. However, at any given vertical level within the lungs, there may also be some increase in the mismatching of perfusion to diffusion. This gives rise to a small increase of arterial unsaturation in vigorous effort. Diffusional problems are exacerbated if there is a poor matching of ventilation to perfusion or frank chest disease.

Venous Oxygenation

If children can be motivated to a good maximum effort, they reach a very low mixed venous oxygen content; this reflects a lesser relative blood flow to the skin and other tissues than would be anticipated in adults, a more active lifestyle than many adults, and possibly a combination of a hypokinetic cardiac output with very active enzymes in the working tissues.

Aging is generally associated with a narrowing of the maximum arteriovenous oxygen difference and a high mixed venous oxygen content. The blood flow to the skin and tissues other than muscle becomes relatively greater with aging; there is usually a decrease of habitual activity, and there may be some loss of function on the part of intramuscular enzymes.[65]

Hemoglobin Concentrations

The blood hemoglobin concentration is relatively low (typically 12 to 13 g per 100 mL) in prepubertal children, to the point that this limits the maximum arteriovenous oxygen difference.[80] However, with the onset of puberty, there is a rapid change toward young adult hemoglobin levels. Some authors have suggested that the elderly become anemic, but this does not seem to be the case unless there is repeated blood loss (for example, from hemorrhoids, peptic ulcer, or gastrointestinal carcinoma), poor iron absorption (vitamin deficiencies, pyloric resection), or a generally inadequate diet.[81]

CARDIAC REGULATION

General Considerations

The cardiac pacemaker has both vagal and sympathetic innervation. In the endurance athlete and other well-trained persons, a strong vagal tone contributes to a slow resting heart rate, and during exercise a part of the rise of heart rate reflects a release of this activity. During exercise there is also an increased sympathetic drive, supplemented at high heart rates by the action of circulating catecholamines and possibly by local effects of left atrial distention (the Bainbridge reflex). Thus, even after a cardiac transplant operation, vigorous exercise is eventually able to induce a substantial increase of heart rate.[82]

The stroke volume is modulated by changes in preloading, after-loading, and myocardial contractility. Exercise tends to increase preloading, partly because of an increase in tone of the peripheral veins, and partly because venous return is encouraged by the pumping action of the contracting muscles. Thus, particularly when exercising in an upright posture, the end-diastolic volume is increased (see above). There may be a very transient muscular vasodilatation as exercise is initiated, but almost immediately there is a sharp increase of afterload, as noradrenaline liberated from the sympathetic nerve terminals produces a general vasoconstriction. In active muscles, this response, in turn, is countered by a more dramatic vasodilatation caused by an effect of adrenaline upon beta-receptors, together with the local influence of increasing intravascular concentrations of potassium and hydrogen ions.[83] The net response to moderate exercise is thus a decrease of peripheral vascular resistance. If effort becomes more intense, the response is complicated, because intramuscular blood vessels are compressed by the contracting muscle fibers (see below). Finally, as maximum effort is approached, sympathetic cholinergic fibers play an important role in redirecting blood flow from the skin and the viscera to the working muscles.[84] Vigorous exercise also induces an increase of myocardial contractility; this typically develops as the anaerobic threshold is passed and blood catecholamine levels begin to rise.[57]

Cardioactive Drugs

Exercise is commonly prescribed for the patient who has sustained a myocardial infarction and is receiving either calcium-blocking or beta-blocking drugs. Many of the studies purporting to justify the use of these drugs have in fact tested healthy young adults rather than "postcoronary" patients; in healthy populations, compensating mechanisms are such that the deterioration of maximum power output is quite small after drug administration.[1] However, it is less clearly demonstrated that these agents have no adverse effects upon the exercise performance of those patients with established hypertension or myocardial ischemia.

Calcium-blocking drugs reduce myocardial contractility;[85] this may be helpful in established hypertension, but in ischemic heart disease the reduction of ventricular power may be sufficient to precipitate cardiac failure, and there have been suggestions that the indiscriminate use of calcium-blocking agents has increased the mortality of "postcoronary" patients.

Beta-blocking drugs abolish the catecholamine-mediated increase of exercise heart rate, complicating the regulation of training intensity by heart rate monitoring.[1] They also counter the increase of myocardial contractility that normally occurs during vigorous effort. Healthy individuals remain able to develop a fairly normal maximum cardiac output by invoking the Frank-Starling mechanism. This option is less likely to be open to a diseased heart; nevertheless, the prognosis of "postinfarct" patients seems to be improved by the use of beta-antagonists (Taylor et al).[86]

Speed of Adaptation to Exercise

Despite the bradycardia while resting, subjects who have been conditioned to athletic competition may demonstrate a very high heart rate during the period of excitement prior to the commencement of exercise. As activity begins, there is further tachycardia, associated with a reduction of vagal tone and an irradiation of impulses from the motor cortex and limb proprioceptors. If the work rate is moderate, a steady-state heart rate plateau is reached within 1 to 2 minutes, but if the exercise is more intense, both heart rate and cardiac output continue to rise slowly, reflecting a rising deep body temperature, a peripheral sequestration of the available blood volume, the secretion of catecholamines, the onset of fatigue with a progressive recruitment of mechanically less efficient muscles, and possible psychological reactions to the continuing activity.[87,88]

The speed of adaptation to exercise is important to the measurement of cardiac output (the "Fick principle" assumes that a steady state has already been reached) and the estimation of oxygen consumption from the power output (for instance, in a simple step or cycle ergometer test). Because sympathetic nerve activity is involved in the various adaptations that occur when exercise is initiated, the time course of the process is slowed after administration of beta-blocking drugs or after cardiac transplantation.

If intensive exercise is begun without allowing sufficient time for a warm-up, the sudden rise of systemic blood pressure could provoke a cardiac arrhythmia.[89] Presumably, both a less intensive sympathetic discharge and a reduced peripheral vascular resistance contribute to an improvement of prognosis if a warm-up is allowed.

Following exercise, both heart rate and cardiac output remain elevated for some minutes; the continuing cardiovascular response reflects partly the time required to clear anaerobic metabolites from the working tissues and partly a continued elevation of core temperature and circulating hormone levels. If the intensity of exercise exceeds the anaerobic threshold, the accumulated oxygen debt may be such that the heart rate shows a transient overshoot in the first few seconds following exercise;[90] nevertheless, there remains a close correlation between the heart rate monitored in the first 10 to 15 seconds following exercise and the immediate end-exercise value, a finding that is exploited in both exercise prescription and the design of simple fitness tests.[91,92]

Vasodilatation after exercise may lead to a sudden drop of blood pressure, particularly if the environment is hot and humid (a poorly ventilated shower and changing area) and if the subject stands without activating the muscle pump by gentle, continued exercise (a warm-down). It is important to avoid such hypotension, because it may cause a cardiac arrhythmia, a transient loss of consciousness, or even sudden death.[93,94]

Systemic Blood Pressure and Cardiac Work Rate

The level of the systemic blood pressure is important from two points of view: first, it is the main determinant of cerebral blood flow and thus of continuing consciousness; and second, it is a major determinant of cardiac work rate and thus of myocardial oxygen consumption.

Most physicians have been content to measure the blood pressure under resting conditions. The average young adult demonstrates resting figures of about 120/80 mm Hg, depending on the technique that has been used. Values are often higher in the anxiety-provoking situation of a doctor's office or a precompetition medical examination than in the home or field laboratory.[95,96] Averages can also be influenced by a rounding of numbers or a preferential reporting of certain digits. An athlete may have a relatively high systolic reading, the increased pulse pressure reflecting a large resting stroke volume;[97] the diastolic pressure may also be better maintained, because this is influenced by the elasticity of the aortic wall. Many authors would regard repeated blood pressure readings of more than 150/90 mm Hg as pathologic; different authors recommend treatment (salt restriction and diuretics to reduce blood volume) at diastolic pressures between 90 and 100 mm Hg.

During vigorous, progressive endurance exercise, the systolic pressure rises progressively, reaching a figure of 180 to 220 mm Hg (24–29 kPa) in the course of 15 minutes or more (Table 2–1).[97] Diastolic pressure is hard to measure during vigorous, rhythmic exercise, but apparently it changes relatively little. The rise of blood pressure probably represents an attempt to sustain perfusion of the working muscles in the face of a rising external impedance.[54] If the myocardium is becoming ischemic, the attending physician may observe the ominous sign of a static or even a falling systolic blood pressure; this reflects a failing myocardium and is an urgent indication to halt exercise. Isometric exercise gives a much more rapid rise of blood pressure;[55] during a sustained isometric contraction, there is a large increase of extravascular impedance and no intercontraction interval when local perfusion can be restored. The elderly are often advised against both

TABLE 2–1 Systolic Blood Pressure in Relation to Age and Work Rate

Age (yr)	Rest (1MET)* (kPa)	Work Rate and Systolic Pressure			
		4 METs* (kPa)	6 METs* (kPa)	8 METs* (kPa)	10 METs* (kPa)
25	16.0	19.3	20.8	22.3	23.8
35	16.3	19.6	21.6	23.5	25.2
45	16.7	20.2	22.4	23.5	24.8
55	17.0	20.9	23.4	25.5	27.5

* MET is the ratio of the observed oxygen consumption to basal metabolic rate. (Based on Data of Dr. S. M. Fox. From Shephard RJ. Exercise physiology. Toronto: BC Decker, 1987: 78.)

isometric exercise and heavy lifting. However, because the rise of blood pressure is a function of the duration of effort, it is possible to arrange brief isometric contractions without inducing an excessive rise of blood pressure.

The tension (T) in the ventricular wall is related to intraventricular blood pressure (P_v) by the Law of Laplace:

$$T = \frac{P_v (R_1 R_2)}{h (R_1 + R_2)}$$

where h is the wall thickness and R_1 and R_2 are the principal radii of the ventricle. Refinements of the formula consider the transverse shear associated with bending; such calculations point to the conclusion that tensions are greatest in the immediate subendocardial region.[98] Because the vessels supplying this part of the heart wall must penetrate the ventricle, this region is in double jeopardy of local ischemia. Note further that any ventricular hypertrophy that is induced by endurance training decreases wall tension, as does any increase of myocardial contractility that decreases cardiac dimensions.

The two main components of cardiac work are attributable to the pumping of blood (the integral of P∂V between the end-diastolic and the end-systolic points) and the maintenance of wall tension (T), also integrated over the contraction phase of the cardiac cycle:

$$\text{Rate of working} = \left(\int_{V_d}^{V_s} P \partial V + \alpha \int_0^t T \partial t \right) f_h$$

where α is a constant to convert tension to units of work, and f_h is the heart rate. The first term may be regarded as "useful" and the second as "wasted" work; unfortunately, the second term is usually much larger than the first, so that the efficiency of cardiac contraction is relatively low.

The corollary of this observation is that it is relatively less costly for a postcoronary patient to induce an increase of cardiac output by exercising than to raise heart rate and blood pressure by sitting at home worrying about the condition of his or her heart!

Clinicians find it useful to correlate symptoms and signs of myocardial ischemia (for example, anginal pain or electrocardiographic ST segmental depression) with the cardiac work rate. The latter is approximated by the double product (systolic pressure × heart rate) or, less frequently, by the triple product (systolic pressure × heart rate × duration of systole).[99] Notice that the double product provides a valid estimate of cardiac work only if stroke volume and contraction time remain constant. During exercise, the second factor is more likely to be constant than the first, and fortunately for the calculation, it is the major component of total work; for this reason, the double product correlates quite well with myocardial oxygen consumption.[100]

REGIONAL BLOOD FLOW

Muscle

Although local vasodilatation increases regional blood flow to the working muscles several-fold during moderate exercise, there is a danger that the forceful contractions of intense effort could restrict muscle perfusion. Isometric contractions begin to limit blood flow when 15 to 20 percent of maximum voluntary force is exerted, and vascular occlusion is complete at about 70 percent of maximum voluntary force (Fig. 2–4).[56,101,102] Maximum rhythmic work on a cycle ergometer typically uses 25 to 35 per-

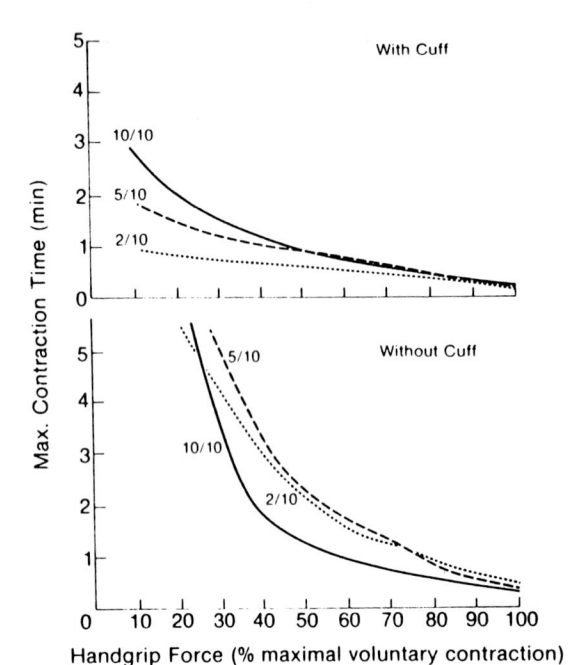

Figure 2-4 Endurance of isometric contraction in relation to force exerted (percentage of maximum voluntary contraction), occlusion of circulation by sphygmomanometer cuff, and intermittency of effort (2 sec of 10 sec, 5 sec of 10 sec, continuous). (Based on data of Shephard.[14] From Physiology and biochemistry of exercise by Roy Shephard. Copyright © 1982 by Praeger Publishers. Reprinted by permission of Praeger Publishers.)

cent of maximum voluntary force, and there is some evidence that the power output in this type of activity is limited by local muscular perfusion.[54,103] Three corollaries may be noted:

1. Vascular occlusion is most likely to occur if effort is sustained by a small muscle group that must contract at a high proportion of its maximum voluntary force.
2. The peak power output during endurance effort can sometimes be improved by training programs that increase muscular strength.
3. Adoption of a slow pace (for example, the use of a high gear on a cycle) requires application of a greater force for a given power output, and thus increases the likelihood of vascular occlusion.

Vigorously contracting muscles assist in circulating the blood. Folkow and associates (1970) have estimated that the working muscles provide up to 30 percent of the cardiovascular energy needed during vigorous exercise, thus relieving the heart somewhat of its workload.[104]

Skin

When performing moderate exercise in extreme heat, the skin blood flow (5–10 L per minute) can account for a third of the maximum cardiac output (Fig. 2–5).[31,105,106,106a] Cutaneous vasodilatation persists to a fairly high work rate, but in all-out effort there is a constriction of both arterioles and cutaneous veins, in an attempt to sustain circulation to the brain and working muscles; this reflects the intense outpouring of catecholamines in near maximal effort.[57] Cutaneous blood flow is restricted by certain "doping" agents such as the amphetamines, and on occasion this has led to fatalities in long-distance cyclists.[18]

If skin blood flow is inadequate to meet the demands of thermal homeostasis, the individual may develop various forms of heat illness, including collapse, thermal shock, and hyperpyrexia.[3,18]

Viscera

At rest, much of the total cardiac output is directed to internal organs such as the kidney and

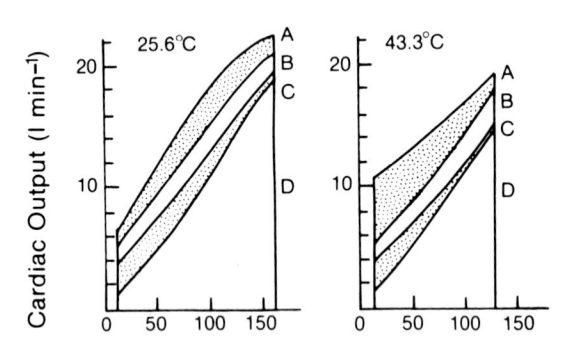

Figure 2-5 Distribution of cardiac output in cool (25.6° C) and hot (43.3° C) environments: (A) skin flow, (B) flow to heart and brain, (C) flow to viscera, (D) muscle flow. (From Physiology and biochemistry of exercise by Roy Shephard. Copyright © 1982 by Praeger Publishers. Reprinted by permission of Praeger Publishers.)

liver (Fig. 2–5). As with the cutaneous circulation, the visceral blood flow provides a reserve that can be called upon in vigorous physical activity. For example, when exercise is performed in the heat, the renal blood flow may drop from its resting value of 1.1 L per minute to only 0.2 L per minute. Although the resulting decrease of renal filtration leads to some diminution in the oxygen consumption of the kidney, the arteriovenous oxygen difference for this organ may thus show a threefold to fourfold augmentation. During combinations of vigorous exercise and heat exposure, the decrease of visceral flow may be sufficient to cause a disturbance of renal function;[107] the mildest expression is a proteinuria, with the appearance of red cells and casts in the urine, but in more severe cases complete renal failure has been described.[108]

Brain

The blood vessels of the brain have little ability to vary their vascular resistance.[109] Flow thus depends largely on the aortic and carotid arterial pressure. To the extent that exercise increases aortic pressure, it may increase cerebral perfusion. There have been occasional reports that physical activity improves mental function, particularly in older individuals in whom the blood supply is becoming marginal.[110]

On the other hand, as maximum exercise is approached, a falling blood pressure may lead to a disturbance of consciousness, with bizarre responses to questioning, a loss of postural control, and eventual unconsciousness.[3,6]

Lungs

Under resting conditions, the pulmonary arterial pressure is quite low (about 25/10 mm Hg). From the cardiovascular viewpoint, three main zones can be distinguished (Fig. 2–6).[111] In the upper part of the lungs, intrapulmonary pressure exceeds pulmonary arterial pressure, and flow is not possible at any time during the breathing cycle. In the second zone, intrapulmonary pressure is intermediate between pulmonary arterial and pulmonary venous pressures. Flow thus occurs when the intrapulmonary

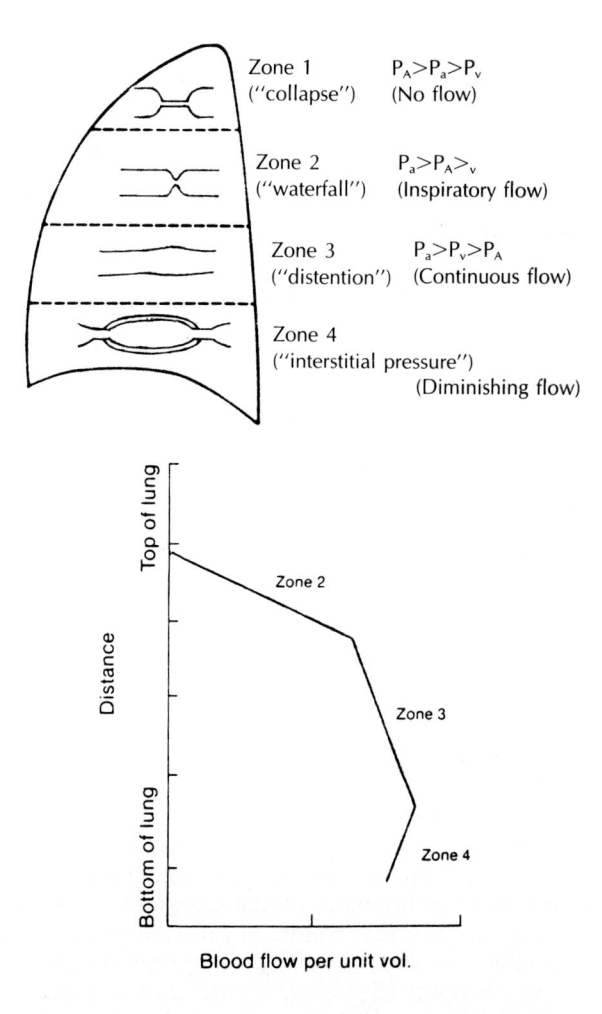

Zone 1 ("collapse") $P_A > P_a > P_v$ (No flow)

Zone 2 ("waterfall") $P_a > P_A > P_v$ (Inspiratory flow)

Zone 3 ("distention") $P_a > P_v > P_A$ (Continuous flow)

Zone 4 ("interstitial pressure") (Diminishing flow)

Figure 2–6 West's (1977) concept of pulmonary blood flow to various regions of the lung. (*Zone 1*) alveolar pressure exceeds pulmonary arterial pressure, and the pulmonary capillaries are collapsed; (*Zone 2*) the alveolar pressure is intermediate between pulmonary arterial and pulmonary venous pressures, so that capillary opening varies during the respiratory cycle; (*Zone 3*) pulmonary venous pressure exceeds alveolar pressure, so that the pulmonary capillaries remain open throughout the breathing cycle; (*Zone 4*) flow is influenced by interstitial pressures. (From Shephard RJ. Exercise physiology. Toronto: BC Decker, 1987: 88.)

pressure falls (during inspiration), but it becomes progressively restricted during expiration. In the third zone, intrapulmonary pressure is less than pulmonary venous pressure throughout the respiratory cycle, and pulmonary blood flow is largely independent of the phase of ventilation. Pulmonary blood flow is thus directed preferentially to the lowest third of the lungs. Under resting conditions, the distribution of alveolar ventilation is also very uneven, with a large part of the inspired gas volume being directed to the upper parts of the lung, and some arterial unsaturation can occur from the mismatching of ventilation and perfusion.

Vigorous exercise helps to correct the mismatching of ventilation and perfusion. The vertical distribution of ventilation becomes more uniform, and at the same time an increase of pulmonary arterial pressure allows perfusion of the upper parts of the lung. There is a substantial increase of the mean ventilation-to-perfusion ratio in maximum effort, but at the same time there is a much smaller scatter of ventilation-to-perfusion ratios about this mean value. Nevertheless, some mismatching persists, both from the top to the bottom of the lung and also at a given level within the lung.

The average time for the passage of a red cell through the pulmonary capillaries is 0.75 seconds at rest, but during vigorous exercise this drops to 0.33 seconds, with the consequence that there may be insufficient time for gas exchange in the shorter pulmonary capillaries.[11]

Vasodilatation allows a twofold to threefold increase of pulmonary blood flow during moderate activity, without any substantial increase of pulmonary arterial pressures. However, the pulmonary arterial pressure must be doubled to accommodate the fourfold to sixfold increase of flow observed during maximum effort.

Heart

The ventricular muscle is supplied by right and left coronary arteries, which arise from the root of the aorta immediately above the aortic valves. A good blood supply is essential not only to normal cardiac function but also to survival of the ventricular muscle, because there is little possibility of anaerobic metabolism in cardiac tissue.[30] Occlusion of the main coronary arteries can occur from either a spasm of the vessel wall or the accumulation of atherosclerotic deposits immediately below the vascular endothelium. According to Poiseuille's law, flow resistance is proportional to the fourth power of vessel radius, so that 70 percent obstruction of an artery must occur before there is a significant blockage of flow. The force of left ventricular contraction is such that coronary blood flow must occur mainly during diastole (Fig. 2–7); the inner part of the myocardium (served by vessels that penetrate the ventricular wall) is particularly vulnerable to ischemia during systole.[98]

Maximum exercise normally induces a fourfold to fivefold increase of coronary flow.[112] However, there is also a relative shortening of the diastolic phase of the cardiac cycle as the heart rate increases, so the blood supply becomes more marginal even in a healthy heart. Ischemia is likely to develop in the patient with atherosclerosis. The oxygen lack may be sensed as an anginal pain, commencing in the midline of the chest, and radiating along the inner aspect of the left arm, or up into the root of the neck. However, sometimes it is "silent," revealed only by electrocardiographic evidence of slow ventricular repolarization (a horizontal or downward sloping depression of the ST segment of the electrocardiogram >0.1 mV).

ENVIRONMENTAL STRESS

Heat

Prolonged exercise is usually associated with a progressive exudation of fluid from the circulation into the peripheral tissues, with a decrease of blood volume and an upward drift of heart rates. Heat exposure exacerbates this tendency, with a substantial fluid loss in sweat (up to 2 L per hour) and a wide dilatation of the peripheral veins.

The normal circulatory demands of the working muscles are supplemented by the requirements of heat dissipation (a skin blood flow of 5 to 10 L per minute). If the heart is in good condition, there may initially be an increase of peak cardiac output relative to the figures observed in a cool environment, but as activity continues, there is increasing difficulty in pumping sufficient blood to the various regions of the body.[17] An inadequate blood supply to the viscera can contribute to renal and adrenal shock.

With repeated exposure to heat, acclimatization occurs. There is some cross-adaptation

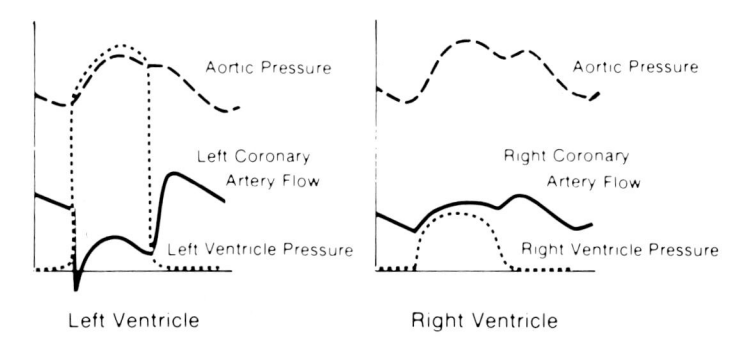

Figure 2–7 Pressure relationships and coronary blood flow over the cardiac cycle. (From Physiology and biochemistry of exercise by Roy Shephard. Copyright © 1982 by Praeger Publishers. Reprinted by permission of Praeger Publishers.)

between heat exposure and endurance training, but for full acclimatization to a hot environment, it is necessary to undertake repeated bouts of vigorous physical activity in the heat. As a result of increased blood volume, greater venous tone, and other adaptations, the core temperature of a heat-acclimated individual is stabilized, with less evidence of circulatory strain (the heart rate is lower for a given combination of heat and exercise, and the blood pressure is better maintained.[3,18]

Cold

Acute cold exposure causes an intense cutaneous vasoconstriction, which works to conserve body heat.[3,113] Recent studies have suggested that flow to the limb muscles is also restricted in very cold situations. As a result, a large temperature differential may develop between the limbs and the core, and too rapid attempts to restore the limb circulation in a victim of hypothermia may flood the heart and other key organs with dangerously cold venous blood.[114]

The corollary of this observation is that vigorous exercise, which increases blood flow to the limbs, decreases the insulation of the body and encourages heat loss in a cold environment.[114] With severe cooling, the vasoconstrictor nerves become paralyzed, and skin flow is increased, further augmenting the rate of heat loss. A "hunting reaction" may be observed, in which warm arterial blood temporarily restores constrictor nerve function, with an alternation of vasoconstriction and vasodilatation.

Cold constriction of the peripheral veins increases central blood volume, encouraging a large cardiac stroke volume and possibly some increase of peak power during vigorous exercise.[115] The arterial constriction, on the other hand, increases after-loading, so that the person with myocardial ischemia typically complains of anginal pain while exercising in the cold.[18] If exposure to the low temperature is sustained, the central blood volume is quite rapidly normalized by a cold diuresis.[3]

High Altitudes

The immediate reaction to moderate exercise at high altitude is a tachycardia, the body's attempt to compensate for the reduced oxygenation of arterial blood.[18] With acclimatization, an increase of ventilation increases arterial oxygen saturation, and the tachycardia is lessened.

Hyperventilation leads to a hypocapnia, with decreased perfusion of both the skin and the brain. The cutaneous vasoconstriction increases the blood pressure response to a given level of physical activity. Because of the cerebral vasoconstriction, there is an optimum level of hyperventilation at any given altitude; excessive hyperventilation may further increase arterial oxygen saturation, but the benefits of this are countered by a decrease in blood flow to the brain.[13]

As exposure to high altitude continues, there

is a compensatory decrease of plasma buffering capacity.[116] Partly for this reason and partly because of the cutaneous vasoconstriction, there is a decrease of maximum stroke volume and cardiac output.[117]

Underwater

The initial response to swimming underwater is influenced by the adoption of a horizontal posture. Consequently, the stroke volume is greater than in upright exercise (particularly at light work rates).[8]

A combination of cold exposure and counterpressure on the leg veins increases central blood volume, inducing a cold diuresis and a reduction of blood volume. With very prolonged underwater activity (> 6 hours), the loss of normal gravitational stimuli reduces the tone of the leg veins; there may thus be a decrease of blood pressure (postural hypotension) on emerging from the water and resuming a normal upright position.[3]

The ratio of regional blood flow to local tissue volume influences the distribution and clearance of inert gases during diving.[118] The pattern of decompression sickness is thus modified by vigorous physical activity.

TYPES OF EXERCISE

Isotonic Exercise

In humans, it is not possible to draw a clear distinction between isotonic and isometric exercise. However, some forms of activity such as uphill treadmill running involve mainly rhythmic isotonic activity of the large muscles, with only a limited postural and isometric component, whereas other types of activity are predominantly isometric.

During rhythmic activity, the body is able to maintain oxygen homeostasis at intensities of exercise below the anaerobic threshold (75 to 80 percent of the mode-specific peak oxygen intake). At higher intensities of effort, muscle blood flow fails to match metabolic demand (possibly because of the external impedance of the most active muscles, such as the quadriceps during cycle ergometry). The systemic blood pressure rises progressively, and if this adaptation does not suffice to restore muscle perfusion, lactic acid accumulates in the working tissues until local concentrations are sufficient to inhibit glycolysis and thus muscular contraction.

The magnitude of the peak oxygen transport is influenced by the volume of active muscle. Values observed during cycle ergometry are only 92 to 93 percent of the maximum for uphill treadmill running, and most subjects achieve only about 70 percent of maximum oxygen intake when carrying out work with the arm and shoulder muscles.[3,6] In this last situation, the problem of perfusing small and vigorously contracting arm muscles is compounded by absence of the leg muscle pump. Central blood volume is thus reduced by a pooling of fluid in the leg veins.

Difficulty in sustaining adequate local perfusion becomes even more severe if the arms are held above the head (for instance when playing tennis, or using a paintbrush on a ceiling).[119] With this type of activity, there is a substantial element of isometric work in sustaining body posture, and the local perfusion pressure is reduced by the height of the limb relative to that of the heart.

Isometric Exercise

Isometric and heavy lifting exercise is a common feature of conditioning programs. In ordinary life, isometric work is performed in sustaining body posture against gravity, in gripping, in lifting heavy loads, and in pushing objects with substantial inertia.

In 1958, Royce investigated the local blood flow through an isometrically contracting muscle. He found that the external impedance of the active muscle fibers first restricted flow at 15 to 20 percent of maximal voluntary force, and that vascular occlusion became complete if the contraction was increased to 70 percent of maximum voluntary force.[56] The implication is that the likelihood of partial or total occlusion of muscle blood flow can be reduced by a strengthening of the relevant muscle groups. Perhaps for this reason, a well-trained competitor is able to exercise relatively close to maximal oxygen intake before there is a significant accumulation of lactate.

Systemic blood pressure begins to rise with the accumulation of anaerobic metabolites.[55] The extent of the rise in pressure is a relatively linear function of the contraction duration. Because significant muscle strengthening seems possible with contractions of only 10 seconds, and blood pressure reverts to normal between contractions, it is possible to conduct an isometric muscle strengthening program without danger to the heart, using intermittent contractions, each held for less than 10 seconds.

Aerobic Exercise

Aerobic exercise implies rhythmic activity at an intensity at which the oxygen demand can be satisfied by an increase of cardiac output. In a brief bout of progressive large muscle exercise, it is possible to move very close to the maximum oxygen intake. However, in more protracted events (duration 30 minutes to 8 hours), it is necessary for the athlete to operate at a progressively smaller fraction of maximum oxygen intake.

There are two main reasons for a progressive limitation of exercise intensity as the duration of activity is extended. First, blood flow is necessarily nonuniform, so that some regions of muscle are underperfused in near maximal effort. Lactate accumulates in these underperfused regions, with a progressive development of fatigue. Second, a rising core temperature, sweating, and an extravascular accumulation of fluid progressively reduce maximum cardiac output. Thus, a person can sustain 75 to 80 percent of maximum oxygen intake during a 3-hour marathon event, but it is difficult to develop more than 50 percent of maximum oxygen intake during an 8-hour bout of activity.[120–122]

Anaerobic Activity

During a single burst of anaerobic activity, performance is essentially limited by local reserves of energy and is thus independent of cardiovascular performance. However, a substantial "oxygen debt" is accumulated, to be repaid during the recovery period. Thus, by an appropriate adjustment of work and recovery cycle length, repetitive bursts of anaerobic activity can provide a cardiovascular stimulus analogous to aerobic exercise.[123]

TRAINING REGIMENS

Aerobic (Endurance) Training

The immediate, short-term response to training in a sedentary person is a 20 to 30 percent increase of maximum oxygen intake.[5] This is achieved largely through an increase of cardiac stroke volume. Maximum heart rate is certainly not increased, and some authors have even described a decrease with training.[21] Likewise, arterial oxygenation is not improved; indeed, Dempsey and associates have suggested that well-trained athletes are particularly vulnerable to arterial oxygen unsaturation during peak effort.[11] Increases of hemoglobin concentration, if any, are quite marginal, but a more effective distribution of cardiac output may also allow some decrease of mixed venous oxygen content.

In a more long-term perspective, rigorous training probably causes some ventricular hypertrophy, although Bouchard and Malina have argued that there are substantial, genetically determined differences among individuals in the ability to increase ventricular wall thickness.[124]

The pattern of training needed to increase cardiac output and encourage ventricular hypertrophy involves some overload of the cardiovascular system. The most important variable is the intensity of activity relative to initial fitness (Fig. 2–8).[5,125] For the average young adult, the initial intensity should be 60 to 70 percent of maximum oxygen intake, but in a very sedentary person (a senior citizen or a patient who has recently sustained a myocardial infarction), 50 to 60 percent of maximum oxygen intake may prove an effective training stimulus.[126] The heart rate, lightly palpated over the carotid artery immediately following exercise, generally provides an effective guide to exercise intensity. However, in a patient who is being treated by beta-blocking drugs, other indices such as the "rating of perceived exertion" may need to be substituted.[127]

Other variables influencing training re-

44 / Scientific Foundations of Sports Medicine

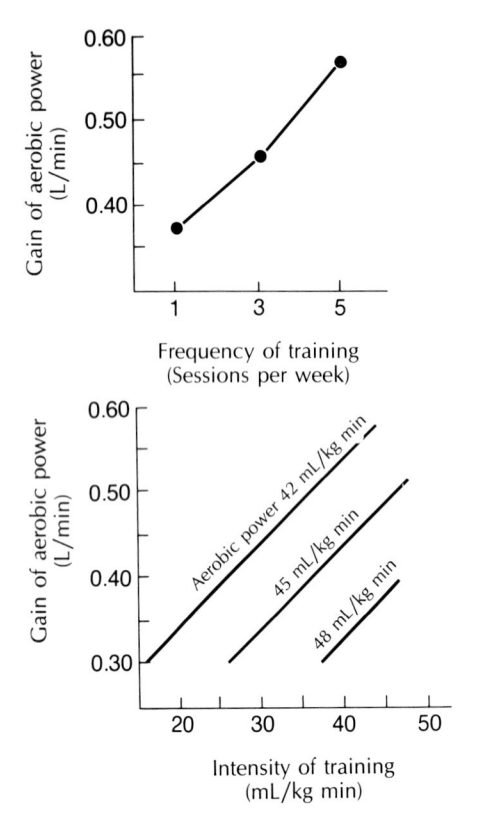

Figure 2–8 Influence of intensity of training, initial fitness, and frequency of training on gains of aerobic power. (From Shephard RJ. Exercise physiology. Toronto: BC Decker, 1987: 130.)

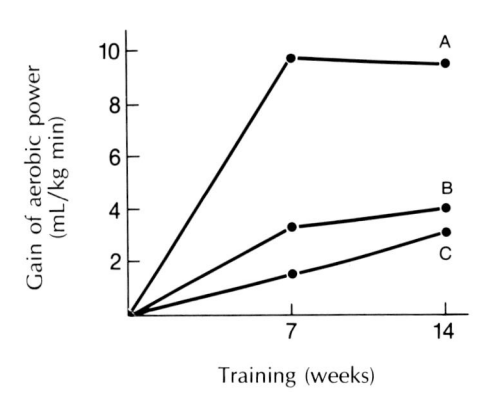

Figure 2–9 The influence of intensity and frequency of training of elderly subjects. (A) 3.3 sessions/wk, pulse 130–140 beats/min; (B) 1.3 sessions/wk, pulse 130–140 beats/min; (C) 3.3 sessions/wk, pulse 120 beats/min. (From Shephard RJ. Exercise physiology. Toronto: BC Decker, 1987: 154.)

sponse are the frequency and duration of activity. The young adult should aim for sessions of at least 20 to 30 minutes' duration, three to five times per week.[5] However, it is worth emphasizing that more prolonged activity can compensate to some extent for a lower intensity. Thus, the frail elderly can obtain some cardiovascular training from prolonged walking (Fig. 2–9).[65]

Muscular Training

Some aerobic training programs take no account of muscle function. This is a mistake. Prolonged jogging can lead to a weakening of the arm muscles, so that if heavy work must later be performed by the arms, the rise of blood pressure (and thus the cardiac work rate) is greater than it would have been before involvement in the training program.[128] Conversely, strengthening of the muscles by isometric or heavy endurance exercise facilitates their perfusion, decreasing the rise of systemic blood pressure and the workload imposed upon the heart.

Specificity of Training

There has been considerable discussion of the specificity of training. The current consensus is that training involving the leg muscles gives some improvement of subsequent arm performance (perhaps a 50 percent transfer), but that arm training does little to augment performance when using the legs.[129]

The most logical explanation of such observations is that the peak power output of the arms is limited largely by perfusion of the working muscles, and that although these muscles are strengthened by arm training, there is little improvement of central cardiovascular function. In contrast, because of the larger active muscle mass, leg exercise is limited by both cardiac and muscle function; in this situation, the cardiovascular component of training can facilitate subsequent performance of arm exercise.

Training and Myocardial Ischemia

Some, but not all animal experiments have suggested that endurance training stimulates the development of collateral blood vessels and thus the oxygen supply to the myocardium after occlusion of a major coronary vessel.[130–132] On the other hand, most authors are agreed that this type of response does not occur in humans after myocardial infarction, perhaps because the intensity of training is insufficient, and perhaps because the deterioration of the vessels is too far advanced.[132,133]

Nevertheless, a program of endurance training is of considerable benefit to the ischemic myocardium. The cardiac work rate at a given power output is substantially reduced by the decrease of systemic blood pressure and slowing of heart rate, whereas a lengthening of the diastolic phase of the cardiac cycle or ventricular hypertrophy allows an easier perfusion of the coronary arteries.

FUNCTIONAL EXERCISE TESTING

General Considerations

Most current cardiovascular tests either measure maximum oxygen intake directly or infer it from the linear relationship between heart rate and oxygen consumption or the equivalent power output. Progressive exercise tests also allow the lactate ("anaerobic") threshold to be predicted from a discontinuity in the relationship between oxygen consumption and ventilation. Myocardial ischemia may be detected by recording the electrocardiogram during and immediately following all-out effort.[134] Finally, an increasing number of laboratories are testing cardiac function more directly, using either echocardiography or CO_2 rebreathing estimates of cardiac output.[131,135,136]

Directly Measured Maximum Oxygen Intake

The maximum oxygen intake reflects the product of maximum cardiac output and maximum arteriovenous oxygen difference. Because the latter is a relatively fixed quantity, there is a close correlation between maximum oxygen intake and cardiac function.

Maximum oxygen intake is best measured directly by a progressive large muscle task such as uphill treadmill running to exhaustion (Fig. 2–10). As the work-rate is increased, a stage is reached at which oxygen consumption plateaus or shows an increase of less than 2 mL per kilogram per minute. With other tasks such as cycle ergometry, the muscle volume involved is smaller; the peak oxygen intake is thus 7 to 8 percent less than the treadmill maximum, and the activity of some subjects is halted by muscular fatigue before a central limitation of performance can be demonstrated (Table 2–2). If there is not an oxygen consumption plateau, other possible signs of maximum effort include a heart rate close to the age-related maximum, a respiratory gas exchange ratio of more than 1.10, and a terminal blood lactate of at least 10 to 11 mmol per liter.[3,5]

When testing an athlete, it is useful to compare the sport-specific peak oxygen transport with the treadmill value. Top level competitors are often able to achieve close to 100 percent of their treadmill maximum while pursuing a simulation of their sport, whereas an indifferent performer falls far short of this achievement.

Submaximal Tests

Although the risks of a direct measurement of maximum oxygen intake are extremely low in a healthy person, a submaximum test is still a little safer and is to be preferred in situations in

TABLE 2–2 Peak Oxygen Intake Observed During Three Types of Ergometer Exercise

Type of exercise	Maximum O_2 intake (L/min)	(%)	Maximum heart rate (beats/min)	Maximum blood lactate (mmol/L)
Treadmill	3.81	100	190	13.6
Cycle ergometer	3.56	93	187	12.4
Bench stepping	3.68	96	188	11.7

Based on data obtained by International Biological Programme working party. (Shephard RJ. Exercise physiology. Toronto, Ontario: BC Decker, 1987: 114.)

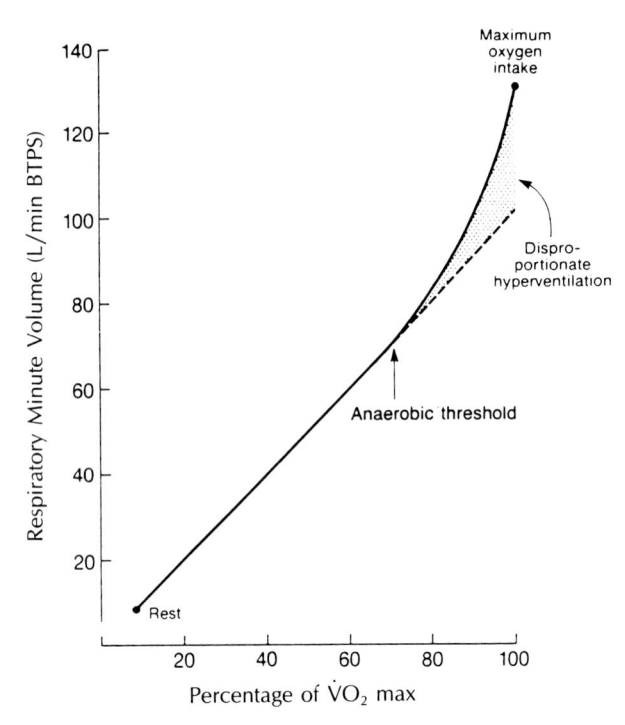

Figure 2–12 The relationship between respiratory minute volumes and oxygen consumption. (*BTPS*) body temperature and pressure, saturated with water vapor. Note onset of disproportionate hyperventilation at so-called "anaerobic threshold." (From Shephard RJ. Exercise physiology. Toronto: BC Decker, 1987: 18.)

Most of the necessary information can be derived from a single unipolar chest lead (CM$_5$). However, many clinicians prefer to examine three unipolar lead placements (CM$_2$, CM$_4$, and CM$_6$). The reference electrode is placed over the manubrium sterni, and the neutral lead is attached to the nape of the neck.[131,133,134]

Given some preliminary skin abrasion and the use of modern lightweight electrodes, there should be little difficulty in recording a clear electrocardiographic signal during exercise. For precise evaluation of ST segmental voltages, electronic averaging devices can also be used to scan 16 or 32 similar electrocardiograph waveforms. Myocardial ischemia is usually diagnosed from a horizontal or downsloping ST depression of 1 mm or more, measured 60 to 80 msec after the QRS complex. Clinical interpretation of this sign is complicated by many "false-negative" and "false-positive" tracings (Tables 2–4 and 2–5).[133,145] The precision of the diagnosis can be increased by considering other features of the electrocardiogram, such as the height of the R waves.

Echocardiography

Echocardiography provides estimates of ventricular wall thickness, the speed of ventricular contraction, and the fraction of the ventricular contents ejected at systole.[135] Moderate exercise can be performed in a semisupine position, but it is difficult to engage in maximum or vigorous submaximum exercise during echocardiography. Moreover, current echocardiographic technique does not allow absolute measurements of cardiac output.

Cardiac Output

The carbon dioxide rebreathing method in essence applies the Fick principle to the exchange of carbon dioxide.[136] Again, there are

(a) Multifocal premature ventricular contractions (B and C) with two normal complexes (A)

(b) Ventricular tachycardia (B) following two normal complexes (A)

(c) Ventricular fibrillation

(d) Wolff-Parkinson-White syndrome Note extremely short PR interval

(e) Downward-sloping ST segmental depression

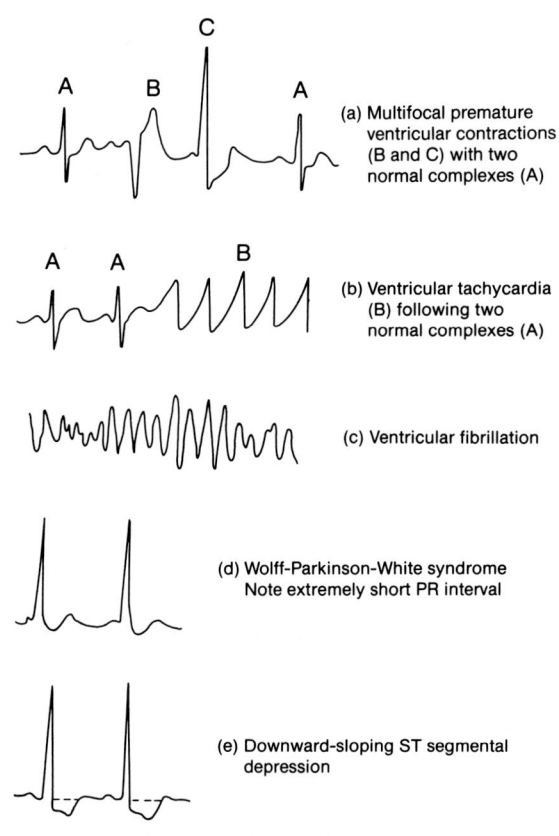

Figure 2–13 Schematic illustration of various adverse effects of hypoxia upon the waveform of the electrocardiogram. (From Shephard RJ. Exercise physiology. Toronto: BC Decker, 1987:81.)

TABLE 2–4 Influence of Disease Prevalence on the Proportion of False-Positive and False Negative Exercise ECG Test Results

Disease Prevalence and Test result	Ischemia Absent	Ischemia Present	Test errors (%)
50 per 1,000 with myocardial ischemia			
Positive	95	40	70.4
Negative	855	10	1.2
425 per 1,000 with myocardial ischemia			
Positive	58	340	14.6
Negative	517	85	14.1

(From Shephard RJ. Exercise physiology. Toronto: BC Decker, 1987: 82.)

a number of problems in making accurate determinations of cardiac output as maximum effort is approached. In theory, the Fick formula assumes a steady state, whereas carbon dioxide output increases rapidly as maximum effort is approached and lactate begins to accumulate. Arterial CO_2 content is estimated from either the end-tidal CO_2 pressure or expired gas concentrations and an assumed dead space. However, with the large CO_2 output of vigorous exercise, the end-tidal concentration may overestimate the mean arterial CO_2 for the entire respiratory cycle, and it is equally difficult to make a reliable estimate of dead space during all-out exercise. The venous CO_2 content is estimated from the plateau observed during the rebreathing of a gas mixture containing a high CO_2 concentration. If a good plateau is achieved before there has been time for a recirculation of blood, it is assumed that the CO_2 tension in the rebreathing bag matches that in mixed venous blood; however, confidence in the procedure is weakened by the need to apply a "downstream" correction of 10 or more torr to allow for the intravascular changes of CO_2 tension that occur during vigorous exercise.[136] Finally, it is necessary to make assumptions about the shape of the CO_2 dissociation curve in the face of exercise-induced changes in both hemoglobin concentrations and alkaline reserve. Despite these various potent theoretical objections, the CO_2 rebreathing method gives very credible figures for exercise cardiac out-

TABLE 2–5 Reasons for False-Positive and False-Negative Exercise Stress Tests

False-positive results	False-negative results
Hyperventilation	Insufficient exercise intensity
Cigarette smoking	ST elevation at rest
Glucose and carbohydrate loads	Abnormalities of ventricular conduction
Diuretics, potassium loss	Nitroglycerine and other vasodilators
Abnormal stress on left ventricle	
ST depression at rest	
Abnormal ventricular conduction (e.g., left ventricular bundle branch block)	
Antidysrhythmic drugs (e.g., procainamide, quinidine)	
Digitalis therapy	

(From Shephard RJ. Exercise physiology. Toronto: BC Decker, 1987: 83.)

put.[136] When cross-validation has been possible, the results have agreed closely with those obtained by other techniques.[146]

Practical Procedures and Interpretation

Careful preparation of the subject is very important prior to exercise testing. Measurements should preferably be made at least 24 hours after the last bout of strenuous exercise and 12 to 14 hours after a meal, cigarettes, alcohol or caffeine-containing drinks.[5] If interpretations of cardiovascular condition are to be based upon the heart rate during submaximal exercise, it is also important to conduct measurements in a room no warmer than 20 to 22° C and to allay anxiety by at least one practice of the required test procedures.[5] A substantial list of absolute and relative contraindications to exercise testing has been noted (American College of Sports Medicine, 1975; Table 2–6). There are also a number of important indications for halting an exercise test, including ST segmental depression of more than 0.2 mV, frequent premature ventricular contractions (for instance, more than three in any 10-second interval), and failure of the systemic blood pressure to show the anticipated rise (Table 2–7).

The clinical value of exercise testing is sometimes overestimated. The absolute figure for an athlete's maximum oxygen intake can be compared with that of the best international competitors in a particular discipline; however, in most types of sport, performance depends as much on efficiency in usage of the available oxygen as in maximization of supply. A competitor who is relatively poorly endowed from the cardiovascular viewpoint may thus achieve a surprisingly good performance on the track or in the pool.

Likewise, it is difficult to prescribe exercise for the average sedentary adult following a stress test. At least a half of the variance in maximum oxygen intake is genetically determined.[124] A mediocre score may thus indicate either a poorly endowed candidate who has already reached his or her potential or a lazy person who needs stimulating to much greater physical activity. It could be argued that the maximum oxygen intake reading gives valuable guidance in setting an appropriate intensity of exercise at the onset of training. A well-performed maximum oxygen intake measurement has a 4 to 5 percent experimental error, and to this must be added a 10 to 20 percent intraindividual variation caused by such factors as recent exercise, alterations of fluid balance, and intercurrent infection.[22] Finally, the energy cost of any prescribed exercise varies substantially from one person to another. At best, a maximum oxygen intake measurement can thus provide no more than a crude guide to the required intensity of exercise. Fine-tuning of the prescription must be based upon the individual's reactions on any given day—the rating of perceived exertion, the exercise heart rate, the extent of sweating, and the level of ventilation; ideally, there should be

TABLE 2–6 Contraindications to Exercise Testing

Absolute contraindications
  Acute infectious disease
  Unstable metabolic disorder
  Significant locomotor disturbance
  Excessive anxiety
  Recent or impending myocardial infarction
  Manifest cardiac failure
  Acute myocarditis
  Aortic stenosis
  Probability of recent pulmonary embolism

Special precautions needed
  Atrial fibrillation or flutter
  Atrioventricular block
  Left bundle-branch block
  Premature ventricular excitation (Wolff-Parkinson-White syndrome)

(From Shephard RJ. Ischemic heart disease and exercise. London: Croom Helm, 1981.)

TABLE 2–7 Indications for Halting an Exercise Test

Increasing chest pain
Severe dyspnea or fatigue
Faintness
Claudication
Signs of cerebrovascular insufficiency (pallor, cold moist skin, cyanosis, staggering gait, confusion)
Excessive rise in blood pressure
Sudden fall in systolic pressure
ST segmental depression >0.2 mV (horizontal or downsloping)
Premature ventricular contractions (more than 3 in 10 seconds, polyfocal, R on T)
Paroxysmal ventricular or supraventricular dysrhythmias
Conduction disturbances other than slight atrioventricular block

(From Shephard RJ. Ischemic heart disease and exercise. London: Croom Helm, 1981.)

some sweating, but the subject should still be able to engage in conversation.

A third suggested justification for stress testing is the ability to detect adverse reactions to exercise, such as deep ST segmental depression or premature ventricular contractions. However, particularly if exercise testing is widely applied to a low-risk population, as many as two-thirds of apparently adverse reactions are false-positive test results.[145] The widespread testing of symptom-free adults thus creates a great deal of unwarranted anxiety about cardiac function. Further investigations such as scintigraphy and angiography can resolve some of the anxiety, but at a substantial cost, and if unnecessary angiograms are performed, there is also some risk to the life of the patient.

Perhaps the most reasonable argument for exercise testing is that the progress of the individual can be followed. The athlete can trace the development of maximum oxygen intake over the course of a training program, the sedentary adult can likewise be motivated to persist with a conditioning program as gains in physical status are demonstrated, and responses to drug therapy or to a rehabilitation program can be monitored. The problem of genetically determined, interindividual differences in aerobic power is overcome if the person serves as his or her own control, but the difficulty of large, day-to-day intraindividual differences of score persists. Perhaps more seriously, particularly if improvements of test score are being used as a basis of motivation, the gains of maximum oxygen intake realized by a given amount of training diminish rapidly as an individual's physical potential is approached.

American physicians have argued the need of an exercise stress test before allowing an increase of physical activity in patients over the age of 35 years.[65,147,148] However, the comments above show that the dividends from such an examination are extremely slender; indeed, in some populations, the proportion of false-positive test results is so large that the majority of warnings against exercise would be erroneous.[145] In addition, insistence on a medically supervised stress test has created the false impression that exercise is something dangerous, rather than a natural form of behavior. For the person without cardiac risk factors, it is preferable to recommend a modest increase of physical activity without formal exercise testing. Gentle weekly progression should be encouraged, with testing reserved for those individuals who develop symptoms in response to such a regimen.[65]

CORONARY HEART DISEASE RISK ASSESSMENTS

Primary Coronary Risk Factors

Paffenbarger (1977) has suggested that reports on habitual activity, cigarette consumption, and blood pressure provide sufficient information to identify a population with an eightfold increase of coronary risk—a much clearer identification, incidentally, than is possible by use of an exercise electrocardiogram.[149]

In terms of voluntary leisure activity, Paffenbarger and colleagues (1986) have found some coronary protection is associated with a weekly energy expenditure of 2 megajoules (MJ), and maximum benefit is seen with a deliberate weekly expenditure of 8 to 9 MJ.[150] The risk caused by cigarette smoking increases with smoke exposure, as measured in pack-years. At one time, it was argued that the blood carbon monoxide levels of a smoker were sufficient to cause a local hypoxia of the vessel walls;[151] this hypothesis has now been largely rejected. Possibly, nicotine has a more direct action upon the heart, increasing myocardial irritability and thus the chances of inducing a cardiac arrhythmia. Hypertension increases cardiac work rate and thus the risk of myocardial ischemia.

The simple risk assessment of habitual activity, smoking habits, and blood pressure is commonly supplemented by some measure of overnutrition. Obesity is well recognized as a cardiac risk factor, although it has also been argued that it provides no independent assessment of risk if allowance is made for its association with hypertension and an adverse lipid profile.[152,153] Body mass is in any event a somewhat fallible indicator of cardiac risk, because a small increase of "weight" may reflect either an active lifestyle (with a good development of lean tissue) or sedentary living (with an accumulation of body fat).[154] Partly because the North American population has become more active over the past decade, actuarial groups have recently found it necessary to revise "ideal weights" in an upward direction.[155,156] More useful information on overnutrition is obtained by measurements of skinfold thicknesses. The "male" pattern of abdominal fat deposition seems to be associated with a higher cardiac risk than the "female" pattern of fat accumulation on the hips and thighs.[157] The total percentage of body fat can also be estimated by underwater weighing, although this approach requires cumbersome apparatus and an experienced investigator.

Cardiac risk has for long been associated with a high serum cholesterol (>270 mg per 100 mL), and if drastic measures are adopted to reduce initially high cholesterol levels (a combination of rigid dieting and regular treatment with cholesterol-lowering drugs), some decrease of future coronary incidents can be achieved.[158] It is now recognized that the most important aspect of the serum lipid profile is the ratio of the scavenging high-density lipoprotein (HDL)-cholesterol—particularly HDL-2—to low-density lipoprotein (LDL)-cholesterol. Regular physical activity (for instance, jogging 18 to 20 km per week) produces a clinically useful increase of high-density lipoprotein (HDL)-cholesterol.[159,160]

Other Risk Factors

The risk of a coronary attack normally increases with age, although it is less clearly established that the increased risk is a necessary accompaniment of aging. Plainly, the nature of atherosclerotic lesions is such that once established, they tend to progress as a person becomes older. The blood pressure also rises somewhat with age, increasing the cardiac work rate and thus exacerbating any tendency to myocardial ischemia.

The risk of a coronary attack is greater in men than in women. However, the cardiac advantage of women is currently lessening in developed countries.[161] Part of the previous difference of risk may have reflected traditional female roles and lifestyle (including a lesser average consumption of cigarettes and a greater concern about obesity). There also seems to be some hormonal influence, in view of three factors: the adverse impact of a "male" distribution of body fat, loss of female protection after the menopause, and the adverse impact of contraceptive medication containing progesterone.

There has been much debate concerning "stress" and heart disease. Russek (1966) indicated that occupational stress was a major determinant of coronary attacks, but others have suggested that cardiac stress is largely confined to the upwardly mobile.[162,163] Likewise, Rosenman (1983) has strongly urged the adverse influence of a time-conscious, type-A personality.[164] Others have cautioned that the main negative component of the type-A personality syndrome is an aggressive hostility; if this feature is absent, then type-A behavior confers no additional disadvantage.

Other cardiac risk factors include a poor glucose tolerance curve, a high serum uric acid, and a family history of premature death from heart disease. Heredity probably has some impact upon ischemic heart disease through such mechanisms as a faulty handling of cholesterol and glucose metabolism, together with a familial propensity for obesity. However, it is quite difficult to disentangle the true effects of heredity from responses to a common home environment, which may include such adverse influences as sedentary living, cigarette smoking, and overeating.

Moderate levels of alcohol consumption have been associated with some increase of HDL-cholesterol and thus a reduced risk of heart attacks.[165] However, most calculations suggest that other risks associated with regular alcohol ingestion outweigh this small advantage, so a moderate consumption of alcohol cannot be commended as a public health measure.

Coronary Risk Assessment

Many authors think of coronary risk assessment primarily in terms of an exercise stress test, and (despite the high incidence of false-positive records) there is a statistical association between exercise-induced ST-segmental depression and the risk of a future heart attack.[3,145] However, the foregoing discussion indicates that there are much simpler procedures for identifying the person at increased risk.[65] If the objective is to identify high-risk patients, then a simple activity and smoking history, together with a clinical determination of resting blood pressure, is already four times more effective than an exercise stress test. The confidence of predictions can be increased further by taking a family history and by making simple observations of body mass relative to height, skinfold distribution, and "Ketostix" urinary sugar estimation.

Finally, it is worth enquiring, "What is the purpose of risk factor assessment?" It is certainly useful to identify patients with hypertension and diabetes (who may require medical treatment), but the advice offered to the remaining patients is rather similar whether they fall into a high- or a low-risk category. They should be encouraged to increase habitual exercise progressively to a deliberate weekly expenditure of 8 to 9 MJ, to stop smoking, to strive for an ideal body mass, and to avoid hostile attitudes either at work or in the family.

REFERENCES

1. Tesch P. Exercise performance and beta blockade. Sports Medicine 1985; 2:389–412.
2. di Prampero PE. Anaerobic capacity and power. In: Shephard RJ, ed. Frontiers of fitness. Springfield, IL: CC Thomas, 1971.
3. Shephard RJ. Physiology and biochemistry of exercise. New York: Praeger Publishing, 1982.
4. Wilkes D, Gledhill N, Smyth R. Effect of acute induced metabolic acidosis on 800-m racing time. Med Sci Sports Exerc 1983; 15:277–280.
5. Shephard RJ. Endurance fitness. 2nd ed. Toronto: University of Toronto Press, 1977.
6. Shephard RJ. Human physiological work capacity. London: Cambridge University Press, 1978.
7. Holmér I. Physiology of swimming man. Acta Physiol Scand (Suppl) 1974; 407:1–55.
8. Rennie DW, Prendergast DR, di Prampero, et al. Energetics of the overarm crawl. Med Sci Sports 1973; 5:65.
9. Seliger V, Pachlopnikova I, Mann M, et al. Energy expenditure during paddling. Physiol Bohemoslov 1969; 18:49–55.
10. Shephard RJ. Science and medicine of canoeing and kayaking. Sports Med 1987; 4:19–33.
11. Dempsey JA, Hanson PG, Henderson KS. Exercise-induced arterial hypoxaemia in healthy human subjects at sea level. J Physiol 1984; 355:161–175.
12. Shephard RJ. Respiratory factors limiting prolonged effort. Can J Sport Sci 1987; 12:45S–52S.
13. Shephard RJ. Altitude training camps. Br J Sports Med 1974; 8:38–45.
14. Saltin B, Hermansen L. Esophageal, rectal, and muscle temperature during exercise. J Appl Physiol 1966; 21:1757–1762.
15. Henry JP. The significance of the loss of blood volume into the limbs during pressure breathing. J Aviat Med 1951; 22:31–38.
16. Asmussen E, Bøje O. Body temperature and capacity for work. Acta Physiol Scand 1945; 10:1–22.
17. Saltin B. Oxygen transport by the circulatory system during exercise in man. In: Keul J, ed. Limiting factors of physical performance. Stuttgart: G Thieme, 1973:235.
18. Shephard RJ. Environment. In: Williams JGP, Sperryn P, eds. Sports medicine. London: Arnold, 1976:76.
19. Åstrand I. Aerobic work capacity in men and women with special reference to age. Acta Physiol Scand 1960; 49 (Suppl 169):1–92.
20. Shephard RJ, Vandewalle H, Boulel E, Monod H. Muscle mass as a factor limiting work. J Appl Physiol 1988; 64:1472–1479.
21. Davies CTM. Commentary. Can Med Assoc J 1967; 96:743–744.
22. Wright GR, Sidney KH, Shephard RJ. Variance of direct and indirect measures of aerobic power. J Sports Med Phys Fitness 1978; 18:33–42.
23. Bevegard S, Holmgren A, Jonsson B. The effect of body position on the circulation at rest and during exercise with special reference to the influence on the stroke volume. Acta Physiol Scand 1960; 49:279–285.
24. Holmgren A, Ovenfors C. Heart volume at rest and during muscular work in the supine and in the sitting position. Acta Med Scand 1960; 167:267–274.
25. Wilson JN, Grow JB, Demong CV, et al. Central venous pressure in optimal blood volume maintenance. Arch Surg 1962; 85:563–578.
26. Niinimaa V, Shephard RJ. Training and oxygen conductance in the elderly. J Gerontol 1978; 33:362–367.
27. Rodeheffer RJ, Gerstenblith G, Becker LC, et al. Exercise cardiac output is maintained with advancing age in healthy human subjects: cardiac dilatation and increased stroke volume compensate for a diminished heart rate. Circulation 1984; 69:201–213.
28. Simmons R, Shephard RJ. Measurement of cardiac output during exercise. Applications of an acetylene rebreathing method to arm and leg exercise. Int Z Angew Physiol, 1971; 29:159–172.
29. Rushmer RF. Constancy of stroke volume in ventricular responses to exertion. Am J Physiol 1959; 196:745–750.
30. Katz AM. Physiology of the heart. New York: Raven Press, 1977.
31. Rowell LB. Circulatory adjustments to dynamic exercise. In: Human circulation regulation during physical stress. New York: Oxford University Press, 1986:213.
32. Chapman CB, Baker O, Franklin D. Mechanisms of cardiac control in exercise. J Clin Invest 1959; 38:1202–1210.
33. Erickson HH, Bishop VS, Kardon MB, Horowitz LD. Left ventricular internal diameter and cardiac function during exercise. J Appl Physiol 1971; 30:473–479.
34. Horowitz LD, Atkins JM, Keshin SJ. Role of the Frank-

Starling mechanism in exercise. Circ Res 1972; 31:868–877.
35. Mitchell JH, Wildenthal JH. Left ventricular function during exercise. In: Larson AO, Malmborg RO, eds. Coronary heart disease and physical fitness. Copenhagen: Munksgaard; Scandinavian University Books, 1970.
36. Vatner SF, Franklin D, Higgins CB, et al. Left ventricular response to severe exertion in untethered dogs. J Clin Invest 1972; 51:3052–3058.
37. Wildenthal K, Mitchell JH. Dimensional analysis of the left ventricle in unanaesthetized dogs. J Appl Physiol 1969; 27:115–119.
38. Braunwald E, Goldblatt A, Harrison DC, Mason DT. Studies on cardiac dimensions in intact, unanaesthetised man. Effects of muscular exercise. Circ Res 1963; 13:460–467.
39. Braunwald E, Ross J, Sonnenblick EH. Mechanisms of contraction of the normal and failing heart. Boston: Little, Brown, 1976.
40. Crawford M, White D, Amor K. Echocardiographic evaluation of left ventricular size and performance during hand grip and supine and upright bicycle exercise. Circulation 1979; 59:1118–1127.
41. Gorlin R, Cohen L, Elliott W, et al. Effect of supine exercise on left ventricular volume and oxygen consumption in man. Circulation 1965; 32:361–371.
42. Sharma B, Goodwin RF, Raphael MJ, et al. Left ventricular angiography on exercise: a new method of assessing left ventricular function in ischemic heart disease. Br Heart J 1976; 38:59–70.
43. Slutsky R, Karliner J, Ricci D, et al. Response of left ventricular volume to exercise in man assessed by radionuclide equilibrium angiography. Circulation 1979; 60:565–571.
44. Sorenson SG, Ritchie JL, Caldwell JH, et al. Serial exercise radionuclide angiography. Validation of count-derived changes in cardiac output and quantitation of maximal exercise ventricular volume change after nitroglycerin and propranolol in normal men. Circulation 1980; 61:600–609.
45. Tebbe U, Hoffmeister N, Sauer G, et al. Changes in left ventricular diastolic function in coronary artery disease with and without angina pectoris assessed from ventriculography. Clin Cardiol 1980; 3:19–25.
46. Bar-Shlomo BB, Druck MN, Morch JE, et al. Left ventricular function in trained and untrained healthy subjects. Circulation 1982; 65:484–488.
47. Steingart RM, Wexler J, Slagle S, Scheuer J. Radionuclide ventriculographic responses to graded supine and upright exercise: critical role of the Frank-Starling mechanism at submaximal exercise. Am J Cardiol 1984; 53:1671–1677.
48. Poliner LE, Dehmer GJ, Lewis SE, et al. Left ventricular performance in normal subjects: a comparison of the responses to exercise in the upright and supine positions. Circulation 1980; 62:528–534.
49. Higginbotham MB, Morris KG, Coleman RE, Cobb FR. Sex-related differences in the normal cardiac response to upright exercise. Circulation 1984; 70:357–366.
50. Boucher CA, Anderson MD, Schneider MS, et al. Left ventricular function before and after reaching anaerobic threshold. Chest 1985; 87:145–150.
51. Isakandrian AS. Nuclear cardiac imaging: principles and applications. Philadelphia: FA Davis, 1987.
52. Little RC. Physiology of the heart and circulation. Chicago: Year Book Medical Publishing, 1985.
53. McLaughlin PR, Morch JE. Myocardial imaging. Don Mills: Addison-Wesley, 1985.
54. Kay C, Shephard RJ. On muscle strength and the threshold of anaerobic work. Int Z Angew Physiol 1969; 27:311–328.
55. Lind AR, McNicol GW. Muscular factors which determine the cardiovascular responses to sustained and rhythmic exercise. Can Med Assoc J 1967; 96:706–712.
56. Royce J. Isometric fatigue curves in human muscle with normal and occluded circulation. Res Quart 1958; 29:204–212.
57. von Euler US. Sympatho-adrenal activity in physical exercise. Med Sci Sports 1974; 6:165–173.
58. Isakandrian AS, Hakki A-H, Kane SA, et al. Quantitative radionuclide angiography to assess circulatory changes during upright exercise in patients with poor left ventricular function. J Cardiac Rehab 1981; 1:423–432.
59. Rerych S, Scholz P, Newman, et al. Cardiac function at rest and during exercise in normals and patients with coronary heart disease. Ann Surg 1984; 187:449–464.
60. Thadani U, Parker JO. Hemodynamics at rest and during supine and sitting bicycle exercise in normal subjects. Am J Cardiol 1978; 41:52–59.
61. Upton MT, Rerych SK, Roeback JR, et al. The effect of acute and prolonged exercise on left ventricular function. Circulation 1978; 58:II-7 (abstr).
62. Weiss JL, Weisfeldt ML, Mason SJ, et al. Evidence of Frank-Starling effect in man during severe semi-supine exercise. Circulation 1979; 59:655–661.
63. Plas F. Guide de cardiologie du sport. Paris: Laboratoires Besins-Iscovesco, 1976.
64. Rost R. Herz und sport. Erlangen: Perimed Fachbuch, 1984.
65. Shephard RJ. Physical activity and aging. 2nd ed. London: Croom Helm, 1987.
66. Millikan GA. Experiments on muscle haemoglobin in vivo; the instantaneous measurement of muscle metabolism. Proc Roy Soc (Biol) 1937; 123:218–241.
67. Chance B. Cellular oxygen requirements. Fed Proc 1957; 16:671–680.
68. de Wijn JF, de Jongste JL, Mosterd W, Willebrand D. Haemoglobin, packed cell volume, serum iron, and iron-binding capacity of selected athletes during training. J Sports Med Phys Fitness 1971; 11:42–51.
69. Ferro-Luzzi A, Topi GC, Caldarone G. Consumi alimentari abituali di atleti italiani probabili olimpici (P.O. 1972). Med dello Sport 1975; 28:109–125.
70. Shephard RJ, Conway S, Thomson M, et al. In: Pawluk J, ed. Nutritional demands of submaximum work: marathon and trans-Canadian events. Warsaw: Polish Sports Federation International Symposium on Athletic Nutrition, 1976.

71. Kiiskinen A, Kemppinen L, Hasen J. Is the anemia following repeated sessions of heavy physical exercise caused by a decreased rate of production of red cells? In: Proceedings of conference, metabolic adaptation to prolonged exercise. Magglingen: Swiss Institute of Sports Medicine, 1973.
72. Verde T, Shephard RJ, Corey P, Moore R. Sweat composition in exercise and heat. In: Bachl N, Prokop L, Suckert R, eds. Current topics in sports medicine. Wien: Urban & Schwarzenburg, 1984: 1056.
73. Davies CTM, Van Haaren JPM. Effect of treatment on physiological responses to exercise in East African industrial workers with iron deficiency anaemia. Br J Ind Med 1973; 30:335–340.
74. Bar-Or O, Shephard RJ, Allen CL. Cardiac output of 10–13 year old boys and girls during submaximal exercise. J Appl Physiol 1971; 30:219–223.
75. Åstrand PO. Experimental studies of physical working capacity in relation to age and sex. Copenhagen: Munksgaard, 1952.
75a. Shephard RJ. Physical activity and growth. Chicago: Year Book Publishers, 1982.
76. Lester FM, Sheffield LT, Trammell P, Reeves TJ. The effect of age and athletic training on maximal heart rate during muscular exercise. Am Heart J 1968; 76:370–376.
77. Sidney KH, Shephard RJ. Maximum testing of men and women in the seventh, eighth, and ninth decades of life. J Appl Physiol 1977; 43:280–287.
78. Weisfeldt ML, Gerstenblith ML, Lakatta EG. Alterations in circulatory function. In: Andres R, Bierman EL, Hazzard WR, eds. Principles of geriatric medicine. New York: McGraw Hill, 1985:248.
79. Kavanagh T, Shephard RJ. The effects of continued training on the aging process. Ann NY Acad Sci 1977; 301:455–465.
80. Shephard RJ. The influence of age on the haemoglobin level in congenital heart disease. Br Heart J 1956; 18:49–54.
81. Shephard RJ. Nutrition and the physiology of aging. In: Young ER, ed. Nutrition, aging, and health. New York: Alan Liss, 1986:1.
82. Kavanagh T, Yacoub MH, Mertens DJ, et al. Responses to progressive exercise training after cardiac transplantation. Circulation, in press.
83. Haddy FJ, Scott JB. Metabolical factors in peripheral circulatory regulation. Fed Proc 1975; 34:2006–2011.
84. Folkow B, Neil E. Circulation. London: Oxford University Press, 1971.
85. Kindermann W. Calcium antagonists and exercise performance. Sports Med 1987; 4:177–193.
86. Taylor JW, Williams MA, Ryschon KL, Fardy PS. Logistic regression to predict risk for early exercise training in cardiac patients. Med Sci Sports Exerc 1982; 14:115 (abstr).
87. Broman S, Wigertz O. Transient dynamics of ventilation and heart rate with changes in work load from different load levels. Acta Physiol Scand 1971; 81:54–74.
88. Jones WB, Finchum RN, Russell RO, Reeves TJ. Transient cardiac output responses to multiple levels of supine exercise. J Appl Physiol 1970; 28:183–189.
89. Barnard RJ, Gardner GW, Diaco NV, et al. Cardiovascular responses to sudden strenuous exercise: heart rate, blood pressure, and ECG. J Appl Physiol 1973; 34:833–837.
90. Yamaji K, Shephard RJ. Heartrate overshoot in running events. Br J Sports Med 1986; 20:62–65.
91. Bailey DA, Shephard RJ, Mirwald RL. Validation of a self-administered home test of cardiorespiratory fitness. Can J Appl Sport Sci 1976; 1:67–78.
92. Cotton FS, Dill DB. On the relationship between the heart rate during exercise and that of the immediate postexercise period. Am J Physiol 1935; 111:554–558.
93. McDonough J, Bruce RA. Maximal exercise testing in assessing cardiovascular function. In: Proc National Conference on Exercise in the Prevention, in the Evaluation and in the Treatment of Heart Disease. JSC Med Assoc 1969; 65 (Suppl 1):26–33.
94. Shephard RJ, Kavanagh T. Predicting the cardiac catastrophe in the "postcoronary" patient. Can Fam Phys 1978; 24:614–618.
95. Shephard RJ, Cox M, Simper K. An analysis of PAR-Q responses in an office population. Can J Public Health 1981; 72:37–40.
96. Young MA, Rowlands DB, Stallard TJ, et al. Effect of environment on blood pressure: home versus hospital. Br Med J 1983; 286:1235–1236.
97. Kavanagh T, Shephard RJ. Physiological data on Masters' Athletes, in preparation.
98. Mirsky I. Review of various theories for the evaluation of left ventricular wall stresses. In: Mirsky I, Ghista D, Sandler H, eds. Cardiac mechanics: physiological, clinical and mathematical considerations. New York: John Wiley & Sons, 1974:381.
99. Blomqvist G. Exercise physiology related to diagnosis of coronary artery disease. In: Fox SM, ed. Coronary artery disease: prevention, detection, rehabilitation with emphasis on exercise testing. Denver, CO: International Medical Corporation, 1974: 2-1.
100. Jorgensen CR, Gobel FL, Taylor HL, Wang Y. Myocardial blood flow and oxygen consumption during exercise. Ann NY Acad Sci 1977; 301:213–223.
101. Maréchal R, Pirnay F, Petit JM. Débit circulatoire pendant le contraction isométrique. Arch Int Physiol Biochem 1973; 81:273–281.
102. Kilböm Å. Circulatory adaptations during static muscular exercise. Scand J Work Environ Health 1976; 2:1–13.
103. Clausen JP. Muscle blood flow during exercise and its significance for maximal performance. In: Keul J, ed. Limiting factors of human performance. Stuttgart: G. Thieme, 1973:253.
104. Folkow B, Gaskell P, Waaler BA. Blood flow through limb muscles during heavy rhythmic exercise. Acta Physiol Scand 1970; 80:61–72.
105. Brouha L, Radford EP. The cardiovascular system in muscular activity. In: Johnson WR, ed. Science and medicine of exercise and sports. 1st ed. New York: Harper & Row, 1960.

106. Rowell LB. Human cardiovascular adjustments to exercise and thermal stress. Physiol Rev 1974; 54:75–159.
106a. Wade OL, Bishop JM. Cardiac output and regional blood flow. Oxford: Blackwell Scientific Publications, 1962.
107. Refsum HE, Strømme SB. Relationship between urine flow, glomerular filtration, and urine solute concentration during prolonged heavy exercise. Scand J Clin Lab Invest 1975; 35:775–780.
108. Wyndham CH, Strydom N. Korperliche Arbeit bei hoher Temperatur. In: Hollmann W, ed. Zentrale Themen der Sportmedizin. Berlin: Springer Verlag, 1972.
109. Zobl EG, Talmers FN, Christensen RC, Baer LJ. Effect of exercise on the cerebral circulation and metabolism. J Appl Physiol 1965; 20:1289–1293.
110. Dustman RE, Ruhling RO, Russell EM, et al. Aerobic exercise training and improved neuropsychological function of older individuals. Neurobiology of Aging 1984; 5:35–42.
111. West JB. Blood flow. In: Regional differences in the lung. New York: Academic Press, 1977:85.
112. Lundgren O, Jodal M. Regional blood flow. Ann Rev Physiol 1975; 37:395–414.
113. Leblanc J. Man in the cold. Springfield, IL: CC Thomas, 1975.
114. Shephard RJ. Adaptation to exercise in the cold. Sports Med 1985; 2:59–71.
115. Bryan AC. Commentary. Can Med Assoc J 1967; 96:804.
116. Kreuzer F. Transport of O_2 and CO_2 at altitude. In: Margaria R, ed. Exercise at altitude. Dordrecht: Excerpta Medica Foundation, 1967:149.
117. Hannon JP, Shields JL, Harris CW. Effects of altitude acclimatization on blood composition of women. J Appl Physiol 1969; 26:540–547.
118. Kidd DJ, Stubbs RA. The use of the pneumatic analogue computer for divers. In: Bennett PB, Elliott DH, eds. Physiology and medicine of diving. London: Baillière, Tindall & Cassell, 1969:386.
119. Åstrand I. Circulatory responses to arm exercise in different work positions. Scand J Clin Lab Invest 1971; 27:293–297.
120. Åstrand I. Degree of strain during building work as related to individual aerobic work capacity. Ergonomics 1967; 10:293–303.
121. Bonjer FH. Relationship between working time, physical work capacity, and allowable caloric expenditure. In: Muskelarbeit und Muskeltraining. Darmstadt: Gentner Verlag, 1968.
122. Hughes AL, Goldman RF. Energy cost of hard work. J Appl Physiol 1970; 29:570–572.
123. Åstrand I, Åstrand PO, Christensen EH, Hedman R. Myohemoglobin as an oxygen store in man. Acta Physiol Scand 1960; 48:454.
124. Bouchard C, Malina RM. Genetics of physiological fitness and motor performance. Exerc Sport Sci Rev 1983; 11:306–399.
125. Shephard RJ. Intensity, duration, and frequency of training as determinants of the response to a training regime. Int Z Angew Physiol 1968; 26:272–278.
126. Sidney KH, Shephard RJ. Frequency and intensity of exercise training for elderly subjects. Med Sci Sports 1978; 10:125–131.
127. Borg G. The perception of physical performance. In: Shephard RJ, ed. Frontiers of fitness. Springfield, IL: CC Thomas, 1971.
128. Hellerstein HK. Limitations to marathon running in the rehabilitation of coronary patients: anatomic and physiologic determinants. Ann NY Acad Sci 1977; 301:484–494.
129. Clausen JP. Effects of physical training on cardiovascular adjustments to exercise in man. Physiol Rev 1977; 57:779–815.
130. Eckstein RW. Effect of exercise and coronary artery narrowing on coronary collateral circulation. Circ Res 1957; 5:230–235.
131. Froelicher VF. Exercise testing and training. Chicago: Year Book Publishers, 1983.
132. Schaper W. Influence of physical exercise on coronary collateral blood flow in chronic experimental two-vessel occlusion. Circulation 1982; 65:905–912.
133. Shephard RJ. Ischemic heart disease and exercise. London: Croom Helm, 1981.
134. Blackburn H. Measurement in exercise electrocardiography. The Ernst Simonson Conference. Springfield, IL: CC Thomas, 1969.
135. Abbasi AS. Echocardiographic interpretation. Springfield, IL: CC Thomas, 1981.
136. Jones NL, Campbell EJM, Edwards RHT, Robertson DG. Clinical exercise testing. Philadelphia: WB Saunders, 1975.
137. Margaria R, Aghemo P, Rovelli E. Indirect determination of maximal O_2 consumption in man. J Appl Physiol 1965; 20:1070–1073.
138. Maritz JS, Morrison JF, Peter J, et al. A practical method of estimating an individual's maximum oxygen intake. Ergonomics 1961; 4:97–122.
139. Von Döbeln W. Human standard and maximal metabolic rate in relation to fat-free body mass. Acta Physiol Scand (Suppl) 1956; 126:1–79.
140. Wahlund H. Determination of physical work capacity. Acta Med Scand 1948; 215 (Suppl 9):1–127.
141. Cotes JE. Occupational safety and health series report 6. Geneva: International Labour Organization, 1966.
142. Shephard RJ. Current status of the Canadian Home Fitness Test. S Afr J Res Sport, Physical Education, and Recreation 1979; 2:19–35.
143. Brooks G. The lactate shuttle during exercise and recovery. Med Sci Sports Exerc 1986; 18:360–368.
144. Wasserman K, Beaver WL, Whipp BJ. Mechanisms and patterns of blood lactate increase during exercise in man. Med Sci Sports Exerc 1986; 18:344–352.
145. Shephard RJ. Prognostic value of exercise testing for ischemic heart disease. Br J Sports Med 1982; 16:220–229.
146. Paterson DH, Cunningham DA. Comparison of methods to calculate cardiac output using CO_2 rebreathing method. Eur J Appl Physiol 1976; 35:223–230.
147. Cooper KH. Guidelines in the management of the exercising patient. JAMA 1970; 211:1663–1667.
148. American College of Sports Medicine. Guidelines

for graded exercise testing and prescription. Philadelphia: Lea & Febiger, 1975.
149. Paffenbarger RS. Physical activity and fatal heart attack: protection or selection? In: Amsterdam EA, Wilmore JH, de Maria AN, eds. Exercise in cardiovascular health and disease. New York: Yorke Books, 1977:35.
150. Paffenbarger RS, Hyde RT, Wing AL, Hsieh CC. Physical activity, all-cause mortality, and longevity of college alumni. N Engl J Med 1986; 314:605–613.
151. Åstrup P, Hellung-Larsen P, Kjeldsen K, Mellemgaard K. The effect of tobacco smoking on the dissociation curve of oxyhaemoglobin. Scand J Clin Invest 1966; 18:450–457.
152. Kannel WB, Brand FN. Cardiovascular risk factors in the elderly. In: Andres R, Bierman EL, Hazzard WR, eds. Principles of geriatric medicine. New York: McGraw-Hill, 1985:104.
153. Keys A, Aravanis C, Blackburn H, et al. Coronary heart disease: overweight and obesity. Ann Intern Med 1972; 77:15–27.
154. Nutrition Canada. National survey. Coordinator: ZI Sabry. Ottawa: Health & Welfare Canada, 1973.
155. Andres R. Mortality and obesity: the rationale for age-specific height–weight tables. In: Andres R, Bierman EL, Hazzard WR, eds. Principles of geriatric medicine. New York: McGraw Hill, 1985:311.
156. Metropolitan Life Insurance. 1983 Metropolitan height and weight tables. Stat Bull Metrop Life Ins Co 1983; 64:2.
157. Björntorp P. Physiological and clinical aspects of exercise in obese persons. Exerc Sport Sci Rev 1983; 11:159–180.
158. Lipid Research Clinics Program. II. Relationship of reduction in the incidence of coronary heart disease to cholesterol lowering. JAMA 1984; 251: 365–374.
159. Kavanagh T, Shephard RJ, Lindley LJ, Pieper M. Influence of exercise and lifestyle variables upon high-density lipoprotein cholesterol after myocardial infarction. Arteriosclerosis 1983; 3:249–259.
160. Williams PT, Wood PD, Haskell WL, Vranizan K. The effects of running mileage and duration on plasma lipoprotein levels. JAMA 1982; 247:2672–2679.
161. Anderson TW, Halliday ML. The male epidemic: 50 years of ischaemic heart disease. Publ Health (Lond) 1979; 93:163–172.
162. Russek HI. Emotional stress, tobacco smoking, and ischemic heart disease. In: Raab W, ed. Prevention of ischemic heart disease. Principles and practice. Springfield, IL: CC Thomas, 1966.
163. Hinckle LE. An estimate of the effects of "stress" on the incidence and prevalence of coronary heart disease in a large industrial population in the United States. Thromb Diath Haemorrh 1972; 51 (Suppl):15–65.
164. Rosenman RH. Psychosomatic risk factors and coronary heart disease: indications for specific preventive therapy. Bern: Hans Huber Publishers, 1983.
165. Castelli WP, Gordon T, Hjortland MC, et al. Alcohol and blood lipids. The cooperative lipoprotein phenotyping study. Lancet 1977; 2:153–155.

Chapter 3
Respiratory Responses and Adaptations to Exercise

TONY G. WALDROP

The respiratory system plays a pivotal role in meeting the demands placed upon the body during exercise. The muscular work of exercise requires increased uptake and delivery of oxygen to the active muscles as well as an increased removal of metabolites such as carbon dioxide. The oxygen uptake ($\dot{V}O_2$) can increase from a basal level of 250 mL per minute to 5 L per minute during severe exercise.[1] This increased oxygen uptake is brought about by large increases in ventilation during exercise. Ventilation can increase from a resting level of 6 L per minute to more than 150 L per minute during exhausting exercise.[1] It is well known that a linear relationship exists between oxygen uptake and ventilation for mild to moderate exercise. Ventilation increases out of proportion to metabolic rate during severe exercise (Fig. 3–1).[1-3]

The respiratory and cardiovascular systems function together to meet the demands imposed by exercise. It is obvious that an increased ventilation must be coupled to an increased cardiac output if the elevated oxygen requirement of the working tissues is to be met. Chapter 2 discusses the cardiovascular responses to exercise in greater detail.

RESPIRATORY RESPONSES TO EXERCISE

Two types of exercise are encountered every day for most individuals. *Static (isometric) exercise* is defined as muscular contraction that produces principally a change in tension with only small changes in the length of the active muscles.[4] Lifting or pushing heavy objects is considered static exercise. *Dynamic (rhythmic) exercise* involves muscular contraction that consists primarily of changes in the length of the muscle with minor changes in tension of the active muscles.[4] Walking, running, swimming, and bicycling are all types of dynamic exercise. The respiratory response is different for these two types of exercise.

Respiratory Responses to Static Exercise

Several investigators have studied the respiratory response to static handgrip exercise in humans.[5-7] These studies have shown that the magnitude of the increase in ventilation is proportional to the tension developed by the contracting muscles. Exercise at 15 percent of the

60 / Scientific Foundations of Sports Medicine

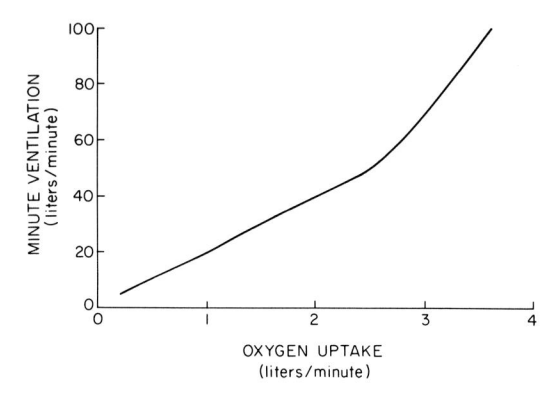

Figure 3-1 Relationship between ventilation and oxygen consumption. Ventilation increases in direct proportion to oxygen consumption up to heavy workloads.

maximal voluntary contraction (MVC) does not elicit a significant change in ventilation. However, static exercise at and above 20 percent MVC produces increases in ventilation that result from an increase in tidal volume without a significant change in the frequency of breathing (Fig. 3-2).[5]

The time course of the respiratory response to static exercise at 20 percent MVC and above consists of a small increase in ventilation at the onset of the exercise with no further change for the next 3 minutes (Fig. 3-2).[5] A rapid and progressive increase in breathing then occurs after approximately 3 minutes of exercise. This ventilatory response is that of hyperventilation, because a significant fall in end-tidal P_{CO_2} occurs after 3 minutes of exercise at 30 percent MVC. In one study, a fall of 6 torr in end-tidal P_{CO_2} was present in subjects after 5 minutes of static exercise at 30 percent MVC.[5]

Respiratory Responses to Dynamic (Rhythmic) Exercise

The respiratory response to dynamic exercise has been well documented. Ventilation increases immediately at the beginning of exercise.[8,9] This initial increase in ventilation within one to two breaths at the onset of exercise is followed by a relatively stable plateau over the next 20 to 40 seconds.[3,8] This level is followed by a gradual increase in ventilation over the next few minutes of exercise until a steady state is achieved (Fig. 3-3). The increased ventilation during dynamic exercise results from increases in both tidal volume and respiratory frequency. The increased respiratory frequency response during dynamic exercise is in contrast to the absence of such a response during static exercise.

The respiratory response to moderate dynamic exercise has long been thought to be an increase in breathing without any changes in arterial P_{CO_2}, i.e., an isocapnic hyperpnea.[2,8] However, this concept has been questioned in recent years. Studies performed in a wide va-

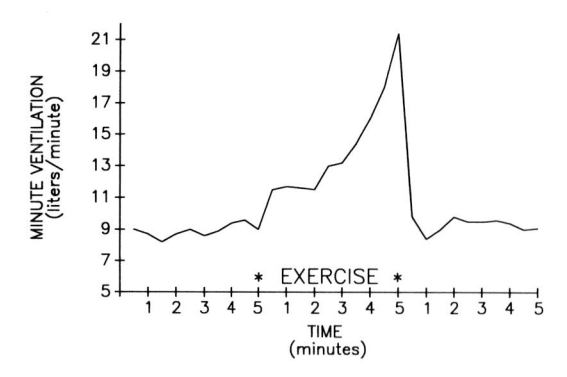

Figure 3-2 Ventilatory response to static (handgrip) exercise. Asterisks denote the beginning and end of the exercise bout. (Adapted from data of Muza SR, Lee LY, Wiley RL, et al. J Appl Physiol 1983; 54:1457–1462.)

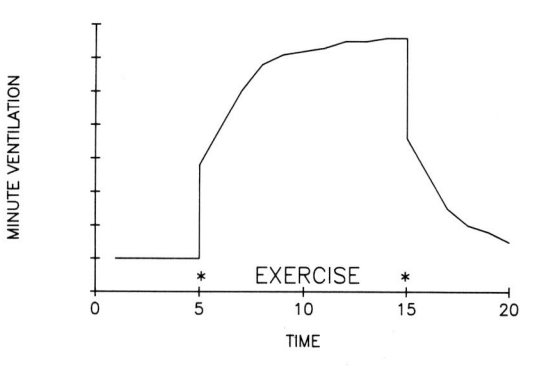

Figure 3-3 Ventilatory response to rhythmic exercise. Asterisks denote the beginning and end of the exercise bout. (Adapted from Dempsey JA, Vidruk EH, Mastenbrook SM. Fed Proc 1980; 39:1498–1505.)

riety of animal species have shown that P_{CO_2} falls during dynamic exercise. The animal species that respond in this manner include dogs, rats, ponies, goats, lizards, birds, and cats.[10-18] Musch and co-workers have shown that a significant fall in arterial P_{CO_2} occurs in dogs running on a treadmill, even during moderate exercise. The magnitude of this hypocapnia remains unchanged despite a rise in body temperature and metabolic acidosis when the exercise intensity is increased.

There is still debate about the possibility of hyperventilation during dynamic exercise in humans. Several studies have documented a slight hyperventilation producing a fall in P_{CO_2} (approximately 3 torr) at the onset of exercise.[19-22] However, this hypocapnia dissipates after 30 seconds of exercise, and P_{CO_2} returns to control levels. Other investigators have not observed this initial fall in arterial P_{CO_2} in human subjects.[8,23,24] Fordyce and colleagues have concluded from a survey of human studies that a fall in P_{CO_2} (hyperventilation) is more pronounced at the onset of treadmill exercise than at the onset of exercise on a bicycle ergometer.

In summary, moderate (more than 15 percent MVC) static exercise increases ventilation because of an increase in tidal volume with no significant change in respiratory frequency. The increased ventilation associated with dynamic exercise results from increases in both tidal volume and frequency of breathing. Hypocapnia develops relatively slowly during static exercise and appears only after 3 minutes of sustained exercise. Hypocapnia develops at the onset of dynamic exercise, at least in some studies, but dissipates rapidly in humans. This hypocapnia is sustained in dogs during treadmill exercise.

Coupling of Breathing and Locomotor Rhythms

A number of studies have concluded that breathing occurs at a frequency related to limb movements during dynamic exercise.[10,25-29] This association between breathing and locomotor movements has been observed in a number of quadrupedal species, including dogs, rabbits, and horses, as well as in bipeds (e.g., humans). The coupling in animals that locomote on all four limbs is a one-to-one relationship during trotting and galloping, i.e., one breath per locomotor cycle (Fig. 3–4).[26] The relationship is not as clear with two-leg locomotion. The breathing rhythm in humans occurs at various multiples of the locomotor rhythm, i.e., 4:1, 3:1, 3:2, and so on (see Fig. 3–4).[26] Moreover, human subjects do not couple their breathing and pedal or stride frequencies at all times during bicycle ergometer or treadmill exercise. Instead, humans go in and out of coupling during any exercise bout. Various reports found that the coupling of rhythms ranges from 25 percent to 94 percent of the exercise duration (see Fig. 3–4).[25,26,28,29] The amount of coupling appears to depend upon a number of factors.[25,28,29] Inexperienced runners seldom couple their breathing to locomotor rhythm. Greater linkage between breathing and stride frequencies occurs when stride (or pedaling) frequency is controlled by listening to a metronome or watching a speedometer. In addition, greater coupling occurs at high than at low exercise intensities.

The tendency to breathe at a rhythm similar to the locomotor frequency indicates neural linkage between the respiratory and locomotor systems. It has been suggested that this coupling results from supraspinal interactions be-

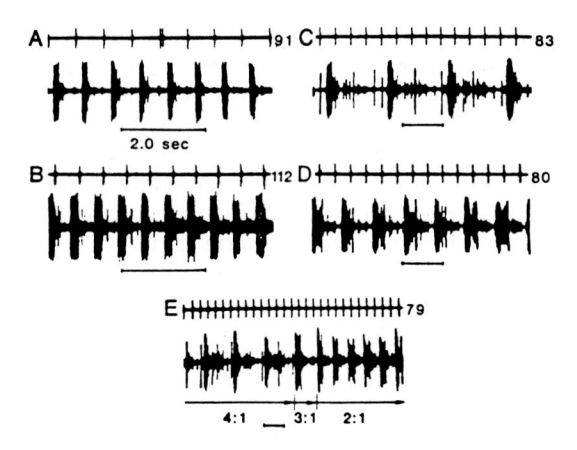

Figure 3–4 Relationship between respiratory and locomotor rates in horses (A and B) and a human (C through E). Upper trace is a measure of footfall of right forelimb in horses or leg in humans. Lower trace is a measure of breathing. The numbers to the right of upper traces are the stride rate per minute. (From Bramble DM, Carrier DR. Science 1983; 219:215–256. Copyright 1983 by the American Association for the Advancement of Science. Reproduced with permission.)

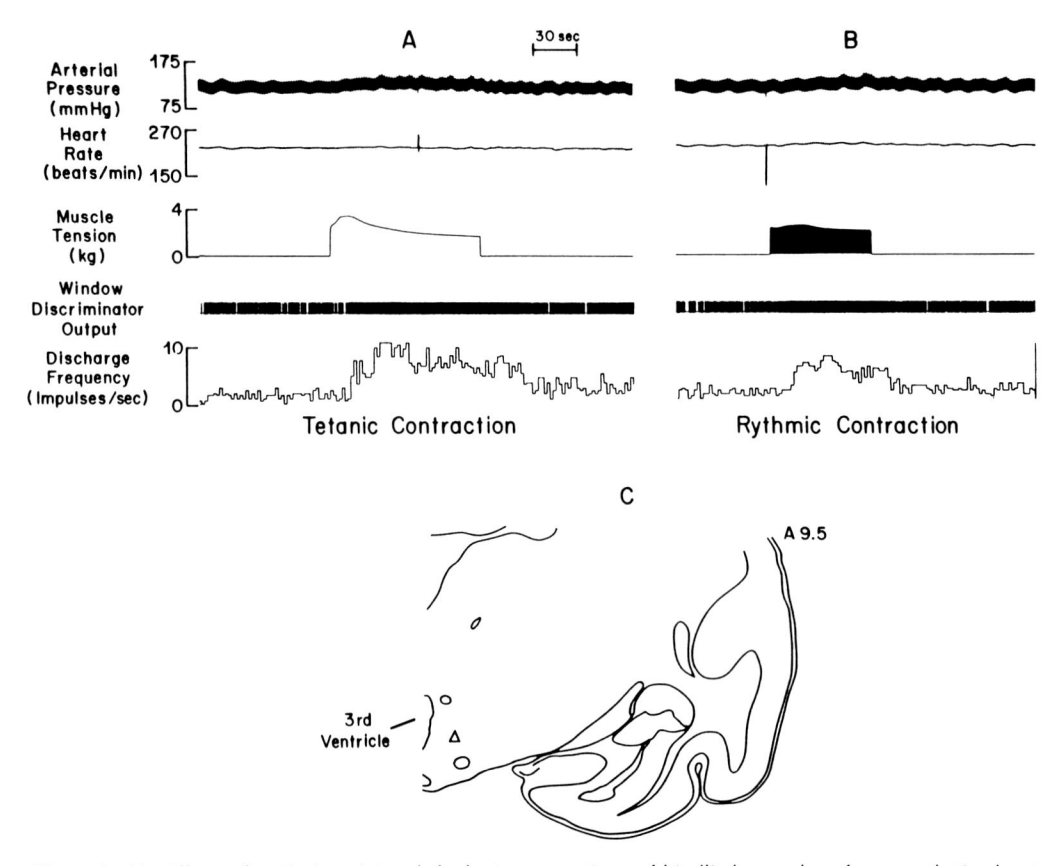

Figure 3-11 Effects of static (tetanic) and rhythmic contractions of hindlimb muscles of an anesthetized cat upon the discharge frequency of a neuron located in the hypothalamic locomotor region. The location of the neuron is denoted by a triangle in the line drawing.

12 weeks of swim training increased the vital capacity, total lung capacity, and functional residual capacity of female varsity swimmers (17 to 21 years old).[72] No change in residual volume was observed.

Training has several effects upon breathing during rest and exercise conditions. Kieper studied three pairs of identical twins who trained 5 days a week for 4 weeks.[74] Training did not alter resting minute ventilation or dead space; however, resting tidal volume was increased and respiratory frequency decreased after training. These effects resulted in a 13 percent increase in alveolar ventilation. It was concluded that training increases the "economy of respiration."[74] In another study, the ventilatory responses to exercise of outstanding endurance athletes were compared to those of nonathletes.[75] The results confirmed other reports that

had concluded that minute ventilation for a given workload is less in the athlete than in the nonathlete.[76] Possible physiologic advantages of this reduced ventilation were discussed by the authors.[75] Slight decreases in the work of breathing and perceived effort, which would be associated with the decreased ventilation, may contribute to endurance performance.

Ventilatory Strength and Endurance

It is well known that training can increase the strength and endurance of limb skeletal muscles. Similar training effects have been reported for diaphragmatic muscle. Leith and Bradley examined the possibility that training would increase the strength and endurance of the respiratory muscles.[77,78] Subjects were studied before and after training that was specific for respiratory muscles. One group performed strength training, which consisted of maximal static inspiratory and expiratory efforts. A second group did endurance training, which involved repeated voluntary hyperventilation to exhaustion. Both groups trained 30 to 45 minutes per day, 5 days per week for 5 weeks. Strength training increased maximal static inspiratory and expiratory pressures, which indicates an increase in the strength of the respiratory muscles. Endurance training increased the maximal voluntary ventilation that could be sustained for 15 seconds.

Other investigators have examined the possibility that normal exercise programs can increase the strength and endurance of respiratory muscles. These studies have shown that ventilatory muscle strength is improved by training programs involving swimming, bicycle ergometer exercise, or running.[72,73,79,80] Figure 3–12 shows the effects of training on a bicycle ergometer upon two measures of respiratory muscle strength. Robinson and Kjeldgaard found that a 15-week training program of running increased the maximal sustainable ventilatory capacity for 15 minutes and the maximal voluntary ventilation of their subjects.[81] They concluded that running improves both respiratory muscle strength and endurance in healthy, previously sedentary individuals. It is also known that intensive swimming and canoeing improve the ventilatory endurance of cystic fibrosis patients.[79]

Biochemical and Contractile Properties of the Diaphragm

Even though the aforementioned studies have shown that training can improve ventilatory strength and endurance, little is known about the mechanisms responsible for these improvements. Training is known to have a number of beneficial effects upon limb skeletal muscles. Endurance training elicits large increases in oxidative enzymatic activity of limb skeletal muscles.[82] It is less clear whether training has a similar effect upon oxidative capacity of the diaphragmatic activity.

Two studies have shown that endurance training can also increase the oxidative capacity of the diaphragm. Ianuzzo and co-workers examined the effects of 12 to 16 weeks of endurance training on a treadmill upon glycolytic and oxidative enzyme activities in the diaphragms of rats.[83] They observed a 23 to 30 percent increase in oxidative enzyme activities and a 20 percent increase in hexokinase (glycolytic enzyme) activity. An increase in the oxidative capacity of the diaphragm after endurance training in rats has also been reported by another laboratory.[84] A 17 percent increase in succinate dehydrogenase activity was observed after training for 8 weeks; however, no further increase was seen with an additional 18 weeks of training. This change in diaphragmatic oxidative capacity was much less than the 44 percent increase in succinate dehydrogenase activity of limb muscle (plantaris) from the same rats (Fig. 3–13).

A recent study reported that endurance training has no effect upon mitochondrial proteins in diaphragm muscles of rats.[85] However, these investigators did observe a 50 percent increase in the mitochondrial protein content of the plantaris muscle and a 13 percent increase in maximal oxygen uptake, indicating a substantial effect of training. It was suggested that the lack of training effect in the diaphragm might have been due to a "preadaptation secondary to the diaphragm's high chronic activity." This possibility is supported by the fact that the oxi-

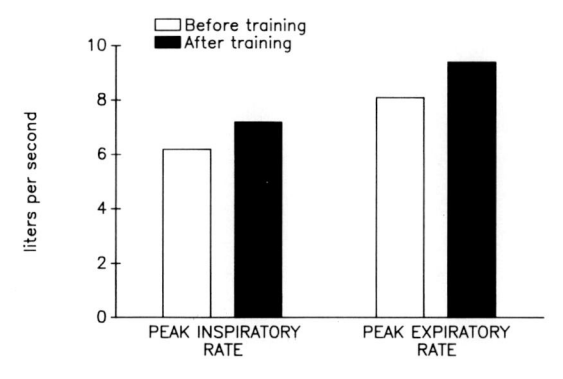

Figure 3–12 Effects of endurance training upon maximal respiratory flows in normal human subjects. Both peak inspiratory and peak expiratory flows were increased after 6 weeks of training. (Drawn from data of Gimenez M, Cereceda V, Teculescu D, et al. Eur J Appl Physiol 1982; 49:379–387.)

SUCCINATE DEHYDROGENASE ACTIVITIES

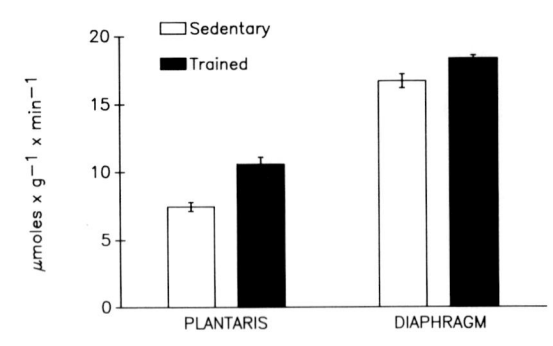

Figure 3–13 Effects of 8 to 12 weeks of endurance training upon succinate dehydrogenase activities of the plantaris and diaphragm muscles of rats. (Drawn from data of Moore RL, Gollnick PD. Pflugers Arch 1982; 392:268–271.)

dative capacity and mitochondrial protein content of the diaphragm before training is approximately two-fold greater than control values for the plantaris muscle. Metzger and Fitts have also reported that endurance training, which increases the oxidative capacity of limb muscles, has no effect upon mitochondrial enzymes in the diaphragm.[86] In addition, these investigators examined contractile properties of diaphragms from trained and untrained rats. Endurance training had no effect upon peak tetanic tension, peak rise in tetanic tension, the ratio of twitch to tetanus, peak twitch tension, peak rise in twitch tension, or contraction time during twitch contraction. Similar findings have been reported by another laboratory.[87]

In summary, only small, if any, training effects occur in the oxidative capacity or contractile properties of the diaphragm as compared to limb skeletal muscles. This lack of effect may be explained by the chronic use of the diaphragm. Because the diaphragm is active continuously from birth, endurance training of this muscle has probably occurred already. Therefore, additional training has only small effects.

Ventilatory Responses to Hypoxia and Hypercapnia

A number of studies have examined the responses of athletes to breathing hypoxic gas mixtures.[71,75,88–90] These studies have shown clearly that athletes have a blunted ventilatory response to hypoxia at rest, compared to the response in sedentary controls (Fig. 3–14). This blunted response has been observed in long-distance runners, swimmers, and cross-country skiers. In addition, the response to hypoxia has been shown to correlate inversely with maximal oxygen uptake.[88] However, the response to hypoxia during exercise does not differ between athletes and nonathletes.[88]

The altered response to hypoxia observed in athletes probably results from genetic characteristics of the athletes rather than from training. Scoggin and co-workers examined the ventilatory response of five outstanding distance runners and their siblings and parents.[90] A decreased response to hypoxia was observed in the runners, as compared to a group of nonathletes. The response of the nonathletic relatives of the runners was also blunted, as compared to the group of sedentary controls. The ventilatory response to hypoxia of the runners did not differ from that of their relatives.

It is not clear whether the respiratory response to hypercapnia of the athlete is different from that of the nonathlete. In one study it was reported that training increases the ventilatory response of rowers to increases in CO_2.[91] This finding contrasts with the results of most other studies. Ohkuma and co-workers found that endurance swimmers tended to have a reduced

RESPONSE TO HYPOXIA

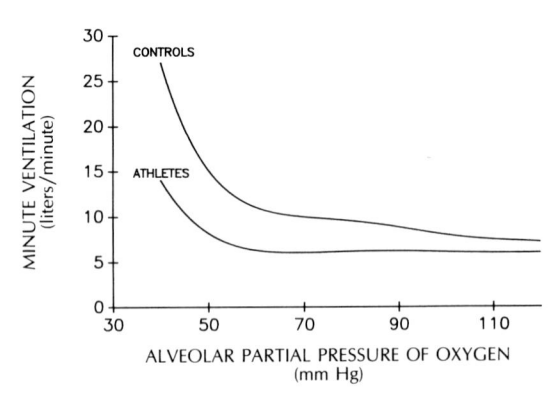

Figure 3–14 A comparison of the ventilatory responses to hypoxia in a group of long-distance runners and a group of nonathletic controls. (Adapted from Scoggin CH, Doekel RD, Dryger MH, et al. J Appl Physiol 1978; 44:464–468.)

response, compared to that seen in sprint swimmers.[92] In addition, the ventilatory response to hypercapnia of the swimmers was less than that of a group of untrained swimmers, although neither of these differences was significant. Heigenhauser and associates also found no significant differences in the ventilatory response to increases in CO_2 among synchronized, speed, and recreational swimmers.[93] The ventilatory response of marathon runners to hypercapnia has also been examined.[94] No significant difference was observed between the runners and untrained controls. In contrast, other studies have found a decreased response to hypercapnia in athletes.[75,88,95,96] It has also been reported that there is a strong similarity between the ventilatory response of swimmers and their siblings to hypercapnia. However, the relationship was not as strong between the swimmers and their parents.[90]

It is not known whether the reduced respiratory response to chemical stimuli is advantageous to the athlete. It has been noted that endurance athletes who have a blunted response to hypoxia ventilate less for a given workload than do nonathletes.[97] It was hypothesized that the low exercise ventilation may link a reduced responsiveness to hypoxia and hypercapnia to athletic performance. Another study noted that there was a close relationship between the ventilatory response to hypercapnia and the level of exercise ventilation in marathon runners.[94] However, their responses to hypoxia and hypercapnia did not correlate with performance in the marathon. Thus, the actual effect of a reduced hypoxic response upon performance has not been determined.

An exaggerated response to hypoxia has been observed in another type of endurance athlete. West reported that mountain climbers who are successful at reaching severe altitudes have above-average increases in ventilation in response to the hypoxia imposed by the reduced barometric pressure of high altitude.[98]

VENTILATORY FATIGUE AND EXERCISE

Fatigue of respiratory muscles has received a great deal of attention in recent years. Respiratory fatigue and its consequences are especially relevant to pulmonary disease.[99] Respiratory fatigue has been defined as "the point at which a subject is unable to generate the predetermined transdiaphragmatic pressure."[100] Breathing becomes irregular and disorganized when this point is reached. Fatigue was observed eventually in healthy humans who were instructed to breathe at a level at which the diaphragm generates 40 percent or more of the maximum inspiratory pressure that can be generated.[100] In contrast, the diaphragm was able to function normally for indefinite periods at less than 40 percent of the maximal pressure. The percent contribution of the diaphragm, intercostals, and accessory respiratory muscles alternated over time once fatigue was present.[101] It has been suggested that this alternation of effort by the respiratory muscles postpones the onset of fatigue.

Several investigators have examined the possibility that respiratory fatigue occurs during exercise. In one study, four male runners were tested before and immediately after completion of a marathon.[102] Significant decreases in maximal inspiratory and expiratory pressures, as well as a reduced maximal voluntary ventilation, were observed in the runners after the prolonged exercise. These findings indicate that both respiratory strength and endurance are depressed after running a marathon, i.e., that running a marathon produces respiratory fatigue. Martin and colleagues have also noted that respiratory fatigue may be one factor influencing performance during severe exercise.[103] Their study examined the effects of voluntary, sustained (2.5 minutes) maximal hyperventilation upon subsequent running performance. Subjects were unable to exercise as long or at as high a workload when the run was preceded by a bout of hyperventilation. These investigators suggested that the hyperventilation induced respiratory fatigue that was responsible for the reduced performance.[103] Bender and Martin have reported that exhausting exercise lasting less than 10 minutes does not alter maximal voluntary ventilation; however 60 minutes of severe exercise did produce a decrement in ventilatory endurance.[104] Thus, it appears likely that fatigue may limit ventilatory performance during sustained severe workloads.

VENTILATORY AND LACTATE (ANAEROBIC) THRESHOLDS

Wasserman and McIlroy described the "anaerobic threshold" in a paper published in 1964.[105] It was noted that breathing increases out of proportion to metabolic rate at exercise intensities at and above approximately 50 percent of maximal oxygen uptake. Wasserman and colleagues have proposed that this increased ventilation results from anaerobic metabolism and a concomitant production of lactic acid in exercising muscles, which leads to elevations in CO_2 and hydrogen ion concentration in the blood.[24] It was thought that the onset of lactic acid production in exercising muscles could be determined by noting the point that ventilation increased out of proportion to metabolic rate. This initial method for determining the anaerobic threshold has been refined by Wasserman and others.[106,107] Extensive criticism of the anaerobic threshold and its relationship to ventilation has been published. The concept of the anaerobic threshold has been critically evaluated and redefined in recent review articles written by Davis and by Brooks.[107,108]

An explanation of the controversy over the anaerobic threshold involves a description of the changes in lactate concentrations that occur during exercise. Blood lactate concentration does not change from resting levels when one exercises at mild to moderate intensities; however, it does increase at more severe exercise levels. The anaerobic threshold has been defined recently as the exercise intensity at which the concentration of lactate in the blood increases over resting levels.[108] Increases in exercise intensity above the anaerobic threshold lead to progressive elevations in blood lactate.

It has been suggested that the increase in lactate that occurs in the blood at the anaerobic threshold results from muscle hypoxia.[24] This explanation suggests that no lactate is produced in exercising skeletal muscles until exercise exceeds the anaerobic threshold. It has been clearly shown that lactate production occurs even at light workloads.[108] Others have correctly noted that both lactic acid production and lactate removal are active processes that function during exercise.[108] A number of body tissues including the heart, liver, and skeletal muscle are known to metabolize lactate. Therefore, the build-up of lactate in the blood that occurs at approximately 50 percent of maximal oxygen uptake results from an imbalance between lactic acid production and lactate removal. Because the build-up of lactate does not result solely from lactic acid production, Brooks has suggested that a more correct term for the anaerobic threshold would be *lactate threshold.*[108]

A number of investigators have questioned whether the build-up of lactate in the blood that begins at the lactate threshold is responsible for the abrupt increase in ventilation (ventilatory threshold) noted at approximately the same time. Several studies have shown that the lactate threshold can be uncoupled temporally from the ventilatory threshold.[109–112] A study of patients with McArdle's disease has provided convincing evidence that the lactate and ventilatory thresholds are not cause and effect.[113] McArdle's patients lack the enzyme necessary for the production of lactic acid; however, these patients do display a hyperventilation (ventilatory threshold) at approximately 70 to 85 percent of maximal oxygen uptake (Fig. 3–15).

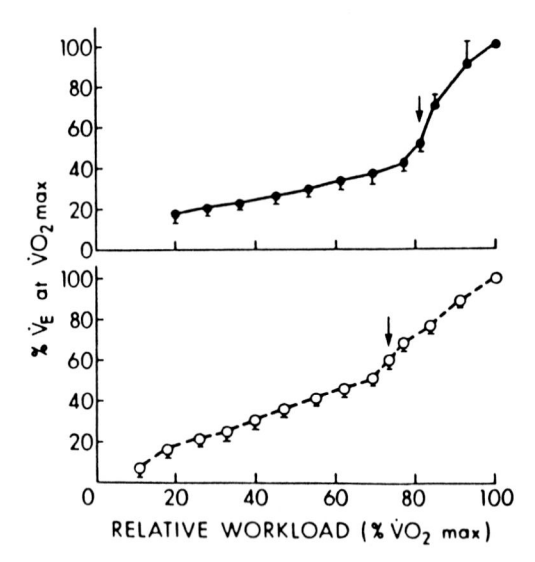

Figure 3–15 A comparison of the ventilatory responses to progressive incremental exercise in normal subjects (*open circles*) and in patients with McArdle's disease (*filled circles*). The arrows denote the points at which ventilation increased out of proportion to metabolic rate in both groups of subjects. (From Hagberg JM, Coyle EF, Carroll JE, et al. J Appl Physiol 1982; 52:991–994. Reproduced with permission of American Physiological Society.)

These results suggest that nonhumoral stimuli are responsible for the abrupt increase in ventilation out of proportion to metabolic rate.

The lactate threshold has been used extensively as a measure of endurance ability and a basis for prescribing of training programs.[107] A number of studies have correlated the ventilatory threshold with endurance capacity of subjects. Athletes possess a much higher lactate threshold than do nonathletes.[107,114] In addition, exercise training increases the point (percent of maximal $\dot{V}O_2$) at which ventilation increases out of proportion to workload. Davis has suggested that an exercise intensity just below the lactate threshold represents the highest workload that can be maintained for long periods of time.[107] Clinicians have used the lactate threshold, approximated by determination of the ventilatory threshold, as one means to assess disease impairment. However, because the actual cause of the lactate threshold is not known, it is uncertain how useful this measure is in evaluating the exact impairment possessed by the patient(s).

In summary, the concept of an anaerobic threshold linked to muscle hypoxia lacks scientific basis. However, a lactate threshold, which results from an imbalance between lactic acid production and lactate removal, is supported by current research. The cause of this imbalance has not yet been determined. It is unlikely that the build-up of lactate and its subsequent chemical reactions are solely responsible for the ventilatory threshold that normally occurs at approximately the same exercise intensity. Even though the exact coupling is unknown, the ventilatory threshold does appear to be related to endurance performance.

REFERENCES

1. Astrand P-O, Rodahl K. Textbook of work physiology: physiological bases of exercise. New York: McGraw-Hill, 1977.
2. Comroe JH. Physiology of respiration. Chicago: Year Book Medical Publishers, 1974.
3. Dempsey JA, Vidruk EH, Mastenbrook SM. Pulmonary control systems in exercise. Fed Proc 1980; 39:1498–1505.
4. Mitchell JH, Wildenthal K. Static (isometric) exercise and the heart: physiological and clinical considerations. Annu Rev Med 1974; 25:369–381.
5. Muza SR, Lee LY, Wiley RL, et al. Ventilatory responses to static handgrip exercise. J Appl Physiol 1983; 54:1457–1462.
6. Myhre K, Andersen KL. Respiratory responses to static muscular work. Respir Physiol 1971; 12:77–89.
7. Wiley RL, Lind AR. Respiratory responses to sustained static muscular contractions in humans. Clin Sci 1971; 40:221–234.
8. Dejours P. Control of respiration in muscular exercise. Handbook of physiology, Section 3: Respiration. Vol. 1. Washington, DC: American Physiological Society, 1971: 631.
9. Krogh A, Lindhard J. The regulation of respiration and circulation during the initial stages of muscular work. J Physiol 1913; 47:112–136.
10. Eldridge FL, Millhorn DE, Kiley JP, Waldrop TG. Stimulation by central command of locomotion, respiration, and circulation during exercise. Respir Physiol 1985; 59:313–337.
11. Favier R, Desplanches D, Frutoso J, et al. Ventilatory and circulatory transients during exercise: new arguments for a neurohumoral theory. J Appl Physiol 1983; 54:647–653.
12. Fregosi RF, Dempsey JA. Arterial blood acid–base regulation during exercise in rats. J Appl Physiol 1984; 57:396–402.
13. Kiley JP, Kuhlman WD, Fedde MR. Respiratory and cardiovascular responses to exercise in the duck. J Appl Physiol 1979; 47:827–833.
14. Mitchell GS, Gleeson TT, Bennett AF. Ventilation and acid–base balance during graded activity in lizards. Am J Physiol 1981; 9:R27–R37.
15. Musch TI, Friedman DB, Haidet GC, et al. Arterial blood gases and acid–base status of dogs during graded dynamic exercise. J Appl Physiol 1986; 61:1914–1919.
16. Pan LG, Forster HV, Bisgard GE, et al. Hyperventilation in ponies at the onset of and during steady state exercise. J Appl Physiol 1983; 54:1394–1402.
17. Powers SK, Beadle RE, Thompson D, Lawler J. Ventilatory and blood gas dynamics at onset and offset of exercise in the pony. J Appl Physiol 1987; 62:141–148.
18. Smith CA, Mitchell GS, Jameson LC, et al. Ventilatory response of goats to treadmill exercise: grade effects. Respir Physiol 1983; 54:331–341.
19. Asmussen E. Ventilation at transition from rest to exercise. Acta Physiol Scand 1973; 89:68–78.
20. Cerretelli P, Sikand R, Farhi LE. Readjustments in cardiac output and gas exchange during onset of exercise and recovery. J Appl Physiol 1966; 21:1345–1350.
21. D'Angelo E, Torelli G. Neural stimuli increasing respiration during different types of exercise. J Appl Physiol 1971; 30:116–121.
22. Fordyce WE, Bennett FM, Edelman SK, Grodins FS. Evidence in man for a fast neural mechanism during the early phase of exercise hyperpnea. Respir Physiol 1982; 48:27–43.
23. Lewis BM. Measurement of arterial blood gases at the transition from exercise to rest. J Appl Physiol 1983; 54:1340–1344.
24. Wasserman K, Whipp BJ, Loyal SN, Beaver WL. An-

aerobic threshold and respiratory gas exchange during exercise. J Appl Physiol 1973; 35:236–243.
25. Bechbache RR, Duffin J. The entrainment of breathing frequency by exercise rhythm. J Physiol 1977; 272:553–561.
26. Bramble DM, Carrier DR. Running and breathing in mammals. Science 1983; 219:251–256.
27. Iscoe S. Respiratory and stepping frequencies in conscious exercising cats. J Appl Physiol 1981; 51:835–839.
28. Jasinskas CL, Wilson BA, Hoare J. Entrainment of breathing rate to movement during work at two intensities. Respir Physiol 1980; 42:199–209.
29. Paterson DJ, Wood GA, Morton AR, Henstridge JD. The entrainment of ventilation frequency to exercise rhythm. Eur J Appl Physiol 1986; 55:530–537.
30. Viala D, Persegol L, Palisses R. Relationship between phrenic and hindlimb extensor activities during fictive locomotion. Neurosci Lett 1987; 74:49–52.
31. Viala D, Vidal C, Freton E. Coordinated rhythmic bursting in respiratory and locomotor muscle nerves. Neurosci Lett 1979; 11:155–159.
32. Garlando F, Koh J, Koller EA, Pietsch P. Effect of coupling the breathing and cycling rhythms on oxygen uptake during bicycle ergometry. Eur J Appl Physiol 1985; 54:497–501.
33. Casaburi R, Storer TW, Ben-Dov I, Wasserman K. Effect of endurance training on possible determinants of $\dot{V}O_2$ during heavy exercise. J Appl Physiol 1987; 62:199–207.
34. Hanson P, Claremont A, Dempsey J, Reddan W. Determinants and consequences of ventilatory responses to competitive endurance running. J Appl Physiol 1982; 52:615–623.
35. Martin BJ, Morgan EJ, Zwillich CW, Weil JV. Control of breathing during prolonged exercise. J Appl Physiol 1981; 50:27–31.
36. Eldridge FL, Millhorn DE, Waldrop TG. Exercise hyperpnea and locomotion: parallel activation from the hypothalamus. Science 1981; 211:844–846.
37. Kao FF. An experimental study of the pathways involved in exercise hyperpnoea employing cross-circulation techniques. In: Cunningham DJC, Lloyd BB, eds. The regulation of human respiration. Oxford: Blackwell, 1963:461.
38. Casey K, Duffin J, McAvoy GV. The effect of exercise on the central-chemoreceptor threshold in man. J Physiol 1987; 383:9–18.
39. DiMarco AF, Romaniuk JR, von Euler C, Yamamoto Y. Immediate changes in ventilation and respiratory pattern associated with onset and cessation of locomotion in the cat. J Phsyiol 1983; 343:1–16.
40. Orlovskii GN. Spontaneous and induced locomotion of the thalamic cat. Biofizika 1969; 6:1095–1102.
41. Waldrop TG, Henderson MC, Iwamoto GA, Mitchell JH. Regional blood flow responses to stimulation of the subthalamic locomotor region. Respir Physiol 1986; 64:93–102.
42. Waller WH. Progression movements elicited by subthalamic stimulation. J Neurophysiol 1940; 3:300–307.
43. Waldrop TC, Mullins DC, Millhorn DE. Control of respiration by the hypothalamus and by feedback from contracting muscles in cats. Respir Physiol 1986; 64:317–328.
44. Waldrop TG, Bauer RM, Iwamoto GA. Microinjection of GABA antagonists into the posterior hypothalamus elicits locomotor movements and a cardiorespiratory activation. Brain Res 1988; 444:84–94.
45. Goodwin GM, McCloskey DI, Mitchell JH. Cardiovascular and respiratory responses to changes in central command during isometric exercise at constant muscle tension. J Physiol 1972; 226:173–190.
46. McCloskey DI, Mitchell JH. Reflex cardiovascular and respiratory responses originating in exercising muscle. J Physiol 1972; 224:173–186.
47. Rodgers SH. Ventilatory response to ventral root stimulation in the decerebrate cat. Respir Physiol 1968; 5:165–174.
48. Waldrop TG, Rybicki KJ, Kaufman MP. Chemical activation of groups I and II muscle afferents has no cardiorespiratory effects. J Appl Physiol 1984; 56:1223–1228.
49. Kaufman MP, Waldrop TG, Rybicki KJ, et al. Effects of static and rhythmic twitch contractions on the impulse activity of group III and IV muscle afferents. Cardiovasc Res 1984; 18:663–668.
50. Mitchell JH, Schmidt RF. Cardiovascular reflex control by afferent fibers from skeletal muscle receptors. Handbook of physiology, Section 2. The cardiovascular system. Vol. 3. Peripheral Circulation. Bethesda, MD: American Physiological Society, 1983:623.
51. Hirche H, Schumacher E, Hagemann H. Extracellular K^+ concentration and K^+ balance of the gastrocnemius muscle of the dog during exercise. Pflugers Arch 1980; 387:231–237.
52. Mizumura K, Kumazawa T. Reflex respiratory response induced by chemical stimulation of muscle afferents. Brain Res 1976; 109:402–406.
53. Rybicki KJ, Kaufman MP, Kenyon JL, Mitchell JH. Arterial pressure responses to increasing interstitial potassium in hindlimb muscle of dogs. Am J Physiol 1984; 247:R717–R721.
54. Rybicki KJ, Waldrop TG, Kaufman MP. Increasing gracilis muscle interstitial potassium concentrations stimulates group III and IV afferents. J Appl Physiol 1984; 58:936–941.
55. Tibes U. Neurogenic control of ventilation in exercise. In: Cerretelli P, Whipp BJ, eds. Exercise bioenergetics and gas exchange. Amsterdam: Elsevier, 1980:146.
56. Stebbins CL, Longhurst JC. Bradykinin-induced chemoreflexes from skeletal muscle: implications for the exercise reflex. J Appl Physiol 1985; 59:56–63.
57. Stebbins CL, Longhurst JC. Bradykinin in reflex cardiovascular responses to static muscular contraction. J Appl Physiol 1986; 61:271–279.
58. Stebbins CL, Maruoka Y, Longhurst JC. Prostaglandins contribute to cardiovascular responses evoked by static muscular contraction. Circ Res 1986; 59:645–654.
59. Kaufman MP, Rybicki KJ, Waldrop TG, Ordway GA. Effect of ischemia on the responses of group III and IV afferents to static muscular contraction. J Appl Physiol 1984; 57:644–650.

60. Coote JH, Hilton SM, Perez-Gonzales JF. The reflex nature of the pressor response to muscular exercise. J Physiol 1971; 215:789–804.
61. Kaufman MP, Rybicki KJ. Muscular contraction reflexly relaxes tracheal smooth muscle in dogs. Respir Physiol 1984; 56:61–72.
62. Longhurst JC. Static contraction of hindlimb muscles in cats reflexly relaxes tracheal smooth muscle. J Appl Physiol 1984; 57:380–387.
63. Kaufman MP, Rybicki KJ, Mitchell JH. Hindlimb muscular contraction reflexly decreases total pulmonary resistance in dogs. J Appl Physiol 1985; 59:1521–1526.
64. Kagawa J, Kerr HD. Effects of brief graded exercise on specific airway conductance in normal subjects. J Appl Physiol 1970; 28:138–144.
65. Wasserman K, Whipp BJ, Castagna J. Cardiodynamic hyperpnea: hyperpnea secondary to cardiac output increase. J Appl Physiol 1974; 36:457–464.
66. Jones PW, Huszczuk A, Wasserman K. Cardiac output as a controller of ventilation through changes in right ventricular strain. J Appl Physiol 1982; 53:218–224.
67. Waldrop TG. Respiratory responses to chemical activation of left ventricular receptors. Respir Physiol 1986; 63:383–393.
68. Waldrop TG, Mullins DC. Cardiorespiratory responses to chemical activation of right ventricular receptors. J Appl Physiol 1987; 63:733–739.
69. Waldrop TG, Mullins DC, Henderson MC. Effects of hypothalamic lesions on the cardiorespiratory responses to muscular contraction. Respir Physiol 1986; 66:215–224.
70. Waldrop TG, Stremel RW. Responses of hypothalamic neurons to tetanic and rhythmic contractions of hindlimb muscles. Proc Cong Int Union Physiol Sci 1986; 16:166.
71. Bjurstrom RL, Schoene RB. Control of ventilation in elite synchronized swimmers. J Appl Physiol 1987; 63:1019–1024.
72. Clanton TL, Dixon GF, Gadek JE. Effects of swim training on lung volumes and inspiratory muscle conditioning. J Appl Physiol 1987; 62:39–46.
73. Gimenez M, Cereceda V, Teculescu D, et al. Square-wave endurance exercise test (SWEET) for training and assessment in trained and untrained subjects. III. Effect on VO₂max and maximal ventilation. Eur J Appl Physiol 1982; 49:379–387.
74. Kieper CH. Effects of endurance training on acid–base status and pulmonary ventilation. Eur J Appl Physiol 1983; 51:295–302.
75. Martin BJ, Sparks KE, Zwillich CW, Weil JW. Low exercise ventilation in endurance athletes. Med Sci Sports Exerc 1979; 11:181–185.
76. Morrison JF, van Malsen S, Noakes T. Evidence for an inverse relationship between the ventilatory response to exercise and the maximum whole body oxygen consumption value. Eur J Appl Physiol 1983; 50:265–272.
77. Bradley ME, Leith DE. Ventilatory muscle training and the oxygen cost of sustained hyperpnea. J Appl Physiol 1978; 45:885–892.
78. Leith DE, Bradley M. Ventilatory muscle strength and endurance training. J Appl Physiol 1976; 41:508–516.
79. Keens TG, Krastins IRB, Wannamaker EM, et al. Ventilatory muscle endurance training in normal subjects and patients with cystic fibrosis. Am Rev Resp Dis 1977; 116:853–860.
80. Martin BJ, Stager JM. Ventilatory endurance in athletes and nonathletes. Med Sci Sports Exerc 1981; 13:21–26.
81. Robinson EP, Kjeldgaard JM. Improvement in ventilatory muscle function with running. J Appl Physiol 1982; 52:1400–1406.
82. Saltin B, Gollnick PD. Skeletal muscle adaptability: significance for metabolism and performance. Handbook of physiology, Section 10. Skeletal muscle. Bethesda, MD: American Physiological Society, 1983:555.
83. Ianuzzo CD, Noble EG, Hamilton N, Dabrowski B. Effects of streptozotocin diabetes, insulin treatment, and training on the diaphragm. J Appl Physiol 1982; 52:1471–1475.
84. Moore RL, Gollnick PD. Response of ventilatory muscles of the rat to endurance training. Pflugers Arch 1982; 392:268–271.
85. Fregosi RF, Sanjak M, Paulson DJ. Endurance training does not affect diaphragm mitochondrial respiration. Respir Physiol 1987; 67:225–237.
86. Metzger JM, Fitts RH. Contractile and biochemical properties of diaphragm: effects of exercise training and fatigue. J Appl Physiol 1986; 60:1752–1758.
87. Farkas GA, Roussos C. Adaptability of the hamster diaphragm to exercise and/or emphysema. J Appl Physiol 1982; 53:1263–1272.
88. Byrne-Quinn E, Weil JV, Sodal IE, et al. Ventilatory control in the athlete. J Appl Physiol 1971; 30:91–98.
89. Godfrey S, Edwards RHT, Copland GM, Gross PL. Chemosensitivity in normal subjects, athletes, and patients with chronic airway obstruction. J Appl Physiol 1971; 30:193–199.
90. Scoggin CH, Doekel RD, Dryger MH, et al. Familial aspects of decreased hypoxic drive in endurance athletes. J Appl Physiol 1978; 44:464–468.
91. Kelly MA, Laufe MD, Millman RP, Peterson DD. Ventilatory response to hypercapnia before and after athletic training. Respir Physiol 1984; 55:393–400.
92. Ohkuma T, Fujitsuka N, Utsuno T, Miyamura M. Ventilatory response to hypercapnia in sprint and long-distance swimmers. Eur J Appl Physiol 1980; 43:235–241.
93. Heigenhauser GJF, Oldridge NB, Jones NL. The CO_2 responsiveness and ventilatory response to leg and arm exercise in female swimmers. Respir Physiol 1983; 53:263–272.
94. Mahler DA, Moritz ED, Loke J. Ventilatory responses at rest and during exercise in marathon runners. J Appl Physiol 1982; 52:388–392.
95. Miyamura M, Yamashima T, Honda Y. Ventilatory responses to CO_2 rebreathing at rest and during exercise in untrained subjects and athletes. Jpn J Physiol 1976; 26:245–254.
96. Saunder NA, Leeder SR, Rebuck AS. Ventilatory response to carbon dioxide in young athletes: a family study. Am Rev Resp Dis 1976; 113:497–502.
97. Martin BJ, Weil JV, Sparks KE, et al. Exercise ventilation correlates positively with ventilatory che-

moresponsiveness. J Appl Physiol 1978; 45:557–564.
98. West J. Everest—the testing place. New York: McGraw-Hill Book, 1985.
99. Derenne J-PH, Macklem PT, Roussos C. The respiratory muscles: mechanics, control, and pathophysiology. Am Rev Resp Dis 1978; 118:581–601.
100. Roussos C, Macklem PT. Diaphragmatic fatigue in man. J Appl Physiol 1977; 43:189–197.
101. Roussos C, Fixley M, Gross D, Macklem PT. Fatigue of inspiratory muscles and their synergic behavior. J Appl Physiol 1979; 46:897–904.
102. Loke J, Mahler DA, Virgulto JA. Respiratory muscle fatigue after marathon running. J Appl Physiol 1982; 52:821–824.
103. Martin B, Heintzelman M, Chen H. Exercise performance after ventilatory work. J Appl Physiol 1982; 52:1581–1585.
104. Bender PR, Martin BJ. Maximal ventilation after exhausting exercise. Med Sci Sports Exerc 1985; 17:164–167.
105. Wasserman K, McIlroy MB. Detecting the threshold anaerobic metabolism in cardiac patients during exercise. Am J Cardiol 1964; 14:844–852.
106. Caiozzo VJ, Davis JA, Ellis JF, et al. A comparison of gas exchange indices used to detect the anaerobic threshold. J Appl Physiol 1982; 53:1184–1189.
107. Davis JA. Anaerobic threshold: review of the concept and directions for future research. Med Sci Sports Exerc 1985; 17:6–18.
108. Brooks GA. Anaerobic threshold: review of the concept and directions for future research. Med Sci Sports Exerc 1985; 17:22–31.
109. Heigenhauser GJF, Sutton JR, Jones NL. Effect of glycogen depletion on the ventilatory response to exercise. J Appl Physiol 1983; 54:470–474.
110. Hughes EF, Turner SC, Brooks GA. Effects of glycogen depletion and pedaling speed on anaerobic threshold. J Appl Physiol 1982; 52:1598–1607.
111. Neary PJ, MacDougall JD, Bachus R, Wenger HA. The relationship between lactate and ventilatory thresholds: coincidental or cause and effect? Eur J Appl Physiol 1985; 54:104–108.
112. Segal SS, Brooks GA. Effects of glycogen depletion and workload on postexercise O_2 consumption and blood lactate. J Appl Physiol 1979; 47:512–514.
113. Hagberg JM, Coyle EF, Carroll JE, et al. Exercise hyperventilation in patients with McArdle's disease. J Appl Physiol 1982; 52:991–994.
114. Vago P, Mercier J, Ramonatxo M, Prefaut CH. Is ventilatory anaerobic threshold a good index of endurance capacity? Int J Sports Med 1987; 8:190–195.

Chapter 4
Temperature Regulation

GEORGE L. BRENGELMANN

BODY TEMPERATURE

Because all living things produce heat, even the simplest forms tend toward a thermal equilibrium in which body temperature is warmer than environmental temperature. *Homeotherms* employ physiologic mechanisms and behavior to adjust that equilibrium as required to maintain constant body temperature.

In humans, the physiologic effectors under control of the neural integrative centers that regulate temperature are shivering, the cutaneous vasculature, and the sweat glands. Shivering changes the rate at which metabolic heat is produced. Control of skin blood flow enables adjustment, in effect, of the insulation afforded by the superficial tissues. Through evaporation of sweat, the body can be cooled. Besides these automatic mechanisms, we use behaviors such as selection of appropriate clothing to extend the range of tolerable thermal conditions.

Normal Body Temperature

"Normal" body temperature in humans is near 37.0° C (98.6° F).* This value was selected on the basis of clinical experience summarized by DuBois in a scale of normal versus abnormal temperatures from which Figure 4–1 was adapted.[1,2] As with blood pressure, pH, or any other regulated physiologic variable, a precise value for "normal" cannot be given. Under identical conditions, different temperatures are found in different individuals. For example, the data in Figure 4–2 were obtained at the same time of day in healthy young men and women allowed ample time to come into equilibrium with a neutral thermal environment.[3] In a larger group, 276 medical students seated in class, mean oral temperature was found to be nearly the same (36.7° C), but with wider dispersion in the data that reflects the relative lack of control; prior to class these people were free to eat, smoke, exercise, and so on.[4]

The difference between oral and rectal temperatures illustrated in Figure 4–2 reveals that the concept of "normal" body temperature is complicated by the fact that temperatures obtained at different sites within the body differ. This would become more apparent if temperatures were available from within the bloodstream, the brain, the liver, and so on. Which measurement site should be used as the reference for "normal"? Which best represents the status of the protected inner "core" of the body? Which is closest to the temperature of the neurons that supply the body temperature control system with information about internal temperature? How would a "mean" body temperature be defined? These questions are addressed below after development of necessary background. First, however, body temperature

---
*Henceforth, temperatures will be specified in degrees Centigrade. A conversion chart to degrees Fahrenheit is included in Figure 4–2.

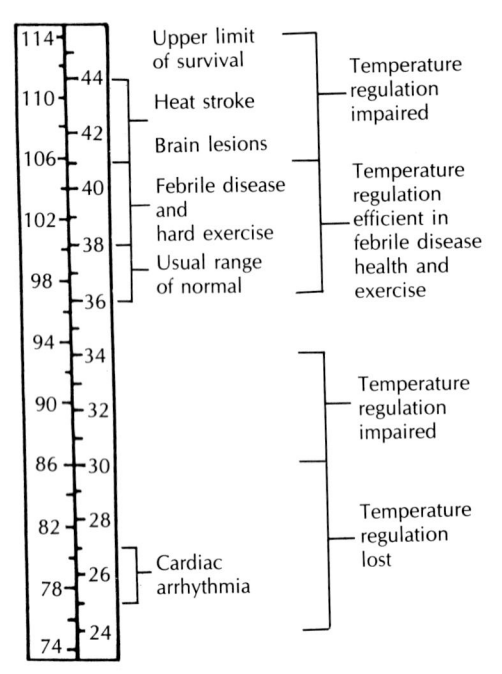

Figure 4-1 Extremes of body temperature. (Redrawn from Brengelmann GL. Temperature regulation. In: Ruch TC, Patton HD, eds. Physiology and Biophysics. 20th ed. Philadelphia: WB Saunders, 1973.)

rhythms and extremes can be discussed in nonspecific terms.

Body Temperature Rhythms

Besides variations among individuals (see Figure 4–2), normal body temperature also varies in a given individual with time. In the 24-hour *circadian* rhythm, temperature ranges from a minimum early in the morning to a peak 0.5 to 1.0° C higher in midafternoon. Also, body temperature cycles through approximately 0.4° C during the 28-day menstrual or *lunar* cycle, with the minimum during the follicular phase and the peak in the luteal phase.

These temperature cycles are not mere reflections of cyclic patterns of activity. They are associated with changes in the properties of the temperature regulation system, so that a different temperature would be maintained at different times under otherwise identical conditions. For example, the relationship between skin blood flow and internal temperature varies with time of day and, in women, with the day of the month.[5,6]

Body Temperature Extremes

In *hyperthermia* body temperature is above normal; in *hypothermia*, it is below. The chart in Figure 4–1 indicates, crudely, the boundaries of the region of tolerable temperatures.

Fatal hyperthermia is associated with symptoms described as *heat stroke*, including weak and rapid pulse, unconsciousness, and convulsions. The skin is often hot and dry, indicating failure of the sweating mechanism. Blood cell abnormalities and disseminated intravascular coagulation may occur. Heat stroke is an extreme medical emergency that does not afford opportunities for deliberate experimental investigation and calibration of equipment. Usually, only measurements of rectal temperature are made; these may inadequately represent temperatures of vital organs (see discussion of the discrepancy between rectal and brain temperature below). The diagnosis of heat stroke has been made with rectal temperatures as low as 40.6° C. Tissue damage occurs in the vicinity of 42° C. (For detailed discussions of heat stroke, see the work of Leithead and Lind and of Hales).[7,8]

Less severe illnesses of hypothermia such as heat exhaustion and heat syncope are not due to high tissue temperature *per se*. Rather, they occur because of the accumulated effects of long periods of sweating and high skin blood flow. Electrolyte imbalance and dehydration hypovolemia are obvious dangers of inadequately or inappropriately compensated sweating. Less obvious is the fact that high skin blood flow not only requires a large cardiac output but also reduces central venous pressure. Thus, both sweating and high skin blood flow can act to deplete the central volume reservoir and reduce capability to maintain normal blood pressure.[7,9]

In hypothermia, temperatures much farther removed from normal temperature are tolerated. Tissue damage in hypothermia, i.e., frostbite, does not occur until cells freeze. However, in terms of function, a person whose core temperature falls below 35.5° C is severely hampered. Uncontrollable spasms of shivering make coordinated motion almost impossible.

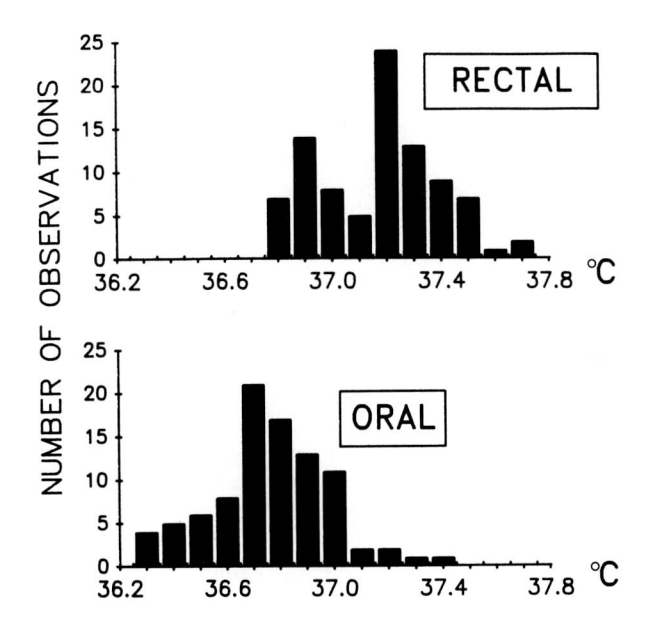

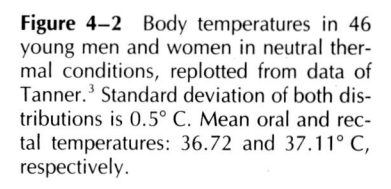

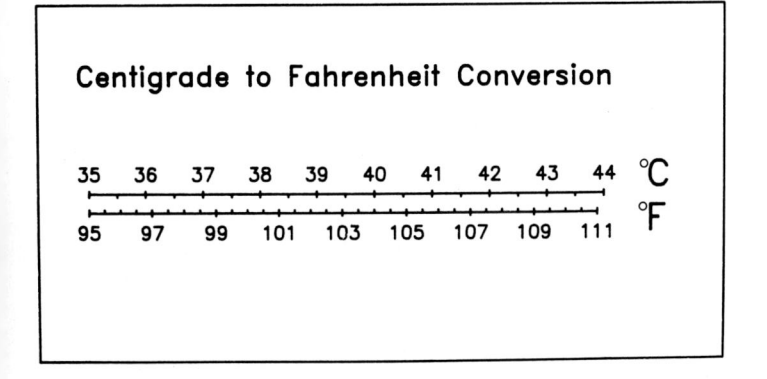

Figure 4–2 Body temperatures in 46 young men and women in neutral thermal conditions, replotted from data of Tanner.[3] Standard deviation of both distributions is 0.5° C. Mean oral and rectal temperatures: 36.72 and 37.11° C, respectively.

Below 35° C, shivering gives way to lassitude and mental confusion; the victim is unable to participate in his or her rescue. But people have recovered, except for frozen superficial tissues, from accidental hypothermia during which body temperatures fell below 20° C. In profound hypothermia, deliberately induced for surgical procedures, core temperature has been taken below 30° C routinely, but with the necessity of dealing with ventricular fibrillation, which is likely to occur when the myocardium is in the 26 to 30° C range. (For a comprehensive discussion of hypothermia, see the work of Keatinge.[10])

BODY HEAT PRODUCTION RATE AND ITS MEASUREMENT

Metabolic energy is released in stoichiometric proportion to the amount of oxygen and substrate consumed. This energy soon degrades to the form of heat within the body, except for whatever fraction leaves the body when external work is done. That fraction is small; the efficiency of the body as an engine for lifting weights, pedaling a bicycle, and other activities is at best less than 30 percent (ratio of energy output to energy expenditure).[11]

Rate of release of energy can be determined by direct calorimetric techniques, but these are cumbersome and impractical. Fortunately, the rate at which oxygen is consumed is easy to measure. Therefore, common practice is to determine energy release from oxygen consumption rate multiplied by the appropriate factor for the current substrate mix. For a normal mixed diet, close to 4.8 kcal of energy[†] is released per liter of oxygen consumed. Heat production rate is computed as energy release rate minus rate of work.

Our concern is with the rate of oxygen consumption at tissue level. What we measure is oxygen consumption at mouth level. These can differ, temporarily, when the amount of oxygen stored in the body changes. For example, if the pattern of respiration is changed so that the functional residual capacity (FRC) of the lungs increases, roughly 20 percent of that volume increase is oxygen which appears, from a mouth level measurement, to have been consumed.

In other words, when we measure oxygen consumption, we simply subtract the amount expired from the amount inspired. An increase in FRC adds to that difference, because more oxygen is contained within the lungs at the end of expiration. This is oxygen that has been consumed in the sense that it is now within the body, but it has not been taken up in metabolism.

The discrepancy between oxygen consumption measured at mouth level versus the true tissue level value is worst over short time spans. "Breath-to-breath" determinations have a high degree of variability if the lung volume at end-expiration fluctuates. Over longer time periods, the average mouth level measurement accurately reflects tissue level oxygen consumption, because the total volume of oxygen stored in the lungs plus the other storage forms (oxygen combined with hemoglobin or myoglobin) is a small reservoir (roughly a liter) relative to the amount consumed over a period of minutes.

Carbon dioxide production rate, although also stoichiometrically related to the rate of energy release at tissue level, is not a practical measure because of the huge amount of carbon dioxide stored within the body in the bicarbonate form. Hyperventilation or hypoventilation can result in several minutes of apparent carbon dioxide production rate far out of match with metabolic production.

In a resting adult, the oxygen consumption rate is typically $3.5 \text{ ml} \cdot \text{min}^{-1} \cdot \text{kg}^{-1}$. With vigorous exercise, the rate increases ten-fold or more. In a study of maximal rates of oxygen consumption, Saltin and Åstrand found that untrained individuals were capable of more than $40 \text{ ml} \cdot \text{kg}^{-1}$; the highest values found in outstanding athletes exceeded $80 \text{ ml} \cdot \text{kg}^{-1}$.[12] To convert these quantities to heat production rate in $\text{kcal} \cdot \text{hr}^{-1}$, multiply by 60 (minutes per hour), divide by 1,000 (ml per liter), and multiply by 4.8 ($\text{kcal} \cdot \text{l}^{-1}$): for example, $3.5 \text{ ml} \cdot \text{min}^{-1} \cdot \text{kg}^{-1}$ equals $1.0 \text{ kcal} \cdot \text{hr}^{-1} \cdot \text{kg}^{-1}$. This easy-to-remember quantity can be kept in mind as the reference level of energy production for adults, e.g., resting heat production in a 70-kg person is near $70 \text{ kcal} \cdot \text{hr}^{-1}$.

Besides muscular activity, metabolic heat production rate can be increased by temperature itself. In the so-called Q_{10} effect, metabolic rate increases approximately 10 percent per degree Centigrade rise in tissue temperature.[13]

THERMAL STRESS RELATED TO BODY HEAT CAPACITY

"Thermal stress," "heat stress," and "cold stress" refer to occasions when the balance between heat production and loss rates is at least temporarily upset. The difference between heat production rate and the rate at which heat is lost to the environment translates into a rate of change of body temperature according to the body heat capacity.

The exact figure for heat capacity of the body is near $0.83 \text{ kcal} \cdot \text{kg}^{-1} \cdot (°C)^{-1}$. In other words, accumulation in 1 kg of body tissue of 1 kcal of heat increases the tissue temperature by nearly 1°C. For the purposes of this chapter, heat capacity is rounded to $1.0 \text{ kcal} \cdot \text{kg}^{-1} \cdot$

[†]Kilocalories (the amount of heat that elevates the temperature of 1 L of water 1° C) are used for heat, on the assumption that readers are familiar with the unit commonly used for energy content of foods; when a food item is described as containing a certain number of calories, say 140 calories in 100 ml of milk, the unit meant is the so-called large calorie, i.e., the kilocalorie. To convert kilocalories to kilojoules, multiply by 4.2. Kilocalories per hour ($\text{kcal} \cdot \text{hr}^{-1}$) and watts are used in references to heat flow rates and power output, depending on the practice of the literature from which the examples were taken. To convert $\text{kcal} \cdot \text{hr}^{-1}$ to watts, multiply by 1.16.

($°$ C)$^{-1}$. This allows the crude approximation that the rate of temperature increase (or decrease) can be numerically equated to the net rate of heat storage (or loss) per kilogram.

Consider the following examples of thermal imbalance:

1. Heat production rate at the normal level of 1 kcal · hr^{-1} · kg^{-1}, but heat loss kept at zero. The estimated rate of body temperature increase is 1.0° C· hr^{-1}. A practical approximation of zero heat loss conditions can be experienced in a normal indoor environment by wearing a thick "wet suit" (a garment of foam rubber designed for protection against intensely cold water).
2. Heat production rate elevated ten-fold, to 10 kcal · hr^{-1} · kg^{-1} but heat loss kept at zero. A practical approximation would result from vigorous exercise in an air environment in a wet suit or in a hot, high-humidity environment. The estimated rate of increase of body temperature is 10° C · hr^{-1}.
3. Heat production rate at a normal resting level, 1 kcal · hr^{-1} · kg^{-1}, but heat loss rate 10 percent greater. The amount of heat in the body would decrease at the rate of 0.1 kcal · hr^{-1} · kg^{-1}. Estimated rate of fall of body temperature is 0.1° C · hr^{-1}. A practical approximation would be a lightly dressed, resting person exposed to a cool environment.

Example 1 above illustrates the potential for endogenous heat stress represented by our rate of heat production at rest. According to the estimate, more than 5 hours of accumulation of the heat produced at rest would be fatal (assuming a starting level of 37° C). From one perspective, this is a long time; the high heat capacity of the body allows us to endure for a few hours the stress of a hot or cold environment in which we could not reach a tolerable steady state. We can afford to delay escape from the environment or to wait until the weather changes.

But the heat capacity of the body is not large in relation to the high rates of heat production of which we are capable during exercise. With the rate of body temperature increase estimated in example 2, estimated survival time falls to 0.5 hour, or less if the Q_{10} effect is considered. Fit individuals can exercise at levels associated with heat production far above the rate used in example 2. Consequently, endogenous heat can accumulate rapidly even with little or no insulation from clothing, if heat loss is restricted by environmental conditions, particularly if high ambient temperatures and humidity combine. In short, the heat production rates associated with severe exercise are potentially dangerous; matching them with comparable heat loss is an urgent physiologic priority.

In the other realm of thermal stress, cold stress, we have of course no comparable endogenous problem that would cause body temperature to fall at high rates. In example 3, the rate of cooling associated with a 10 percent excess of heat loss over heat production could be tolerated for hours. No serious impediment to performance would develop until the internal temperature fell below 35.5° C. Humans who tolerate exposure to cold environments for a long time, such as aborigines who sleep lightly clad through the cold desert night, tend to do so without reaching a steady state in which physiologic measures accomplish thermal balance; rather, they benefit from the high heat capacity of the body and slow cooling rate that occurs with a modest excess of heat loss over production, and they endure until conditions change.[11] High cooling rates and survival times measured in minutes occur with extreme convective cooling, such as in the pressurized gas mixture air of a deep sea chamber or immersion in cold water.[11]

MEAN BODY TEMPERATURE

The temperature inside the body is not uniform (see discussion of core temperature below). The distribution changes in different thermal conditions. Therefore, the rates of temperature change calculated in the above analyses of thermal imbalance are not necessarily correct for some particular site of core temperature measurement, such as the mouth or rectum. The correct temperature to use in relating body heat capacity and heat storage rates is *mean body temperature* (T_{mb}). The body is in thermal balance when the rate of change of T_{mb} is zero.

In theory, to determine T_{mb} we would partition the body into segments small enough to be of uniform temperature, compute the product of temperature and heat capacity of each segment, take a sum of all these, and, finally, divide by the total heat capacity. In other words, T_{mb} is an average weighted according to heat capacity.

In practice, crude approximations are substituted, based on experimental measurements of heat loss and, usually, on one core temperature and an average skin temperature calculated as the area-weighted average of several temperatures obtained at representative portions of the body surface. For example, T_{mb} might be calculated as 0.67 times rectal temperature plus 0.33 times average skin temperature. Unfortunately, these estimations of mean body temperature are grossly inaccurate in all but the exact conditions for which they were defined.[14]

Therefore, mean body temperature is more useful as a concept than as a practical means of analyzing thermal balance. Heat content may differ in two thermal states associated with equal values of conveniently measured core and skin temperature. For example, after exercise, a relative excess of heat content may be concealed in internal tissues that are not accessible for temperature measurement and that are slow to cool, despite recovery to preexercise levels of rectal and skin temperature.

CORE TEMPERATURE

Convective Distribution of Heat and Uniformity of Core Temperature

Inside the body, heat moves by conduction and convection. Heat transfer by conduction is analogous to transport of solutes by diffusion, with temperature gradient equivalent to concentration gradient. Convective heat transport is analogous to the bulk transport of materials by the blood, with the temperature difference between arterial and venous blood being equivalent to concentration difference. In the tissues of the organs deep within the body, convective heat transport prevents development of large temperature gradients.

In a well-perfused tissue, no cell is far from a capillary in which blood flows. Therefore, small temperature differences suffice for conductive transfer of heat from cells to capillaries. Once in the blood, the heat is carried away convectively; the temperature of venous blood is practically indistinguishable from tissue temperature and is only tenths of a degree above the temperature at which arterial blood entered the tissue. Arterial blood temperature is uniform throughout the major arteries except in the arms and legs. Combined with this fact, the small increments of venous over arterial temperature and equilibrium of tissue temperature with venous temperature add up to near uniformity of temperatures deep inside the body. These are the factors that underlie the concept of "core" temperature; the convective action of the circulation results in a nearly uniform temperature deep within the trunk and head.

In Table 4–1 are quantitative estimates of temperature differences within the body core. The organs are assumed to be in a steady thermal state, i.e., all the metabolic heat produced is balanced by an equal rate of heat transfer out of the organ so that temperatures throughout the organ are steady. Heat transfer out of the organ is assumed to be entirely by convection. Tissue temperature is assumed to be equal to the temperature of venous blood leaving the organ.

Given these assumptions, the increment in venous temperature relative to the temperature of the inflowing arterial blood depends on the ratio of the rate of heat production to the rate of perfusion. The quantity of heat transported by the blood equals the temperature difference times the heat capacity of the blood times the blood flow rate. The specific heat of blood is 0.92 $kcal \cdot kg^{-1} \cdot (°C)^{-1}$; the specific gravity is 1.06. Therefore, the quantity of heat that changes the temperature of 1 L of blood by 1° C is 0.98 kcal. For practical purposes, this can be rounded to 1.0 $kcal \cdot (°C^{-1})$.

Thus, the ratio of the heat production rate (calculated from oxygen consumption) to the perfusion rate of an organ numerically estimates the arteriovenous temperature difference. That ratio, of course, is also in proportion with the arteriovenous difference in oxygen content. The bigger the difference between arterial and venous oxygen concentration, the bigger the difference between venous and arterial temperature.

The computed increments in Table 4–1 predict that the mass of the body represented by the organs in the list is at uniform temperature within a few tenths of a degree, in steady-

TABLE 4–1 Core Temperature Uniformity, Calculated Temperature Difference for Organs in a Resting 70-kg Human

Body part	Blood flow (ml/min)	Oxygen consumption (ml/min)	Heat production (kcal/min)	Temperature difference (°C)
Splanchnic	1,500	60	.29	.19
Kidneys	1,200	14	.07	.06
Brain	750	60	.29	.38
Coronary	250	35	.17	.67
Total*	3,700	169	.81	.22
Skin	500	10	.05	.10
Muscle	1,000	60	.29	.29
Lungs[†]	5,500		.18 (heat lost)	.03

Blood flow and oxygen consumption data are from Rowell.[9] Heat production is based upon 4.8 kcal/L of oxygen consumed. The temperature difference, equal to the elevation in venous blood temperature relative to arterial temperature, is calculated with the specific heat of blood approximated as equal to $1.0 \text{ kcal} \cdot (°C \cdot 1)^{-1}$.
Temperature differences calculated for the noncore organ systems, skin and muscle, 0.10 and 0.29° C, respectively, are meaningless because of the large effect in superficial tissues of heat exchange with the environment.
* Combined blood flow of these organs, 3,700 ml/min, is 67% of cardiac output; proportion of total oxygen consumption is 68%. Calculated overall temperature difference is based upon combined blood flow and oxygen consumption of the four organs.
[†] Flow through the lungs is the entire cardiac output. Heat loss is taken as 15% of total heat production, the typical rate of evaporative heat loss from the lungs. Calculated temperature difference refers to temperature of mixed venous blood (pulmonary artery) minus temperature of blood in aorta.

state conditions. These estimates agree with the limited number of measurements that have been made in humans of intraorgan and intravascular temperature.[15,16]

An organ left out of Table 4–1 is the uterus. In pregnancy, the heat produced by the fetus must be removed by way of the placenta and the uterine circulation. Obviously, fetal body temperature is elevated above that of the mother, and this elevation increases if uterine blood flow falls, as it may in exercise and hyperthermia, just those conditions in which the arterial inflow is already at an elevated temperature.

Temperature Difference Associated with Heat Lost from the Lungs

The computation for the lungs in Table 4–1 is not derived from pulmonary heat production. The heat removed convectively from the lungs is much greater than locally produced metabolic heat. The lungs are ventilated with ambient air and are the route for loss, through evaporation, of an appreciable fraction of the total body heat production, (see discussion of evaporation below). Nonetheless, pulmonary temperature deviates little from other core tissues. The heat lost through the lungs is removed from the enormous blood supply represented by the entire cardiac output; therefore temperature in the aorta is only a few tenths of a degree above that in the pulmonary artery.

Core Temperature Uniformity When Organ Blood Flow Changes

Various stresses result in cardiovascular reflexes that change organ blood flow. Specifically, flow is reduced in the kidneys and splanchnic region as part of the response to exercise or hyperthermia. However, the heat production rate is not reduced. The increased ratio of the heat production rate to the blood flow rate results in increased temperatures.

An upper limit to the increment in venous over arterial temperature can be estimated from the maximal possible oxygen extraction. Suppose that all the oxygen available in a sample of arterial blood, say 200 ml per liter of blood, were completely extracted in aerobic metabolism. At 4.8 kcal per liter of oxygen, the amount of heat released would be 0.96 kcal. Therefore, under the severest limitation of flow, the increment of organ temperature over arterial temperature is limited to less than 1° C. (Note that organ temperature increment relative to arterial temperature is roughly numerically equal to the fraction of oxygen extraction.)

This estimate assumes a steady state. An organ deprived of flow altogether would briefly continue to produce heat anaerobically and attain higher temperatures. But in any situation lasting longer than minutes, metabolism is oxidative, organ flow is no less than the minimum necessary to supply sufficient oxygen, and the limit of 1° C must apply. Strictly, the estimated 1° C difference applies to the arteriovenous difference. With low perfusion, the assumption that tissue and venous blood temperatures are in equilibrium may be inaccurate; appreciable gradients may develop within the tissue.

Effect of External Energy Sources

A greater increment of deep tissue temperature over arterial blood temperature can develop through liberation of nonmetabolic heat. This is possible, for example, through the absorption of microwave or radiofrequency (diathermy) energy. For skeletal muscle, an additional possibility is heat liberated as external work is done, as when descending stairs (see discussion of temperatures in active muscle below).

As long as an external energy source supplies heat to a tissue, local temperature increments greater than that associated with the metabolism:perfusion ratio can persist. The resulting increase in venous blood temperature increases the temperature of mixed venous blood and, in turn, temperatures of arterial blood and tissues elsewhere. After the energy source is removed, temperature falls toward the steady-state level dictated by metabolism and perfusion. The time required for equilibration depends on the ratio of total mass to perfusion rate and would be long, for example, in a muscle in which blood flow had fallen to resting levels along with cessation of activity.

TEMPERATURES IN SUPERFICIAL TISSUES

Superficial tissue temperature is (usually) lower than that of incoming arterial blood, because heat is dissipated from the body surface to the environment. After passage through the microcirculation, blood and tissue temperatures are equilibrated, and venous blood leaves at a temperature lower than arterial blood. At thermal equilibrium, this convective supply of heat plus local tissue heat production balance the rate at which heat leaves at the surface.

At the body surface, skin temperature is at a level set by the rate at which heat is supplied from the body interior and the thermal characteristics of the environment (see section on thermal interaction with the environment below). Progressively higher temperatures are found in successively deeper layers of skin, fat, and muscle.[17] This gradient pattern varies with skin blood flow (Fig. 4–3) and with the level of activity in underlying muscle.

When a temperature gradient exists, heat flow by conduction down the gradient necessarily occurs. However, the gradient in the superficial tissues is set by the inherent conductivity of the tissues only in the extreme of zero blood flow. Otherwise, the thermal profile is dominated by convective heat exchange among the layers. Deeper layers are cooled by venous blood returning in small vessels from the skin. In turn, blood bound for the skin in small arteries is cooled in transit.

Cold Stress

When the thermoregulatory system acts to reduce heat loss, alpha-adrenergic vasoconstriction reduces skin blood flow. The proportion of convective relative to conductive heat transfer in superficial layers falls. With the reduced rate of delivery of heat to superficial tissues, the influence of low environmental temperature penetrates deeper (see Fig. 4–3). The temperature profile tends towards the limit associated with the intrinsic insulating property of unperfused tissue (roughly equal to cork). Individuals with a thick layer of subcutaneous fat have an advantage in the cold, because the insulation of this poorly perfused tissue adds to that of the skin.

The precooling that occurs as blood bound for the skin gives up heat to surrounding tissue that has been cooled by venous blood draining more superficial layers is an example of what is termed *countercurrent transfer of heat*. The advantageous consequence is that heat is con-

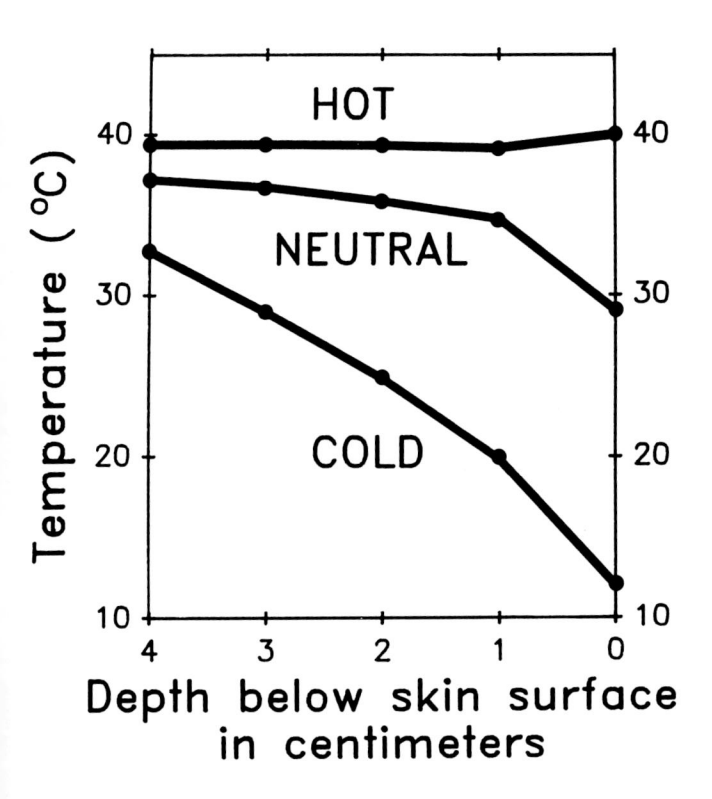

Figure 4–3 Thermal profiles under three conditions between extremes of skin blood flow, replotted from data of Sargeant.[17] Temperatures were obtained from thermocouples inserted to the indicated depths on the lateral surface of the quadriceps, midthigh. The line labeled "neutral" was obtained with the subject in a neutral environment, with no clothing over the thigh. In "hot" and "cold" conditions, the leg was immersed in water to obtain the indicated skin temperature.

served; a blood supply adequate for cutaneous nutrition can be maintained without resulting in the rate of heat loss that would occur if arterial blood arrived near the surface at core temperature. In other words, countercurrent exchange is like a thermal short circuit acting to preserve the heat content of the body core. It is a major feature of the adaptation to cold conditions in various animal species.[11]

The countercurrent exchange in superficial layers is brought about by the equilibration of temperature inside small vessels with the surrounding tissue. In larger vessels, just a few generations up from arterioles or venules, less surface is available for heat exchange relative to the blood flow rate; consequently, equilibration is incomplete.[18] Nonetheless, some heat can be exchanged across the walls of arteries or veins large enough to have names. In measurements made in human volunteers exposed to cold, radial artery temperature was well below that in the brachial artery.[19] In some individuals, the brachial vein nearly envelops the brachial artery; this anatomy suggests optimization for heat transfer.

In the arms and legs, the influence of environmental cooling penetrates deeper than in the trunk. A longitudinal gradient develops along the long axis, i.e., more distal skin is cooler and so are the more distal deeper tissues. The interior temperature of the fingers and toes falls far below core temperature. This pattern relates to the simple geometric relationship between surface area and volume.

The trunk, extremities, and fingers and toes are roughly cylindrical, in descending order of radius. The ratio of surface area to volume of a cylinder varies inversely with radius. Thus, the fingers have many times more surface area per unit of volume than the trunk. Heat is produced in volume and is lost from surface—the more surface area per unit volume, the more readily a segment is cooled.

This geometric fact means that the problem of defending against cooling differs enormously in degree for smaller animals, such as rodents. Even among humans, those of smaller dimensions (low birth-weight infants are the extreme example) and of greater overall surface to area ratio, are more affected by a cool environment.

Heat Stress

The gradient in superficial tissues is minimal, i.e., temperatures are closer to core temperature, when skin blood flow is high as a result of active vasodilatation (active cutaneous vasodilatation depends on an unknown vasodilator transmitter substance possibly liberated by fibers associated with the activation of sweat glands).[9] At maximal levels of this response, specific flow or blood flow per unit mass of skin may exceed 300 ml·min^{-1}·g^{-1}, matching maximal rates that can be reached even in the kidney.

Equally high flow develops in regions of skin that are heated directly. This can be seen in the reddening of an area soaked in hot water. This vasomotor response is intrinsic to the cutaneous vasculature; it is not a reflex mediated by the sympathetic nervous system, and it occurs even in regions of skin that have lost their nerve supply. The increase in local convection due to increased skin blood flow does minimize the superficial gradient, but note that it acts to increase heat transfer into the body if the locally warmed skin is above core temperature. Nonetheless, the response can be seen as beneficial if confined to a limited area of skin, in that the effect is to conduct heat away from an area that might otherwise reach excessive local temperatures.

When a large fraction of the whole skin area is directly heated, as in immersion in a hot tub, the locally mediated blood flow increase in the skin plus reflex-driven active cutaneous vasodilatation lead to more rapid rates of core temperature increase and to mounting cardiovascular stress associated with supplying several liters of blood per minute to the cutaneous vasculature.[9]

Temperatures in Active Muscle

During exercise, active skeletal muscle in the extremities becomes the major source of metabolic heat. In steady states of exercise, active muscle metabolism is aerobic. Therefore, according to the estimated maximal temperature difference calculated above, muscle temperature would not rise more than 1° C above the temperature of the arterial supply *unless heat is gained from a nonmetabolic source.*‡

This estimate is borne out by measurements that have been made in active muscle in human volunteers. A few are available that can be compared with simultaneous measurements of arterial blood temperature or another core temperature that would closely approximate arterial blood temperature. For example, Saltin and Hermansen found that temperature within the quadriceps femoris muscle exceeded esophageal temperature (which closely approximates arterial temperature) by roughly 0.4° C during exercise on a bicycle ergometer (see Fig. 4–14), over a range of oxygen consumption from 25 to 75 percent of maximal.[20] Äikäs and coworkers found that quadriceps femoris (vastus lateralis) temperature rose rapidly with the onset of exercise and soon equilibrated at 0.7° C above esophageal temperature.[21]

Nadel and associates recorded a muscle temperature of 41.6° C in a subject doing simulated downhill pedaling on an ergometer;[22] under these conditions of "negative work" exercise, external work done on the muscle adds heat beyond that produced metabolically.

In short, with the exception of situations in which negative work or other heat sources such

---

‡The calculation is at least a slight overestimate, because in reality oxygen extraction is less than 100 percent, and some of the energy released is converted to external work.

as diathermy or high temperature in the skin overlying active muscle add nonmetabolic heat, active skeletal muscle temperature does not deviate far above that of the body core.[23]

Skin Temperature and Increased Local Heat Dissipation Over Active Muscles

Some of the heat produced by active muscle is carried convectively to the overlying skin through preheating of arterial blood bound for the skin, and there it is dissipated to the environment. This local heat transfer phenomenon is similar to the countercurrent process described above, but in reverse; the benefit is that less of the heat liberated during exercise needs to be transported into the central core of the body.

Blood bound for the skin overlying muscle makes its way through arterial branches that have arborized to nearly arteriolar dimensions within the muscle—no artery of appreciable dimensions supplies the skin. These small dimensions are associated with high surface area per unit volume of vessel, which permits effective heat transfer from the muscle cells to the cutaneous arterial supply.[18] Consequently, arterial blood warms up on the way to the skin, increases skin temperature locally, and thus enhances heat loss to the environment. Possibly, the fact that cutaneous vessels vasodilate when warmed adds to the efficiency of this process through directing skin blood flow to areas influenced by muscle heat. In contrast to the circulatory pattern associated with countercurrent conservation of heat, much of the venous blood from the skin collects in large surface veins and makes the transit back through deeper (and hotter) levels through vessels with relatively small surface-to-volume ratios that take up little heat, compared to the tiny vessels of the arterial supply.

This phenomenon would account for the observations of Aulick and co-workers, who found only a slightly higher temperature in the femoral vein than in the femoral artery of subjects exercising hard (up to 61 percent of maximal oxygen consumption) on a treadmill.[24] Also, direct evidence of elevated skin temperatures above active muscles was obtained by Cooper and colleagues.[25]

CORE–SHELL THERMAL MODEL OF THE BODY

Body Shell and Clothing As Insulators

A simple view of heat transfer within the body is the old concept of an inner "core" at uniform temperature (T_{co}) and an outer "shell" with a gradient from core temperature on the inside down to a uniform skin temperature (T_{sk}) on the outer surface. The shell is treated as a layer of insulation of variable thickness—thick in the cold, thin in the heat (representing the effect of reduction or increase of skin blood flow). The internal organs, physically within the core, benefit from a uniform thermal environment maintained over a wide range of endogenous and exogenous heat stress; the tissues of the shell must endure a wider range of temperature (see Fig. 4–3).

The core–shell model of the body has no practical value in the sense of enabling precise predictions of particular body temperatures in particular environments. Both T_{co} and T_{sk} are fictions that conceal the actual complexity of patterns of internal and superficial temperatures; the inherent insulation of body tissues is not variable; heat transfer across superficial tissues is not simple conduction through a layer of insulating material. But the model is useful for semiquantitative treatments of the effects of changes in skin blood flow and the insulation qualities of clothing. Also, when combined with the simplified quantitative treatments of heat exchange with the environment, described below, it aids in understanding how core and skin temperatures relate to ambient conditions.

Insulation and Conductivity of the Shell and of Clothing

The insulating property of a slab of material is defined as the ratio of the temperature difference between the opposite faces and the rate of heat flow. For a given rate of heat flow and thickness of material, the greater the insulation, the larger the temperature difference. In a well-insulated house, the large temperature difference between the warm inside and the cold outside surfaces is associated with only small rates of heat loss. Analogously, shell insulation (I_{sh}) is defined as follows:

$$I_{sh} = \frac{T_{co} - T_{sk}}{H_{sh}} \quad (1)$$

(H_{sh} refers to the heat that passes through the shell tissues, i.e., total heat production less the heat loss through the respiratory tract.)

Unlike a house, the insulation defined for the body in equation 1 is variable, because a change in skin blood flow varies the amount of heat transported to the body surface for a given ($T_{co} - T_{sk}$).

Clothing insulation (I_{cl}) is defined as follows (assuming that all the heat that leaves the body through the shell conducts across the clothing):

$$I_{cl} = \frac{T_{sk} - T_{su}}{H_{sh}} \quad (2)$$

(T_{su} refers to clothing surface temperature.)

These may be rewritten as follows:

$$T_{co} = T_{sk} + H_{sh} \cdot I_{sh} \quad (3a)$$

$$T_{sk} = T_{su} + H_{sh} \cdot I_{cl} \quad (3b)$$

A useful rearrangement of equation 1 is this:

$$H_{sh} = (I_{sh})^{-1} \cdot (T_{sk}) \quad (4)$$

The reciprocal of insulation is given the name "conductivity." The better the insulation, the less the conductivity. Representing the conductivity of the shell tissues as $K_{sh} = (I_{sh}^{-1})$, we arrive at the following equation:

$$H_{sh} = K_{sh} \cdot (T_{co} - T_{sk}) \quad (5)$$

Analysis of Thermal Balance in Terms of the Core–Shell Model

In a steady-state, the heat lost through the shell tissues equals the total amount of heat produced minus the amount lost directly from the core through the respiratory tract. Surface temperature equilibrates at a level determined by H_{sh} and environmental conditions (see summary of the section on thermal interaction with the environment). From equations 3a and 3b, the relationships that occur in a steady state are clear: T_{co} is necessarily elevated above T_{sk} by an amount equal to the product of H_{sh} and I_{sh}. The variable "insulation" of the shell makes possible maintenance of a fixed T_{co} for a broad spectrum of levels of T_{sk} and H_{sh}.

In neutral or cool environments, we select clothing to achieve a T_{sk} that is comfortable, near 33.5° C. In terms of equation 3b, I_{cl} is chosen for a given level of H_{sh} to obtain a T_{sk} that is perceived as comfortable. This is associated with a T_{co} set by H_{sh} and I_{sh}.

In cold environments, I_{cl} must be large; otherwise, in the extreme with $I_{cl} = 0$, the naked skin is necessarily at the temperature (T_{su}) (equation 3b) determined by the environmental conditions and H_{sh} (see equation 10 below). If maximal I_{sh}, i.e., minimal K_{sh}, cannot support a big enough ($T_{co} - T_{sk}$), the only possibility for obtaining a sufficient elevation of T_{co} above T_{sk} (equation 3a) is increase in H_{sh} (by shivering or voluntary exercise).

The warmer the environment, the more we reduce I_{cl} to a socially acceptable minimum, driven by the desire to maintain T_{sk} at a comfortable level. If the environment and level of metabolism make this impossible, even with I_{cl} at zero, then I_{sh} must decrease (K_{sh} increase); otherwise, T_{co} would rise in parallel with T_{sk} (assuming that heat production rate is constant). With severe exogenous heat stress, the increase in skin blood flow is so great that insulation is virtually zero and ($T_{co} - T_{sk}$) approaches zero (equation 1).

Exogenous heat stress becomes intolerable when equilibrium T_{sk} is pushed up to the point at which T_{co} exceeds the upper limit of the range of tolerable internal temperatures; it is physically impossible for ($T_{co} - T_{sk}$) to be less than zero in a steady state, because H_{sh} is always positive (equation 3a). With still further increase in T_{sk}, an additional increase in skin blood flow is not only futile but actually makes things worse, because the high rate of convective heat transfer only increases T_{co}.

Thus, if we take 42° C as the point of irreversible thermal damage, an environment in which T_{sk} is forced to 42° C or above is clearly intolerable. The actual safe upper limit is lower—recall that temperature increments exceed those in Table 4–1 as a result of visceral vasoconstriction necessitated by the enormous skin blood flow.

Take particular note that, no matter how great the physiologic thermoregulatory response, T_{co} cannot be brought below T_{sk}. True, we can tolerate environments with temperatures far above tolerable T_{co}. Blagden and Fordyce demonstrated this in 1775 by personally enduring the environment of a baker's oven hot enough to cook a steak they brought in with them.[26] But this depends entirely on the efficacy of the sweating mechanism in reducing T_{sk} below ambient temperature (see section on evaporation below). In an environment in which humidity is so high that evaporative heat loss is impossible, T_{co} must exceed ambient temperature.

Relationship Between Skin Blood Flow Rate and Shell Conductivity

Equation 5 has the same form as the equation used to obtain the arterial-to-venous temperature differences listed in Table 4–1. If we assume that the heat that leaves the body surface arrives convectively through blood that reaches the skin at core temperature and leaves it at skin temperature, then the following describes H_{sh} in terms of skin blood flow (SkBF) and the heat capacity of blood (K_b):

$$H_{sh} = K_b \cdot SkBF \cdot (T_{co} - T_{sk}) \quad (6)$$

The similarity between equations 6 and 5 formally shows the conductivity of the shell (K_{sh}) as equal to the product of the skin blood flow rate (in liters·min^{-1}) and blood heat capacity (in kcal · L^{-1}, numerically approximated as 1.0). In the core–shell model, then, changes in skin blood flow are equivalent to changes in the conductivity of the shell tissues.

The approximations behind equation 6 are indeed crude. Arterial blood does not arrive in cutaneous arterioles at core temperature, nor does departing venous blood equilibrate with skin surface temperature. The equation generally underestimates skin blood flow. Nonetheless, the relationship is adequate for studying the consequences of changes in environmental conditions or skin blood flow. The reader can benefit from exploring the qualitative implications of this relationship, with questions such as the following examples (chosen to correspond to the conditions of the examples in the final section of the chapter).

1. **Skin Blood Flow at Rest: Neutral Environment.** In a person weighing 70 kg, with metabolic rate at a resting level, 70 kcal · hr^{-1}, neutral conditions would be associated with core and skin temperature near 36.5° C and 34° C, respectively. Taking heat loss from the respiratory tract as 18 kcal · hr^{-1} (25 percent of total heat production), the heat loss through the shell is 52 kcal · hr^{-1}, (70–18), equal to 0.87 kcal · min^{-1}. The ratio of this H_{sh}—expressed as kcal · min^{-1} to the core–shell temperature difference, 2.5° C—is 0.347, i.e., skin blood flow is estimated as 0.347 L · min^{-1}, not an unreasonable estimate, compared with accepted values.[9]

2. **Skin Blood Flow During Exercise: Neutral Environment.** A person exercising at a power output level of 150 W, with H_{sh} 345 kcal · hr^{-1} and with ambient temperature at 21° C would reach thermal equilibrium with skin temperature at 27° C and core temperature at 38.0° C. Skin blood flow, computed as H_{sh} divided by 60 times (38–27), is estimated as 0.52 L · min^{-1}. The requirement for skin blood flow increase relative to rest is reduced by the widened core–shell difference.

3. **Skin Blood Flow During Exercise: Warm Environment.** The same individual at the same power output level and H_{sh} but with ambient temperature at 31° C would stabilize at nearly the same core temperature but with skin temperature near 33° C. Skin blood flow, computed as above, is estimated as 1.15 L · min^{-1}. With further increase in ambient temperature, the core–skin gradient

flex redistribution or cardiac output that occurs in exercise or hyperthermia, nor is cerebral metabolism.[§] Consequently, the offset between arterial and brain temperature, estimated as 0.38° C in Table 4–1, should be identical in those conditions with what exists in unstressed conditions.

Therefore, because perfusion of the rectal region is markedly influenced by exercise and heat stress, rectal temperature becomes proportionately poorer as an indicator of brain temperature and progressively slower to respond to changes. Reports of rectal temperatures above 43° C in individuals who have survived heat stroke cannot be taken as evidence that the brain or other organs reached the same temperature.[8]

THERMAL INTERACTION WITH THE ENVIRONMENT

Convection

Air acts as a heat transfer fluid. Heat is carried away from the body convectively as air close to the surface of the skin or clothing absorbs heat, changes density, and rises. Like a candle, the body creates a rising column of heated air (natural convection). With increased relative movement, as when we run or are exposed to wind, the rate of heat transfer increases (*forced convection*). In quantitative terms:

$$H_c = A_c \cdot K_c \cdot (T_{su} - T_{amb}) \quad (7)$$

In this relationship, H_c is the amount of convective heat and T_{su} and T_{amb} are, respectively, surface and air (ambient) temperatures. The difference between T_{su} and T_{amb} can be viewed as the driving force for convection (T_{su} refers to skin temperature when the skin is naked). A_c refers to the total area of the body exposed for convective heat exchange, typically less than the total body surface area because some areas, such as under the arms, are not exposed. A_c can be reduced by deliberate behaviors, such as when a cat sleeps curled up in a cold environment.

The remaining parameter, K_c, expresses the characteristics of the environment; the greater the relative velocity between the air and the skin surface, the greater the value. The relationship can be described empirically in terms of velocity raised to a fractional power near 0.5; values listed in Table 4–2 are based on the practical approximation recommended by Kerslake.[32]

In an indoor environment, the surface to air temperature difference is, typically, 4° C. For a 70-kg individual of average build, A_c would be near 1.5 m². Thus with K_c at 5.2 kcal·(hr·m²·°C)$^{-1}$ (the indoor environment value listed in Table 4–2), $H_c = 1.5 \cdot 5.2 \cdot 4 = 31.2$ kcal·hr^{-1}, less than half of the resting level of heat production (typically 70 kcal·hr^{-1} for a person of this size). However, the entries in Table 4–2 for higher air velocities show that total convective heat loss increases greatly; for the same surface–air difference, winds at gale force would increase heat loss more than seven-fold, so that what was a comfortable air temperature would represent a dangerous cold stress. Other entries in Table 4–2, based on velocities of walking or running, show how the relative wind that develops helps dissipate the elevated heat produced by exercise.

Equation 7 is one of the bases of "wind-chill" indices. The effect of the greater K_c associated with a particular velocity of air at a particular temperature is represented by computing a lower temperature, the "wind-chill" temperature, that would result in the same rate of convective heat loss for a still-air value of K_c. In other words, the temperature difference driving convection is represented as the actual temperature difference times the ratio of the actual K_c to that associated with still air.

Water is enormously more effective as a medium for convective heat transport. The temperature difference between the skin surface and well-stirred water is so small it is difficult to measure. Another medium with high K_c is the high-pressure gas mixture used for deep diving.[11]

[§]This assumption of constant cerebral perfusion assumes normal ventilation, i.e., normal partial pressures of oxygen and carbon dioxide. In extreme hyperthermia, humans begin to hyperventilate.[9] This presumably causes brain blood flow to fall because of the reduction in the arterial concentration of carbon dioxide. The magnitude of the resulting increase in cerebral relative to arterial temperature is unknown.

TABLE 4–2 Heat Transfer Coefficient at Various Air Velocities*

Condition	Air velocity (m·s⁻¹)	K_c in W·(m²·°C)⁻¹	K_c in kcal·(hr·m²·°C)⁻¹
Typical indoor	.5	5.9	5.24
Walking, 4 mi·hr⁻¹	1.8	11.1	9.94
2 h, 36 min marathon	4.5	17.6	15.7
4-min mile	6.7†	21.5	19.2
60 mph gale	27†	43.1	38.5

* Based on $K_c = 8.3 \cdot V^{0.5}$ for units of W·(m²·°C)⁻¹ $K_c = 7.4 \cdot V^{0.5}$ for units of kcal·(hr·m²·°C)⁻¹. Empirical relationship taken from Kerslake.[32]
† Extrapolated figures—data compiled by Kerslake extend to 5 m·sec⁻¹.

Finally, note that heat can move convectively in either direction depending on which temperature—surface or ambient—is the greater. *When environmental temperature exceeds body surface temperature, we gain heat by convection.*

Radiation

We gain heat by radiation when we are exposed to intense radiant sources of heat, e.g., the sun, or heat lamps. We also exchange heat by radiation with surrounding surfaces, either gaining or losing heat depending on whether surface temperatures are higher or lower than the temperature of the exposed body surface. A precise description of the rate at which heat is radiated away from a surface at a given temperature involves the fourth power of the temperature, but in the range of ordinary room and skin temperatures, the following is an adequate description of radiative heat exchange in an enclosed environment where the enclosing surfaces are at a uniform temperature (T_r).

$$H_r = A_r \cdot K_r \cdot (T_{su} - T_r) \quad (8)$$

Here, K_r is a constant with the same units as K_c; it includes the factor that approximates what remains when $(T_{su}^4 - T_r^4)$ is divided by $(T_{su} - T_r)$. In the limited range of ordinary indoor temperatures, K_r can be taken as 6 W·(m²·°C)⁻¹, or 5 kcal·(hr·m²·°C⁻¹). A_r refers to the area available for exchange, again less than total body surface area to the extent that certain body areas are shielded from exchange. T_{su} equals skin temperature when the skin is naked. Note that, as with convection, we gain or lose heat by radiation depending on which temperature—surface or skin—is greater.

Equation 8 does not apply, of course, to radiation received from intense sources like the sun or heat lamps. We gain heat from them at a rate that depends on their radiant output and the amount and emissivity of the body surface area exposed. For example, in the direct rays of the sun, the incident energy is approximately 1,000 W·m⁻². Most of the energy is in the range of wavelengths in which virtually none is reflected, regardless of skin color, in the visible range of the spectrum. This subject is treated in detail in Kerslake's book.[32]

Equation 8 is also invalid for low T_r and for environments in which T_r is nonuniform. For example, in a room with large windows on a clear night with the walls and air at what is ordinarily a comfortable temperature, the occupants feel cold because of greater H_r. The infrared radiation from the body surface passes through the glass, and none is returned.

Evaporation

Water that evaporates absorbs roughly 600 kcal of heat (700 W·hr) per liter in the change of state from liquid to gas, the so-called *latent heat of vaporization*. The possible rates of evaporation from the body surface represent large quantities of heat relative to body heat capacity and even maximal rates of heat production.

Inevitable Water Loss

Our expired air is saturated with water vapor evaporated from the surfaces of the respiratory tract. Also, a much smaller amount of water leaves the body by diffusion across the skin, the *insensible perspiration*. Together, these typically amount to a total of 1 L per day. For a person who expends 2,400 kcal of energy per day, this evaporative heat loss accounts for 25 percent of the total heat transferred to the environment. Because ventilation increases in proportion to intensity of exercise, so does the rate of respiratory heat loss; the fraction of the total heat loss remains in the 10 to 25 percent range.

At altitude, the total volume of air expired increases inversely with barometric pressure. Though total pressure is less, the saturation partial pressure of water vapor at core temperature is not. Therefore, altitude hyperpnea increases respiratory heat loss, a factor that compounds mountain climbers' problems of maintaining thermal balance.

Respiratory heat loss can be reduced if hot humid air is inspired, a technique that has some benefit in rewarming victims of hypothermia.[33] In keeping with the old saying, "It's not the heat, it's the humidity," the heat supplied by the heat capacity of air is of trivial significance compared with the prevention of evaporation. Heat can actually be gained by condensation during ventilation with humid air if the dew point of the inspired air exceeds body temperature.

Sweating

When the sweat glands are activated, the rate of secretion over the whole body can increase the rate at which water is evaporated from the body from the baseline rate of tens of milliliters per hour, from respiration, to the range of liters per hour ($L \cdot hr^{-1}$). Robinson recorded 1.44 $L \cdot hr^{-1}$ (10 percent respiratory water loss) in an elite athlete running uphill on a treadmill in severe heat;[34] 1.8 $L \cdot hr^{-1}$ has been recorded over a 2-hour run, also in hot laboratory conditions.[35] Measurements in the field have shown that rates exceeding 1 $L \cdot hr^{-1}$, maintained throughout the race, are typical for marathon runners.[36]

This output of the sweat glands, *sensible perspiration*, has enormous potential for removal of metabolic heat. The high rates of heat production that occur during exercise can be balanced by evaporation of sweat at rates that can be maintained almost indefinitely, provided that adequate water intake replaces the loss.

For a quantitative description of evaporative heat loss, the following formulation is accurate enough for present purposes:

$$H_e = 600 \cdot (SR) \qquad (9)$$

(SR refers to the combined rate of respiratory water loss and sweat secretion, in $L \cdot hr^{-1}$, and 600 refers to the approximate latent heat of evaporation of sweat, in $kcal \cdot L^{-1}$.

The potential of this mechanism for heat loss can be realized *provided that all the secreted sweat evaporates*. Sweat that drips on the floor or is absorbed in a towel has no cooling effect on the body. For equation 9 to be correct, the rate of evaporation of sweat rather than the rate of secretion should be used. Whether secreted sweat evaporates depends upon the humidity and convective characteristics of the environment. Better quantitative descriptions of evaporative heat loss than equation 9 have been developed.[32] These incorporate the partial pressures of water in ambient air and at the skin surface and a convection coefficient to account for the effectiveness of air movement in enhancing evaporation.

In warm dry air, particularly if air moves relative to the body, as during running, all secreted sweat evaporates. The skin is dry, and a runner may speak of "not working up a sweat," even though evaporation of liters of sweat was what kept him or her alive.

The opposite extreme is an environment with warm air and 100 percent humidity. Evaporation is possible only to the extent that the vapor pressure of water at the skin surface exceeds the vapor pressure in the adjacent air. Unevaporated sweat drips off the body. Sweating is obvious, but because no change of state from liquid to vapor has occurred, the sweat that leaves the body in liquid form has no effect on body temperature. The individual complains of sweating although sweat rates are actually lower, inhibited by the wetness of the skin (hidromeiosis; see below).

In an environment with 100 percent humidity at air temperatures in excess of body temperature, heat loss by evaporation is impossible, even from the respiratory surfaces where surface temperature is near core temperature. Condensation would occur, so, in principle, heat can be gained in this way. Such an environment is intolerable, whereas we can tolerate heat gains by convection and radiation almost indefinitely, provided that sufficient sweat can be evaporated.

Factors that Interfere with Evaporative Heat Loss

Dehydration

Sweating inadequately compensated by drinking results in progressive dehydration. Water loss associated with high sweat rates amounts to more than 1 percent of total body weight per hour; this loss of hypotonic solute results in plasma hyperosmolarity as well as hypovolemia in all the body fluid compartments. Dehydration beyond 1 or 2 percent of body weight results in a decline of sweat rate. The corresponding reduction in rate of heat dissipation results in increased temperatures of the core and skin. These are signals that tend to restore sweat rate but that worsen the state of dehydration.

Dehydration, inhibition of sweating, and reduced heat dissipation progress in an accelerating spiral toward intolerable hyperthermia. Prolonged exercise, particularly endurance events such as marathons, entails this risk even in mildly warm weather. For prevention, adequate fluid replacement is imperative. See the position statement of the American College of Sports Medicine entitled "Prevention of Thermal Injuries During Distance Running."[37]

In an experimental analysis of this process, Ekblom and associates found that rectal temperatures in three men were approximately 1° C higher after an hour of hard exercise (equivalent to 60 percent of the maximum level of which they were capable) with no fluid replacement, than in a previous session in which they drank enough tap water to prevent weight loss.[38] Total weight loss in the dehydration session was near 1 percent. Numerous studies of the effects of hypohydration on resting and exercising subjects, with weight loss from 4 to 7 percent, has been summarized by Sawka and colleagues.[39]

Dehydration resulting from loss of water by routes other than sweating also inhibits sweating. Fortney and colleagues found that an isotonic hypovolemia equivalent to reduction of total body water by 3 percent of total body weight, induced by diuretics, altered the control of sweating, as reflected in the relationship between sweating rate at various points on the body surface and core temperature.[41]

Hidromeiosis

Sweat secretion rate falls in areas of the skin that remain wet for extended periods. For example, during an 8-hour walk in moist heat, sweat rate fell steadily after reaching a peak near 1 L·hr^{-1} in the first hour. A similar pattern occurs in persons immersed in hot baths. Such declines are not caused by dehydration, because the sweat rate immediately increases if the skin is dried. The phenomemon, called *hidromeiosis*, seems to reflect a physical interference with sweat gland function caused by the water content of the stratum corneum, rather than any decline in output from reduced neural stimulation or "fatigue" of the secretory mechanism.[42]

Inappropriate Evaporative Heat Loss

We do not have to sweat to experience a major effect of evaporation on our thermal balance. In weather that is only cool in temperature, people who get wet may suffer hypothermia as a consequence of evaporation of water from the body surface. Even the high rates of heat production in heavy exercise do not balance the heat loss rates that occur in only mildly cool,

---

Readers interested in this problem should be aware that comparisons in exercising subjects are complicated by the fact that ingested fluids may not be completely absorbed. In other words, body weight loss underestimates dehydration if unabsorbed fluid remains in the digestive tract. (For an introduction to the literature, see Brouns and co-workers.[40])

but wet, conditions, particularly when wind promotes evaporation. Thus, although the natural preoccupation with those responsible for marathon races is the danger of hyperthermia, some cases of collapse in races run on rainy days have been due to hypothermia.[43]

In clinical fluid loss, we are inclined to focus on the cardiovascular consequences and electrolyte imbalance and overlook the thermal consequences. But if the fluid has evaporated from the body surface, the associated cooling may have radically affected thermal balance. A spectacular example is the high evaporative heat loss experienced by patients who have extensive burns and who lose many liters of water each day from the portions of the body where the stratum corneum, the normal barrier against diffusion of water, has been destroyed.

Summary

Total heat loss is the sum of the evaporative, radiative, and convective components plus direct conduction to solid objects with which the body is in contact (usually a negligible fraction). In indoor environments without forced convection or intense radiant sources, the nonevaporative portion of total heat loss is roughly equally divided between convection and radiation. Secretion of sweat makes it possible to take advantage of the large latent heat of water in dissipation of heat to protect against hyperthermia.

Equations 7 through 9 enable completion of the development of relationships between body and ambient temperatures and heat loss from the body surface that begin with equations 1 through 5 when radiant and air temperatures (and areas exposed for convection and radiation) are identical:

$$H_{sh} = A_c \cdot (K_c + K_r) \cdot (T_{su} - T_{amb}) \quad (10)$$

The total amount of heat lost via the skin is represented by H_{sh} (total heat production less evaporative heat loss from the respiratory tract). A_c refers to the exposed surface area, and the definition of T_{amb} is broadened to represent the equal radiant and air temperatures. The equation may be rearranged as follows:

$$T_{su} = T_{amb} + \frac{H_{sh} - H_e}{A_c \cdot (K_c + K_r)} \quad (11)$$

Equation 11, together with equations 3a and 3b, describes the successive steps that link ambient and core temperature (see Fig. 4–8 for specific examples). These and other applications of the principles of this section are developed below in the sections on body temperature, effector activity, and thermal balance in specific environments.

CONTROL OF THERMAL BALANCE

Effector Systems

Two physiologic mechanisms with powerful capability to modify heat loss have been introduced. Sweating and skin blood flow are under control of the sudomotor and vasomotor outflow to the skin, respectively, from the sympathetic division of the autonomic nervous system. Sudomotor fibers are cholinergic. The vasomotor fibers that exert a vasoconstrictor influence on cutaneous vessels are alpha-adrenergic. These equip the cutaneous vasculature with the capability to modulate flow between a minimum level (so low that our measuring techniques cannot detect it) and a maximum associated with complete removal of vasoconstrictor activity. Far greater flow rates occur during hyperthermia; therefore, cutaneous vascular smooth muscle must also be subject to the influence of a vasodilator transmitter, perhaps from a separate set of vasomotor fibers, possibly a co-transmitter released in conjunction with activation of sweat glands. (For a discussion of properties of the cutaneous vasculature, see the monograph by Rowell.[9])

These motor outflows, sudomotor and vasomotor, with preganglionic neurons in the spinal cord, are under control of descending influence from integrative centers in the hypothalamus, in the typical pattern of autonomic reflexes such as those that regulate blood pressure.

The third automatic effector, shivering, is also under control of the thermoregulatory centers in the hypothalamus. Obviously, this departs from the typical pattern of an autonomic motor function presided over by the hypothalamus, in that the skeletal muscles that are activated are under voluntary control.

Central Integration

The control signals that set the activity level of the effectors of thermoregulation represent the output, so to speak, of integrative centers in the hypothalamus that process input information related to core and skin temperature. A decerebrate animal with all hypothalamic tissue removed is poikilothermic (i.e., having no control of thermoregulatory effectors, as in cold-blooded species). However, in a high decerebration that does not remove the hypothalamus or interfere with its descending connections, the thermoregulatory system appears to be intact; normal body temperature is maintained. Thus, although voluntary behavior and descending signals from other higher levels in the brain can influence the integrative centers in the hypothalamus, the hypothalamic level of integration is sufficient for regulating body temperature.

Cutaneous Thermoreception

Among cutaneous sensory fibers are two populations with activity strongly dependent upon skin temperature, "warm" and "cold" fibers. Neither class appears to have specialized receptive structures; they terminate as naked fibers. In "warm" fibers, firing rate increases when the receptive area is warmed, and vice versa (Fig. 4–4).[44] However, in both populations the temperature–firing rate relationship turns downward after reaching a maximum. Thus a "warm" or "cold" fiber can exhibit the same average frequency at two different temperatures.

How can these temperatures be discriminated? How can integrative neural mechanisms tell whether a given frequency represents one temperature or another on the other side of the peak? The answer is not known. One possibility is that the pattern of impulses might differ for two impulse trains with the same average frequency and that this sensory coding conveys the necessary information. Another possibility lies in the extraordinary dynamic characteristics of these rapidly-adapting fibers. As shown in Figure 4–5, the discharge rate of temperature-sensitive fibers overshoots when the temperature changes.[44] For example, as the temperature stimulating a warm fiber increases, the discharge frequency is temporarily much higher than the ultimate level achieved after temperature stabilizes.

These dynamic properties (see Fig. 4–5) can be compared with two observations from everyday psychophysiologic knowledge. First, we adapt to and become unaware of a fixed temperature, but we perceive the slightest change. Second, if the hands are placed in warm and cold water, respectively, and then plunged into neutral-temperature water, the sensation from the hand that was cold is warm, and the sensation from the hand that was warm is cold. Clearly, information in the discharge pattern that is related to the direction and rate of temperature change has major significance in the decoding of the input from cutaneous thermoreceptors, which underlies our conscious awareness of skin temperature.

That skin temperature information is supplied to the hypothalamic integrative neurons has been verified by direct recordings in animals. The information is undoubtedly incorporated in control. All three effectors are influenced by skin temperature, especially when it changes rapidly. Perhaps information from particular areas is given particular weight; the distribution of receptor sites is far from uniform; the face is richly supplied, other areas, less so. (For a comprehensive treatment of the subject of cutaneous thermoreception by an outstanding contributor to the research literature on this subject, see the monograph by Hensel.[44])

Core Temperature Thermoreception

The hypothalamic neurons of thermoregulation are also supplied with information related to internal temperature. The actual sites of thermosensitivity in humans have never been determined experimentally. Nor are they likely to be found with anatomical techniques, because thermosensitivity is associated with no known structural characteristic.

Physiologists have searched for thermosensitive regions in the body core much as one might undertake to locate the thermostat of a

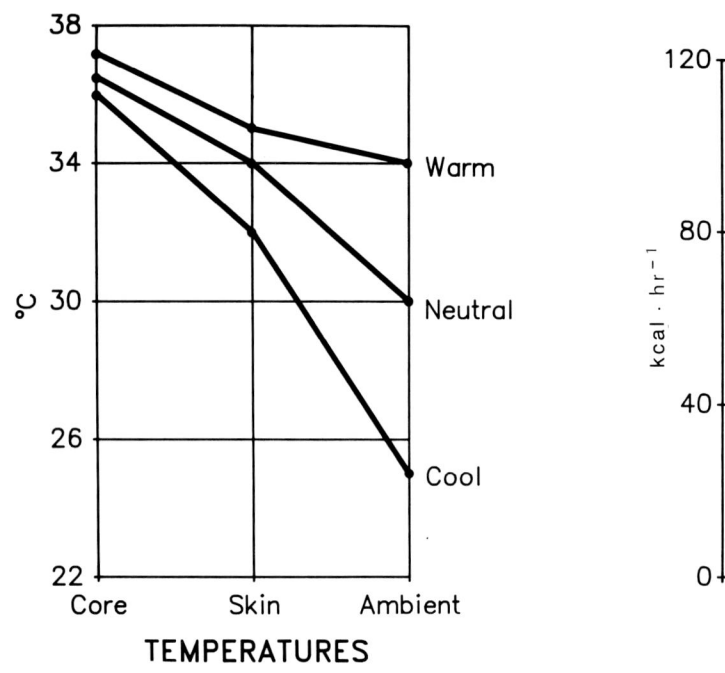

Figure 4-8 Temperatures and heat loss in environments in and bordering the zone of vasomotor regulation. Based on data obtained in experiments with near-naked supine subjects in calorimetric experimental chambers.[52,53]

Neutral Environment

The data points joined by the line labeled "neutral" in Figure 4-8 are ambient temperature, 30° C; skin temperature, 34° C; and core temperature, 36.5° C. These are compatible with a steady state that could be maintained indefinitely; it is neutral in the sense that core temperature would not change and the environment would be perceived as comfortable.

In a thermal steady state, heat loss and heat production are balanced; thus, the right panel in Figure 4-8 (bar labeled "neutral") shows total heat loss equal to 70 kcal·hr^{-1}. Since baseline evaporative heat loss rate is 18 kcal·hr^{-1}, the balance (70 − 18 = 52) equals the sum of radiative and convective heat loss, individually calculated below:

$$H_c = 1.5 \cdot 3.7 \cdot (34 - 30) = 22 \text{ kcal} \cdot \text{hr}^{-1}$$
$$H_r = 1.5 \cdot 5.0 \cdot (34 - 30) = 30 \text{ kcal} \cdot \text{hr}^{-1}$$
$$\text{Combined total:} \quad\quad\quad\quad\quad 52 \text{ kcal} \cdot \text{hr}^{-1}$$

Note that radiation accounts for the larger proportion of the nonevaporative heat loss. This is typical in indoor environments with little or no forced air movement. K_c is less than K_r until air velocity reaches roughly 0.5 m·sec^{-1}.[32]

Borders of the Zone of Vasomotor Regulation

What is the range of environmental conditions over which thermoregulation is accomplished through vasomotor regulation only? In our examples, for near-naked subjects, lying quietly in a calorimeter, the air temperature boundaries of the zone were roughly 25° and 30° C. However, it is pointless to describe this zone in terms of air temperature. Humans choose clothing to achieve thermal comfort; in a space suit, the most extreme cold is tolerated. The question is better phrased in terms of skin temperatures, because the end result of the interaction between the environment, clothing, and the level of heat production is a particular distribution of skin temperature. Two environments that are radically different but equally comfortable, given the appropriate clothing, have in common the same comfortable skin temperatures.

Range of Skin Temperatures in the Zone of Vasomotor Regulation

The range of skin temperatures over which thermal balance in a resting person is maintained without resorting to increased metabolism or sweating is narrow, less than 1° C (centered on 34° C) in the calorimetric studies on which Figure 4–8 is based. This narrow range has been confirmed in studies in which subjects were immersed in water, which makes skin temperature uniform so that it can be defined unequivocally.[54]

People from different geographical areas and different histories of exposure to thermal stress choose 33.5° C (area-weighted average) as the skin temperature associated with the sensation of optimal thermal comfort.[44] Evidently, the point at which we are most comfortable is in the middle of the skin temperature range associated with the zone of vasomotor regulation.

Range of Core Temperatures in the Zone of Vasomotor Regulation

Keep in mind that some decline or elevation in core temperature accompanies the skin temperature changes within the boundaries of the zone of vasomotor regulation (see the sequential approach to new equilibrium below). The data available from the calorimetric studies on which Figure 4–8 is based are limited to rectal temperature, which spanned less than 0.2° C. But the experiments may not have been long enough to reveal slight thermal imbalances (see above discussion of the consequences of thermal stress related to heat capacity).

Presumably, control of skin blood flow in this zone depends upon the combined stimulus from both skin and core temperature, acting synergistically according to a scheme like that illustrated in Figure 4–7 for control of sweat rate and shivering. However, quantitative information on this interaction has not yet been obtained.

Heat Stress

The data on the line and bar labeled "warm" in Figure 4–8 represent a steady-state response to a mild heat stress with ambient temperature at 34° C and skin temperature, 35° C. The level at which core temperature would stabilize is estimated below.

Sequential Approach to New Equilibrium

When ambient temperature is increased, skin temperature does not instantaneously follow. Therefore, the driving force ($T_{sk} - T_{amb}$, in terms of equations 7 and 8) for convective and radiative heat loss falls. Also, in these first moments following the ambient temperature change, nothing occurs that would alter evaporative heat loss. Total heat loss, therefore, is initially reduced in amount equal to the decrement in convective plus radiative transfer. Neither has a signal developed that would call for change in skin blood flow; therefore, the rate of delivery of heat to the skin surface has not changed. The reduced rate of heat loss and unabated rate of heat delivery result in accumulation of heat in the skin; consequently skin temperature is driven upward. That, in turn, leads to elevation of core temperature, perhaps over a period measured in hours (again see consequences of thermal stress related to heat capacity).

As this process continues, the increased core and skin temperatures activate reflex responses. An increase in skin blood flow may be sufficient to prevent further temperature increases during mild heat stress. The higher skin temperature that develops (both because greater skin blood flow puts skin temperature closer to core temperature and because core temperature has risen) is sufficient to bring convective plus radiative heat loss back to the steady-state level. Such a heat stress, in other words, would be within the range handled in the zone of vasomotor regulation.

In our present example, skin temperature would have to climb to 38° C (34 + 4) to restore nonevaporative heat loss, because the given convective and radiative characteristics of the environment require a 4° C skin-to-ambient difference for the transport of 52 kcal·hr⁻¹ to the environment. A tolerable equilibrium with skin temperature at 38° C is possible; conceivably, skin blood flow could rise to the point that internal temperature would be only slightly above skin temperature.

But, on the way toward that potential equilibrium at high skin temperature, the combined thermal input derived from cutaneous and core thermoreceptors passes the threshold beyond which reflex activation of sweat glands occurs. Thereafter, if environmental humidity permits, increased evaporation accounts for an increasing share of total heat loss. In the particular environmental conditions in which the data in Figure 4–8 were obtained, the skin–ambient temperature difference stabilized at 1° C. In this steady state, evaporation made up for the large reduction in convective and radiative heat loss. The sweat rate necessary for this equilibrium can be calculated as follows. First, nonevaporative heat loss is determined from the skin and ambient temperatures:

$$H_c = 1.5 \cdot 3.7 \cdot (35 - 34) = 5.5 \text{ kcal} \cdot \text{hr}^{-1}$$
$$H_r = 1.5 \cdot 5.0 \cdot (35 - 34) = 7.5 \text{ kcal} \cdot \text{hr}^{-1}$$
Combined total: $13 \text{ kcal} \cdot \text{hr}^{-1}$

Thus, evaporative heat loss had to amount to 57 kcal·hr⁻¹ (70 − 13), of which heat loss caused by evaporation from the respiratory tract and transcutaneous diffusion account for 18 kcal·hr⁻¹, the same as in the neutral environment (this assumes that ventilation did not change). Heat loss due to evaporation of sweat, then, equals 39 kcal·hr⁻¹ (77 − 18), for which the minimum sweat rate necessary (equation 9) is as follows:

$$\frac{39 \text{ kcal} \cdot \text{hr}^{-1}}{600 \text{ kcal} \cdot \text{L}^{-1}} = 0.065 \text{ L} \cdot \text{hr}^{-1}$$

How does this sweat rate relate to the core and skin temperatures in the new steady state? To answer this correctly, we would need a functional description of the particular individual's control of sweating like that in Figure 4–9.[55] Individuals differ markedly in their sweat rate versus core and skin temperature relationship, but Figure 4–9 is representative of published data and serves for this illustration. First, we need sweat rate in the appropriate units.

Sweat rate in Figure 4–9 is expressed in terms of mg per minute per square cm of body surface area, as is conventional. To convert 0.065 L·hr⁻¹ into these units, divide by the body surface area (1.7 m² = 17,000 cm²), and apply conversion factors for hours to minutes and liters to mg (1 L = 1 kg = 1,000,000 mg).

$$\frac{0.065 \cdot 1,000,000}{60 \cdot 17,000} = 0.064 \text{ mg} \cdot \text{min}^{-1} \cdot \text{cm}^{-2}$$

To locate this point on the graph in Figure 4–9, find the intersection between a horizontal line at 0.064 and the appropriate skin temperature line. The point plotted in the figure necessarily falls on the line corresponding to the given skin temperature, 35° C. The intersection is at 37.064° C on the core temperature axis, because the slope of the lines in Figure 4–9 is 1.0 mg·min⁻¹·cm⁻² per degree centigrade and the 35° C line intersects the axis at 37° C.

Summary

The temperatures in Figure 4–8 and the slopes of the lines connecting them show the contrast between thermal balance in a neutral and a warm environment. The reduced slope of the segment connecting the warm environment core and skin temperatures reflects the increased skin blood flow; the reduced slope of the segment connecting skin and ambient temperature reflects the reduced convective and radiative heat loss. The line separating the shaded and the unshaded portion of the bar graph moves downward with progressive increase in ambient temperature; thermal equilibrium can be established even with ambient temperature above skin temperature, provided that evaporation can take up the entire body heat production plus the heat gained at the surface by convection and radiation. The higher core and skin temperatures that develop in a warm environment combine synergistically to elicit adequate effector responses in an interaction at least qualitatively similar to that illustrated in Figure 4–9.

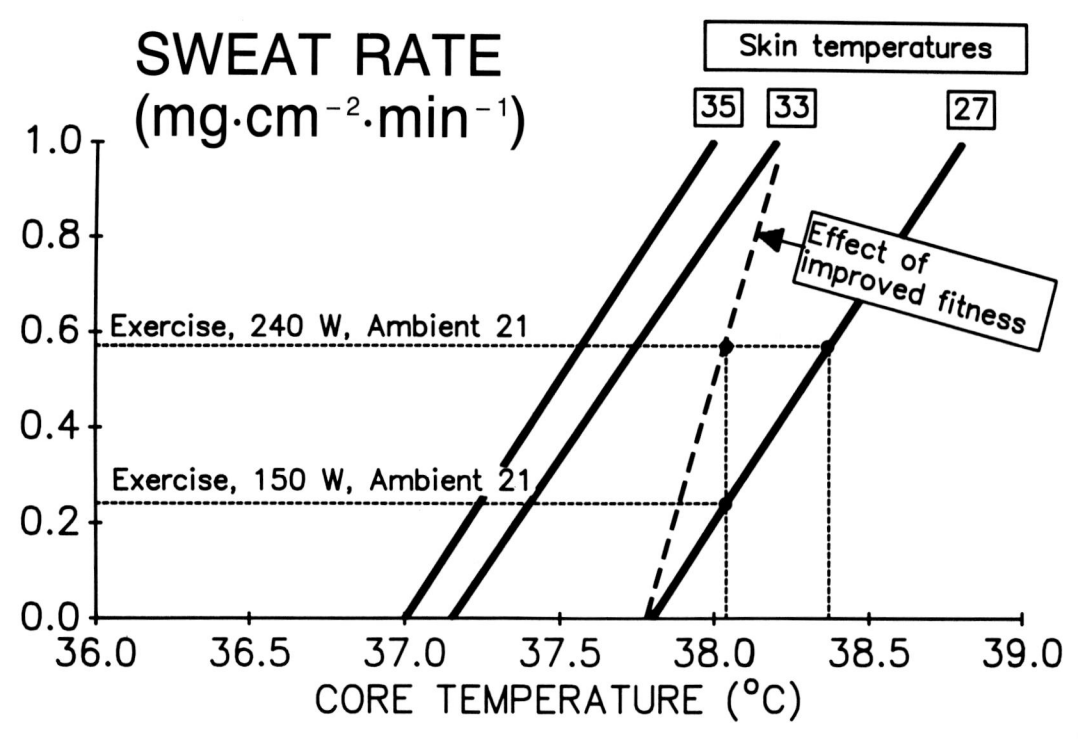

Figure 4–13 Sweat rate versus core and skin temperature; effects of change in power output level and of change in fitness. The solid skin temperature lines are identical to those in Figure 4–12. The dashed line represents data obtained by Roberts and associates of subjects before and after training.[63] This representation simplifies the effect of increased fitness as a rotation of the 27° C skin temperature line. In reality, a slight leftward shift of threshold was also observed.

conditions were fixed, with moderate forced convection and temperature near 21° C.

In agreement with previous observations, core temperature in a given individual stabilized after 10 to 20 minutes of exercise at a level related to power output level and characteristics of the individual, i.e., it was lower for a more fit individual at a given level of exercise.[57,62] But when the core temperatures for different individuals were plotted against oxygen consumption expressed as a fraction of the maximal oxygen consumption of which he or she was capable, the individual differences were resolved. In other words, two people exercising at the same fraction of maximal oxygen consumption stabilize at nearly the same core temperature even if they differ greatly in fitness and, therefore, have corresponding differences in rate of heat production. Saltin and Hermansen also found that individuals stabilized at the same skin temperature at the same fraction of maximal oxygen consumption.[20]

This phenomenon, too, can be better understood with the conceptual foundation of Figure 4–13. Assume that the skin temperature at which an exercising individual stabilizes with ambient temperature at 21° C is 27° C, as it was in Nielsen's study (see Fig. 4–11). With changes in workload, the point (see Fig. 4–13) defining the individual's sweat rate moves along the 27° C skin temperature line (ignoring the small changes in skin temperature that accompany changes in workload in a fixed environment). How much change in core temperature occurs for a given change in workload, then, depends upon the slope of that line as illustrated in the preceding section. Slope changes with the level of fitness.

The bold dashed line is based upon data obtained in a study of the effects of training.[63] No appreciable change in the origin of the sweat rate–core temperature line for a given skin temperature occurred, but the slope increased after a period of training sufficient to increase fitness level. Obviously, higher sweat rate oc-

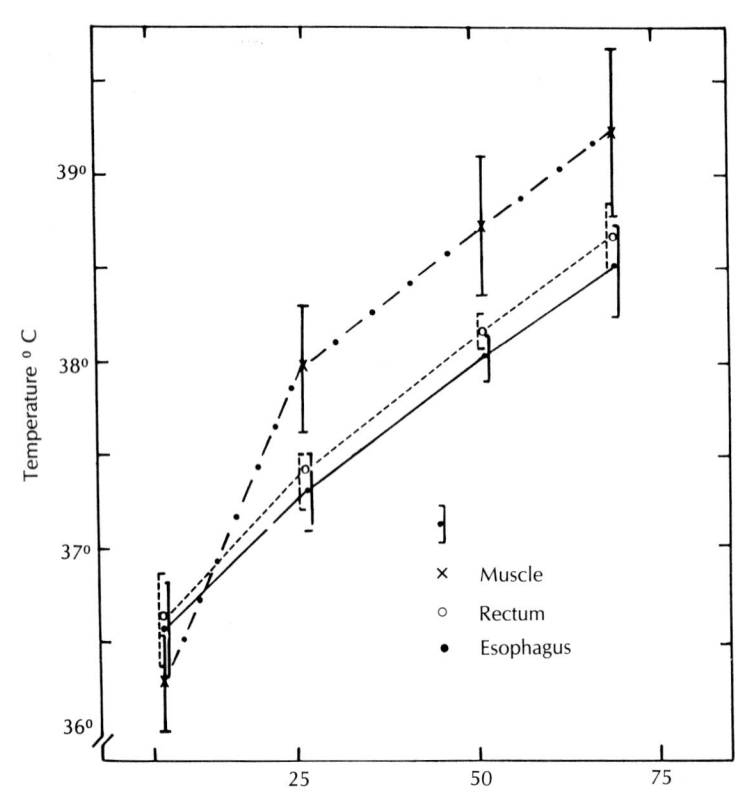

Figure 4-14 Body temperatures observed by Saltin and Hermansen in exercising subjects, plotted against fraction of maximal oxygen consumption. Average temperature measured simultaneously in the esophagus, the rectum, and the working muscle in relation to the oxygen uptake in percent of the individual's maximal oxygen uptake. Seven subjects worked for 60 min on a bicycle ergometer. To the left, data obtained at rest. SD = standard deviation. (From Saltin B, Hermansen L. J Appl Physiol 1966; 21:1757–1762.)

curs for the same core and skin temperatures in given ambient conditions in a person who is more fit. In other words, if the solid and the dashed lines for 27° C skin temperature represent the control of sweating in a given individual before and after increasing his or her maximal level of oxygen consumption, the difference must work out so that the increased sweat rate associated with a given core temperature just matches the increase in heat production associated with the greater power output level of which the person becomes capable. The rotation of the dashed line relative to the solid one must be in proportion to the increase in maximal oxygen consumption.

These examples have been made as close to real-life situations as possible. Readers who grasp the physical principles of heat exchange and the physiology of the effector systems that adjust thermal balance will be able to make at least crude practical analyses of other real situations. However, the best guide for what happens in a real situation is experimental data from matching conditions.

The research literature in the field of temperature regulation is full of useful information on responses of human subjects—male and female, young and old—to a great variety of combinations of ambient conditions and levels and types of exercise. The reference list accompanying this chapter is only a small sample.

(To pursue a particular line of interest, look for recent symposia and reviews. The *Journal of Applied Physiology* and *Medicine and Science in Sports and Exercise* are valuable sources of information. These plus two European journals, *Pflüger's Archiv* and *Acta Physiologica Scandinavica,* contain most of the articles that have contributed to the present structure of knowledge in the field.)

Acknowledgement

Much of this chapter was written during sabbatical leave spent in the laboratory of Dr. Greg Gass at the Cumberland College of Health Sciences, Lidcombe, N.S.W., Australia. Discussions with Dr. Gass and his colleagues and students shaped new ideas that radically affected the contents. Support from the College and the Cumberland College Foundation is gratefully acknowledged.

REFERENCES

1. DuBois EF. Fever and the regulation of body temperature. Springfield, IL: Charles C Thomas, 1948.
2. Brengelmann GL. Temperature regulation. In: Ruch TC, Patton HD, eds. Physiology and biophysics. Vol III. 20th ed. Philadelphia: WB Saunders, 1973:105.
3. Tanner JM. The relationships between the frequency of the heart, oral temperature and rectal temperature in man at rest. J Physiol (Lond) 1951; 115:371–390.
4. Ivy AC. What is normal or normality? Bull Northwestern Univ Med School 1944; 18:22–32.
5. Stephenson LA, Wenger CB, O'Donovan BH, Nadel ER. Circadian rhythm in sweating and cutaneous blood flow. Am J Physiol 1984; 246:R321–R324.
6. Stephenson LA, Kolka MA. Menstrual cycle phase and time of day alter reference signal controlling arm blood flow and sweating. Am J Physiol 1985; 249:R186–R191.
7. Leithead CS, Lind AR. Heat stress and heat disorders. Philadelphia: FA Davis, 1964.
8. Hales JRS, ed. Thermal physiology. New York: Raven Press, 1984.
9. Rowell LB. Human circulation: regulation during physical stress. New York: Oxford University Press, 1986.
10. Keatinge WR. Survival in cold water. Oxford: Blackwell Scientific Publications, 1969.
11. Slonim NB, ed. Environmental physiology. St. Louis: CV Mosby, 1974.
12. Saltin B, Åstrand P. Maximal oxygen uptake in athletes. J Appl Physiol 1967; 23:353–358.
13. Brown AC. Energy metabolism. In: Ruch TC, Patton HD, eds. Physiology and biophysics. Vol III. 20th ed. Philadelphia: WB Saunders, 1973:85.
14. Colin J, Timbal J, Houdas Y, et al. Computation of mean body temperature from rectal and skin temperatures. J Appl Physiol 1971; 31:484–489.
15. Eichna LW, Berger AR, Rader B, Becker WH. Comparison of intracardiac and intravascular temperatures with rectal temperatures in man. J Clin Invest 1951; 30:353–359.
16. Graf W. Patterns of human liver temperature. Acta Physiol Scand 1959; 46 (Suppl 160):1–135.
17. Sargeant AJ. Effect of muscle temperature on leg extension force and short-term power output in humans. Eur J Appl Physiol 1987; 56:693–698.
18. Lemons DE, Chien S, Crawshaw LI, et al. Significance of vessel size and type in vascular heat transfer. Am J Physiol 1987; 253; 253:R128–R135.
19. Bazett HC, Love L, Newton M, et al. Temperature changes in blood flowing in arteries and veins in man. J Appl Physiol 1948; 1:3–19.
20. Saltin B, Hermansen L. Esophageal, rectal, and muscle temperature during exercise. J Appl Physiol 1966; 21:1757–1762.
21. Äikäs E, Karvonen MJ, Piironen P, Ruosteenoja R. Intramuscular, rectal and oesophageal temperature during exercise. Acta Physiol Scand 1972; 54:366–370.
22. Nadel ER, Bergh U, Saltin B. Body temperatures during negative work exercise. J Appl Physiol 1972; 33:553–558.
23. Davies CTM. The effects of different levels of heat production induced by diathermy and eccentric work on thermoregulation during exercise at a given skin temperature. Eur J Appl Physiol 1979; 40:171–180.
24. Aulick LH, Robinson S, Tzankoff SP. Arm and leg intravascular temperatures of men during submaximal exercise. J Appl Physiol 1981; 51:1092–1097.
25. Cooper T, Randall WC, Hertzman AB. Vascular convection of heat from active muscle to overlying skin. J Appl Physiol 1959; 14:207–211.
26. Blagden C. Experiments and observations in a heated room. Phil Trans Roy Soc (Lond) 1775; 65:111–123.
27. Shiraki K, Konda N, Sagawa S. Esophageal and tympanic temperature responses to changes in core blood temperature during hyperthermia. J Appl Physiol 1986; 61:98–102.
28. Brengelmann GL, Johnson JM, Hong PA. Electrocardiographic verification of esophageal temperature probe position. J Appl Physiol 1979; 47:638–642.
29. Cooper KE, Cranston WI, Snell ES. Temperature in the external auditory meatus as an index of central temperature changes. J Appl Physiol 1964; 19:1032–1035.
30. Brengelmann GL. Dilemma of body temperature measurement. In: Shiraki K, Yousef MK, eds. Man in stressful environments. Springfield, IL: Charles C Thomas, 1988:5.
31. Shiraki K, Yousef MK, eds. Man in stressful environments. Springfield, IL: Charles C Thomas, 1988.
32. Kerslake D McK. The stress of hot environments. Cambridge: Cambridge University Press, 1972.
33. Hayward JS, Eckerson JD, Kemna D. Thermal and cardiovascular changes during three methods of resuscitation from mild hypothermia. Resuscitation 1984; 11:21–33.
34. Robinson S, Meyer FR, Newton JL, et al. Relations between sweating, cutaneous blood flow, and body temperature in work. J Appl Physiol 1965; 20:575–582.
35. Gisolfi CV, Copping JR. Thermal effects of prolonged treadmill exercise in the heat. Med Sci Sports Exerc 1974; 6:108–113.
36. Pugh LGCE, Corbett JL, Johnson RH. Rectal temperatures, weight losses, and sweat rates in marathon running. J Appl Physiol 1967; 23:347–352.
37. American College of Sports Medicine Position Statement. Prevention of thermal injuries during distance running. Phys Sportsmed 1984; 12:43–47.
38. Ekblom B, Greenleaf CJ, Greenleaf JE, Hermansen L. Temperature regulation during exercise dehydration in man. Acta Physiol Scand 1970; 79:475–483.
39. Sawka MN, Francesconi RP, Young AJ, Pandolf KB. Influence of hydration level and body fluids on exercise performance in the heat. JAMA 1984; 252:1165–1169.
40. Brouns F, Saris WHM, Rehrer NJ. Abdominal complaints and gastrointestinal function during long-lasting exercise. Int J Sports Med 1987; 8:175–189.
41. Fortney SM, Nadel ER, Wenger CB, Bove JR. Effect of blood volume on sweating rate and body fluids in exercising humans. J Appl Physiol 1981; 51:1594–1600.
42. Brown WK, Sargent F II. Hidromeiosis. Arch Environ Health 1965; 11:442–452.
43. Maughan RJ, Leiper JB, Thompson J. Rectal tempera-

ture after marathon running. Br J Sports Med 1985; 19:192–195.
44. Hensel H. Thermoreception and temperature regulation. London: Academic Press, 1981.
45. Freund PR, Brengelmann GL, Rowell LB, Halar E. Attenuated skin blood flow response to hyperthermia in paraplegic men. J Appl Physiol 1984; 56:1104–1109.
46. Tam H-S, Darling RC, Cheh H-Y, Downey JA. The dead zone of thermoregulation in normal and paraplegic man. Can J Physiol Pharmacol 1978; 56:976–983.
47. Brown AC, Brengelmann GL. The interaction of peripheral and central inputs in the temperature regulation system. In: Hardy JD, ed. Physiological and behavioral temperature regulation. Springfield, IL: Charles C Thomas, 1970:684.
48. Cooper KE, Cranston WI, Snell ES. Temperature regulation during fever in man. Clin Sci 1964; 27:345–356.
49. Zeisberger E. The roles of monoaminergic neurotransmitters in thermoregulation. Can J Physiol Pharmacol 1986; 65:1395–1401.
50. Gagge AP, Winslow CEA, Herrington LP. The influence of clothing on the physiological reactions of the human body to varying environmental temperatures. Am J Physiol 1938; 124:30–50.
51. Johnson JM, Brengelmann GL, Hales JRS, et al. Regulation of the cutaneous circulation. Fed Proc 1986; 45:2841–2850.
52. Hardy JD, Soderstrom GF. Heat loss from the nude body and peripheral blood flow at temperatures of 22° C to 35° C. J Nutr 1938; 16:493–509.
53. DuBois EF. Heat loss from the human body. Bull NY Acad Med 1939; 15:143–173.
54. Craig AB, Dvorak M. Thermal regulation during water immersion. J Appl Physiol 1966; 21:1577–1585.
55. Nadel ER, Bullard RW, Stolwijk JAJ. Importance of skin temperature in the regulation of sweating. J Appl Physiol 1971; 31:80–87.
56. Benzinger TH, Kitzinger C, Pratt AW. The human thermostat. In: Hardy JD, ed. Temperature: its measurement and control in science and industry. Vol 3. Part 3. New York: Reinholdt Publishing, 1963:637.
57. Nielsen M. Die Regulation der Körpertemperatur bei Muskelarbeit. Skand Arch Physiol 1938; 68:215–227.
58. Adams WC, Fox RH, Frey AJ, McDonald IC. Thermoregulation during marathon running in cool, moderate, and hot environments. J Appl Physiol 1975; 38:1030–1037.
59. Saltin B, Gagge AP, Stolwijk JAJ. Muscle temperature during submaximal exercise in man. J Appl Physiol 1968; 25:679–688.
60. Davies CTM. Influence of skin temperature on sweating and aerobic performance during severe work. J Appl Physiol 1979; 47:770–777.
61. Davies CTM, Brotherhood JR, ZeidiFard E. Temperature regulation during severe exercise with some observations on the effects of skin wetting. J Appl Physiol 1976; 41:772–776.
62. Nielsen B. Regulation of body temperature and heat dissipation at different levels of energy and heat production in man. Acta Physiol Scand 1938; 68:215–227.
63. Roberts MF, Wenger CB, Stolwijk JAJ, Nadel ER. Skin blood flow and sweating changes following exercise training and heat acclimation. J Appl Physiol 1977; 43:133–137.

Chapter 5
Menstrual Dysfunction in the Female Athlete

CHARLOTTE F. SANBORN

A substantial proportion of female athletes develop menstrual irregularities or secondary amenorrhea. The fact that the highest frequencies have been noted primarily among distance runners and ballet dancers has led to the most popular explanation, the fat hypothesis. It has been widely believed that when body weight, or more specifically, body fat, falls below a critical level, the athlete becomes amenorrheic. Consequently, the majority of the initial research in athletic amenorrhea has been directed toward testing the first logical piece of the puzzle. However, in the course of examining the role of body fat, confounding factors have emerged as additional causes of athletic amenorrhea. To understand athletic amenorrhea, it is important to clarify its prevalence and its etiology. These aspects must be examined thoroughly before treating menstrual dysfunction.

PHYSIOLOGY OF THE MENSTRUAL CYCLE

Beginning at puberty, human females undergo reproductive cycles involving a complex interaction of the hypothalamus, pituitary gland, ovaries, and uterus. These reproductive cycles can be divided further into two separate cycles that together prepare the reproductive system for pregnancy. The cyclic changes that occur in the ovaries is known as the *ovarian cycle;* those occurring in the endometrium constitute the uterine cycle, commonly referred to as the *menstrual cycle.*

Ovarian Cycle

The ovary is a complex organ with a dual function: production and release of ova, and production of hormones (estrogen and progesterone). The ovarian cycle can be simplistically divided into two phases: preovulatory and postovulatory. The *preovulatory phase,* also known as the follicular phase, is characterized by ovarian follicular enlargement and maturation. The development of follicles is induced by cyclic release of the gonadotropic hormones—follicle stimulating hormone (FSH) and luteinizing hormone (LH)—from the anterior lobe of the pituitary. Gonadotropic releasing hormone (GnRH), synthesized in the hypothalamus, causes this cyclic release of FSH and LH. The early development of the follicles is induced by FSH, but after a few days, one follicle begins to mature rapidly while the others begin to involute. The maturing follicle produces increasing amounts of estrogen, which is believed to be the stimulus for the sharp peak in both LH and FSH just before ovulation. Around midcycle (day 14), the follicle undergoes a sudden growth spurt under the influence of FSH and LH.

The culmination of the follicular phase is ovulation, the rupture of the follicular wall with the release of the ovum into the peritoneal cavity. The ovum begins its migration to the uterus, where it is discarded with the next menstruation if fertilization does not occur. Meanwhile, the empty follicle becomes filled with luteal cells and forms a new glandular structure called the corpus luteum. Under the influence of LH, the corpus luteum secretes mainly progesterone and some estrogen. The high circulating levels of progesterone and estrogen inhibit the release of FSH and LH from the pituitary. The corpus luteum then degenerates, leading to a sharp decrease in the levels of the ovarian hormones. As this occurs, a new cycle of follicle maturation begins with a rise in concentration of FSH.

Menstrual Cycle

Ovarian hormones cause the cyclic changes in the endometrium. The menstrual cycle is divided into three phases: the menstrual phase, the proliferative (follicular) phase, and the secretory (luteal) phase. The first day of menstruation is counted as the beginning of the menstrual cycle. The functional layer of the uterine wall is sloughed off and discarded during menstruation. The proliferative phase (days 6 to 14) coincides with the development of the ovarian follicles. The endometrium increases two- to threefold during this phase of repair and proliferation. The secretory phase (days 15 to 28) coincides with the formation and secretion of the corpus luteum. If fertilization does not occur, the thickened endometrium enters an ischemic or premenstrual phase. Toward the end of this phase the superficial layers of the endometrium are shed, and another menstrual cycle is begun.

PREVALENCE OF MENSTRUAL IRREGULARITIES

Menstrual cycles have been classically defined as regular if the length of the cycle is 28 days with a menses of 5 days. However, "it has been stated that the only regular aspect of the menstrual cycle is that it is irregular."[1] Menstrual cycle disturbances or irregularities may take the form of any of the following:

1. Length: an increase or decrease in number of days of the cycle or menses
2. Dysmenorrhea: painful or difficult menstruation
3. Late menarche: delayed onset of the first menses
4. Oligoamenorrhea: few or scanty menstrual cycles
5. Amenorrhea: the absence of menses, further classified as
   a. primary amenorrhea: menses has never occurred
   b. secondary amenorrhea: cessation of menses after menarche has occurred

This list could be expanded, but it illustrates how varied the term menstrual irregularity can be. Use of any of these definitions could lead to noting irregularities in any female population, not just in athletes. Do athletes have an increased prevalence of menstrual irregularities in comparison to nonathletes?

More than 2 decades ago, studies introduced data that training might be associated with menstrual irregularities.[2,3] In 1954, irregular menstrual cycles were reported to be prevalent among 47 Olympic athletes questioned (12.8 percent).[2] Anecdotes were also provided of athletes whose menstrual irregularities were believed to coincide with training and competition.

Erdelyi was the first, in 1963, to report a possible association between intense training and amenorrhea.[3] In a survey of 557 Hungarian female athletes, "unfavorable" menstrual cycle changes occurred in 62 (11 percent) of the athletes. Some of the menstrual disorders listed were dysmenorrhea, irregular periods, and amenorrhea. Amenorrhea occurred more frequently in athletes who participated in strenuous activities such as tennis, rowing, and skiing. An association was also noticed between age and menstrual irregularities. A higher prevalence was found in the athletes between 15 and 17 years of age than in those 18 years and older.

However, only recently has amenorrhea among distance runners, ballet dancers, and other athletes been formally described (Table

5–1). In 1977, 400 women from the top 25 teams at the National Cross-Country Championships were surveyed, resulting in a final sample of 128 women.[4] Athletes who had experienced three or fewer periods per year were classified as having amenorrhea, and all other subjects were classified as "regular." The incidence of secondary amenorrhea was high, 24 percent. The following year, 38 female athletes were surveyed who participated in the 1978 National Cross-Country Championships.[5] Approximately half of the respondents reported having only one period within the preceding 3 months, and 2.6 percent reported having no periods within the last 6 months. A high incidence of amenorrhea (zero to five menses per year) was also found among women who had run the Avon International Women's Marathon (n = 168).[6] These runners were divided into two groups: runners, those who ran more than 30 miles per week; and joggers, those who ran 5 to 30 miles per week. The frequency of amenorrhea was higher in the runners (24 percent) than in the joggers (14 percent).

Contradictory results have been found in three surveys of large populations of women runners.[7-9] In a survey of almost 900 women runners in Portland, Oregon, only 6 percent of the women developed secondary amenorrhea after they started running.[7] The exact definition of amenorrhea was not provided, and the runners, on the average, ran less than 20 miles per week. In the second survey, questionnaires were distributed to over 1,800 women who entered the 1979 New York City Marathon.[8] Amenorrhea was defined as having no more than one period in the last 10 months. Of the 270 women who had regular menstrual cycles before training, only 1 percent became amenorrheic during training. Another strict definition of amenorrhea was used in a study of 350 women who had run either the 1980 Boston Marathon or a 10-km race in Minneapolis.[9] Amenorrhea was defined as having no menstrual cycles in the past year. Only 3.4 percent of the sample had amenorrhea by this definition.

Dancers not only experience secondary amenorrhea but also have a high incidence of primary amenorrhea. In a survey of 89 young ballet dancers, 20 had not undergone menarche.[10] Of the remaining 69 dancers, 19 percent reported secondary amenorrhea (no menses for at least 3 consecutive months), and 30 percent reported irregular menstrual cycles. Using the same definition, other authors also reported a high frequency of secondary amenorrhea (37 percent) among professional ballet dancers.[11]

A question arising from these studies was whether amenorrhea was prevalent among athletes participating in all sports. The prevalence of amenorrhea was reported for long distance

TABLE 5–1 Prevalence of Secondary Amenorrhea

Population	Number	Percent	Definition	Reference
Controls				
College	500	2.3	> 2 months no periods	57
Swedes	2,000	3.3	< 3 periods/yr	81
Runners				
Cross-country	128	24.0	≤ 3 periods/yr	4
Cross-country	38	44.7	No periods previous 3 mo	5
> 30 mi/wk	89	24.0	0–5 periods/yr	6
5–30 mi/wk	22	14.0	0–5 periods/yr	6
NY marathon	270	1.0	< 1 period previous 10 mo	8
Joggers	885	~6.0	No definition provided	7
Marathon	237	25.7	≤ 3 periods/yr	12
Ballet dancers				
Students	69	18.8	At least 3 mo no periods	10
Professional (29) + students (5)	34	44.0	At least 3 mo no periods	41
Professional	32	36.7	At least 3 mo no periods	11
Athletes				
College varsity	140	12.1	No periods previous 3 mo or < 4 periods/yr	13
Swimmers	197	12.3	≤ 3 periods/yr	12
Cyclists	33	12.1	≤ 3 periods/yr	12

runners, collegiate swimmers, and national caliber cyclists.[12] The incidence of amenorrhea was higher in all three groups when compared to controls. However, the runners had a significantly higher incidence (25.7 percent) than the swimmers (12.3 percent) or cyclists (12.1 percent). A large sample of collegiate varsity athletes was also surveyed using a definition of no menstrual cycles in the previous 3 months, or four or fewer periods per year.[13] Among the 140 athletes surveyed, 17 (12.1 percent) had secondary amenorrhea.

Short Luteal Phase

The frequency of menstrual irregularities and amenorrhea in athletes typically has been obtained from menstrual cycle histories. Thus, the identification of normal or regular cycles has been based on the occurrence of menses and cycle length, not on an endocrinologic basis. Using basal body temperatures as a marker for ovulation, 14 women runners were studied as they trained for a marathon.[14] While their cycle lengths remained normal throughout training, one-third of the runners had monophasic cycles and another third had a short premenstrual phase. In addition, several studies have found that athletes usually have a short luteal phase.[15–17] In the study by Bonen and colleagues, four teenage swimmers were compared to a control group of teenagers and a group of fertile adult women.[15] Blood samples were collected daily throughout one complete menstrual cycle. The follicular phase and luteal phase lengths were determined from the peak value of luteinizing hormone. The swimmers had a very short luteal phase (4.5 days) relative to the two control groups (7.8 days for the teenage group and 13.4 days for the adult group; $p < 0.05$). Further, the failure of progesterone to rise in the luteal phase suggested that the swimmers experienced anovulatory menstrual cycles. However, because only one menstrual cycle was evaluated, the frequency of anovulatory menstrual cycles could not be determined. Although the teenage control subjects had a shorter luteal phase than the adult controls, an endocrine profile indicated normal ovulatory cycles.

A negative correlation has been found between running mileage and luteal phase length.[16,17] A 30-year-old woman was followed for 18 consecutive cycles.[16] The luteal phase was the length between a change observed in cervical mucus and the beginning of the next menses. Menstrual cycles remained unaltered throughout the training program. However, the length of the luteal phase slowly decreased with an increase in running mileage (Fig. 5–1). Similar findings were described in two runners using daily basal body temperatures to determine the length of the luteal phase.[17] As training mileage increased, the length of the luteal phase decreased. In one runner the length of the luteal phase decreased from 12 to 8 days and evolved into anovulatory cycles. Once training decreased, these changes were reversed.

Results from these studies indicate that classifying menstrual cycles based only on menstrual histories can be erroneous. This suggests that the incidence of amenorrhea reported so far is conservative, particularly if "menstrual irregularities" are included.

Defining Amenorrhea

The fact that these studies vary in the frequency of amenorrhea reported may be related to the different definitions of amenorrhea or differences in athletic populations surveyed. The following criteria are recommended for standard definitions:

1. Regular menstruation
   a. 12 periods per year at intervals of 28 ± 5 days

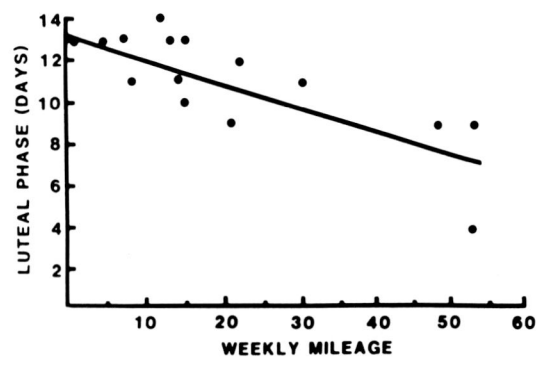

Figure 5–1 The length of the luteal phase decreased as the training mileage increased ($r = -0.81$; $p < 0.001$). (From Shangold MM, Freeman R, Thysen B, Gatz M. Fertil Steril 1979; 31:130–133.)

b. Duration of each menses 3 to 7 days
   c. Ovulatory cycle(s) with a normal luteal phase length
2. Athletic amenorrhea
   a. Three or fewer periods per year with no more than one period in the previous six months
   b. Regular menstrual cycles established within 18 months following menarche
   c. Training begun before development of amenorrhea
   d. Discontinued taking birth control pills for at least 6 months before amenorrhea developed
   e. Negative gynecologic screen: complete medical history, physical examination, and laboratory evaluation, and other causes of secondary amenorrhea, e.g., hyperandrogenism, pituitary tumor, ovarian failure, and pregnancy, ruled out

ETIOLOGY OF ATHLETIC AMENORRHEA

The high frequency of athletic amenorrhea observed among runners and ballet dancers has provided insight into the possible mechanism(s). These athletes characteristically have low body weight and a low percentage of body fat.[10,18] Both activities involve strenuous training, emotional stress, and training at a young age, often before menarche. All of these factors have been implicated in the etiology of athletic amenorrhea (Table 5–2).[19] The most popular theory has been related to low body weight or, more specifically, low body fat—the "fat hypothesis."

Fat Hypothesis

Frisch and associates at Harvard advanced the hypothesis that a direct relationship exists between a critical amount of body fat and the onset and maintenance of menstruation.[20–25] The theory was based on the observation that menarche occurs at a critical weight rather than a specific age.[21,23,24] Further arguments used by Frisch and her associates to support their hypothesis were: first, that puberty in rats was reached at a specific body weight rather than a critical age;[26] second, that the steady decrease in age at menarche in the past century has been attributed to reaching the critical weight at an earlier age because of better nutrition than in the past;[27,28] third, that clinically observed amenorrhea in patients with anorexia nervosa and in patients with simple weight loss was reversed upon regaining weight;[29–31] and fourth, that aromatization of androgens to estrogen occurs in adipose tissue, providing an extragonadal source of estrogen.[32]

Several criticisms have been directed at this hypothesis.[33,34] The major one arises from the manner in which percent of body fat was estimated by these investigators, using a height–weight equation rather than a direct measurement.[35] The critical values predicted by Frisch and co-workers can be seriously questioned, but the fat hypothesis, nevertheless, merits consideration.

Female athletes are an excellent test for the fat hypothesis, especially runners and ballet dancers because of their typically low body fat levels. Competitive distance runners have been shown to have body fat levels as low as 5.9 percent.[18] Preliminary findings in surveys of athletes tended to support the critical weight theory. Menstrual irregularities and amenorrhea were found most commonly in runners who weighed less than 115 pounds and who lost more than 10 pounds after beginning training.[7] Shangold and Levine also found amenorrheic runners were significantly lighter in body weight than regularly menstruating women (50 kg versus 55 kg respectively, $p < 0.05$).[8]

Data from ballet dancers further support the fat hypothesis. Ballet students with primary and secondary amenorrhea weighed less than the regularly menstruating ballet dancers, 43.5 kg, 44.9 kg, and 47.0 kg, respectively.[10] Professional ballet dancers with secondary amenorrhea also weighed less than regularly menstruating ballet dancers.[11] Although average body weights were not provided, amenorrheic professional ballet dancers had a significantly lower percent of ideal weight than dancers without menstrual irregularities (84.3 percent and 88.6 percent, respectively, $p < 0.05$).

However, low body weight is not always synonymous with low body fat. Many athletes may initially lose weight while training, but weight usually stabilizes. Body fat may con-

TABLE 5-2 Proposed Causes of Athletic Amenorrhea

Low body weight or fat	Immature reproductive axis
Absolute weight loss	Young athlete
Critical level, set point	Nulliparity
Late menarche	Prior menstrual irregularities
Training before menarche	Psychological stress
Diet	Multiple factors
Energy drain–caloric deficit	Others?
Hormonal alterations	
Acute hormonal response	
Chronic hormonal response	

tinue to decrease, resulting in a change in the ratio of lean mass to body fat. For example, in one study, women training for a marathon had a decrease in percent of fat without a change in body weight.[36] A complex relationship exists between exercise and body composition. Thus, weights and heights are not an accurate predictor of body composition for athletes.

Several studies have compared either predicted or measured percent of body fat of amenorrheic and regularly menstruating athletes. Schwartz and associates compared amenorrheic runners (no menses for at least 4 months preceding the study) to three groups: regularly menstruating runners who ran more than 30 miles per week, regularly menstruating runners who ran 5 to 30 miles per week, and nonrunning controls.[37] Mean percent of body fat and weight were significantly lower in the amenorrheic runners in comparison to the other groups ($p < 0.01$). Body fat was estimated from skinfold thicknesses and was 18.2 percent for the amenorrheic runners, approximately 23 percent for both groups of regularly menstruating runners, and 27.4 percent for the controls. However, opposite findings have been reported.[5,38] The average percent of body fat, as estimated from skinfold thickness, has been found not to be statistically different between amenorrheic (14.1 percent) and regularly menstruating runners (17.7 percent).[38] In addition, no significant differences in mean body weight or sum of skinfold thicknesses have been reported between amenorrheic and regularly menstruating collegiate cross-country runners.[5]

The results of the body weight and body fat studies are conflicting. However, the different methods used in determining body fat in the athletes—skinfold thickness versus hydrostatic weight—might contribute to the varied findings. Predicting body density from anthropometric variables such as skinfold measurements can result in large errors, because the prediction equations are population specific.[39] Hydrostatic weighing is one of the most accurate methods for measuring body density. However, actual measurement of the residual lung volume is crucial for computing body densities. Predicted values for residual volumes have a greater standard error than actual measured volumes (±500 mL versus ±100 mL, respectively).[40] For a 55-kg woman the estimation of body fat could have an error of plus or minus 5 percent (using a predicted residual volume) versus plus or minus 1 percent (using an actual value).

Using the hydrostatic weighing method and estimated residual volumes, no difference in percent of body fat was found between dancers with and without menstrual irregularities.[41] Opposite results were found in a group of 42 female athletes selected from college varsity sports (track and field, swimming and diving, tennis, and volleyball), high school varsity track and field, and a general population of distance runners.[42] Percent of body fat was measured by the hydrostatic weighing technique using a helium dilution method to calculate residual volume. The amenorrheic athletes (no menses in the previous 3 months, or four periods in the previous year) had a significantly lower percent of body fat, 13.1 percent, than the regularly menstruating athletes, 16.3 percent ($p < 0.05$). However, there was considerable overlap between the two groups (Fig. 5–2). Because of the wide range in percent of body fat within and between the groups, these authors concluded that body fat was not the explanation for athletic amenorrhea.

Recently we have measured the body fat of distance runners using hydrostatic weighing with residual volumes measured.[43] Distance

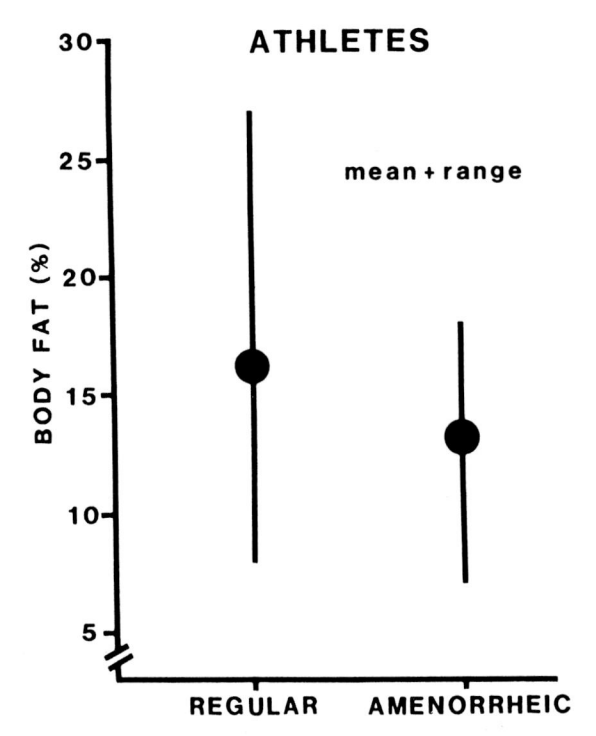

Figure 5–2 Mean (± range) percent of body fat of amenorrheic and regularly menstruating athletes. (From Carlberg KA, Buckman MT, Peake GT, Riedesel ML. Med Sci Sports Exerc 1983; 15:215–217.)

runners were selected who trained more than 40 miles per week. Based on strict criteria, athletes were classified as amenorrheic if the following criteria were met: not more than three periods per year, not more than one period in the 6 months prior to the study, regular menstrual cycles were established within 18 months following menarche, and the menses were present up to the time that training began. To ensure that amenorrhea would be related to training and not to other causes, the amenorrheic subjects were evaluated by a board-certified reproductive endocrinologist. The second, regularly menstruating, group had 12 periods per year, at intervals of 23 to 33 days, with a duration of 3 to 7 days, and with cycles that were shown to be ovulatory on at least one occasion in each runner. The regularly menstruating and amenorrheic runners were similar in weight, height, age, menarcheal age, weekly training mileage, days per week of training, years of training, and maximum oxygen uptake. Percent of body fat for the two groups was the same:

17.7 plus or minus 2.1 percent for the amenorrheic athletes and 17.4 plus or minus 1.2 percent for the regularly menstruating athletes (Fig. 5–3A). The final groups were small (n = 7 in each) owing to the stringent selection criteria used. To explore whether trends found in the strictly selected groups were present in larger groups, the selection criteria were relaxed. The amenorrheic group was expanded to 20 by adding 13 subjects in the following categories: lower training mileages (n = 5), irregular menstrual cycles prior to athletic amenorrhea (n = 3), not screened by reproductive endocrinologist (n = 3), parous (n = 1), and amenorrhea occurring after discontinuing oral contraceptives but persisting longer than 6 months (n = 1). Of the 14 subjects added to the expanded regularly menstruating group (n = 21), nine were not confirmed to have had ovulatory cycles and five had lower training mileage. Even when the criteria were relaxed slightly to include more subjects, the mean percent of body fat was not statistically different between the groups (Fig. 5–3B). Thus, current research does not support the idea that low body fat in itself causes athletic amenorrhea. Whether each athlete has her own critical body fat level or set point for becoming amenorrheic is not known at this time.[42]

The finding of osteopenia (low bone mass) in amenorrheic athletes in comparison to reg-

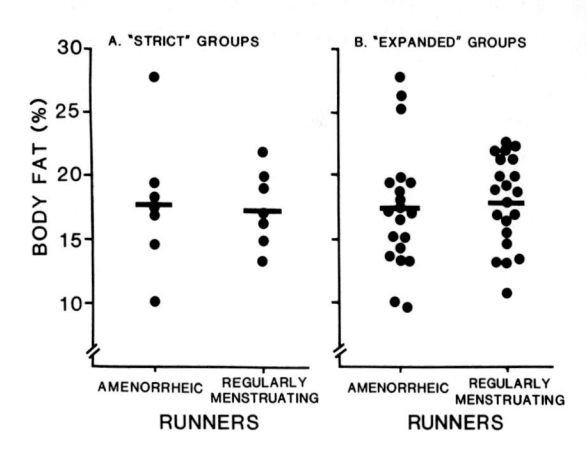

Figure 5–3 (A) Percent of body fat from strictly selected amenorrheic and regularly menstruating distance runners. Group means are not significantly different. (B) Data from strictly selected groups plus additional subjects chosen with slightly relaxed selection criteria. Means for expanded groups are not significantly different. (From Sanborn CF, Albrecht BH, Wagner WW Jr. Med Sci Sports Exerc 1987; 19:210.)

ularly menstruating athletes presents a methodologic problem in underwater weighing of the female athlete.[44–46] Percent of body fat would be overestimated when the bone mineral content was lower than the reference standard. Following a criticism of Sanborn and colleagues' study, the percent of body fat data were recalculated assuming that the amenorrheic athlete had a 15 percent reduction in spinal skeletal mass.[47] Despite the manipulation of the data, the results did not change; there was no difference in body fat between the two groups. The difficulty of understanding the relationship of body fat and body weight to athletic amenorrhea is further complicated by other variables. The following variables have appeared alone or in various combinations with athletic amenorrhea: late menarche, intense training prior to menarche, prior menstrual irregularities, intense training, nulliparity, young age, and psychological stress. Because these factors continually surface, each has been implicated in the onset of amenorrhea in athletes.

Late Menarche

A later age of menarche has been reported for athletes than for nonathletes.[48] The mean age of menarche was 13.6 years for 66 college track and field athletes and 12.2 years for 30 nonathletes, a significant difference. It has also been reported that Olympic volleyball athletes have a significantly later age at menarche (14.2 years) when compared with high school and collegiate athletes (13.0 years) and controls (12.3 years).[49]

The cause of late menarche in some athletes is not known. Does athletic training delay menarche, or do late maturers choose to be in certain sports?[49] It has been suggested that for each year of training before menarche, the onset of menstruation is delayed by 5 months.[50] Other investigators found not only that intense sports activity alone could delay menarche but also that a synergistic effect occurred between sports participation and thinness in delaying menarche.[51]

The link between late menarche and athletic amenorrhea is not known. Ballet dancers with secondary amenorrhea also have delayed menarche. Menarche occurred at a mean age of 14 years in two groups of amenorrheic ballet dancers and at an even later age (15 years) in another study.[10,41,52]

Among amenorrheic runners the findings have been diverse. Feicht and colleagues reported significantly delayed menarche in amenorrheic middle distance runners (14.1 years) compared with regularly menstruating runners (13.3 years). A similar difference was reported by Wakat, Sweeney, and Rogol between their amenorrheic (14.3 years) and regularly menstruating runners (12.9 years).[5] Baker and associates also found that the age at menarche was significantly higher in amenorrheic runners (13.8 years) than in regularly menstruating runners (12.2 years).[38] On the other hand, three studies on runners have found the age at menarche to be similar between the two groups.[8,37,43] Schwartz and co-workers reported no statistical difference in mean menarcheal age between amenorrheic and regularly menstruating runners, and Shangold and Levine found menarche occurring at age 12.2 years for a group of amenorrheic runners and at 12.7 years for a group of regularly menstruating runners.[8] In the study by Sanborn and colleagues mentioned above, the groups of runners, defined by strict criteria, were not statistically different in menarcheal age.[43] However, when the groups were expanded, the only variable that was significantly different between the two groups was menarcheal age. Overall, the amenorrheic runners had a later average age at menarche by 1 year than the regularly menstruating group.

The differences between these studies might be due to the age at which these athletes began training. The athletes who had a later menarche had begun their training at a very young age or around menarche, whereas the women who began training in their mid-20s had menarcheal ages comparable to nonathletes.[5,8,10,37,41]

Does late menarche suggest that the reproductive system is "fragile" and that any added stress, i.e., training, results in menstrual dysfunction?[5] To date, this question remains unanswered.

Intense Training Prior to Menarche

In only one study has a direct relationship been found between intense training prior to menarche and athletic amenorrhea.[50] Swimmers and runners who began training prior to menarche had four times the incidence of amenorrhea (no menses for 6 months) than did those who began training after menarche. However, another study found no association between training before menarche and amenorrhea.[43]

Prior Menstrual Irregularity

It has been proposed that reproductive maturity, as demonstrated by age, pregnancy, early age of menarche, and regular menstrual cycles, protects an athlete from menstrual irregularity.[6,19,38] Conversely, reproductive immaturity (nulliparity, late menarche, and prior irregular menstrual cycles) has been hypothesized to predispose an athlete to becoming amenorrheic.[6,19,38] Secondary amenorrhea has been reported to be more common in athletes who had a history of prior menstrual irregularity. Shangold and Levine stated that the single best predictor of amenorrhea in their sample of runners was the presence of prior menstrual irregularity.[8] Further, Schwartz and co-workers found that more than 50 percent of their amenorrheic runners had past menstrual cycle irregularity.[37] To date, the possibility cannot be ruled out that these women may be constitutionally predisposed to developing athletic amenorrhea.

Quantity of Training

Is the amenorrhea experienced in athletes a direct result of training and a distinct entity, i.e., athletic amenorrhea, or is the pathogenesis multifactorial and is training just one piece of the puzzle? The frequency of amenorrhea has been positively correlated with the number of miles run per week.[4] The incidence steadily increased from 6 percent in those running less than 10 miles per week to 43 percent in those running more than 60 miles per week. In a later study, runners, cyclists, and swimmers were surveyed to determine the incidence of amenorrhea in these endurance sports.[12] Again, weekly training mileage was correlated to amenorrhea among the runners; however, no such relationship could be shown for the swimmers and cyclists (Fig. 5–4). An association between training and frequency of menstrual dysfunction in distance runners was substantiated by Dale, Gerlach, and Wilhite.[6] In this study runners were divided into two groups: those who ran more than 30 miles per week (runners), and those who ran 5 to 30 miles per week (joggers). Four percent of the controls (n = 54) were amenorrheic (zero to five periods per year) in comparison to 14 percent of the joggers and 24 percent of the runners. Finally, support for an association was reported by Frisch and colleagues, who found that the prevalence of amenorrhea in swimmers (n = 21) and runners (n = 17) increased during the training season in comparison to preseason.[50]

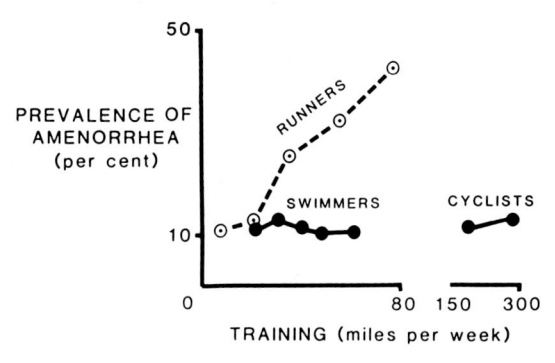

Figure 5–4 The prevalence of amenorrhea increased linearly as training mileage increased in runners (p < 0.001). Swimmers and cyclists had a 12 percent incidence regardless of training mileage. (From Sanborn CF, Martin BJ, Wagner WW Jr. Am J Obstet Gynecol 1982; 143:859–861.)

Contradictory results have been reported by other investigators who found no association between training mileage and the prevalence of amenorrhea.[5,7,38] Disagreement is probably a result of study design. To investigate the correlation between prevalence of amenorrhea and training mileage, the following criteria should be met: a large random sample, a wide range of training mileage, and dichotomous groups. The groups should be divided by specific mileage, with equal numbers of subjects in each cell. In the Feicht and co-workers, and Sanborn and co-workers studies, these criteria were met.[4,12] In the Wakat and colleagues study, each point on the graph was selected based on intervals of 15 miles run per week (20 to 35, 36 to 50, 51 to 65, and 66 to 80) (Fig. 5–5).[5] The number of athletes represented for each point is not known. Further, the range of

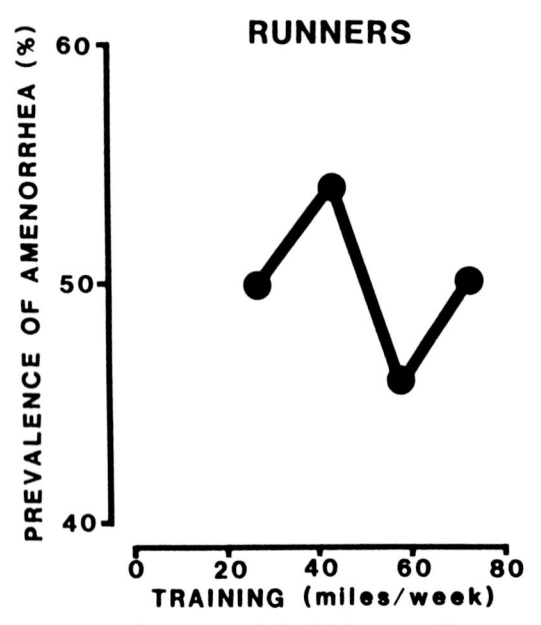

Figure 5–5 There was no relationship between miles run per week and prevalence of amenorrhea in runners. (Adapted from Wakat DK, Sweeney KA, Rogol AD. Med Sci Sports Exerc 1982; 14:265.)

weekly training was from 20 to 80 miles and did not include lower training mileages. Speroff and Redwine also found no correlation between weekly running mileage and amenorrhea.[7] However, few of their women ran more than 20 miles per week. In the study by Baker and associates, a higher prevalence of amenorrhea was found in the runners who ran less than 40 miles per week than in the athletes who ran more than 40 miles per week (37.5 percent and 26.6 percent, respectively); however, the sample sizes were small, and the groupings were not specific.

All of these studies have examined quantity of training, miles per week, days per week, weeks, and months of training. None has examined the intensity of training, i.e., at what percentage of maximum oxygen uptake the athletes train. More work is required to determine whether certain characteristics of training cause amenorrhea.

Hypothalamic Maturity

Dale, Gerlach, and Wilhite were the first to note that prior pregnancy appeared to protect an athlete from developing amenorrhea.[6] Fifty percent of the runners who had never borne children (nulliparous) had menstrual irregularity, whereas only 20 percent of the parous runners developed irregularities. The maturity of the hypothalamic-pituitary-ovarian system has also been related to the age of the athletes. In the previous study comparisons were not made between the ages of the amenorrheic and regularly menstruating runners or the ages of the nulliparous or parous runners. Baker and coworkers found that amenorrhea occurred more often in runners who were 18 to 30 years of age (67 percent) than in those 30 years of age or older (9.0 percent).[38] The nulliparous runners in this study had a higher prevalence of amenorrhea than the parous runners; however, they were also younger. These findings suggest that younger nulliparous runners may be more susceptible to athletic amenorrhea because of an immature hypothalamic-pituitary-ovarian axis.

Psychological Stress

An alternative cause of athletic amenorrhea could be psychological stress stemming from intense training and competition. Amenorrheic middle distance runners have subjectively rated the months they trained per year as more intense than the regularly menstruating group has done.[4] This finding was substantiated by Schwartz and associates.[37] Four psychological tests were administered to the athletes to assess depression, anxiety, compulsive behavior, hypochondriacal tendencies, and overall stress. No significant differences were found between the groups in any of these tests. However, the amenorrheic athletes subjectively reported more stress associated with running than did the regularly menstruating group. According to the authors, the tests were not as sensitive as the subjective ratings in picking up subtle psychological differences.

Some male "obligatory runners" have been shown to have psychological profiles similar to those of women with anorexia nervosa.[54] Recently, anorexia nervosa, a psychological eating disorder, has been reported in female runners and in ballet dancers.[55,56] In the former study, 90-minute psychiatric interviews were structured to explore the nature and extent of psychiatric differences between amenorrheic and regularly menstruating runners.[55] Eating disorders were diagnosed in 62 percent of the amenorrheic runners but in none of the regularly menstruating runners. Low food intake, ritualized dietary habits, caloric deficits through heightened energy expenditures, and compulsive behaviors were several other parallels observed between the amenorrheic group and patients with anorexia nervosa. Major affective disorders in either first-degree or second-degree relatives were prevalent in the amenorrheic runners (77 percent) and were virtually absent in the regularly menstruating runners (5 percent). Although there were obvious limitations to the study (single interviewer and the subject reporting family history), these data suggest a link between athletic amenorrhea, major affective disorders, and eating disorders.

In the study of ballet dancers, 55 dancers from national and regional classical ballet companies were given a variety of questionnaires to assess menstrual status, eating behavior, and psychological profile.[56] Delayed menarche (at or after age 14 years) was found in 55 percent of the ballet dancers, and 19 percent had amenorrhea for 5 months or longer. Prolonged amenorrhea was associated with eating disorders and anorexia nervosa. The authors concluded that eating problems (anorexia nervosa and restricted caloric intake) may play an important role in the pathogenesis of amenorrhea in athletes. There is little doubt that extreme cases of starvation caused by severe illness or wartime conditions can cause amenorrhea.[57] However, as in the current publications, it is impossible to differentiate between amenorrhea caused by malnutrition and psychogenic amenorrhea.

Diet

There is evidence that nutritional status and diet can affect the reproductive system. Although the mechanisms are unknown, poor dietary habits are often cited as the explanation for amenorrhea in anorexia nervosa. The diets of amenorrheic and regularly menstruating athletes have been found to be different in nutrient composition and in total caloric consumption.

Amenorrheic runners have been found to be primarily vegetarian, whereas their regularly menstruating counterparts were not.[58] The regularly menstruating runners ate five times more meat than the amenorrheic group ($p < 0.05$) (Fig. 5-6). Vegetarianism was defined as consuming less than 200 g per week of meat (any combination of red or white). Using this classification, 82 percent of the amenorrheic runners were considered vegetarian, whereas only 13 percent of the regularly menstruating runners were vegetarian. Other dietary survey studies have found that amenorrheic athletes consume significantly less fat and carbohydrates than the regularly menstruating athletes.[46,58,59]

A surprising finding has been the low total caloric intakes reported by these athletes re-

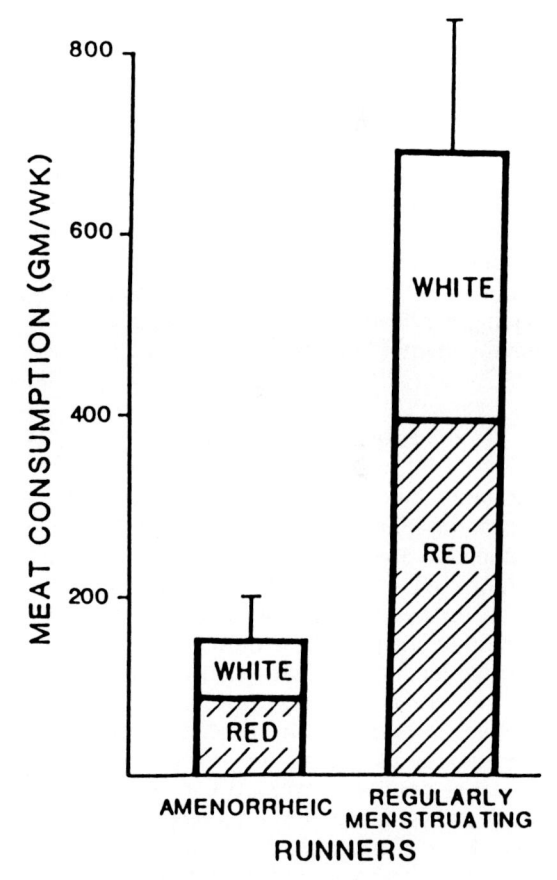

Figure 5-6 Weekly total meat consumption, white meat (poultry and fish) and red meat, of amenorrheic and regularly menstruating runners. (From Brooks SM, Sanborn CF, Albrecht BH, Wagner WW Jr. Lancet 1984; 1:559-560.)

gardless of menstrual status. The total calories consumed by many female athletes are below the recommended values even for nonexercising women. Sedentary women aged 25 to 55 should consume 1,800 to 2,200 kcals per day.[60] In fact, the mean total caloric consumption for female athletes has been reported from as low as 1,272 kcals per day to as high as 2,397 kcals per day.[45,59] These athletes would appear to be in negative caloric balance when their high caloric expenditures are compared to these low caloric intakes. The daily caloric intake of women running 10 miles a day should approach 2,600 kcals to maintain energy balance.[61] Therefore, the question arises whether a negative caloric balance or "caloric energy drain" might explain amenorrhea in athletes. As is true of the previous theoretical causes of athletic amenorrhea, a clear-cut answer cannot be given. Amenorrheic runners have been found to have significantly lower caloric intakes, borderline lower values, and similar caloric consumptions when compared with regularly menstruating runners.[44-46] However, virtually all of the athletes, regardless of menstrual status, could be considered to be eating too few calories. Caution needs to be taken in extrapolating these findings, but the pattern of restricted nutritional intake along with a "compulsive" obsession with training and leanness continually surfaces in the female amenorrheic athlete.

Hormonal Alterations

The interrelationship within the hypothalamic-pituitary-ovarian axis is responsible for the events that lead to a normal menstrual cycle. The sole purpose of this cycle is the development of the ovum for fertilization: the ovarian cycle. Disruption of any part of the intricate negative and positive feedback system of this axis can lead to menstrual dysfunction. Exercise-induced changes in hormones have been implicated in the etiology of athletic amenorrhea. The hormonal responses to exercise can be examined in two ways: acute hormonal responses after a short bout of exercise, and chronic responses to long-term exercise. An in-depth review of the literature concerning hormonal alterations in exercising females has been written by Loucks and Horvath.[62]

Acute Response

Briefly, the effect of exercise on gonadotropins (follicular stimulating hormone and luteinizing hormone) and steroid hormones (estrogen and progesterone) is difficult to interpret. Problems may stem from the fact that hormonal changes can reflect an increased production, hemoconcentration resulting from shifts in plasma volume during exercise, or a decreased clearance of the hormone in the blood.[63] However, prolactin response to an acute bout of 40 minutes of running at 80 percent $\dot{V}O_2$max and at $\dot{V}O_2^+$max was not greater in amenorrheic runners than in regularly menstruating runners.[64,65] Further, no significant differences were found between the two groups in basal serum prolactin or in the serum prolactin response to thyrotropin releasing hormone.[65] The similarities of prolactin response to acute bouts of exercise between amenorrheic and regularly menstruating runners suggest that hyperprolactinemia is not the cause of athletic amenorrhea.

The initial findings of a rise in testosterone with short-term exercise raised the possibility that hyperandrogenism might be the reason for the noted amenorrhea.[63,66,67] When corrections were made for plasma volume shifts, serum testosterone concentrations were found to be similar at rest and during an acute bout of exercise between matched amenorrheic and regularly menstruating runners.[64,65]

The initiation of the menstrual cycle is dependent upon the pulsatile release of gonadotropin releasing hormone (GnRH), which is demonstrated as an elevation in luteinizing hormone (LH). The baseline LH pulse amplitude has been found to be significantly low in amenorrheic runners (Fig. 5-7).[68] Further, acute exercise (60 minutes at 60 percent $\dot{V}O_2$max) has been found to have an inhibitory effect on LH pulsatile release in regularly menstruating runners.[69] In amenorrheic runners, an exaggerated gonadotropin response to GnRH hormone has been observed. A similar response is found in women who have hypothalamic, psychogenic, or stress-related amenorrhea.[65] Conversely, a reduced gonadotropin response to GnRH hormone is often found in amenorrhea associated with weight loss.[65] In view of these facts, Yahiro and associates have hypothesized that athletic amenorrhea may develop as a re-

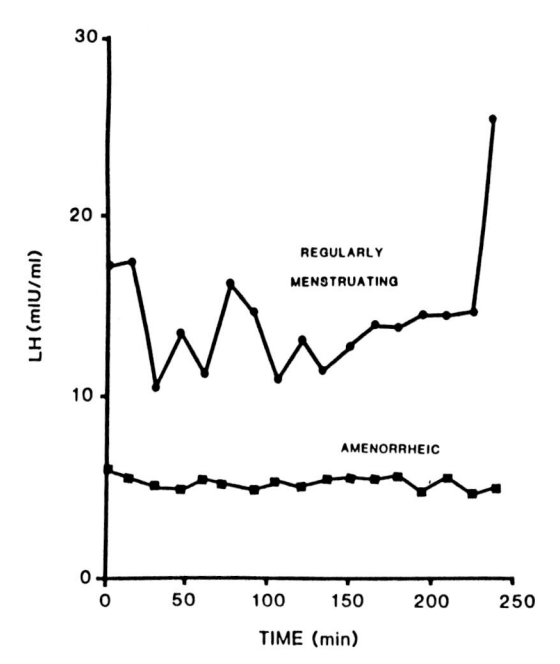

Figure 5–7 LH pulse frequency and amplitude of a regularly menstruating and an amenorrheic runner. (From Fisher EC, Nelson ME, Frontera WR, et al. J Clin Endocrinol Metab 1986; 62:1232–1236.)

sult of reduced GnRH hormone secretion, an increased pituitary sensitivity to estrogens, or both.[65]

Chronic Hormonal Response

Luteinizing hormone and follicular stimulating hormone levels have been found to be low and noncyclic in amenorrheic distance runners.[66] In comparison to a normal ovulatory cycle (Fig. 5–8), the values of serum estradiol and progesterone were always suppressed and showed no cyclic changes (Fig. 5–9).

Preliminary findings suggest that the pituitary is functioning and that the most probable level of menstrual dysfunction in the athlete is at the hypothalamus or above. A GnRH stimulation test in a small sample of amenorrheic athletes has resulted in normal secretions from the pituitary and ovaries.[70]

Three studies have followed regularly menstruating athletes as they undergo an exercise training program.[71–73] The effect of endurance training on the menstrual cycle was studied in 19 regularly menstruating women.[71,72] After approximately 13.5 months of training, the subjects were averaging 63.4 miles of running per week. Menstrual changes occurred in all but one subject. The major change was a decrease in the amount of menstrual flow or a decrease in number of days of menstruation. None of the subjects developed amenorrhea. Although total body weight did not change, there was a significant decrease in percent of body fat from 25 to 22 percent. With the exclusion of estradiol concentrations, in all of the hormones measured (thyroid hormone, thyroid-

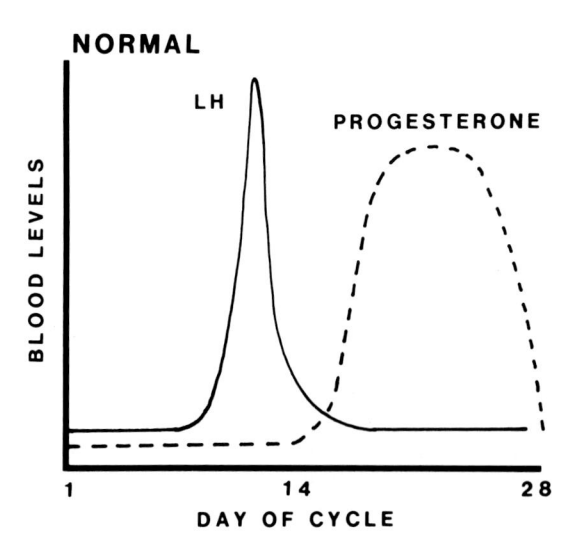

Figure 5–8 Hormonal profile of a normal ovulatory non-runner control. (From Dale E, Gerlach DH, Martin DE, Alexander CR. Phys Sportsmed 1979; 7:83–95.)

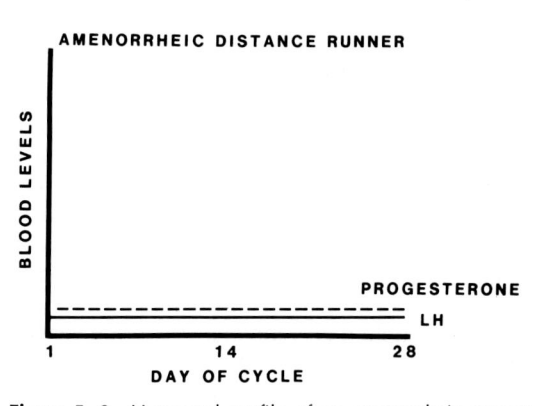

Figure 5–9 Hormonal profile of an amenorrheic runner with an anovulatory cycle. (From Dale E, Gerlach DH, Martin DE, Alexander CR. Phys Sportsmed 1979; 7:83–95.)

TABLE 5–3 Therapeutic Approach to the Amenorrheic Athlete

Problem	Therapeutic Options
Absent menstrual flow	Evaluation to rule out disease
	Explanation and reassurance
	Medroxyprogesterone 10 mg/d on days 16–25 monthly whether or not withdrawal bleeding occurs
Risk for osteoporosis	Increase oral calcium
	Medroxyprogesterone 10 mg/d for 10 d/mo
	Cyclic estrogens and progesterone
	Medroxyprogesterone 10 mg/d on days 16–25
Infertility	Decrease exercise intensity by 10 percent
	Gain 1–2 kg weight
	Monitor basal temperature for 3 mo
	After 3 mo, if ovulation has not occurred, give progesterone vaginal suppositories
	Further reduce exercise, weight, and stress
	Ovulation induction measures

(From Prior JC, Vigna Y. Gonadal steroids in athletic women: contraception, complications, and performance. Sports Med 1985; 2:287–295.)

their performance; therefore, decreasing training and gaining weight are often not even considered as a potential therapy regimen.

Acknowledgment

My sincere appreciation to W. W. Wagner Jr. for invaluable guidance, and to S. G. Engsberg for helpful criticism of the manuscript.

REFERENCES

1. Ruch TC, Patton HD, eds. Physiology and biophysics. 19th ed. Philadelphia: WB Saunders, 1965:1185.
2. Bausenwien I. Zur Frage Sport und Menstruation. Deutsche Medizinische Wochenschrift 1954; 79:1526–1532.
3. Erdelyi GJ. Gynecological survey of female athletes. J Sports Med Phys Fitness 1963; 2:174–179.
4. Feicht CB, Johnson TS, Martin BJ, et al. Secondary amenorrhoea in athletes. Lancet 1978; 2:1145–1146.
5. Wakat DK, Sweeney KA, Rogol AD. Reproductive system function in women cross-country runners. Med Sci Sports Exerc 1982; 14:263–269.
6. Dale E, Gerlach DH, Wilhite AL. Menstrual dysfunction in distance runners. Obstet Gynecol 1979; 54:47–53.
7. Speroff L, Redwine DB. Exercise and menstrual function. Phys Sportsmed 1980; 8:42–52.
8. Shangold MM, Levine HS. The effect of marathon training upon menstrual function. Am J Obstet Gynecol 1982; 143:862–869.
9. Lutter JM, Cushman S. Menstrual patterns in female runners. Phys Sportsmed 1982; 10:60–72.
10. Frisch RE, Wyshak G, Vincent L. Delayed menarche and amenorrhea in ballet dancers. N Engl J Med 1980; 303:17–19.
11. Cohen JL, Kim CS, May PB, Ertel NH. Exercise, body weight, and professional ballet dancers. Phys Sportsmed 1982; 10:92–101.
12. Sanborn CF, Martin BJ, Wagner WW Jr. Is athletic amenorrhea specific to runners? Am J Obstet Gynecol 1982; 143:859–861.
13. Carlberg KS, Buckman MT, Peake GT, Riedesel ML. A survey of menstrual function in athletes. Eur J Appl Physiol 1983; 51:211–212.
14. Prior JC, Cameron K, Ho Yuen B, Thomas J. Menstrual cycle changes with marathon training: anovulation and short luteal phase. Can J Appl Sport Sci 1982; 7:173–177.
15. Bonen A, Belcastro AN, Ling WY, Simpson AA. Profiles of selected hormones during menstrual cycles of teenage athletes. J Appl Physiol 1981; 50:545–551.
16. Shangold MM, Freeman R, Thysen B, Gatz M. The relationship between long-distance running, plasma progesterone, and luteal phase length. Fertil Steril 1979; 31:130–133.
17. Prior JC, Yuen BH, Clement P, et al. Reversible luteal phase changes and infertility associated with marathon training. Lancet 1982; 2:269–270.
18. Wilmore JH, Brown C. Physiological profiles of women distance runners. Med Sci Sports 1974; 6:178–181.
19. Baker ER. Menstrual dysfunction and hormonal status in athletic women: a review. Fertil Steril 1981; 36:691–696.
20. Frisch RE. Weight at menarche: similarity for well-nourished and under-nourished girls at differing ages and evidence for historical constancy. Pediatrics 1972; 50:445–450.
21. Frisch RE. A method of prediction of age of menarche from height and weight at ages 9 through 13 years. Pediatrics 1974; 53:384–390.
22. Frisch RE, McArthur JW. Menstrual cycles: fatness as a determinant of minimum weight for height necessary for their maintenance or onset. Science 1974; 185:949–951.
23. Frisch RE, Revelle R. Height and weight at menarche and a hypothesis of critical body weights and adolescent events. Science 1970; 169:397–399.
24. Frisch RE, Revelle R. The height and weight of girls

and boys at the time of initiation of the adolescent growth spurt in height and weight and the relationship to menarche. Hum Biol 1971; 43:140–159.
25. Frisch RE, Revelle R, Cook S. Components of weight at menarche and the initiation of the adolescent growth spurt in girls: estimated total water, lean body weight, and fat. Hum Biol 1973; 45:469–483.
26. Kennedy GG, Mitra J. Body weight and food intake as initiating factors for puberty in the rat. J Physiol (Lond) 1963; 166:408–418.
27. Tanner JM. Growth at adolescence. 2nd ed. Oxford: Blackwell Scientific Publications, 1962.
28. Wyshak G, Frisch RE. Evidence for secular trend in age of menarche. N Engl J Med 1982; 306:1033–1035.
29. Knuth UA, Hull MGR, Jacobs HS. Amenorrhea and loss of weight. Br J Obstet Gynecol 1977; 84:801–807.
30. McArthur JW, Johnson L, Hourihan J, Alonso C. Endocrine studies during the refeeding of young women with nutritional amenorrhea and infertility. Mayo Clin Proc 1976; 51:607–616.
31. Wentz A. Body weight and amenorrhea. Obstet Gynecol 1980; 56:482–487.
32. Yen SC, Jaffe RB, eds. Reproductive endocrinology. Philadelphia: WB Saunders, 1978.
33. Reeves J. Estimating fatness. Science 1979; 204:881.
34. Trussell J. Statistical flaws in evidence for the Frisch hypothesis that fatness triggers menarche. Hum Biol 1980; 52:711–720.
35. Mellits EB, Cheek DB. The assessment of body water and fatness from infancy to adulthood. Monogr Soc Res Child Devel 1970; 35:12–26.
36. Boyden TW, Pamenter RW, Grosso D, et al. Prolactin responses, menstrual cycles, and body composition of women runners. J Clin Endocrinol Metab 1982; 54:711–714.
37. Schwartz B, Cumming DC, Riordan E, et al. Exercise-associated amenorrhea: a distinct entity? Am J Obstet Gynecol 1981; 141:662–670.
38. Baker ER, Mathur RS, Kirk RF, Williamson HO. Female runners and secondary amenorrhea: correlation with age, parity, mileage, and plasma hormonal and sex-hormone-binding globulin concentrations. Fertil Steril 1981; 36:183–187.
39. Jackson AS, Pollock ML. Prediction accuracy of body density, lean body weight, and total body volume equations. Med Sci Sports 1977; 9:197–219.
40. Wilmore J. The use of actual, predicted, and constant residual volumes in the assessment of body composition by underwater weighing. Med Sci Sports 1969; 1:87–89.
41. Calabrese LH, Kirkendall DT, Floyd M, et al. Menstrual abnormalities, nutritional patterns, and body composition in female classical ballet dancers. Phys Sportsmed 1983; 11:86–98.
42. Carlberg KA, Buckman MT, Peake GT, Riedesel ML. Body composition of oligo/amenorrheic athletes. Med Sci Sports Exerc 1983; 15:215–217.
43. Sanborn CF, Albrecht BH, Wagner WW Jr. Athletic amenorrhea: lack of association with body fat. Med Sci Sports Exerc 1987; 19:207–212.
44. Drinkwater BJ, Nilson K, Chesnut CH, et al. Bone mineral content of amenorrheic and eumenorrheic athletes. N Engl J Med 1984; 311:277–281.
45. Marcus R, Cann C, Madvig P, et al. Menstrual function and bone mass in elite women distance runners. Ann Intern Med 1985; 102:158–163.
46. Nelson ME, Fisher EC, Catsos PD, et al. Diet and bone status in amenorrheic runners. Am J Clin Nutr 1986; 43:910–916.
47. Sanborn CF, Wagner WW Jr. Rebuttal to letter. Med Sci Sports Exerc 1987; 19:621–622.
48. Malina RM, Haper AB, Avent HH, Campbell DE. Age at menarche in athletes and nonathletes. Med Sci Sports 1973; 5:11–13.
49. Malina RM, Spirduso WW, Tate C, Baylor AM. Age at menarche and selected menstrual characteristics in athletes at different competitive levels and in different sports. Med Sci Sports 1978; 10:218–222.
50. Frisch RE, Gotz-Welbergen AV, McArthur JW, et al. Delayed menarche and amenorrhea of college athletes in relation to age of onset of training. JAMA 1981; 246:1559–1563.
51. Vandenbroucke JP, van Laar A, Valkenburg HA. Synergy between thinness and intensive sports activity in delaying menarche. Br Med J 1982; 284:1907–1908.
52. Warren MP. The effect of exercise on pubertal progression and reproductive function in girls. J Clin Endocrinol Metab 1980; 51:1150–1156.
53. Wigglesworth J, Hatler L, Stager J. Interpreting the relationship between age of menarche and prepubertal training. Med Sci Sports Exerc 1987; 19:S4 (abstr).
54. Yates A, Leehey K, Shisslak CU. Running—an analogue to anorexia? N Engl J Med 1983; 308:251–255.
55. Gadpaille WJ, Sanborn CF, Wagner WW Jr. Athletic amenorrhea, major affective disorders, and eating disorders. Am J Psychiatry 1987; 144:939–942.
56. Brooks-Gunn J, Warren MP, Hamilton LH. The relation of eating problems and amenorrhea in ballet dancers. Med Sci Sports Exerc 1987; 19:41–44.
57. Drew F. Epidemiology of secondary amenorrhea. J Chronic Dis 1961; 14:396–406.
58. Brooks SM, Sanborn CF, Albrecht BH, Wagner WW Jr. Diet in athletic amenorrhea. Lancet 1984; 1:559–560.
59. Deuster PA, Kyle SB, Moser PB, et al. Nutritional intakes and status of highly trained amenorrheic and eumenorrheic women runners. Fertil Steril 1986; 46:636–643.
60. Food and Nutrition Board. Recommended dietary allowances. Washington, DC: National Academy of Sciences, National Research Council, 1980.
61. Deuster PA, Kyle SB, Moser PB, et al. Nutritional survey of highly trained women runners. Am J Clin Nutr 1986; 45:954–962.
62. Loucks AB, Horvath SM. Athletic amenorrhea: a review. Med Sci Sports Exerc 1985; 17:56–72.
63. Cumming DC, Rebar RW. Exercise and reproductive function in women. Am J Ind Med 1983; 4:113–125.
64. Loucks AB, Horvath SM. Exercise-induced stress responses of amenorrheic and eumenorrheic women. J Clin Endocrinol Metab 1984; 59:1109–1120.
65. Yahiro J, Glass AR, Fears WB, et al. Exaggerated gonadotropin response to luteinizing hormone-releasing hormone in amenorrheic runners. Am J Obstet Gynecol 1987; 156:586–591.
66. Dale E, Gerlach DH, Martin DE, Alexander CR. Phys-

ical fitness profiles and reproductive physiology of the female distance runner. Phys Sportsmed 1979; 7:83–95.
67. Shangold MM, Gatz ML, Thysen B. Acute effects of exercise on plasma concentrations of prolactin and testosterone in recreational women runners. Fertil Steril 1981; 35:699–702.
68. Fisher EC, Nelson ME, Frontera WR, et al. Bone mineral content and levels of gonadotropins and estrogens in amenorrheic running women. J Clin Endocrinol Metab 1986; 62:1232–1236.
69. Cumming DC, Vickovic MM, Wall SR, et al. The effect of acute exercise on pulsatile releasing of luteinizing hormone in women runners. Am J Obstet Gynecol 1985; 153:482–485.
70. McArthur JW, Bullen BA, Beitins IZ, et al. Hypothalamic amenorrhea in runners of normal body composition. Endocr Res Commun 1980; 7:89–91.
71. Boyden TW, Pamenter RW, Stanforth P, et al. Evidence for mild thyroidal impairment in women undergoing endurance training. J Clin Endocrinol Metab 1982; 53:53–56.
72. Boyden TW, Pamenter RW, Stanforth P, et al. Sex steroids and endurance running in women. Fertil Steril 1983; 39:629–632.
73. Bullen BA, Skrinar GS, Beitins IZ, et al. Endurance training effects on plasma hormonal responsiveness and sex hormone excretion. J Appl Physiol 1984; 56:1453–1463.
74. Laatikainen T, Virtanen T, Apter D. Plasma immunoreactive beta-endorphin in exercise-associated amenorrhea. Am J Obstet Gynecol 1986; 154:94–97.
75. Galle PC, Freeman EW, Galle MG, et al. Physiologic and psychologic profiles in a survey of women runners. Fertil Steril 1983; 39:633–639.
76. Gray DP, Dale E. Variables associated with secondary amenorrhea in women runners. J Sports Sci 1983; 1:55–67.
77. Stager JM, Ritchie-Flanagan B, Robertshaw D. Reversibility of amenorrhea in athletes. N Engl J Med 1984; 310:51–52.
78. Sanborn CF, Albrecht BH, Wagner WW Jr. Medically induced reversal of infertility in athletic amenorrhea. Med Sci Sports Exerc 1987; 19:S5 (abstr).
79. Prior JC, Vigna Y. Gonadal steroids in athletic women: contraception, complications, and performance. Sports Med 1985; 2:287–295.
80. Shangold MM. Athletic amenorrhea. Clin Obstet Gynecol 1985; 28:664–669.
81. Fries H, Nillius SJ, Petterson F. Epidemiology of secondary amenorrhea. Am J Obstet Gynecol 1974; 118:473–479.

Chapter 6
Osteoporosis, Diet, and Exercise

JACQUELINE R. BERNING
CHARLOTTE F. SANBORN
WILTZ W. WAGNER

Osteoporosis is the most common disorder of the human skeleton.[1] The condition is characterized by a decreased bone mineral content, increased porosity of the bone, and a decreased resistance to fracture. A moderate degree of osteoporosis is an expected occurrence of the aging process. The pathogenesis of osteoporosis involves many factors, including age, hormones, nutrition, and exercise. An understanding of both the dynamic interaction of each factor and precise and accurate bone measurement are necessary for proper diagnosis and treatment of osteoporosis.

BONE MASS MEASUREMENTS

The techniques used for bone mass measurements include radiogrammetry, photon absorptiometry, x-ray photo densitometry, and computed tomography (CT). Radiogrammetric measurements can be performed quite precisely, especially if multiple metacarpals are measured, but they do not very accurately reflect the amount of bone that is present.[2] According to Mazess, Cameron, and Sorenson, radiogrammetry of the hands does not reflect actual bone mass or intracortical porosity and consistently underestimates bone loss by 20 to 30 percent.[3] Nevertheless, such measurements are probably valid indices of change in skeletal mass in large studies, because loss of cortical bone in the metacarpals is likely to be associated with loss elsewhere, although relative loss may be quantitatively different from site to site.[4]

Single photon absorptiometry provides a measure of peripheral bone mass with a precision error less than 3 percent.[3] This technique is widely available and provides an accurate index of changes in cortical bone. Single photon absorptiometry measures net changes on all envelopes of cortical and trabecular bone, but it does not distinguish between them. Even though single photon densitometry is quite sensitive, 25 percent of the subjects under the age of 70 years who show normal bone mineral content using single photon densitometry have low axial skeleton bone mineral content when measured by dual photon densitometry.

Dual energy photon absorptiometry measures changes in the entire vertebra, both cortical and trabecular bone (Figs. 6–1 and 6–2).[4] It is reproducible to 3 to 4 percent, and it detects all subjects with low trabecular bone mass.

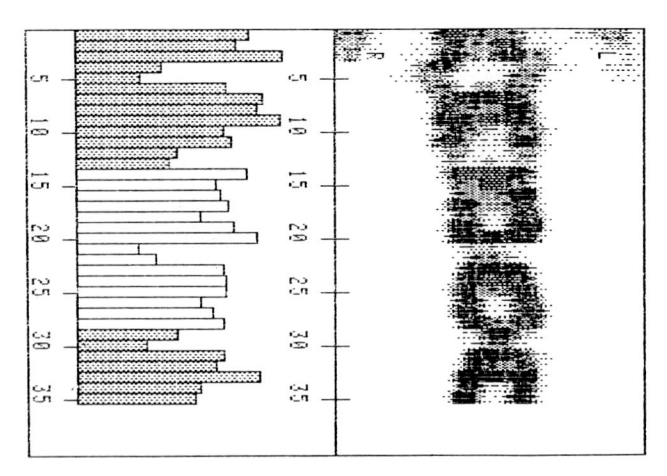

136 / Scientific Foundations of Sports Medicine

Figure 6–1 Bone mass of a 35-year-old regularly menstruating athlete as determined by dual photon absorptiometry. Fracture risk, normal; lines 9 through 29 correspond to the second and fourth lumbar vertebrae (L2 and L4).

CT can be used to measure the trabecular bone within verterbral bodies. Cost, accessibility, and radiation dose limit the wide use of this technique. CT scans have been documented as very precise for repeated measurements, but accuracy is adversely affected by a reciprocal change in marrow fat content.[5]

All measures of the skeletal mineral suffer from the inherent difficulty that bone loss is not uniform throughout the skeleton.[6] Measurements of one bone cannot be extrapolated with confidence to another bone or, indeed, to other sites of the same bone. Loss in the axial skeleton may differ markedly from that in the appendicular skeleton. Loss of trabecular bone with aging has been reported to occur both more slowly and more rapidly than loss of cortical bone.[4,5]

AGE-RELATED OSTEOPOROSIS

Three major etiologic factors are believed to be responsible for the higher incidence of osteoporosis in women: lower peak bone mass of women compared with men of similar age,

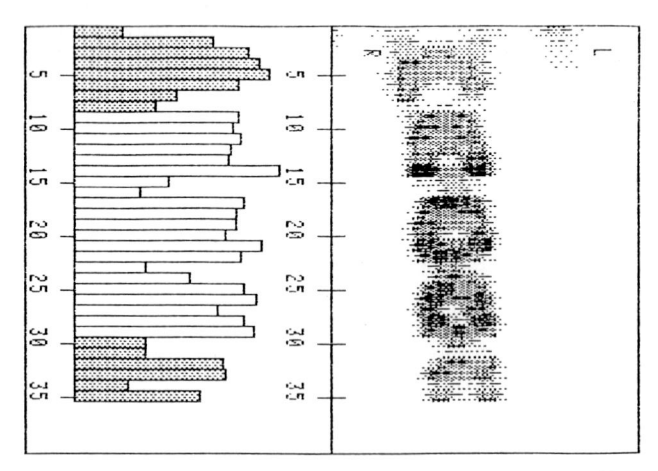

Figure 6–2 Bone mass of an amenorrheic athlete as determined by dual photon absorptiometry. Fracture risk, mild; lines 14 through 28 correspond with third and fourth lumbar vertebrae (L3 and L4).

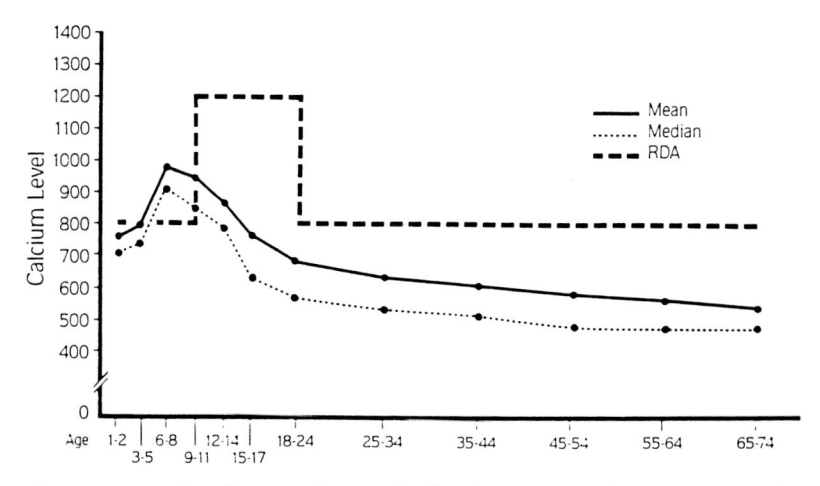

Figure 6–5 Daily calcium intake (mg) for females, U.S. population 1976 to 1980. The mean daily intake of calcium is below the RDA. (From Abraham S, Carroll MD, Dresser CM. Dietary intake findings. USA 1976–1980. Hyattsville, MD: National Center for Health Statistics, U.S. Department of Health and Human Services Publication No. (PHS) 83-1681, 1980.)

bone loss with age was roughly the same among the various groups, namely, about 0.8 percent per year among women and 0.3 percent per year among men. Individuals with an average calcium intake of 300 to 500 mg per day showed no difference in bone density from persons consuming 900 to 1,500 mg per day. The data did not confirm a relationship between habitual calcium intake and either the magnitude of bone mass or its rate of loss. Thus, Garn and co-workers concluded that a high-calcium diet does not promote integrity of compact bone, nor does a low-calcium diet speed bone loss either on a population basis or on an individual basis.

A challenge to Garn and associates' position has recently been presented by Matkovic and co-workers who compared bone status and fracture rate in two regions of Yugoslavia.[28] The populations were matched for ethnic origin, physical activity, living conditions, age, and weight. Further anthropometric determinations such as height and weight were identical. The only difference between the two regions was in habitual calcium intake (800 to 1,100 mg per day versus 350 to 500 mg per day). The higher calcium district had 159,446 inhabitants (82,891 females and 76,555 males). The low-calcium district had 174,250 inhabitants (88,508 females and 85,742 males). Calcium consumption was determined by replicate administration of an extensive questionnaire and chemical analysis of local foodstuffs. The population consuming the higher calcium diet exhibited a significantly greater ($p < .001$) cortical bone density as measured by radiograms and bone morphometry and a reduced incidence of proximal femur fractures at all ages for both sexes. In the population consuming the higher amounts of calcium, milk and dairy products were the main source, whereas in the population consuming less calcium, most of the calories and nutrients were of vegetable origin, and the main sources of calcium were cereals and vegetables.

The effects of calcium supplementation on various indices of change in bone mass have been reported by several groups. Both Recker, Saville and Heaney, and Horsman and associates studied normal postmenopausal women placed on calcium supplements that yielded a total intake of approximately 1,500 mg per day.[29,30] In both studies radiogrammetry of three metacarpals and photon absorptiometry of the distal forearm were used to measure change in bone mass. The first study consisted of 60 postmenopausal women between the ages of 55 and 65. They were randomly divided into three groups: group I was the control, group II was given conjugated estrogen, and group III was given 2,600 mg of calcium carbonate daily. All patients were studied for 2 years. Bone mass, as determined by single photon absorptiometry, decreased by 2.88 percent per year in the control group, by 0.73 percent per year in the hormonal group, and by 1.83 percent per year in the calcium-supplemented group. Comparisons among the groups showed that both calcium carbonate and hormone treatment resulted in significantly less loss of metacarpal thickness than occurred in the control group ($p < .05$).

Recker and associates concluded that calcium carbonate appeared to reduce bone loss in postmenopausal women. Although the effect was not as strong as with estrogen therapy, it certainly could be safely recommended.[29] In the second study Horsman and associates supplemented the normal diet of 24 postmenopausal women with 800 mg of calcium per day for 2 years.[30] Bone loss from the distal radius was reduced, although the retardation in the radius was not statistically significant. The mean rate of decrease in the thickest area of the metacarpals was less than half that of the control group, with the difference approaching statistical significance ($p < .10$).

In other research looking at the effect of calcium supplementation on bone mass, Lee, Lawler, and Johnson studied 20 elderly osteoporotic women and measured bone density of the phalanx from a hand roentgenogram taken with a standard aluminum wedge.[31] No controls were followed. The subjects added three slices of processed cheese and three capsules of dibasic calcium phosphate with vitamin D to their diet each day for 6 months. Eleven subjects had increased bone density, three had no appreciable changes, and six had decreased bone density. The mean bone density increased by 10 percent from the initial values ($p < .05$). The results suggest that, even with a mean age of 70 years, some elderly women can benefit from supplementary calcium and calcium-rich foods to improve bone density. Albanese and associates reported an increase in bone density, determined radiographically, among older female subjects receiving calcium supplements.[22] Twelve subjects (average age 80 years) were maintained on 450 mg of calcium per day; 17 others (average age 82 years) received a calcium supplement of 750 mg per day with 375 IU of vitamin D. Each subject's metacarpal density was determined using radiogrammetry. After 36 months the average density of the supplemented group, expressed in arbitrary units based on an aluminum wedge, increased from 90.1 to 96.1 units, whereas the density of the controls decreased from 90.3 to 84.2 units. Albanese and co-workers state that they "support the use of calcium supplements as a safe and effective modality for the management of incipient or advanced osteoporosis."[32] Results similar to those of Albanese and co-workers were reported by Smith, Reddan, and Smith.[33] They followed a group of elderly females for 3 years using the photon absorption technique in the radius. The women received 750 mg of calcium and 400 IU of vitamin D daily for 36 months. They reported a decline in bone mineral content of 3.29 percent in the control group, and an increase of 2.29 percent among women receiving the calcium and vitamin D.

In summary, it appears there is no direct relationship between calcium consumption and bone mass; however, bone loss may be retarded with calcium supplementation.

Bioavailability

Effective calcium intake depends not only on dietary intake, but also on the availability of the calcium once ingested. Various nutrient interactions influence calcium utilization.

Phosphorus

The ready availability of phosphorus in commonly consumed foodstuffs and its widespread use in food processing have focused attention on the possible deleterious effects of its excessive intake. Animal studies have shown that high intakes of phosphorus can initiate a series of homeostatic adjustments that may result in bone loss.[34] Excessive dietary phosphorus causes an increase in plasma phosphorus and a decrease in serum calcium. The resulting hypocalcemia stimulates secretion of PTH, which in turn increases the rate of bone resorption.[6]

Diets rich in phosphates have led to progressive bone resorption in mice, rats, dogs, rabbits, and pigs.[35-39]

Although high phosphate intake has been shown to increase bone loss in experimental animals, the validity of extrapolating these findings to humans has been questioned. What seems reasonably well established is that dietary phosphorus and urine calcium are inversely correlated, even within the range of usual dietary phosphorus intake.[40] These observations have been interpreted to suggest that mild phosphatemia associated with increased intake binds circulating calcium, which leads to increased release of PTH and consequent increase in bone resorptive activity, which is presumed to be undesirable.

Calcium to Phosphorus Ratio

There is insufficient evidence to establish an optimal calcium to phosphorus ratio, or indeed to determine whether this ratio is of dietary significance in humans.[6] A calcium to phosphorus ratio of 1 to 1 or 2 to 1 has been recommended for humans, but additional studies seem necessary to validate this recommendation.[41] The average American diet has a calcium to phosphorus ratio of 1 to 1.6.[25]

Loss of bone mass by humans due to a low calcium to phosphorus ratio has not been demonstrated. Zemel and Linkswiler maintained eight young male subjects for consecutive 15-day periods on diets with differing calcium to phosphorus ratios.[42] High phosphorus intake (1,835 mg per day) stimulated parathyroid secretion as indicated by increased urinary excretion of cyclic adenosine monophosphate, both with low (399 mg per day) and high (1,199 mg per day) intakes of calcium, and resulted in 0.2 and 0.65 calcium to phosphorus ratios, respectively. Bone resorption, measured by urinary hydroxyproline, was not affected by high phosphorus intakes. With high-calcium, high-phosphorus diets, such as high soft drink consumption, both urinary cyclic adenosine monophosphate and hydroxyproline decreased, suggesting a decrease in parathyroid-mediated bone resorption.

The excessive use of soft drinks could alter the calcium to phosphorus ratio of the diet. Massey and Strang evaluated 13 soft drinks for phosphorus and found levels ranging from 44 to 70 mg per 12-ounce serving, with cola having the most.[43] They estimated that the average college student consumed two 12-ounce colas per day and that the colas contributed 140 mg of phosphorus to the total daily intake. They assumed that the total phosphorus intake for Americans averaged 1.2 g and that the colas contributed about 17 percent of the total dietary phosphorus. They concluded that, although soft drinks are not a major contributor to the dietary phosphorus intake, if they are substituted for milk, the overall effect is low calcium consumption.

Protein

Although high-protein diets have been shown repeatedly to induce hypercalciuria in both humans and animals, questions remain concerning the magnitude, duration, mechanism, and significance of this effect.[6] It appears that high protein intake increases the urinary excretion of calcium at all levels of calcium ingestion. Linkswiler, Joyce, and Anand studied calcium balance in young adult males receiving three levels of protein (47, 95, and 142 g per day) at three levels of calcium intake (500, 800, and 1,400 mg per day).[44] Each experimental period was 15 days, and each subject served as his own control. Phosphorus intakes were the same as those of calcium or slightly greater in each case. Complete 24-hour urine and feces collections were tested for calcium excretion. At the lowest protein intake (47 g per day), the subjects remained in calcium balance at all levels of calcium intake ($p < .05$). At the intermediate protein level (95 g per day), all subjects who received 500 mg of calcium per day were in negative calcium balance, but those receiving 800 mg of calcium per day were in slightly positive balance. Further improvements in calcium balance did not occur when 1,400 mg calcium was given. When the highest level of protein was ingested (142 g per day), all subjects were in negative balance on a daily calcium intake of either 500 mg or 800 mg per day. At 1,400 mg of calcium per day, 12 of the 15 subjects had negative calcium balances. Urinary calcium was significantly affected by the levels of protein intake. Subjects excreted less calcium when given the low-protein diet than when given the medium levels, with the exception of two subjects; they excreted less when given the medium amounts than the high amounts. An increase in dietary protein caused a rapid increase in urinary calcium excretion. The increase in calciuria translates into a negative calcium balance, which could enhance bone loss and thereby increase the risk of osteoporosis.

Even more striking effects on urinary calcium excretion were noted by Margen and co-workers in subjects consuming different amounts of protein.[45] All dietary components other than protein were kept constant. Dietary levels of protein from protein or amino acid supplements were administered for a period of 12 to 15 days. Determination of urinary calcium was made on 24-hour collections or 3-day pooled samples using an atomic absorption spectrophotometer. Subjects (n = 4) receiving 2.3 g calcium and an average intake of 12 to 13 g nitrogen (about 80 g protein) daily excreted an average of 80 mg of calcium per day. When the protein intake was raised to 90 g nitrogen (about 560 g protein), subjects (n = 4) excreted almost five times (380 mg) as much calcium as they had on the low-protein diet (p < .01). Other subjects (n = 6), receiving 1.6 g per day of calcium, excreted 46 mg of calcium in the urine on an essentially protein-free diet (1 g per day nitrogen), but 318 mg of calcium when they received 62 g per day nitrogen (about 390 g protein) (p < .01).

The long-term effect of high-protein diets on bone structure is still unknown. Wachman and Bernstein suggested that long-term ingestion of high-protein diets imposes a continuous demand on the buffering capacity of bone and might thus be a factor in human osteoporosis.[46] Wachman and Bernstein hypothesized that, because bone responds to an acid load by dissolution of its basic salts (calcium and phosphorus), and because high meat consumption produces a predominantly acid urine, perhaps the increasing incidence of osteoporosis is a result of life-long utilization of the buffering capacity of the basic salts of bone for the constant assault against pH homeostasis. Acting on this suggestion, Ellis, Holesh, and Ellis, using x-ray densitometry, compared the bone density of fingers of vegetarians (n = 25) with that of omnivores (n = 25).[47] Bone density was determined by roentgenograms of the third metacarpal medulla and the proximal phalanx using a Baldwin Radiological Densitometer. They reported a greater bone density for both sites among the vegetarian group (p < .001). However, a later survey by the same investigators using improved techniques and a larger group of subjects failed to confirm the original observations.[48]

Vitamin D

It is well established that a severe and prolonged deficiency of vitamin D leads to osteomalacia (adult rickets), a condition in which there is defective mineralization of newly forming bone.[49] More recently, it has been speculated that subtle disturbances in the vitamin D endocrine system may participate in some way in the development of age-related osteoporosis. The plasma levels of hormonal vitamin D (calcitriol) in postmenopausal, osteoporotic women are about 30 percent lower than in age- and sex-matched controls. Administration of small amounts (0.5 mg per day) of calcitriol to postmenopausal women caused an increased intestinal absorption of calcium and improved calcium balance.[50]

Fiber

Interest in a possible relationship between fiber intake and osteoporosis stems from the observation that various plant components (e.g., phytate, oxalate, cellulose, uronic acid, sodium alginate), as well as dietary fiber, have a chelating effect on calcium. The mineral, therefore, would not be available for absorption, and a negative calcium balance could occur. A major source of calcium in the American diet is dairy products, which supply about 75 percent of intake. Fruits and vegetables contribute about 12 percent. However, it appears that the consumption of fruits and vegetables may impair the absorption of calcium from other foods. Kelsay, Behall, and Prather observed six men who consumed a diet containing fruits and vegetables (high fiber, 45.8 g) and six men who consumed a diet containing fruit and vegetable juices (low fiber, 21.0 g) for 26 days each.[51] During the last 7 days of the 26-day period, all urine and feces were collected, and daily food composites of the two diets were made. Urinary excretions of calcium did not differ significantly on the two diets, but fecal calcium was 38 percent greater on the high-fiber diet. The mean calcium balance was positive on the low-fiber diet and negative on the high-fiber diet, and the difference was significant (p < .01). The data indicate that diets high in fiber may result in negative calcium balance. McCance and Widdowson found that calcium absorption is greater when consuming less fiber in the diet.[52] Four men and four women consumed 40 to 50 percent of their total calories from either a high-fiber brown flour (214 mg per 100 g) or a low-fiber white flour (56 mg per 100 g) diet for 3 weeks each. The remainder of the diets were regular diets, except that cheese was forbidden and milk was restricted. Urine and feces samples were collected on each subject and were analyzed for calcium excretion. Mineral absorption was taken to be the amount in the food minus the amount in the feces. The researchers found that subjects absorbed 38 percent of the ingested calcium when consuming a diet containing white bread, but only 7 percent on a similar diet with the same amount of brown bread. This suggests that dietary fiber may impair calcium absorption, a situation that may lead to a negative calcium balance.

The presence of oxalates in spinach, kale, rhubarb, cocoa, and other foodstuffs has also evoked concern that calcium absorption might be seriously reduced, especially among individuals on restricted diets. Johnston, McMillian, and Falconer compared fecal calcium excretion in six women who consumed a basal diet before and after adding spinach.[53] The basal diet included 800 mg calcium and met the RDA for all other nutrients. Each subject consumed the basal diet for 4 weeks; then for 8 weeks a 120-g serving of spinach containing 0.6 g oxalic acid and 160 mg calcium was added. Analysis for calcium was made on the feces and urine on the basal diet. The mean intake of calcium for the six subjects was 820 ± 3.7 mg per day. After the addition of spinach, calcium intake rose to 975 ± 5.4 mg for 4 weeks, then to 982 ± 3.9 the last 4 weeks. On the basal diet, two subjects were in calcium balance, but after the addition of spinach only one was in positive calcium balance. The mean daily calcium balance on the basal diet was −26 mg, on the diet containing spinach, −30 mg for the first 4 weeks and −51 mg for the last 4 weeks. The addition of spinach did not significantly alter the calcium balance. The authors concluded that the amount of calcium found in spinach failed to be absorbed.

The question of whether long-term intake of high dietary fiber as consumed by certain individuals is a risk factor for osteoporosis remains unanswered. The evidence of an undesirable effect of fiber on calcium balance merits concern in view of the current trend encouraging greater fiber intake.

In a recent study Recker and associates studied the calcium absorbability from milk products, an imitation milk, and calcium carbonate.[54] The calcium in these products was labeled with radioactive calcium and administered as a series of test meals to 10 healthy postmenopausal women. The mean absorption values for all six sources were tightly clustered between 21 and 26 percent, and none was significantly different from the others using one-way analysis of variance. The authors concluded that none of the sources was significantly superior or inferior to the other.

EXERCISE

An interesting and puzzling cause of osteoporosis is immobilization. Normal, functioning osteoblasts require stimulation, such as that provided the skeletal tissues by muscle pull.[55] Like muscle, bone becomes stronger as greater demands are placed upon it. When subjected to inactivity and immobilization, there is a decrease in bone density and strength.[56-58]

Human data on the affects of immobilization are limited to astronauts, patients with paralytic disease, and normal volunteers on bed rest. Donaldson and co-workers studied three males, ages 21 to 22 years, who underwent 30 and 36 weeks of bed rest.[58] Data obtained during bed rest were compared with those of 3-week ambulatory periods before and after. In addition to calculating mineral content of the diets by standard tables, analysis of the diet was obtained during the study by preparing aliquots of the foods eaten and analyzing them for calcium content. All subjects consumed a mean value of 908 mg of calcium daily. Bone min-

also significantly lower in the amenorrheic group compared to eumenorrheic runners ($p < .01$). The dietary intake of the two groups were similar and there was no difference in calcium intake, either through diet alone or through diet plus supplements in either group. Both groups exceeded the current recommended dietary allowance of 800 mg per day. Because Drinkwater and associates found no difference in bone mass in the radius among the two groups, but significant difference in bone mineral content in the vertebrae among amenorrheic and eumenorrheic runners, they recommend that a site having a high proportion of trabecular bone, such as the lumbar vertebrae, be included in an evaluation of the effect of diminished estrogen stimulation on the bone mineral content of amenorrheic athletes.

Linnell et al evaluated bone mineral content and menstrual regularity in 10 amenorrheic runners, 12 runners with regular menstrual cycles, and 15 nonathletic women with regular menstrual cycles.[65] Twenty-nine of 37 subjects submitted 4-day diet records that were evaluated for daily consumption of calcium and phosphorus using a computer program based on the USDA Nutrient Handbook 8. Six of the subjects submitted 7-day records that were analyzed using a similar program. Two subjects chose not to complete the diet records. Bone mineral content was measured at two sites and was determined by direct photon absorptiometry using a Norland Digital Bone Densitometer. There were no significant differences among the three groups in bone density at either the wrist or the forearm measuring site ($p < .05$). However, a significant relationship was noted between bone mineral content and body fatness in the amenorrheic runners ($r = 0.77$). Within the amenorrheic sample, the five thinnest runners had significantly lower mean trabecular bone mineral content values than the five runners with higher relative body fatness ($p < .05$). There was no significant difference in calcium or phosphorus intake or in the calcium to phosphorus ratio among the three groups of subjects. Linnell and co-workers concluded that amenorrhea, independent of body composition, was not related to reduced bone mineral content in female runners.[65] However, the combination of excessive thinness and amenorrhea may predispose female athletes to lose bone mass.

Marcus and associates designed a study to determine whether severe exercise training might reduce or even reverse deleterious skeletal effects of athletic amenorrhea.[66] Subjects were recruited from a university track team and running organizations in Northern California. Female athletes were included in the study if they were able to run a marathon within 3 hours and ran at least 65 km per week. Seventeen women satisfied the criteria. Six subjects had regular menstrual cycles (11 to 12 periods per year with no interruption since menarche), and 11 were classified as amenorrheic (no periods for 1 to 7 years mean $\pm$ SEM 4.5 years). Spinal density as determined by CT in the amenorrheic runners was lower than that found in the regularly menstruating runners and also lower than in age-matched nonathletic controls. However, the amenorrheic runners had a higher spinal density than runners with secondary amenorrhea of similar duration, but whose exercise was not so severe.[63] Three-day dietary records showed unexpectedly low caloric intake in both groups of runners. In addition, 50 percent of the regularly menstruating subjects consumed less than two-thirds of the RDA for calcium. These researchers concluded that "high-mileage" athletes are able to exercise sufficiently to make up in part for the deleterious skeletal effects of amenorrhea, and that female athletes who train to the degree that menstrual function is compromised should increase calcium consumption to 1,500 mg per day.

In a recent study Nelson and associates evaluated the relationship of diet, exercise, and menstrual status to bone mineral content of female athletes.[67] Eleven athletes were classified as amenorrheic, and 17, as having regular menstrual cycles. Lumbar bone mineral density was measured by dual photon absorptiometry and was found to be significantly lower ($p < .02$) in the amenorrheic athletes. Circulating estradiol was also significantly lower in these athletes. Data from the dietary histories suggested that the amenorrheic women consumed inadequate calories. However, dietary intake for calcium was similar for both groups and on average was higher than the US RDA of 800 mg per day. No correlation was found between calcium consumption and bone mineral content of the lumbar spine. The researchers stated that the low estrogen levels and caloric deficit in the amenorrheic athletes could markedly affect calcium metabolism. The authors suggest that amenorrhea in athletes may have a deleterious effect on the mineral content of trabecular bone. In addition, their data suggest that abnormally low reported food intake forms an integral part of this disorder (Table 6–2).

On a positive note, Drinkwater and colleagues studied a group of previously amenorrheic runners who resumed menses and found that vertebral density was markedly increased from previously reported low levels.[68] Nine of the original group of 14 amenorrheic athletes were retested.[64] Seven of the original 14 regained menses within 1 to 10 months of the initial test, two remained amenorrheic, three moved from the area, one did not wish to participate, and one had become pregnant. The two women who remained amenorrheic showed a further decrease in vertebral bone mineral, whereas the seven athletes who regained menses had a significant increase in spinal density of 0.071 g per square centimeter as determined by dual photon densitometry. Six of the seven women reported a decrease in training mileage or activity, and five women reported a weight gain and an increase in calcium consumption. The researchers commented that the reduction in training and/or activity, as well as the increase in body weight, preceded resumption of menses. The authors concluded that resumption of menses was the primary factor responsible for the significant increase in vertebral bone mineral density of the formerly amenorrheic athletes.

CONCLUSION

The influence of exercise on bone mineral content has been well established. People who are physically active, especially in weight-bearing activity, have more bone mass than those with a sedentary lifestyle. The clinical importance of these observations rests with the fact that eliminating or reducing the number of risk factors associated with osteoporosis may offer some protection during the postmenopausal years.

The importance of preventing osteoporosis was addressed in a consensus conference sponsored by the National Institutes of Health.[69] A number of measures for reducing bone loss were suggested, including use of estrogen replacement therapy, and calcium intake for premenopausal women of 1,000 mg per day and for postmenopausal women of 1,500 mg per day. The consensus panel also suggests weight-bearing activity as a strategy for preventing osteoporosis.

In summary, osteoporosis is a major health concern, especially for women. Although the disease has been regarded as an elderly women's problem, young females, especially those

TABLE 6–2 Comparison of Female Athletes' Bone Mass from Various Studies

	Single photon g/cm²		Dual photon g/cm²
	S_1*	S_2†	
Drinkwater			
Amenorrheic	.53 ± .02	.67 ± .02	1.12 ± .04
Regular	.54 ± .01	.67 ± .02	1.30 ± .03
Marcus			
Amenorrheic	—	.694 ± .01	151‡ ± 8
Regular	—	.720 ± .01	182‡ ± 4.9
Nelson			
Amenorrheic	—	.701 ± .022	1.09 ± .022
Regular	—	.708 ± .01	1.196 ± .025
Linnell			
Amenorrheic	.508 ± .08	.707 ± .07	—
Regular	.529 ± .04	.700 ± .06	—

* S_1 = distal radius
† S_2 = radial shaft
‡ mg/cm³

who have had interrupted menstrual function, may be at risk for decreased bone mass. Although there is still much to be discovered about the cause of osteoporosis, three major risk factors have been identified: hormonal status, particularly estrogen deficiency; calcium consumption; and physical activity.

A lack of estrogen appears to play a major role in the development of osteoporosis. In the past, estrogen therapy has been prescribed in an effort to reverse the effects of osteoporosis in the postmenopausal woman. However, the risks and benefits of estrogen therapy must be fully understood by client and health professional. Estrogen therapy for young amenorrheic athletes must be designed to minimize risks caused by long-term estrogen use.

An increasing amount of evidence implicates calcium deficiency as a contributing factor in the development of osteoporosis. Effective calcium intake depends not only on dietary consumption but also on the bioavailability of the calcium ingested. Calcium requirements for humans still continue to be controversial. However, the National Institute of Health has recommended that premenopausal women consume 1,000 mg per day and postmenopausal women consume 1,500 mg per day.

Studies have shown that mechanical stress or weightbearing activities can lead to an increase in bone mass. Contrary to these findings, intense physical training that interrupts menstrual function in young female athletes may lead to a reduction in bone mass. More research is necessary to draw any firm conclusions on the effects of exercise and athletic amenorrhea on osteoporosis. However, it is recommended that these young female athletes consume a nutritionally balanced diet that includes adequate calories and calcium.

REFERENCES

1. Albanese AA. Bone loss: causes, detection, and therapy. Current topics in nutrition and disease. Vol 2. New York: Alan R. Liss, 1977.
2. Horsman A, Kirky PA. The geometric properties of the second metacarpal. Calcif Tiss Res 1972; 10:289–301.
3. Mazess RB, Cameron JR, Sorenson JA. A comparison of radiological methods for determining bone mineral content. Progress in methods of bone mineral measurements. Washington, DC: US Department of Health, Education, and Welfare, Superintendent of Documents, 1970: 455.
4. Heaney RP, Gallagher JC, Johnston CC, et al. Calcium nutrition and bone health in the elderly. Am J Clin Nutr 1982; 36:986–1013.
5. Gonzalez ER. Prolonged amenorrhea from exercise or endocrine disorders linked to premature osteoporosis. Medical World News, JAMA 1982; August: 81–82.
6. Chinn HI. Effects of dietary factors on skeletal integrity in adults; calcium, phosphorus, vitamin D, and protein. Report for FDA contract 223-78-2275. Bethesda, MD: Life Sciences Research Office, FASEB, 1981.
7. Krane SM, Holick MF. Metabolic bone diseases. In: Isselbacher KF, Adams RD, Braunwald E, et al, eds. Harrison's principles of internal medicine. 9th ed. New York: McGraw-Hill, 1980: 1849.
8. Nordin BEC, Gallagher SC, Aaron JE, Horsman A. Postmenopausal osteopenia and osteoporosis. In: Horsman A, ed. Frontiers in hormone research. Vol. 5. Estrogens in the postmenopause. New York: Karger, 1975:131.
9. Hammond CB, Maxson WS. Physiology of the menopause. Current concepts. The Upjohn Company, 1983.
10. Meema S, Meema HE. Menopausal bone loss and estrogen replacement. Isr J Med Sci 1976; 12:601–606.
11. Morgan B. Osteomalacia, renal osteodystrophy, and osteoporosis. Springfield, IL: Charles C Thomas, 1973.
12. Aitken JM, Hart DM, Anderson JB, et al. Osteoporosis after oophorectomy for nonmalignant disease in premenopausal women. Br Med J 1973; 2:325–328.
13. Albright F, Smith PH, Richardson AM. Postmenopausal osteoporosis. JAMA 1941; 22:2465–2474.
14. Heaney RP. A unified concept of osteoporosis. Am J Med 1965; 39:877–880.
15. Meema HE, Bunker ML, Meema S. Loss of compact bone due to menopause. J Obstet Gynecol 1965; 3:333–342.
16. Aitken JM, Hart DM, Lindsay R. Oestrogen replacement therapy for prevention of osteoporosis after oophorectomy. Br Med J 1973; 3:515–526.
17. Lindsay R, Aitken JM, Anderson JB, et al. Long-term prevention of postmenopausal osteoporosis by oestrogen. Lancet 1976; 1:1038–1045.
18. Lindsay R, Hart DM, Maclean A, et al. Bone response to termination of oestrogen treatment. Lancet 1978; 2:1325–1327.
19. Gordan GS, Picchi J, Roof BS. Antifracture efficacy of long-term estrogens for osteoporosis. Trans Assoc Am Phys 1973; 86:326–332.
20. Burch JC, Byrd BF, Vaughn WK. The effects of long-term estrogen administration to women following hysterectomy. Front Hor Res 1975; 3:208–214.
21. Nachtigall LE, Nachtigall RH, Nachtigall RD, Beckman EM. Estrogen replacement therapy: a 10-year prospective study in the relationship to osteoporosis. Obstet Gynecol 1979; 53:277.
22. Albanese AA, Edelson AH, Lorenze EJ, et al. Problems of bone health in elderly: ten year study. J NY State Med Assoc 1975; 75:326–336.
23. Seeman E, Riggs BL. Dietary prevention of bone loss in the elderly. No. 9. Geriatrics 1981; 36:71–79.
24. Goldring SR, Krane SM. Metabolic bone disease: os-

teoporosis and osteomalacia. Disease-a-Month 1981; 27:1–103.
25. Abraham S, Carroll MD, Dresser CM. Dietary intake findings, United States, 1976–80. Hyattsville, MD: National Center Health Statistics, US Department of Human Services Publication No. (PHS) 83-1681, 1980.
26. Nordin BEC. International patterns of osteoporosis. Clin Orthop Rel Res 1966; 45:17–30.
27. Garn SM, Rohmann CG, Wagner B, et al. Population similarities in the onset and rate of adult endosteal bone loss. Clin Orthop Rel Res 1969; 65:51–59.
28. Matkovic V, Kostial K, Simonovic I, et al. Bone status and fracture rates in two regions of Yugoslavia. Am J Clin Nutr 1979; 32:540–548.
29. Recker RR, Saville PD, Heaney RP. Effect of estrogens and calcium carbonate on bone loss in postmenopausal women. Ann Intern Med 1977; 6:649–655.
30. Horsman A, Gallagher JC, Simpson M, Nordin BEC. Prospective trial of oestrogen and calcium in postmenopausal women. Br Med J 1977; 2:789–792.
31. Lee CJ, Lawler OS, Johnson GH. Effects of supplementation of the diets with calcium and calcium-rich foods on bone density of elderly females with osteoporosis. Am J Clin Nutr 1981; 34:819–823.
32. Albanese AA, Lorenze EJ, Edelson AH, et al. Effects of calcium supplements and estrogen replacement therapy on bone loss of postmenopausal women. Nutr Rep Int 1981; 24:409.
33. Smith EL, Reddan W, Smith PE. Physical activity and calcium modalities for bone mineral increase in aged women. Med Sci Sports Exerc 1981; 13:60–64.
34. Krook L. Dietary calcium-phosphorus and lameness in the horse. Cornell Vet 1968; 58:59–73.
35. Krishnara GVG, Draper HH. Influence of dietary phosphate on bone resorption in senescent mice. J Nutr 1972; 102:1143–1145.
36. Draper HH, Sie T, Bergan JG. Osteoporosis in aging rats induced by high phosphorus diets. J Nutr 1972; 102:1133–1141.
37. LaFlamme GH, Jowsey J. Bone and soft tissue changes with oral phosphate supplements. J Clin Invest 1972; 51:2834–2840.
38. Jowsey J, Balasubramaniam P. Effect of phosphate supplements on soft-tissue calcification and bone turnover. Clin Sci 1972; 42:289–299.
39. DeLuca HF, Castillo L, Jee W, et al. Studies on high phosphate diets. Food Research Institute Annual Report. Madison, WI: University of Wisconsin, 1976: 394.
40. Heaney RP, Recker RP. Effects of nitrogen, phosphorus, and caffeine on calcium balance in women. J Lab Clin Med 1982; 99:46–55.
41. National Research Council, Food and Nutrition Board, National Academy of Sciences. Recommended dietary allowances. Washington, DC: 1980.
42. Zemel MB, Linkswiler HM. Calcium metabolism in the young adult male as affected by level and form of phosphorus intake and level of calcium intake. J Nutr 1981; 111:315–324.
43. Massey LK, Strang MM. Soft drink consumption, phosphorus intake, and osteoporosis. J Am Diet Assoc 1982; 80:581–583.
44. Linkswiler HM, Joyce CL, Anand CR. Calcium retention of young adult males as affected by level of protein and of calcium intake. Trans NY Acad Sci 1974; 36:333–340.
45. Margen S, Chu JY, Kaufman NA, Calloway DH. Studies in calcium metabolism. I. The calciuretic effect of dietary protein. Am J Clin Nutr 1974; 27:584–589.
46. Wachman A, Bernstein DS. Diet and osteoporosis. Lancet 1968; 1:958–959.
47. Ellis FR, Holesh S, Ellis JW. Incidence of osteoporosis in vegetarians and omnivores. Am J Clin Nutr 1972; 25:555–558.
48. Ellis FR, Holesh S, Sanders TAB. Osteoporosis in British vegetarians and omnivores. Am J Clin Nutr 1974; 27:721–722.
49. Parfitt AM, Gallagher JC, Heaney RP, et al. Vitamin D and bone health in the elderly. Am J Clin Nutr 1982; 36:1014.
50. DeLuca HF. The vitamin D system in the regulation of calcium and phosphorus metabolism. Nutr Rev 1979; 37:161–193.
51. Kelsay JL, Behall KM, Prather ES. Effect of fiber from fruits and vegetables on metabolic responses of human subjects. II. Calcium, magnesium, iron, and silicon balances. Am J Clin Nutr 1979; 32:1876–1880.
52. McCance RA, Widdowson EM. Mineral metabolism on dephytinized bread. J Physiol (Lond) 1942; 101:304–313.
53. Johnston FA, McMillian TJ, Falconer GD. Calcium retained by young women before and after adding spinach to the diet. J Am Diet Assoc 1952; 28:933–938.
54. Recker RR, Bamm AR, Barger-Lux MJ, Heaney RP. Calcium absorbability from milk products, an imitation milk, and calcium carbonate. Am J Clin Nutr 1988; 47:93–99.
55. Spencer H. Osteoporosis: goals of therapy. Hosp Pract 1982; 2:133–148.
56. Birkhead ND, Blizzard JJ, Daly JW, et al. Cardiodynamics and metabolic effects of prolonged bed rest. AMR-TDR-63-47. Wright Patterson Air Force Base, 1963.
57. Deitrick JE, Whedon GD, Schorr E. Effects of immobilization upon various metabolic and physiologic functions of normal man. JAMA 1948; 4:3–36.
58. Donaldson CL, Hulley SB, Vogel JM, et al. Effects of prolonged bed rest on bone mineral. Metabolism 1970; 19:1071–1084.
59. Vogel JM, Whittle MW. Bone mineral content changes in skylab astronauts. AJR 1976; 126:96–97.
60. Aloia JF, Cohn SH, Ostuni JA, et al. Prevention of involutional bone loss by exercise. Ann Intern Med 1978; 89:356–358.
61. Williams JA, Wagner J, Wasnich R, Heilbrun L. The effect of long-distance running upon appendicular bone mineral content. Med Sci Sports Exerc 1984; 3:223–227.
62. Emiola L, O'Shea JP. Effects of physical activity and nutrition on bone density measured by radiographic techniques. Nutr Rep Int 1978; 6:668–681.
63. Cann CE, Martin MC, Genant HK, Jaffe RB. Decreased spinal mineral content in amenorrheic women. JAMA 1984; 5:626–629.
64. Drinkwater BL, Nilson K, Chesnut CH, et al. Bone mineral content of amenorrheic and eumenorrheic athletes. N Engl J Med 1984; 5:180–277.
65. Linnell SL, Stager JM, Blue PW, et al. Bone mineral

content and menstrual regularity in female runners. Med Sci Sports Exerc 1984; 4:343–348.
66. Marcus R, Cann C, Madvig P, et al. Menstrual function and bone mass in elite distance runners. Ann Intern Med 1985; 102:158–163.
67. Nelson ME, Fisher EC, Catsos PD, et al. Diet and bone status in amenorrheic runners. Am J Clin Nutr 1986; 43:910–916.
68. Drinkwater BL, Nilson K, Ott S, Chestnut CH. Bone mineral density after resumption of menses in amenorrheic athletes. JAMA 1986; 256:380–382.
69. Osteoporosis: consensus conference. JAMA 1984; 252:799–802.
70. Cann CE, Genant HK, Ettinger B, Cordon GS. Spinal mineral loss in oophorectomized women. JAMA 1980; 244:2056–2059.
71. Cann CE, Martin MC, Genant HK, Jaffe RB. Decreased spinal mineral content in amenorrheic women. JAMA 1984; 5:626–629.

Chapter 7
Effect of Exercise on the Digestive System

BRUCE J. MARTIN

Exercise has an unusual history. In the developed world today it has achieved a popular acceptance as an adjunct to mental and physical health that would have flabbergasted our great-grandparents. In earlier years in America, exercise was viewed as a pernicious necessity, evidence that one struggled in the lower classes, where unremitting toil left scant physical resources for indulgence in pleasure. To move from the scandalously overworked women and children of the early industrial age to the aerobic fitness classes of today is to undergo an attitudinal revolution: from exercise as a cause of disease to a means of preventing disease.

These views of exercise and health are of course primarily cultural, often shifting without sufficient scientific evidence. Exercise consequently is one branch of medical science that typically lags behind public opinion; when the cultural votes are in, proclaiming exercise a panacea, scientists may still be fumbling for a first proof of efficacy.

Despite the prevailing cultural myth and willingly voiced opinions on the subject, there is in fact very little known about how exercise influences the digestive system. The purpose of this chapter is to describe what we do know. However, because so much remains unknown in this field, considerable attention is also paid to what we need to know. The following are the major reasons why the effects of exercise on the gastrointestinal tract are so poorly understood:

1. The gastrointestinal tract remains an area of low public perception and interest.[1] Perhaps this stems from taboos against discussion of many aspects of gastrointestinal function in American society today.[1]
2. Development of suitable techniques for measuring digestive system variables has been slow. The inaccessibility of the gastrointestinal tract makes it resistant to study. For example, contrast the difficulty of measuring flow of air in the respiratory tract, which requires merely a mouthpiece and bag, and measuring flow of liquid in the gastrointestinal tract, which requires a complex and invasive intubation.[2]
3. Researchers have long assumed that changes occurring in the digestive tract during exercise are minor compared with the full-blown responses of the cardiovascular, respiratory, and musculoskeletal systems. Contributing to this perception was the notion that exercise, with its clear-cut sympathetic activation of the heart, was simultaneously minimizing digestive activity

through parallel shifts in autonomic control.[3] Actually, this remains a complex area for further study.

With these caveats in mind, let us now consider in sequence how exercise influences function of each portion of the digestive system.

SALIVARY SECRETION

No one has ever studied the effects of acute or chronic exercise on the volume or composition of saliva. Because parasympathetic nerves innervate salivary glands and control their output, any shift from parasympathetic to sympathetic autonomic dominance would decrease saliva production in exercise. This could be one factor in the obvious behavioral phenomenon that humans always choose to eat when at rest. Another factor contributing to the difficulty of food ingestion during work is the hyperpnea that intensifies as exercise severity increases. Because swallowing inhibits respiration and chewing involves some blockage of the upper airway, both become intolerable as ventilatory demands intensify. The competition between respiration and the chewing and swallowing stages of food assimilation is apparent in patients with emphysema, who show oxygen desaturation of arterial blood hemoglobin while eating.[4]

GASTROESOPHAGEAL REFLUX

Does exercise provoke gastroesophageal reflux? A preliminary study arrives at that conclusion, at least for susceptible individuals, although the data as presented cannot satisfactorily establish the role of exercise.[5] At least 20 percent of patients with demonstrated reflux list exercise as the major precipitator.[6] If exercise does cause reflux, most likely after a meal and in a sensitive person, it would contribute both to esophagitis and to chest pains often confused with those of cardiac origin. This last effect, though apparently fairly rare, would obviously confound interpretation of treadmill exercise tests for the presence of coronary artery disease.[6]

The mechanism by which exercise might cause reflux remains unknown. Most episodes are related to relaxation of the lower esophageal sphincter, which in humans is under both myogenic and cholinergic vagal neural control.[7-9] If exercise, through either hormonal or neural changes, reduces lower esophageal sphincter tone, the way is clear for enhanced backflow of gastric contents. In addition, the increased inspiratory and expiratory muscle activity that generates hyperpnea in exercise greatly widens abdominal and intragastric pressure swings, once again in proportion to exercise intensity.[10] These higher pressures obviously promote reflux of gastric contents into the esophagus and must be countered by rising lower esophageal sphincter pressure. In fact, there is evidence that increased gastric pressure, generated by phase-III fasting gastric contractions, reflexively increases lower esophageal sphincter tone.[11] Increases in intra-abdominal pressure may leave sphincter tone unaltered;[12] this point remains controversial. Although we do not know if the high intra-abdominal and intragastric pressures that are phasically developed as a by-product of hyperpnea in heavy work elevate sphincter pressure, sphincter pressure is greater immediately after 2 hours of work at 50 percent of $\dot{V}O_2$max than in preexercise readings.[13]

There is little information about the influence of exercise on esophageal motility. One preliminary study found that proximal and mid-esophageal peristalsis continued unabated throughout short-term graded exercise to exhaustion, whereas distal esophageal peristalsis was blunted in some and abolished in most subjects.[14] Although 2 minutes of subsequent rest restored active waves in most persons, one subject revealed an absence of distal esophageal peristaltic activity for more than 15 minutes after exercise. How these effects are mediated, and their functional significance, remain unclear.

GASTRIC EMPTYING

The question of how exercise alters rates of gastric emptying of liquid is, obviously, critically important for endurance athletes, for workers in the heat, and perhaps for trauma victims, whose stress may be analogous to that caused by exercise. Consequently, this question has received persistent attention. William Beaumont noted 150 years ago "that mild exercise hastened, and severe exercise slowed, gastric emptying,"[15] and this viewpoint to some extent persists today. The 1920s and 1930s saw several fluoroscopic studies of emptying time: some found no effect, others a slowing or hastening, depending upon which exercise intensity was used.[16,17] These early studies are understandably hampered by small samples for analysis, the nonphysiologic nature of the barium meals utilized, and poor control of exercise intensity and duration.[16,17] A study of mice showed that the first quarter-hour of moderate exercise accelerated gastric emptying, although milder work or longer durations obscured the effect.[18] None of these studies can replace direct measurements on humans, utilizing removal at fixed intervals of gastric residue after oral feeding.[19] The most widely quoted study in this area used these techniques to show that cycle ergometer exercise at intensities up to and including 60 percent $\dot{V}O_2$max did not change gastric emptying rate of a glucose meal.[19] At 70, 80, and 90 percent $\dot{V}O_2$max (each sustained for 15 minutes after fluid ingestion), gastric residue increased such that emptying rate fell by half between 60 percent and 90 percent of $\dot{V}O_2$max. The sample size of 15 subjects was sufficient to firmly establish this conclusion. Prolonged work at 70 percent of $\dot{V}O_2$max for 2 hours showed equivalent gastric emptying rates throughout, although the small sample of three subjects leaves this question unresolved.[19] As the authors themselves note in discussing these results, the presence of a gastric residue says nothing directly about gastric emptying, because that residue represents a balance between fluid secretion into the stomach, fluid absorption from the stomach, and fluid passage into the duodenum. Without a nonabsorbable marker included with the ingestate, the source of the gastric residue is unknown.

Confirmation of the retarding by heavy exercise of gastric emptying comes from a study during exercise at 71 percent of $\dot{V}O_2$max that followed ingestion of 750 mL of tap water. In four subjects, measurably more water (perhaps 50 to 100 mL) was present after 1 hour of exercise than at rest. This volume included both the immediate gastric aspirate and a correction for a nonabsorbable marker, so that the small additional H_2O volume present in the stomach probably represents a real difference.[20] Another study used both gastric aspirates and dilution of a phenol red marker to determine gastric emptying, and showed in four of six subjects that 20 minutes of work at the highest load selected (750 kpm per minute on a bicycle ergometer) retarded gastric emptying.[21] On the other hand, others have found identical emptying rates of a polyethylene glycol marker added to a 560 kcal, mixed, blenderized meal after 2 hours of work at 60 percent $\dot{V}O_2$max.[22] However, by waiting 2 hours, the stomach was virtually empty; perhaps an earlier exercise effect was missed.

In summary, the available evidence suggests that gastric emptying of liquids is slowed when exercise is severe. This effect is naturally less evident after the first hour of exercise when gastric residue is very small. There are no data to indicate, at any exercise intensity or duration, an acceleration in gastric emptying, at least in humans, although this apparently does occur in mice.

What is the mechanism by which exercise slows gastric emptying? It is possible that, analogous to cardiovascular control in work, exercise simply causes extrinsic parasympathetic nervous system withdrawal and hence diminishes gastric motility. However, it is not at all clear that the autonomic nerves behave this way. Part of the confusion about the autonomic nervous system response to exercise concerns the relationship of exercise to the classic "fight or flight" response described by Cannon and de la Paz.[23] That response, a fear or anxiety reaction, involves a generalized sympathetic discharge, apparent in any innervated organ.[24] Exercise is involved in both "fight" and "flight" and consequently can clearly take place (and may well be facilitated) by fear or anxiety. In modern life, such exercise vividly occurs in athletic competition, which mixes maximal exercise with intense emotional arousal, and in forced labor in which external demands may add powerful feelings of fear or hostility to heavy or prolonged physical tasks. Although these reactions are certainly common, it is also true that much if not most exercise is performed by persons in placid psychological states. Here, presumably, a generalized sympathetic discharge is replaced by one tuned to those organ systems critical to maintenance of homeostasis during work.

My hypothesis, then, is that central neural control of the gastrointestinal tract is altered both by exercise per se and by the emotional context of that exercise. This notion, although straightforward, has not been systematically studied. We simply do not know how much exercise alters extrinsic nervous system control of the digestive system, even when it is devoid of fear or anxiety. Also, because stimulation of adrenal medullary catecholamine release and spillover from activated adrenergic nerves cause circulating epinephrine and norepinephrine levels to soar when exercise is severe or prolonged, this hormonal and neuroendocrine effect could dwarf extrinsic nerve influences.[25] Finally, we come full circle: central neural control of the gastrointestinal tract may be insignificant compared with local myogenic and neurogenic activity, particularly in the fed state, so that an exercise effect on central control may be relatively unimportant anyway.[26]

Although the importance of local controls of gastric emptying cannot be denied, these factors remain complex, confusing, and very difficult to interpret even at rest, so their consideration in exercise is largely speculative. Two possibilities emerge. First, exercise could conceivably alter intestinal feedback inhibition of gastric emptying. This inhibition is accomplished by sensory receptors in the proximal bowel that respond to acid, fat, glucose, and various other osmolytes.[27] The inhibition appears to be load dependent, with the amount, not the concentration, of nutrient entering the small bowel determining the gastric emptying rate.[28] Does heavy exercise alter sensory thresholds or enhance feedback signals at a given nutrient load? Because most of the available evidence suggests that neural, not hormonal, mechanisms (they are abolished by truncal vagotomy) mediate the inhibition, exercise would have to act by directly altering an enterogastric reflex.[29] Second, exercise could reduce the gastric emptying rate by a hormonal mechanism. Although hormones obviously influence gastric motility, the overall importance of hormonal regulation or, even more, the impact of a single agent is anybody's guess.[27] Adding to the confusion is the fact that a single hormone that stimulates contractility (e.g., gastrin at the antrum) may paradoxically retard gastric emptying.[27,30,31] We do know that exercise elevates serum gastrin, which should slow emptying, and it dramatically elevates vasoactive intestinal peptide, somatostatin, secretin, and glucagon, all of which lower intragastric pressure.[22,27,32-35]

GASTRIC ACID SECRETION

Slowing gastric emptying during heavy exercise prolongs stomach distention in the fed state and should powerfully stimulate acid secretion in that situation. It is consequently surprising that no study finds increased gastric acid secretion during work, and some even record decreases. One series of studies that found either unchanged or reduced acid output during heavy exercise may be flawed by using gastric aspiration without correcting for recovery of a nonabsorbable marker.[36-39] Incomplete aspiration or variable amounts of ingestate entering the duodenum would introduce error. These authors interpret reduced acid output as a consequence both of water and electrolyte depletion (an unlikely occurrence unless work is prolonged in the heat) and of reduced gastric mucosal blood flow, a possibility that remains controversial. Two other studies have used recovery of nonabsorbable markers to correct volumes obtained through aspiration and to show contrasting results. One found a sizable fall in acid output, in rough proportion to exercise intensity, that reached a near 50 percent decline after 20 minutes of the heaviest work.[21] This was in spite of slowed stomach emptying at this work intensity. The other study found no hint of changed acid production throughout 2 hours of cycle ergometer exercise at 60 percent $\dot{V}O_2$max following ingestion of a solid meal.[22] These last experiments, employing polyethylene glycol as a nonabsorbable marker for gastric aspirates taken after exercise, used in-vivo gastric titration to pH 5 to determine acid secretion rate during the work. Although in-vivo titration yields higher acid secretion values than aspiration, probably because it distends the stomach, it should not introduce error when used identically at rest and in exercise.[40] In keeping with the notion that single hormonal levels can yield confusing information in whole-animal studies, serum gastrin was elevated by exercise without a consequent acid output increase.[22]

EXERCISE AND PEPTIC ULCER

The relationship between regular physical activity and the incidence of ulcer disease is unknown. We do not know how chronic exercise or intense physical training alters any of the variables thought to contribute to gastric or duodenal ulcer. These include gastric mucosal blood flow, the amount and nature of mucus production, long-term gastric acid output, and emotional stress. On this last point, our culture now insists that exercise be taken in regular doses to reduce stress: presumably either the physical or psychological benefits of exercise allow the rage or humiliation provoked by various life events to be ameliorated. This entire concept, although attractive, remains unproven.

At the same time, the concept of stress ulcer is established in humans, as induced by trauma, sepsis, serious illness, or burn injury, and the role of exercise as stress in this sense is not clear. For rats exercising in cages, such a definition may be apt. There is an extensive literature devoted to the topic of activity-stress ulcers in rats.[41-45] When rats are housed in regular cages and allowed to feed 1 hour each day, they do not develop gastric lesions. However, if they are housed in a cage modified to allow running, those that do choose to run develop gastric ulcers in proportion to total energy expended.[44,45] It is unclear whether the ulcers are produced by the stress associated with the exercise, because other stressful manipulations such as immobilization or electric shock also produce them, or whether they result from energy expenditure during work.[44,46,47] If the cause is energy expenditure, the available data do not allow discrimination between activity per se and a relative starvation incurred over several active days, because food intake in the active rats was not quantified and starvation by itself causes gastric mucosal erosion in rats.[43,44]

Can a human get an activity-stress ulcer? As before, we must separate exercise from its emotional framework and answer that in some instances exercise may indeed take place in a milieu of extreme psychological arousal. Nonetheless, it remains sheer speculation that exercise could in this way provoke a stress ulcer. If high-energy expenditure per se can cause the lesion, it is surprising that not even an anecdote about the phenomenon is available in the voluminous literature on highly trained athletes.

GASTROINTESTINAL TRACT BLOOD FLOW DURING EXERCISE

Reference has already been made to gastric mucosal blood flow, and as we peruse the scanty information that we possess concerning exercise and the small and large bowel, similar questions about blood flow control in those organs will arise.

What is the functional significance for motility or, perhaps most important, for absorption of nutrients that any change in blood flow might have? Blood flow at the absorptive site, the villi of the small intestine, is in general directly related to absorption at that site.[48-50] However, of the two—blood flow and absorption—it is not clear which is cause and which is effect, and in fact this may vary under differing laboratory or in-vivo conditions. For our purposes, it is critical to realize that absorptive site blood flow (that is, in the small intestine, villous blood flow) is only one of four parallel flows to muscularis, submucosa, and crypts, as well as to villi. This means that measurements of overall gut blood flow or even of total flow to a single organ are too nonspecific for confident conclusions about effects on absorptive site blood flow. There is no generally accepted technique for measuring blood flow at the absorptive site, so even the basic relationship between villous blood flow and absorption is not well understood.[49] A further stricture on interpretation of the research we are about to consider is that luminal nutrients rapidly increase gut blood flow by as much as 100 percent, so fed and fasted states may have radically different physiology.[49] Finally, there is the cautionary evidence obtained from regional sympathetic nerve stimulation in anesthetized cats.[51] In those experiments, arterial blood pressure rose (as it does in exercise), and overall splanchnic blood flow decreased (as it does in exercise). However, these changes were associated with increased, not decreased, net water reabsorption from the gut.[51] This paradox indicates again how complex the relationship between flow and absorption can be, and it should dissuade us from forming firm conclusions about the physiologic impact of any blood flow change that may occur in exercise.

Gut blood flow studies during exercise have been made in both humans and dogs. Although dogs offer both sufficient size for flow measurement and a willingness to run, they nonetheless may not be ideal for quantitative modeling of human cardiovascular dynamics.

Four dog studies of acute exercise of less than 5 minutes' duration found that superior mesenteric arterial flow was unaltered by exercise.[52-55] Electromagnetic flow meter and radioactive microsphere data are alike in this respect. The hyperemia in the postcibal state was unaltered as well, so that mesenteric arterial flow was much greater during postfeeding exercise than it was at rest before meal ingestion.[52] In all of these acute experiments, exercise was mild; cardiac output rose from rest by about 80 percent. Longer-term mild exercise for as much as 2 hours also failed to alter intestinal blood flow.[56]

Only one study has been devoted to organ-specific flow measurements during exercise. Exercise required 75 percent of the maximal heart rate, and microsphere injections were made during a relatively steady-state portion of that exercise and at exhaustion. Although flows varied widely from organ to organ, gastric fundic, pyloric, duodenal, ileal, pancreatic, hepatic, and colonic flows all were reduced during steady-state exercise.[57] Oddly, decreased flow seen during steady-state work was absent at exhaustion, so that flow at rest and at exhaustion were identical. The most convenient explanation for greater splanchnic vasoconstriction in this particular study, as compared to those discussed earlier, was the more severe level of exercise employed: cardiac output increased 300 percent above control versus an 80 percent increase in the more acute studies. However, at exhaustion cardiac output was increased 400 percent relative to control, yet splanchnic blood flow was equal to that at rest. One possible, albeit entirely speculative, explanation is that sympathetically mediated vasoconstriction dominates in moderate work and is counterbalanced in severe exercise by the vasodilatory influence of epinephrine from the adrenal medulla.[58]

The necessity of separating exercise from emotional arousal, as mentioned earlier, is brought home forcefully in a study of baboons.[59] Both exercise and excitement (induced by washing the cage) doubled heart rate and increased blood pressure, but whereas exercise only marginally altered mesenteric arterial flow, excitement decreased that flow by over 50 percent and increased mesenteric vascular resistance ten-fold.[59] These visceral vascular effects of excitement were equally potent postprandially.[59]

Human studies of blood flow to the gastrointestinal tract during exercise have of course used indirect methods.[60] Using bromosulphalein clearance at the liver, a 1956 study found that recumbent exercise (2½ minutes of leg lifts) reduced estimated splanchnic blood flow by about a third, with splanchnic $\dot{V}O_2$ falling as well.[61] A more definitive study of upright humans, using hepatic clearance of indocyanine green dye, was able to estimate splanchnic flow over the entire range of exercise intensity in 10 young men.[62] Splanchnic blood flow fell in direct proportion to exercise intensity (5 minutes at each intensity), so work at 50 percent $\dot{V}O_2$max reduced flow 30 percent below resting levels, and work at 90 percent $\dot{V}O_2$max reduced it 75 percent below control.[62] These results, if not tainted by systematic error, clearly show that the human splanchnic vasoconstrictive response to exercise is much more pronounced than that of the dog. Because these human results have been amply confirmed by many indirect techniques, there is no reason to suggest that they are invalid.[60,62-66] Instead, one is left to consider why humans and dogs differ so. It may be that dogs simply use less sympathetic nervous system vascular control than humans do, and it has been shown that after compromising cardiac output by heart block, the dog's mesenteric vasoconstriction is sharply increased and resembles that of humans.[60,67,68]

It is physiologic dogma that the mesenteric blood flow changes with exercise are critically important for cardiovascular system control during that exercise.[60] Less well understood is how a meal, particularly a large one, could change mesenteric flow and consequently alter cardiac output, heart rate, or blood pressure in subsequent exercise. Ingestion of 1,000 kcal 20 minutes before mild supine exercise slightly elevated exercise heart rate without changing oxygen uptake or cardiac output.[69,70] The frequent question of how an immediately prior large meal alters cardiovascular responses to severe exercise has never been investigated.

SMALL INTESTINAL MOTILITY, TRANSIT, AND ABSORPTION DURING EXERCISE

Because of its relative inaccessibility, the small intestine—its motility, rates of material transit, or absorption—has been little studied in exercise. Direct measures of intestinal motility are difficult to make and more difficult to interpret. Adding exercise compounds the difficulty. A single preliminary study of motility in exercise exists at this time. Dogs instrumented with jejunal electrodes had intestinal myoelectrical activity recorded during mild (30 percent of the heart rate reserve) and heavy (70 percent of heart rate reserve) exercise. The dogs were fed, then exercised, and although jejunal slow waves were equally frequent before, during, and after exercise, spike bursts were less frequent when work was hard. At the same time, the duration of each spike burst was longer, suggesting that jejunal contractions during exercise are less frequent but more forceful.[71]

It is of course unclear how such changes might alter movement or absorption of material in the small intestine. Myoelectrical activity or motility and actual flow of contents in the small intestine are obviously related, but the relationship is quite complex.[72] During the fed state, flow can vary by an entire order of magnitude while motility patterns appear identical.[2]

Rates of movement of material in the small intestine can be measured with several techniques, all of which offer some interpretative difficulties. The two that have been used in exercise involve tracer substances. Hence, what is actually measured is tracer movement, not movement of food that may accompany tracer ingestion.[72] In one study, after 10 people ingested beads labeled with ^{99}Te, radioactivity over the stomach and colon was monitored to determine proportional loss and accumulation, respectively.[73] This technique allowed study of movement of the entire tracer. The 5-hour postprandial period involved seated rest, intermittent walking, or a mixture of strenuous cycling and walking. Although there was no further documentation of exercise levels, obviously these procedures produced wide differences in metabolic rate. Neither level of activity altered gastric emptying or colonic accumulation of radiolabeled material.[73] Another study of small-bowel transit measured hydrogen (H_2) production after ingestion of a nonabsorbable carbohydrate marker that was mixed into a solid meal.[74] This technique allows detection of the first portion of marker that arrives at the cecum; however, mean transit cannot be quantified. In seven subjects, intermittent heavy exercise failed to change transit time of the marker from mouth to large intestine.[74] In contrast, when nonabsorbable carbohydrate was mixed into a liquid meal and ingested during exercise at 30 percent $\dot{V}O_2$max, exercise accelerated transit by nearly 25 percent.[75] Clearly, much more needs to be done in this area before the exercise–transit relationship is understood.

Although rapid transit can cause malabsorption, there is no absolute correlation between the two, so linking them is not always justified.[76,77] Consequently, assumptions that unchanged transit means unaltered absorption may not be valid. So little is known about intestinal absorption in exercise that the field is essentially open. A 1967 study has been regarded by many as definitive: a triple-lumen catheter was placed in the small bowel in five persons, and glucose, urea, xylose, and tritiated water absorption were compared in exercise (71 percent $\dot{V}O_2$max) and rest.[20] The finding that tritiated water (N = 2), urea (N = 2), xylose (N = 5), and glucose (N = 4) absorption rates in the jejunum were unchanged by exercise has been extensively quoted and, of course, may well be correct.[20] However, this study has been placed in question for more than its small sample size, because it is now known that the catheter itself markedly alters small intestinal motility and transit rates.[78]

One indirect study of sugar absorption in six soldiers found that mild exercise in a hot environment halved 5-hour urinary 3-0-methylglucose output and reduced blood levels of this nonmetabolizable sugar as well.[79] Because urinary output and blood levels of xylose were unaffected, the authors suggest that active, but not passive, carbohydrate transport is impaired during exercise.[79] Although provocative, these findings are confounded by numerous interpretative difficulties, including the unmeasured influence of exercise on both peripheral metabolism and renal clearance of these sugars.

In rats, 1 to 3 weeks of exercise leads to decreased lysine and alanine transport across a segment of intestine in vitro.[80] The mechanism of this change is completely unknown. This isolated result highlights our minimal knowledge of how training might influence intestinal absorption, which I discuss more fully in the section on colonic function in exercise.

PANCREATIC SECRETION DURING EXERCISE

Pancreatic enzyme and bicarbonate secretion has been classically thought to be under three phases of control: cephalic, gastric, and intestinal.[81] The exact brain centers that mediate the cephalic phase (which integrates the sight, smell, and taste of food) are unknown.[81] It is an intriguing possibility that exercise influences this integration, but this area has not been studied. The gastric and intestinal phases of pancreatic secretory control include stimulation of pancreatic exocrine secretion by the presence of duodenal acid (when pH falls below 4.5), amino acids, and emulsified or micellar fatty acids.[82-84] If exercise decreases gastric acid production rate or the rate of gastric emptying, the pH, amino acid, and fatty acid intraduodenal stimulus to pancreatic secretion ought to be reduced, especially in severe exercise. Surprisingly, the two extant studies of exercise pancreatic secretion find decreased bicarbonate and fluid output even in response to a fixed duodenal acid, meat meal, or secretin stimulus.[85,86] In dogs, this depression by exercise was profound and persisted during a subsequent rest period.[85]

Does depression of pancreatic secretion occur in humans during exercise? Is any depression that might occur severe enough to provoke maldigestion or malabsorption of ingested food?

In this area, as in so many others, we are left with only fragmentary, limited evidence concerning the phenomenon of an exercise effect, no information at all about mechanisms, and only our own speculations about functional significance. Clearly, if exercise does diminish pancreatic secretion in response to a fixed duodenal signal, then it must alter the mediation of this stimulus. This could occur hormonally (through secretin or cholecystokinin), neurally by changing vagovagal reflexes, or by other, more obscure neural or paracrine factors.[81] The direct neural effect remains, as we have seen, an open possibility. The traditional hormonal influences are more problematic, because prolonged mild exercise causes peripheral plasma secretin levels to rise, not fall, to 20 times the control level after 3 hours of exercise.[34] Finally, predictably, we know nothing of how exercise might alter paracrine influences on the pancreas.

BILIARY SECRETION DURING EXERCISE

Can acute or chronic exercise in either healthy or diseased persons ever change bile secretion enough to alter absorption of dietary fat? Can exercise change rates of formation of cholesterol or pigment gallstones? These questions have never been thoroughly studied and cannot yet be answered. The one study we do have says simply that acute exercise by a dog does not change volume or composition of bile output;[85] other preliminary work suggests that, after exercise in rats, bile flow and acid output are reduced.[87] Another important unknown is the relationship between exercise and regulation of the plasma cholesterol and the lipoprotein or lipid profile. Most studies agree that regular physical activity protects against coronary artery disease, in part by augmenting high-density lipoprotein (HDL) cholesterol without changing total circulating cholesterol.[88,89] This last effect is presumably mediated at the level of skeletal muscle and adipose tissue.[90] We have no idea whether exercise can change cholesterol excretion, either as fecal sterols or fecal bile acids.[91]

Two studies have measured changes during exercise in a number of hormones or candidate hormones that are purportedly important for regulation of the gastrointestinal tract. The results are intriguing. Besides elevating secretin, as previously noted, 3 hours of work at 40 percent $\dot{V}O_2$max produces huge increments in peripheral plasma vasoactive intestinal peptide (VIP), pancreatic polypeptide (PP), and somatostatin levels.[34] In another study, a 30-km run by seven trained athletes elevated their peripheral plasma motilin, gastrin, VIP, and PP concentrations.[35] These changes took place in concert with the established hormonal changes induced by heavy or prolonged work: decreased insulin, elevated epinephrine and norepinephrine, and increased glucagon. Interpretative problems with these results come in three layers. First, we do not know whether peripheral plasma levels are a meaningful reflection of what is happening at the organ of interest. Second, we do not know the importance, for gastrointestinal function, of a change in concentration of a single hormone, much less the aggregate influence of numerous hormonal changes, some of which may excite, while others inhibit, at any single site. Third, even if an integrated hormonal influence could be totaled, we do not know the overall importance of this aspect of gastrointestinal regulation.[27,72]

EXERCISE AND THE COLON

Several aspects of colonic function in exercise have enormous basic biological as well as clinical significance. First mention here goes to the question of colonic (as well as small intestinal) adaptation to chronic exercise. It is clear that several mammalian species respond to increased energy demands by increasing small and large intestinal mass.[92] These adaptations permit absorption and fermentation of greater amounts of food, so that either the volume or the extraction of calories from ingesta increases to meet energy demand.[92-94] Can similar processes occur in humans? Apparently our own evolution has, over millennia, reduced our colon size and increased small intestinal length in response to a diet maximizing food value per meal.[93,94] Does radically increasing our caloric needs through prolonged daily exercise also influence our gut morphology? We know that some organ systems and processes (e.g., capillarization of skeletal muscle, endurance of heart muscle, bone density, sweat rate, strength of tendons) show remarkable adaptation to training, whereas others (e.g., lung capillary transit time, elasticity of lung tissue) apparently cannot adapt despite high demands imposed by exercise. We know little of the stresses (although we know caloric intake must rise as much as four-fold above sedentary levels), and nothing of the adaptation, that may take place either at the microscopic or gross level in the gut with physical training. Nevertheless, both transport processes and mucosal mass can adapt to numerous stimuli, notably surgical resection and lactation.[95,96] Finally, gastrin has been proposed to regulate adaptation, to be responsible for mucosal growth in both colon and duodenum, such that its action as a growth factor may be more important than its immediate impact upon digestive function.[95,97] An acute period of exercise increases circulating gastrin; can chronic exercise cause a serum gastrin rise large enough and persistent enough to act as a growth factor in humans?

Constipation, some scientists say, is alleviated by regular exercise.[98] Although this notion is embedded in popular thinking to the extent that many gastroenterologists recommend regular exercise for their constipated patients, the role of exercise has, in fact, never been studied. Because as much as 10 percent of the American population qualifies as constipated in some surveys, this is a question with very broad applicability.[99]

Unfortunately, there is minimal understanding, even in healthy persons, of the relationship of exercise to large bowel residence time or whole-gut transit. In one study using radioactive markers to examine colonic movement of material, subjects who were "somatically active" showed more propulsive movements than did those who lay still.[100] Myriad other uncontrolled variables preclude interpretation of this as an indictment of inactivity. Three other more relevant studies, two of them preliminary, measured whole-gut transit of radiopaque pellets or of dyes and found conflicting results: several weeks of moderate daily exercise on a diet fixed in fiber content normalized whole-gut transit time to an intermediate value in one study, accelerated transit in the second study, and had no effect in the third.[101-103] No doubt the last word on this topic has yet to be written!

Gastrointestinal secretory function during physical exercise. Acta Physiol Pol 1975; 25:215–219.
37. Markiewicz K, Cholewa M, Gorski L. Maximal gastric secretion during exertion and restitution. Acta Med Pol 1978; 19:479–484.
38. Markiewicz K, Lukin M. Reserpine effect on gastric secretion during exercise and restitution in healthy subjects. Acta Physiol Pol 1982; 33:209–214.
39. Markiewicz K, Lukin M, Jazdzewski B, Cholewa M. Furosemide effect on gastric basal secretion during exercise and postexercise restitution in healthy subjects. Acta Physiol Pol 1982; 33:295–303.
40. Feldman M. Comparison of acid secretion rates measured by gastric aspiration and by *in vivo* intragastric titration in healthy human subjects. Gastroenterology 1979; 76:954–957.
41. Dairman WM, Juhasz L. A study in mice of benzodiazepine–anticholinergic interaction: protection against restraint-immersion and forced exertion induced gastric mucosal erosion. Pharmacology 1978; 17:104–112.
42. Paré WP. Oral nicotine ingestion and incidence of activity-stress ulcer in the rat. Biochemical Med 1975; 14:51–56.
43. Paré WP, Houser VP. Activity and food-restriction effects on gastric glandular lesions in the rat: the activity-stress ulcer. Bull Psychon Soc 1973; 2:213–214.
44. Paré WP. The influence of food consumption and running activity on the activity-stress ulcer in the rat. Dig Dis 1975; 20:262–273.
45. Robert A, Northam JI, Nezamis JE, Phillips JP. Exertion ulcers in the rat. Dig Dis 1970; 15:497–507.
46. Brodie DA, Hanson HM. A study of the factors involved in the production of gastric ulcer by the restraint technique. Gastroenterology 1960; 38:353–360.
47. Caul WF, Buchanan DC, Hays RC. Effects of unpredictability of shock on incidence of gastric lesions and heart rate in immobilized rats. Physiol Behav 1972; 8:669–672.
48. Donowitz M, Wicklein D, Reynolds DG, et al. Effect of altered intestinal water transport on rabbit ileal blood flow. Am J Physiol 1979; 236:E482–E487.
49. Mailman D. Relationships between intestinal absorption and hemodynamics. Annu Rev Physiol 1982; 44:43–55.
50. Winne G. Influence of blood flow on intestinal absorption of drugs and nutrients. J Pharmacol Ther 1979; 6:333–393.
51. Brunsson I, Eklund S, Jodal M, et al. The effect of vasodilation and sympathetic nerve activation on net water absorption in the cat's small intestine. Acta Physiol Scand 1979; 106:61–68.
52. Burns GP, Schenk WG. Effect of digestion and exercise on intestinal blood flow and cardiac output. Arch Surg 1969; 98:790–794.
53. Fronek K, Fronek A. Combined effect of exercise and digestion on hemodynamics in conscious dogs. Am J Physiol 1970; 218:555–559.
54. Pannier JL, Leusen I. Regional blood flow in response to exercise in conscious dogs. Eur J Appl Physiol 1977; 36:255–265.
55. Vatner SF, Higgins CB, Millard RW, Franklin D. Role of the spleen in the peripheral vascular response to severe exercise in untethered dogs. Cardiovasc Res 1974; 8:276–282.
56. Bülow J, Tøndevold E. Blood flow in different adipose tissue depots during prolonged exercise in dogs. Pflugers Arch 1982; 392:235–238.
57. Sanders TM, Werner RA, Bloor CM. Visceral blood flow distribution during exercise to exhaustion in conscious dogs. J Appl Physiol 1976; 40:927–931.
58. Greenway CV, Lawson AE. The effects of adrenaline and noradrenaline on venous return and regional blood flow in the anesthetized cat with special reference to intestinal blood flow. J Physiol (Lond) 1966; 186:579–595.
59. Vatner SF. Effects of exercise and excitement on mesenteric and renal hemodynamics in conscious, unrestrained baboons. Am J Physiol 1978; 234:H210–H214.
60. Rowell LB. Human cardiovascular adjustments to exercise and thermal stress. Physiol Rev 1974; 54:75–159.
61. Wade OL, Combes B, Childs AW, et al. The effect of exercise on the splanchnic blood flow and splanchnic blood volume in normal man. Clin Sci 1956; 15:457–463.
62. Rowell LB, Blackmon JR, Bruce RA. Indocyanine green clearance and estimated hepatic blood flow during mild to maximal exercise in upright man. J Clin Invest 1964; 43:1677–1690.
63. Clausen JP, Trap-Jensen J. Effects of training on the distribution of cardiac output in patients with coronary artery disease. Circulation 1970; 42:611–624.
64. Hultman E. Studies on muscle metabolism of glycogen and active phosphate in man with special reference to exercise and diet. Scand J Clin Lab Invest 1967; 19 (Suppl 94):1–63.
65. Rowell LB, Blackmon JR, Martin RH, et al. Hepatic clearance of indocyanine green in man under thermal and exercise stresses. J Appl Physiol 1965; 20:384–394.
66. Rowell LB, Murray JA, Brengelman GL, Kraning KK. Human cardiovascular adjustments to rapid changes in skin temperature during exercise. Circ Res 1969; 24:711–724.
67. Scher AM, Ohm WW, Bumgarner K, et al. Sympathetic and parasympathetic control of heart rate in the dog, baboon, and man. Fed Proc 1972; 31:1219–1225.
68. Vatner SF, Higgins CB, White S, et al. The peripheral vascular response to severe exercise in untethered dogs before and after complete heart block. J Clin Invest 1971; 50:1950–1960.
69. Chou CC. Splanchnic and overall cardiovascular hemodynamics during eating and digestion. Fed Proc 1983; 42:1658–1661.
70. Jones WB, Thomas HD, Reeves TJ. Circulatory and ventilatory responses to postprandial exercise. Am Heart J 1965; 69:668–676.
71. Kenney MJ, Flatt A, Summers RW, Gisolfi CV. Intestinal motility changes in fed dogs with exercise. Fed Proc 1986; 45:1045 (abstr).
72. Weisbrodt NW. Motility of the small intestine. In: Johnson LR, ed. Physiology of the gastrointestinal tract,

Vol 1. 2nd ed. New York: Raven Press, 1987:631.
73. Ollerenshaw KJ, Norman S, Wilson CG, Hardy JG. Exercise and small intestinal transit. Nucl Med Commun 1987; 8:105–110.
74. Cammack J, Read NW, Cann PA, et al. Effect of prolonged exercise on the passage of a solid meal through the stomach and small intestine. Gut 1982; 23:957–961.
75. Keeling WF, Martin BJ. Gastrointestinal transit during mild exercise. J Appl Physiol 1987; 63:978–981.
76. Cann PA, Read NW, Brown C, et al. Irritable bowel syndrome: relationship of disorders in the transit of a single solid meal to symptom patterns. Gut 1983; 24:405–411.
77. Krejs GJ. Effect of somatostatin and atropine infusion on intestinal transit time and fructose absorption in the perfused human jejunum. Diabetes 1984; 33:548–551.
78. Read NW, Al-Janabi MN, Bates TE, Barber DC. Effect of gastrointestinal intubation on the passage of a solid meal through the stomach and small intestine in humans. Gastroenterology 1983; 84:1568–1572.
79. Williams JH, Mager M, Jacobson ED. Relationship of mesenteric blood flow to intestinal absorption of carbohydrates. J Lab Clin Med 1964; 63:853–863.
80. Dugas MC, Hazelwood RL, Lawrence AL. Influences of pregnancy and/or exercise on intestinal transport of amino acids in rats. Proc Soc Exp Biol Med 1970; 135:127–131.
81. Soloman TE. Control of exocrine pancreatic secretion. In: Johnson LR, ed. Physiology of the gastrointestinal tract, Vol 2. 2nd ed. New York: Raven Press, 1987:1173.
82. Meyer JH, Way LW, Grossman MI. Pancreatic bicarbonate response to various acids in the duodenum of the dog. Am J Physiol 1970; 219:964–970.
83. Go VLW, Hoffman AF, Summerskill WHJ. Pancreozymin bioassay in man based on pancreatic enzyme secretion: potency of specific amino acids and other digestive products. J Clin Invest 1970; 49:1558–1564.
84. Meyer JH, Jones RS. Canine pancreatic responses to intestinally perfused fat and products of fat digestion. Am J Physiol 1974; 226:1178–1187.
85. Konturek SJ, Tasler J, Obtulowicz W. Effect of exercise on gastrointestinal secretions. J Appl Physiol 1973; 34:324–328.
86. Kuznetsov AP. Effect of muscular exercise on gastric and pancreatic secretory function. Fiziol Cheloveka 1983; 9:946–955.
87. Gimmon Z, Kelley RE, Simko V. Exercise affects bile flow and total bile acid output in rats. Gastroenterology 1981; 80:1156 (abstr).
88. Powell KE, Thompson PD, Casperson CJ, Kendrick JS. Physical activity and the incidence of coronary heart disease. Annu Rev Public Health 1987; 8:253–287.
89. Seals DR, Allen WK, Hurley BF, et al. Elevated high-density lipoprotein cholesterol levels in older endurance athletes. Am J Cardiol 1984; 54:390–393.
90. Wood PD, Haskell WL. The effect of exercise on plasma high density lipoproteins. Lipids 1979; 14:417–427.
91. Rigott NA, Thomas GS, Leaf A. Exercise and coronary heart disease. Annu Rev Med 1983; 34:391–412.
92. Gross JE, Wang Z, Wunder BA. Effects of food quality and energy needs: changes in gut morphology and capacity of *Microtus ochrogaster*. J Mamm 1985; 66:661–667.
93. Milton K. Digestive physiology in primates. News in Physiological Sciences 1986; 1:76–79.
94. Milton K. Food choice and digestive strategies of two sympatric primate species. Am Nat 1981; 117:496–505.
95. Johnson LR. Regulation of gastrointestinal growth. In: Johnson LR, ed. Physiology of the gastrointestinal tract. 2nd ed. New York: Raven Press, 1987:301.
96. Fell BF, Smith KA, Campbell RM. Hypertrophic and hyperplastic changes in the alimentary canal of the lactating rat. J Pathol Bacteriol 1963; 85:179–188.
97. Johnson LR, Aures D, Yuen L. Pentagastrin-induced stimulation of protein synthesis in the gastrointestinal tract. Am J Physiol 1969; 217:151–154.
98. Jones FA, Gummer JWP, Lennard-Jones JE. Clinical gastroenterology. 2nd ed. Oxford: Blackwell, 1968:69.
99. Thompson WG, Heaton KW. Functional bowel disorders in apparently healthy people. Gastroenterology 1980; 83:529–534.
100. Holdstock DJ, Misiewicz JJ, Smith T, Rowland EN. Propulsion (mass movements) in the human colon and its relationship to meals and somatic activity. Gut 1970; 11:91–99.
101. Harrison RJ, Leeds AR, Bolster NR, Judd PA. Exercise and wheat bran: effect on whole gut transit. Proc Nutr Soc 1980; 39:22A (abstr).
102. Cordain L, Latin RW, Behnke JJ. The effects of an aerobic running program on bowel transit time. J Sports Med 1986; 26:101–104.
103. Bingham SA, Cummings JH. The effect of exercise on large intestinal function. Gastroenterology 1987; 92:1317 (abstr).
104. Vena JE, Graham S, Zielezny M, et al. Lifetime occupational exercise and colon cancer. Am J Epidemiol 1985; 122:357–365.
105. Garabrant DH, Peters JM, Mack TM. Job activity and colon cancer risk. Am J Epidemiol 1984; 119:1005–1014.
106. Winawer SJ, Sherlock P. Malignant neoplasms of the small and large intestine. In: Sleisenger MH, Fordtran JS, eds. Gastrointestinal disease. Philadelphia: WB Saunders, 1983:1220.
107. Schrumpf E, Gjone E. Physical activity and the gastrointestinal tract. Scand J Soc Med 1981; Suppl 29:69–70.
108. Lorber SH. Exercise medicine: physiological principles and clinical application. New York: Academic Press, 1983:279.
109. Sullivan SN. The effect of running on the gastrointestinal tract. J Clin Gastroenterol 1984; 6:461–465.
110. Worobetz LJ, Gerrard DF. Gastrointestinal symptoms during exercise in Enduro athletes: prevalence and speculations on the aetiology. N Z Med J 1985; 98:644–646.
111. Sharman IM. Gastrointestinal disturbances in runners. Br J Sports Med 1982; 16:179.
112. Fogoros RN. Gastrointestinal disturbance in runners.

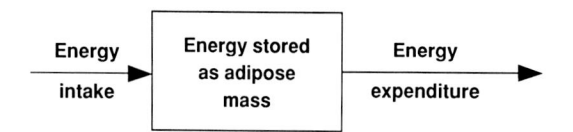

Figure 8–1 Energy balance equation. The change in stored energy is related to the net difference between energy intake and expenditure.

per day) with the same results.[3] These studies were followed, in 1967, by the work of Miller and Mumford, who discovered that pigs fed a very low protein diet would overeat to maintain an adequate protein intake, and that they would waste the excess energy they consumed as heat, thus not gaining as much weight as predicted.[4] The now classic Vermont study by Sims and colleagues similarly demonstrated that certain normal-weight prisoners had tremendous difficulty gaining weight, despite conscious overeating (up to 10,000 kcal per day).[5] In contrast, as is discussed further below, a significant reduction in caloric intake is associated with a fall in overall energy expenditure that might work to resist any hoped-for weight loss. Together these studies provide evidence that energy expenditure can be regulated (up and down) by intake and must be considered an important variable in the energy balance equation. The role that exercise may play in regulating energy expenditure is described more fully below. However, first we present the evidence that reduced exercise-associated energy expenditure is an important determinant of obesity.

ACTIVITY, ENERGY EXPENDITURE, AND THE DEVELOPMENT OF OBESITY

There are several lines of reasoning leading to the conclusion that lower levels of exercise energy expenditure may be important in the pathophysiology of at least some types of obesity in modern humans. Large epidemiologic surveys agree that caloric intake is not greater, and may be less, in the obese than in normal-weight persons.[6] As reviewed by Brownell and Stunkard, there is somewhat conflicting evidence about whether obese children are less active than their normal-weight counterparts, but most studies agree that obese adults are less active.[7] One such study noted that obese adults were more likely to use an escalator than to walk up stairs.[8] In this study, simply putting up a sign encouraging the use of steps had a significant positive impact on this behavior; removal of the sign was quickly followed by the return to greater escalator use. However, just because obese adults are less active, it cannot necessarily be inferred that they in fact expend less energy, because the energy expenditure to complete a given task is greater with increased body weight.[9] Although this is especially true of weightbearing exercise, even nonweightbearing exercise expenditure (i.e., bicycling) may be increased because of the need to move heavier limbs.[10] The distribution of excess adiposity may also affect the energy required merely for postural stability. This increase in energy expended for a given task in the obese is caused by increased work and should not be misunderstood to be secondary to a reduction in true muscular work efficiency. There appears to be little variation among individuals in the energy required to perform a given known unit of muscular work.[11,12] At this time no studies have measured total daily energy expenditure in a free-living environment to determine whether there is a difference between obese and normal-weight subjects that might account for the obesity. A new technique for measuring energy expenditure over a 2-week period by using doubly labeled water ($H^2H^1O^{18}$) is now being evaluated for this purpose and may in the near future shed light on this important question.[13]

EFFECT OF EXERCISE ON BODY WEIGHT AND ADIPOSITY

The effect of spontaneous or enforced exercise on body weight in rats has been studied extensively.[14] Most of these studies demonstrate a lower final body weight or a reduction in adiposity in the chronically exercised animals. However, there is considerable variability in the findings, depending on the sex of the animals (weight loss is more consistent in males) and the species studied (little effect noted in genetically obese animals). A meta-analysis of 13 studies in humans (on a total of 37 separate groups), evaluating the effects of aerobic exercise on body weight, found a mean decrement in weight of .11 to .30 lbs per week, depending on the individual group studied.[6] This weight reduction, although meager compared to the weight loss frequently associated with severe caloric restriction, is nonetheless deceiving, because the changes in body composition are quite different when dietary weight loss and exercise training are compared. In one recent study, 12 male subjects on a 1,200-kcal mixed weight reduction diet for 3 months lost 13.1 kg of weight but only 9.5 kg of fat (28 percent of the weight loss was as fat-free mass).[15] A well-matched group of 14 male subjects participated in a 3-month supervised aerobic exercise program (at 70 to 85 percent of their heart rate reserve) three times per week, with no conscious change in their dietary intake. The exercise group lost only 2.8 kg of body weight but lost 3.5 kg of fat mass and had a small (.7 kg) increment in fat-free mass. Thus, the absolute weight lost during an aerobic exercise program underestimates the true loss of fat because of the accretion of even small amounts of relatively heavy fat-free mass.

Although most studies in normal-weight subjects have been able to detect significant reductions in body fat after an aerobic exercise program, the same may not be true in all subgroups of obese subjects.[16,17] Several attempts have been made to try to classify the heterogeneous population of obese patients better. One of the more helpful and widely used classification systems divides obese patients into subgroups according to their number of fat cells. The most common group, the "hypertrophic obese," have an enlarged mean fat cell size but a normal number of total body fat cells. Hypertrophic obesity is most often moderate in severity (less than 200 percent ideal body weight—IBW), is of adult onset, and is associated with a central distribution of excess adiposity (middle-age spread). The less common "hyperplastic obese" have both an enlarged mean fat cell size and a tremendous increase in total fat cell number (four to ten times normal). Typically, these hyperplastic obese patients have a juvenile onset of their obesity (often but not necessarily before puberty) and a generalized distribution of the excess adiposity. The severity of obesity is also greater in the hyperplastic obese (greater than 180 percent IBW).

The massive, hyperplastic obese have been noted to lose little or even to gain fat with exercise, despite improving their maximum aerobic capacity and their metabolic status.[18] The reasons for the difference in the effect of exercise training in this group are not clear. It has been suggested that the potential for fat loss is limited by a minimum attainable fat cell size. When very active men are studied, the variation in mean fat cell size among subjects is very small despite considerable differences in total body fat.[19] This concept is further supported by a recent study in which ex-obese long distance runners with 14.3 percent body fat were found to have a smaller mean fat cell size than a group of endurance athletes with only 9.5 percent body fat who had no previous history of obesity.[20] Thus, at some minimum fat cell size, the total amount of body fat seemed to depend mainly on the total number of fat cells. In any case, most obese patients do not suffer from massive hyperplastic obesity and thus should significantly reduce their fat mass with aerobic exercise training.

Recent studies show that the distribution of fat may be as or more important metabolically than the total amount of fat. Moderately obese subjects with an upper body or central distribution of body fat not only have a greater number of medical complications associated with their obesity, but also seem to respond with more fat loss and subsequent medical benefit after exercise training.[21,22] This upper body distribution of fat is the most common type of obesity occurring in adult males and is also seen in some adult females.

Other variables may also play a prominent role in determining the body fat response to exercise training. These include intensity, duration, frequency of exercise, and starting weight. As might be expected, those subjects with the highest starting weights have been found to lose the most weight during an exercise training program.[6] A review of exercise studies found that significant weight loss required an exercise frequency of three or more sessions a week, and that weight loss was directly related to the number of calories expended during exercise.[6] In addition, it appears that an exercise duration of 30 or more minutes per day is more likely to be associated with significant weight loss.[17] Low intensity, long duration exercise might be expected to be favorable for fat loss, because

generally accounts for approximately 20 percent of total daily energy expenditure, but it can increase greatly in persons doing heavy exercise for long durations either as recreation or at work.

Recently, investigators have found another curious form of energy expenditure that most properly fits as part of the thermic effect of exercise despite the fact that no useful work is accomplished. This is the energy expended "fidgeting" while a subject is ostensibly at rest.[28] This spontaneous fidgeting activity varied widely in the subjects studied, accounting for between 100 and 800 kcal a day. There is preliminary evidence that fidgeting is a familial trait.

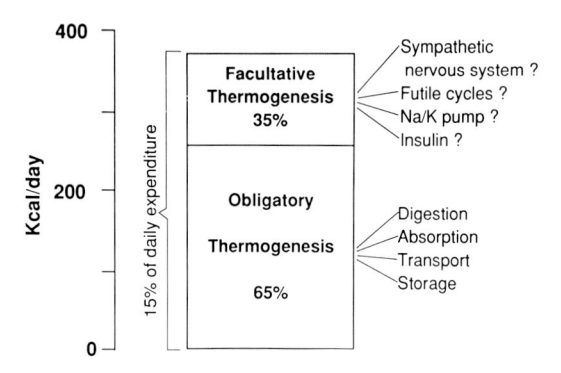

Figure 8-4 Sub-components of the thermic effect of feeding in man and the major determinants of each.

Thermic Effect of Feeding

The thermic effect of feeding is defined as the energy expenditure above resting metabolic rate that occurs following the ingestion of a meal. The exact duration of this effect is unknown, but it has been shown that energy expenditure remains elevated above resting levels for at least 6 hours after the ingestion of food.[29] Despite the fact that the thermic effect of feeding accounts for only 10 to 15 percent of daily energy expenditure, it is of great interest because it varies greatly depending upon the characteristics of the individual. Although there is some disagreement, investigators have demonstrated that the thermic effect of feeding is reduced with age, obesity, and in patients with diabetes mellitus.[30] The thermic effect of feeding also varies with the composition of the diet, being greater after carbohydrate or protein consumption than after consumption of fat.[29] Because the thermic effect of feeding increases when more calories are consumed, it is best expressed as a percentage of calories ingested.

The thermic effect of feeding can be further partitioned into "obligatory" and "facultative" components (Fig. 8-4). The obligatory component accounts for about 66 percent of the thermic effect of feeding and represents the energy expended digesting, absorbing, transporting, and storing the substrates ingested.[31] The exact amount of the obligatory component varies depending on what is eaten, as well as on the metabolic state and storage needs of the individual. Flatt estimates that 23 percent of the caloric value of carbohydrate is utilized for obligatory thermogenesis if carbohydrate is converted to triglyceride (de-novo lipogenesis) and then stored as fat. However, de-novo lipogenesis is felt to occur seldom under normal circumstances in humans, and thus fat that is stored generally comes from fat consumed in the diet.[32] Carbohydrate can also be stored as glycogen at a cost of only 7 percent or may be utilized "on-line" as glucose at a cost of only 5 percent. Fat can be stored as triglyceride in adipose tissue quite efficiently, with an obligatory energy cost of only 3 percent. Because of the high energy costs of protein synthesis, gluconeogenesis, and ureogenesis, the obligatory thermogenesis following ingestion of protein is higher than the other substrates at 25 percent.

The facultative component accounts for only 33 percent of the thermic effect of feeding or 5 percent of total daily energy expenditure.[31] This expenditure of energy produces no work and is felt to be accounted for by metabolic inefficiency caused by loose coupling or uncoupling of oxidative phosphorylation, or by stimulation of inefficient or "futile cycles."[33] An example of uncoupling exists in brown adipose tissue in small mammals, where a specific uncoupling protein disrupts the normal proton conductance pathway in mitochondria.[34] Uncoupling in brown adipose tissue is initiated by sympathetic nervous system stimulation brought on by either cold exposure or overfeeding. The existence of brown adipose tissue in humans is controversial. Huttunen and colleagues found indirect evidence of its existence in adult lumberjacks who were chronically exposed to cold temperatures at work.[35] Furthermore, the uncoupling protein, felt to be specific to functional brown adipose tissue, has been detected by two groups in the adipose tissue of adult humans.[36,37] Newsholme suggests that the "futile" cycling of substrates may not be futile at all.[38] He argues that increasing the rate of bidirectional cycling of substrates through important reactions might increase sensitivity and decrease the response time to a given stimulation. It would in some ways be analogous to revving the engine in a race car in preparation for a starting signal.

EFFECT OF EXERCISE ON THE COMPONENTS OF DAILY ENERGY EXPENDITURE

As alluded to above, the potential increase in energy expenditure due to exercise is greater than can be accounted for merely by the thermic effect of exercise. One well-known effect of exercise training is the accretion of additional fat-free mass (muscle mass). Because fat-free mass accounts for 85 percent of the variance in resting metabolic rate, the increase in fat-free mass associated with training should also be associated with an increment in resting metabolic rate.[28] Although the percentage increase might be small, any increment in this largest component of daily energy expenditure can have significant impact over time. Recent studies demonstrate tremendous variation in the resting metabolic rate response to training, with high and low responders.[39] The reasons for the difference between the groups is not fully understood, but it may be at least partly inherited.[39]

A single bout of exercise may also acutely effect resting metabolic rate. This carry-over effect of acute exercise has usually been found following very strenuous exercise, and it may last for many hours. Bielinski and associates found that resting metabolic rate was increased by almost 5 percent even 18 hours after a 3-hour exercise session at 50 percent of maximal aerobic capacity.[40] This finding has been supported by Devlin and Horton, who found a similar increment in resting metabolic rate more than 12 hours after intermittent exercise to exhaustion at 85 percent of maximal aerobic capacity.[41] The morning after exercise, basal glucose oxidation was reduced, and increases were noted in both lipid oxidation and nonoxidative glucose disposal (glycogen storage). Other groups have failed to find a significant sustained increase in resting metabolic rate following a single bout of exercise.[42,43]

The effect of exercise on the thermic effect of feeding has been studied extensively in animals. Studies in several species have found an increase in the thermic effect of feeding in exercise-trained animals when compared to sedentary controls.[44,45] Studies in humans have been less consistent. In cross-sectional studies, Davis and co-workers found that the thermic effect of feeding was significantly related to maximal aerobic capacity in young subjects.[46] Later, Lundholm and associates also noted that the thermic effect of feeding was 56 percent higher in elderly trained men than in sedentary controls.[47] Acute intense exercise was found to increase the thermic effect of a 100-g glucose meal (given 2 hours later) more than two-fold, when compared to the same meal on a sedentary day.[48] However, others have found that the thermic effect of feeding was actually reduced in trained subjects.[49,50] Studies supporting an enhanced thermic effect of feeding with exercise training point to an increase in the facultative component, with the potential explanation being a heightened sensitivity to catecholamines. Studies that find the thermic effect of feeding reduced after exercise training suggest that reduction is due to both reduced catecholamine responses to the meal and lessened obligatory expenditure as glucose is efficiently used to replace depleted glycogen stores. It is likely that differences in the intensity of training, composition of the meal, and timing of the studies after the last training session may all be important factors in explaining these discrepancies.

Recent studies in humans have noted a synergistic effect of exercising after a meal on the thermic effect of exercise. Segal and Gutin noted an additional increment in exercise energy expenditure when exercise followed a meal.[51] They also demonstrated that this additional energy expenditure was significantly greater in lean subjects than in obese subjects. Thus, there appears to be a defect in the synergistic relationship between eating and exercising in obese subjects. Further studies by Segal and colleagues in subjects of similar relative weights but very different body composition (body builders versus the sedentary obese) found that the increase in the thermic effect of exercise following a meal was greater in the body builders and was related to their greater fat-free mass.[52]

EFFECT OF EXERCISE ON DIETARY WEIGHT LOSS PROGRAMS

One of the unwelcome but well-described consequences of dietary weight loss is a significant reduction in resting metabolic rate.[53,54] The possible reasons for this reduction include a decline in triiodothyronine concentration, a fall in sympathetic nervous system activity as measured by norepinephrine kinetics, and, most importantly, a significant loss of fat-free mass.[15,54–57] As described in one recent study, 28 percent of the total weight lost during 3 months on a 1,200 kcal mixed weight reduction diet was as fat-free mass.[15] These results can be contrasted with a well-matched exercise group that lost only 2.8 kg of total weight but 3.5 kg of fat and had a small (nonsignificant) increase in fat-free mass. Leibel and Hirsch looked at the effect of dietary weight loss on energy expenditure by carefully assessing (in a Clinical Research Center setting) the caloric requirement for weight stability in very obese patients who lost considerable weight through caloric restrictions.[58] They found a 28 percent fall in the required weight stabilization calories (per meter square) after weight reduction. Because the subjects were in caloric balance when the measurements were made, energy expenditure would be equal to energy intake. Although much of the fall in 24-hour energy expenditure may have been caused by a reduction in resting metabolic rate or the thermic effect of feeding, some may also have been secondary to reduced exercise. Others have documented a fall-off of spontaneous activity with caloric restriction, as well as a reduction in the energy cost of a given activity.[54,59] The observed reduction in caloric requirements in the reduced obese patient may be of critical importance in explaining the high recidivism rate in dietary weight loss programs.

Another possible untoward consequence of low calorie diets is their negative impact on exercise capacity. As reviewed by Horton, there is evidence that changes in both the macronutrient as well as the caloric content of the diet can affect exercise performance.[60] Several studies have noted that performance was improved by high-carbohydrate feeding and worsened with a high-fat, low-carbohydrate diet. In one well-controlled study, although time to subjective exhaustion at 65 to 70 percent of maximal aerobic capacity was reduced by 21 percent after 1 week of a very low carbohydrate diet (700 kcal per day), it rebounded to 55 percent above the original baseline after 6 weeks on the diet.[61] This was interpreted as being due to either adaptation to the ketogenic state or less "hobbling" in the weight-reduced state. A follow-up study compared the effect of equicaloric weight reduction diets (800 kcal per day) of either low or moderate carbohydrate content on intermittent high-intensity bicycle exercise time to exhaustion.[62] There was a 50 percent reduction in the muscle glycogen content in the low-carbohydrate group and a similar 50 percent decline in exercise time to exhaustion. Thus, although a low-calorie, low-carbohydrate diet may not greatly affect moderate exercise capacity, it can dramatically reduce muscle glycogen-limited, high-intensity exercise.

Recently studies have compared the effect of diet plus exercise versus diet alone on weight loss and body composition. In one study investigators produced an overall caloric deficit of 500 kcal per day, in three groups of middle-aged women, by: (1) a 500 kcal per day dietary restriction, (2) a 500 kcal per day increase in exercise expenditure, or (3) a daily 250 kcal per day restriction in intake coupled with a daily 250 kcal increase in exercise expenditure.[63] After 16 weeks, total weight loss was not different among the three groups, but because the two exercise groups lost less fat-free mass, significantly more of their weight loss was as fat. A similar paradigm was used by Belko and colleagues, who compared a 50 percent reduction in caloric intake to a 25 percent reduction in caloric intake combined with a 25 percent increment in exercise expenditure.[64] After 6 weeks they found a greater total weight reduction in the diet-only group (7.8 versus 5.7 kg) but no difference in the amount of fat loss (5.1 versus 4.7 kg). Thus, a smaller percentage of the lost weight was as fat-free mass (and more as fat) in the group combining diet plus exercise. The ability of exercise to help maintain fat-free mass while on a weight reduction diet was also demonstrated by Pavlou and co-workers.[65] After 8 weeks on an 800 kcal per day diet with or without exercise, there was no significant change in total weight loss between the two groups, but 95 percent of the weight loss in the exercise group was as fat mass, compared to 57 percent in the diet-only group. A study by Bogardus and associates of obese subjects with either type II (noninsulin-dependent) diabetes mellitus or glucose intolerance found no significant differences in total weight or body composition changes after 12 weeks of either a low-calorie diet (450 kcal per day per square meter) alone or a diet in combination with an aerobic exercise program.[66] However, the distribution of fat loss was different, with the exercise group losing more central fat (a significant reduction in the waist-to-hips ratio). This may account for the greater increase in peripheral insulin sensitivity found in the exercise group, as reflected by greater insulin-mediated (nonoxidative) glucose disposal. As noted above, a central distribution of adiposity (high waist-to-hips ratio) is associated with greater obesity-related complications.

OTHER BENEFICIAL METABOLIC EFFECTS OF EXERCISE

Beyond the overwhelming evidence that exercise training is associated with reductions in adiposity in the large majority of obese persons, there are other substantial metabolic benefits to recommend exercise for the obese. Some of the most common metabolic complications of obesity—glucose intolerance, diabetes mellitus, hyperinsulinemia, hypertension, and hyperlipidemia—have all been demonstrated to improve with exercise. Although each of these disorders is important by itself, together their significance is even greater, because they are each major independent risk factors for atherosclerotic cardiovascular disease. In this section, I emphasize the effects of exercise on glucose and insulin homeostasis and on the plasma lipid profile. With respect to treatment of hypertension, aerobic exercise can be used safely as a first step or as adjunctive therapy in subjects with mild hypertension. The reader is referred to several good recent reviews on exercise and hypertension.[67–70]

Glucose and Insulin Homeostasis

The evidence that glucose and insulin homeostasis is improved by exercise is quite impressive and includes animal studies as well as large epidemiologic, retrospective, and prospective studies in humans. In addition, inactivity or detraining have been shown quickly to result in both insulin insensitivity and glucose intolerance.[71]

The improvement in glucose metabolism induced by exercise is not related to increased insulin secretion, because in fact circulating insulin and c-peptide concentrations are both reduced following acute exercise or chronic exercise training.[71] A steady or improved glucose tolerance in the face of a fall in insulin levels (and insulin release by the beta cells) necessitates a state of enhanced insulin sensitivity. The etiology of this improved insulin sensitivity remains obscure. Although some studies find an increase in insulin binding to its receptors after training, others are unable to find any change.[72–74] Loss of adiposity may enhance insulin sensitivity, but fat loss is not necessary for the exercise effect. Improved insulin sensitivity has been demonstrated to occur after exercise training in the absence of measurable losses of fat.[74] The importance of redistribution of fat after exercise training (away from central depots) has not been studied. It is unlikely that an increased aerobic capacity is the critical determinant for enhanced glucose and insulin homeostasis, because these changes have been documented to occur after training despite no increase in maximal aerobic capacity. Improvement in glucose and insulin homeostasis can even occur acutely after a single bout of exercise.[71] In fact, it is unclear whether the improvements in glucose and insulin homeostasis, which are found with long-term exercise, are due to some specific chronic training effect or, as stated earlier, merely to overlapping effects of single bouts of exercise.

Although exercise has been suggested as useful in the treatment of diabetes since the time of the Indian physician Sushruta (600 B.C.) and has long been strongly advocated by many esteemed diabetologists, the scientific evidence of its usefulness in humans has been substantiated only slowly. Even in type II (noninsulin-dependent) diabetes mellitus, in which obesity and insulin resistance are known to play important roles in causing the disease, early studies of the effect of exercise were inconclusive. Studies by Saltin and associates demonstrated a reduction in basal insulin concentration and normalization of oral glucose tolerance in middle-aged men with mild chemical type II diabetes after a 3-month aerobic exercise program.[75] However, the interpretation of this study is clouded because the subjects also received dietary counseling, and it is unclear whether the improvement in glucose tolerance was due solely to training. Ruderman and co-workers aerobically trained six obese middle-aged men with type II diabetes and found a significant fall in basal insulin concentration and a 30 percent improvement in intravenous glucose tolerance but no change in oral glucose tolerance.[76] Bogardus and colleagues was able to show little if any further improvement in glucose tolerance when exercise training was added to a dietary weight loss program in subjects with either type II diabetes or glucose intolerance.[66] However, in each of these negative studies, the interval between the last bout of exercise and the metabolic measurements of glucose tolerance was at least 3 days. It is likely that at least some of the benefit of exercise may be from its acute effects, so the timing of these studies may explain their negative results. More recent studies in which the postexercise training tests were done within 48 hours of the last bout of exercise have demonstrated significant benefits of exercise on several measures of glucose tolerance in type II diabetics, including improved fasting glucose concentrations, lower glycosylated hemoglobin concentrations, and enhancement in both oral and intravenous glucose tolerance, as well as insulin sensitivity.[74,77–79]

Another possible benefit of the improvement in insulin homeostasis following exercise is the reduction in plasma insulin concentration. Several studies now report that insulin concentration is an independent risk factor for atherosclerotic cardiovascular disease.[80] The reduction in fasting and postprandial insulin concentrations associated with exercise may independently improve the atherosclerosis risk profile in obese hyperinsulinemic patients.

Plasma Lipid and Lipoprotein Concentrations

Abnormalities in the plasma lipid profile are very common metabolic concomitants to obesity. The abnormalities that have been consistently described include: elevations in plasma very low-density lipoprotein (VLDL) and triglyceride concentrations, elevations in low-density lipoprotein (LDL) concentrations, reductions in high-density lipoprotein (HDL) concentrations, and elevations in the LDL-to-HDL ratio.[81] Each of these derangements has been demonstrated to be reversed by exercise training, although there is disagreement about whether the effects of exercise are due to some specific training effect or merely to the loss (or redistribution) of adiposity.[15,82]

In cross-sectional studies, aerobic exercise training has been associated with reduced plasma triglyceride concentrations.[83,84] Similar findings have been demonstrated in some but not all prospective longitudinal training studies.[85–88] The triglyceride lowering effect of exercise has been explained by the increase in lipoprotein lipase-mediated removal of triglyceride rich (VLDL) particles.[89] Although total cholesterol concentrations have also been found to be reduced with aerobic exercise training in some studies, this too has been quite variable.[82,87,90] Some of the discrepancy may be explained by the offsetting effects of exercise on HDL and LDL cholesterol. A small but significant fall in LDL cholesterol (the cholesterol most closely associated with atherosclerosis) might be missed because of a concomitant increase in HDL cholesterol (inversely related to atherosclerosis; see below). For this reason a ratio of LDL to HDL cholesterol may be a more sensitive marker of the response to exercise.

Because of the importance of HDL as a protective factor against atherosclerosis, the effects of exercise on these particles have received particular attention.[91] Both cross-sectional and prospective studies have demonstrated an increase in HDL cholesterol concentration after exercise training.[84,88,90,92] This effect has been found less consistently in women, in studies in which the training is not associated with weight loss, and with anaerobic exercise training.[82,93,94] Indeed, weight loss alone can significantly increase HDL cholesterol concentrations in obese subjects, and there is considerable controversy about whether it is training or the loss of adiposity that is responsible for the observed increment in HDL concentration with exercise.[84,88,92] Because the activity of the enzyme lipoprotein lipase is increased after either dietary weight loss or exercise training and this enzyme appears to be an important determinant of HDL concentration, it may play a central role in the HDL response to exercise.[89,95,96] Others have recently postulated that the increase in high-density lipoproteins associated with training is to a great extent secondary to a fall in the catabolic rate of these particles.[97]

Recently, Schwartz compared the effects of either dietary weight loss or aerobic training for 3 months on high-density lipoproteins in young obese men.[88] Both interventions produced significant increases in total HDL cholesterol, but only the exercise subjects demonstrated an increment in the important, less dense HDL_2 subfraction and in the critical structural protein apolipoprotein A–I. A substantial part of the inverse relationship between plasma HDL concentration and the risk of atherosclerosis seems to reside in the HDL_2 subfraction and may depend on the ability of apolipoprotein A–I to activate the enzyme lecithin cholesterol acyl transferase (LCAT), and thereby to initiate the process of reverse cholesterol transport (away from peripheral cells to the liver, where it is excreted in bile). A follow-up study found similar HDL and apolipoprotein A–I changes in a group of elderly subjects who were aerobically trained for 3 months, despite significantly less improvement in maximal aerobic capacity then was achieved by the young subjects.[98] Thus, improvement in cardiovascular fitness, as reflected by maximal aerobic capacity, may not be the most important determinant of the HDL response to training.

COMPLIANCE WITH EXERCISE PROGRAMS

In this chapter I have discussed possible effects that exercise may have as a treatment modality for obesity either alone or in combination with dietary regimens. However, if an exercise program is to be successful in aiding weight loss, sustaining weight loss, or modifying some of the metabolic abnormalities associated with obesity, the exercise must be maintained. There is a great deal of literature substantiating the difficulty that obese individuals have in maintaining weight loss, but much less is known about long-term adherence to exercise programs. Based on the results of even short-term studies, in which more than 50 percent of enrolled subjects dropped out within a few months, adherence to exercise programs also appears quite poor.[99] Interestingly, the results have been little better in secondary prevention trials with post-myocardial infarction patients who might be expected to be quite motivated.[100] The problem of adherence to exercise programs has been recently reviewed in detail.[99] In this review Martin and Dubbert listed the factors most closely related to a high risk for poor compliance as low self-motivation, depression, and anxiety. Behavioral factors that predicted poor compliance include smoking, blue-collar vocational status, and inactive leisure-time pursuits. The most consistent biological factor for poor compliance was obesity. Environmental and social factors have also been found to be good predictors for dropping out of an exercise program. A negative or even neutral attitude toward exercise by the spouse was associated with twice the drop-out rate than when the spouse was described as actively supportive. Major life changes such as family problems or changes in job or residence have also been noted to have a negative impact on adherence to an exercise program. The design of the exercise program can also affect compliance. Subjects prefer to exercise in groups rather than alone. Convenience factors such as location and the availability of parking can be important. High-intensity exercise that produces great fatigue has a negative impact on adherence and may also predispose to injury-related relapses.

There have been relatively few studies that

32,000-Mr uncoupling protein. Biosci Rep 1983; 3:775–780.
37. Lean MEJ, James WPT. Uncoupling protein in human brown adipose tissue mitochrondria. Isolation and detection by specific antisera. FEBS Lett 1983; 163:235–240.
38. Newsholme EA. A possible metabolic basis for the control of body weight. N Engl J Med 1980; 302:400–405.
39. Poehlman ET, Tremblay A, Nadeau A, et al. Heredity and changes in hormones and metabolic rate with short-term training. Am J Physiol 1986; 250:E711–E717.
40. Bielinski R, Schutz Y, Jequier E. Energy metabolism during the postexercise recovery in man. Am J Clin Nutr 1985; 42:69–72.
41. Devlin JT, Horton ES. Glucose metabolism and thermogenesis in lean, obese, and noninsulin-dependent men following exercise. In: Berry EM, Blondheim SH, Eliahou HE, Shafrir E, eds. Recent advances in obesity research: V. London: John Libbey, 1987:365.
42. Tremblay A, Fontaine E, Nadeau A. Contribution of postexercise increment in glucose storage to variations in glucose-induced thermogenesis in endurance athletes. Can J Physiol Pharmacol 1985; 63:1165–1169.
43. Freedman-Akabas S, Colt SE, Kissileff HR, Pi-Sunyer FX. Lack of sustained increase in VO_2 following exercise in fit and unfit subjects. Am J Clin Nutr 1985; 41:545–549.
44. Miller DS, Mumford P, Stock MJ. Gluttony. II. Thermogenesis in overeating man. Am J Clin Nutr 1967; 20:1223–1229.
45. Gleeson M, Brown JF, Waring JJ. The effects of physical exercise on metabolic rate and dietary-induced thermogenesis. Br J Nutr 1982; 42:173–181.
46. Davis JR, Tagliaferro AR, Kertzer R, et al. Variations in dietary-induced thermogenesis and body fatness with aerobic capacity. Eur J Appl Physiol 1983; 50:319–329.
47. Lundholm K, Holm G, Lindmark L, et al. Thermogenic effect of food in physically well trained elderly men. Eur J Appl Physiol 1986; 55:486–492.
48. Ruderman NB, Balon T, Zorzano A, Goodman M. The postexercise state: altered effects of insulin on skeletal muscle and their physiologic relevance. Diabetes Metab Rev 1986; 1:425–444.
49. Tremblay A, Cole J, LeBlanc J. Diminished dietary thermogenesis in exercise-trained human subjects. Eur J Appl Physiol 1983; 52:1–4.
50. LeBlanc J. Thermogenesis in relationship to feeding and exercise training. Int J Obesity 1985; 9(Suppl 2):75–79.
51. Segal KR, Gutin B. Thermic effects of food and exercise in lean and obese women. Metabolism 1983; 32:581–589.
52. Segal KR, Gutin B, Nyman AM, Pi-Sunyer FX. Thermic effect of food at rest, during exercise, and post-exercise in lean and obese men of similar body weight. J Clin Invest 1985; 76:1107–1112.
53. Bray GA. Effect of caloric restriction on energy expenditure in obese patients. Lancet 1969; 2:397–399.
54. Ravussin E, Burnand B, Schutz Y, Jequier E. Energy expenditure before and during energy restriction in obese patients. Am J Clin Nutr 1985; 41:753–759.
55. Danforth E Jr. The role of thyroid hormones and insulin in the regulation of energy metabolism. Am J Clin Nutr 1983; 38:1006–1017.
56. O'Dea K, Esler M, Leonard P, et al. Noradrenaline turnover during under- and overeating in normal weight subjects. Metabolism 1982; 31:896–899.
57. Schwartz RS, Veith RC, Jaeger LF, et al. Effect of aerobic training on norepinephrine kinetics. Clin Res 1985; 33:66A.
58. Leibel RL, Hirsch J. Diminished energy requirements in reduced obese patients. Metabolism 1984; 33:164–170.
59. Gorsky RD, Calloway DH. Activity pattern changes with decreases in food energy intake. Hum Biol 1983; 55:577–586.
60. Horton ES. Metabolic aspects of exercise and weight reduction. Med Sci Sports Exerc 1986; 18:10–18.
61. Phinney SD, Horton ES, Sims EAH, et al. Capacity for moderate exercise in obese subjects after adaptation to a hypocaloric ketogenic diet. J Clin Invest 1980; 66:1152–1161.
62. Bogardus C, LaGrange BM, Horton ES, Sims EAH. Metabolic fuels and the capacity for exercise during low calorie diets with or without carbohydrate. J Clin Invest 1981; 68:399–404.
63. Zuti WB, Golding LA. Comparing diet and exercise as weight reduction tools. Phys Sportsmed 1976; 4:49–53.
64. Belko AZ, Van Loan M, Barbieri TF, Mayclin P. Diet, exercise, weight loss, and energy expenditure in moderately overweight women. Int J Obesity 1987; 11:93–104.
65. Pavlou KN, Steffee WP, Lerman RH, Burrows BA. Effects of dieting and exercise on lean body mass, oxygen uptake and strength. Med Sci Sports Exerc 1985; 17:446–471.
66. Bogardus C, Ravussin E, Robbins DC, et al. Effects of physical training and diet therapy on carbohydrate metabolism in patients with glucose intolerance and noninsulin-dependent diabetes mellitus. Diabetes 1984; 33:311–318.
67. Seals DR, Hagberg JM. The effect of exercise training on human hypertension: a review. Med Sci Sports Exerc 1984; 16:207–215.
68. Tipton CM. Exercise training and hypertension. Exerc Sport Sci Rev 1984; 144:1045–1057.
69. McMahon M, Palmer RM. Exercise and hypertension. Med Clin North Am 1985; 69:57–70.
70. Sims EAH. Exercise and energy balance in the control of obesity and hypertension. In: Horton ES, Terjung R, eds. Exercise, nutrition, and energy balance. New York: Macmillan 1988.
71. Schneider SH, Kang H. Clinical aspects of exercise and diabetes mellitus. In: Winick M, ed. Nutrition and exercise. Current concepts in nutrition. New York: John Wiley & Sons, 1986:145.
72. Soman VR, Koivisto VA, Deibert D, et al. Increased insulin sensitivity and insulin binding to monocytes after physical training. N Engl J Med 1979; 301:1200–1204.
73. Crettaz M, Horton ES, Wardzala LT, et al. Physical

training of Zucker rats: lack of alleviation of muscle insulin resistance. Am J Physiol 1983; 244:E414–E420.
74. Krotkiewski M, Lonnroth P, Mandroukas K, et al. The effects of physical training on insulin secretion and effectiveness and on glucose metabolism in obesity and type 2 (noninsulin-dependent) diabetes mellitus. Diabetologia 1985; 28:881–890.
75. Saltin B, Lindgarde F, Houston M, et al. Physical training and glucose tolerance in middle-aged men with chemical diabetes. Diabetes 1979; 28(Suppl 1):30–32.
76. Ruderman NB, Ganda OP, Johansen K. The effect of physical training on glucose tolerance and plasma lipids in maturity-onset diabetes. Diabetes 1979; 28(Suppl 1):89–92.
77. Trovati M, Carta Q, Cavalot F, et al. Influence of physical training on blood glucose control, glucose tolerance, insulin secretion, and insulin action in noninsulin-dependent diabetic patients. Diabetes Care 1984; 7:416–420.
78. Reitman JS, Vasques B, Klimes I, Nagulesparan M. Improvement of glucose homeostasis after exercise training in noninsulin-dependent diabetes. Diabetes Care 1984; 7:434–441.
79. Schneider SH, Amorosa LF, Khachadurian AK, Ruderman NB. Studies on the mechanism of improved glucose control during regular exercise in type 2 (noninsulin-dependent) diabetes. Diabetologia 1984; 26:355–360.
80. Stern MP, Haffner SM. Body fat distribution and hyperinsulinemia as risk factors for diabetes and cardiovascular disease. Arteriosclerosis 1986; 6:123–130.
81. Garrison RJ, Wilson PW, Castelli WB, et al. Obesity and lipoprotein cholesterol in the Framingham Offspring study. Metabolism 1980; 29:1053–1060.
82. Goldberg L, Elliot DL. The effect of physical activity on lipid and lipoprotein levels. Med Clin North Am 1985; 69:41–55.
83. Bjorntorp PM, Fahlen G, Grimby A, et al. Carbohydrate and lipid metabolism in middle-aged, physically well-trained men. Metabolism 1972; 21:1037–1044.
84. Wood PD, Haskell WL, Stern MP, et al. Plasma lipoprotein distributions in male and female runners. Ann NY Acad Sci 1977; 301:748–763.
85. Holloszy JO, Skinner JS, Toro G. Effects of a 6-month program of endurance exercise on serum lipids in middle-aged men. Am J Cardiol 1964; 14:753–760.
86. Krotkiewski M, Mandroukas K, Sjostrom L, et al. Effects of long-term physical training on body fat, metabolism, and blood pressure in obesity. Metabolism 1979; 28:650–658.
87. Wood PD, Haskell WL, Blair SN, et al. Increased exercise level and plasma lipoprotein concentrations: a 1-year randomized controlled study in sedentary middle-aged men. Metabolism 1983; 32:31–39.
88. Schwartz RS. The independent effects of dietary weight loss and aerobic training on high density lipoproteins and apolipoprotein A-I concentrations in obese men. Metabolism 1987; 36:165–171.
89. Nikkila EA, Taskinen M-R, Rehunen S, Harkonen M. Lipoprotein lipase activity in adipose tissue and skeletal muscle of runners: relation to serum lipoproteins. Metabolism 1978; 27:1662–1667.
90. Wood PD, Terry R, Haskell WL. Metabolism of substrates: diet, lipoprotein metabolism, and exercise. Fed Proc 1985; 44:358–363.
91. Gordon T, Castelli WP, Hjortland MC, et al. High-density lipoprotein as a protective factor against coronary disease: the Framingham Study. Am J Med 1977; 62:707–714.
92. Hartung GH, Foreyt JP, Mitchell RE, et al. Relation of diet to high-density lipoprotein cholesterol in middle-aged marathon runners, joggers, and inactive men. N Engl J Med 1980; 302:357–361.
93. Vu Tran Z. Differential effects of exercise on serum lipid and lipoprotein levels seen with changes in body weight. JAMA 1985; 254:919–924.
94. Lehtonen A, Viikari J. Serum lipis in soccer and ice hockey players. Metabolism 1980; 29:36–39.
95. Schwartz RS, Brunzell JB. Increase of adipose tissue lipoprotein lipase activity with weight loss. J Clin Invest 1981; 67:1425–1430.
96. Nikkila EA, Taskinen M-R, Kekki M. Relation of plasma high density lipoprotein cholesterol to lipoprotein lipase activity in adipose tissue and skeletal muscle of man. Atherosclerosis 1978; 29:497–501.
97. Herbert PN, Bernier DN, Cullinane EM, et al. High-density lipoprotein metabolism in runners and sedentary men. JAMA 1984; 252:1034–1037.
98. Schwartz RS. The effect of aerobic exercise training on lipid profiles in young and older men. Clin Res 1988; 36:97A.
99. Martin JE, Dubbert PM. Adherence to exercise. Exerc Sport Sci Rev 1985; 13:137–167.
100. Oldridge NB. Compliance and exercise in primary and secondary prevention of coronary heart disease: a review. Prev Med 1982; 11:56–70.
101. Haskell W. Physical activity and health: need to define the required stimulus. Am J Cardiol 1985; 55:4D–9D.

Section III
Musculoskeletal Components

Chapter 9
Skeletal Muscle Physiology

PHILIP D. GOLLNICK
BENGT SALTIN

Skeletal muscles are aggregates of muscle fibers that can be controlled individually or collectively. The multiplicity of movement patterns produced by man in daily life testifies to the intricate control that the nervous system has over the muscles and indicates the diverse characteristics of the muscle fibers. The same muscle or muscle group can respond and adapt to the need for either fine control, short intense effort, or prolonged activity.

The individual motor units that unite to form an entire muscle have different characteristics. The adaptive responses seen in muscle may therefore depend on a combination of the types of motor units contained in the muscle and the pattern or patterns of activity in which they engage. This chapter begins with a brief description of the motor unit and the basis for classification by fiber type that is used throughout to enable the reader to understand our approach to the subject of adaptations to use or disuse. The topic of motor unit properties has been reviewed in depth by Close[1] and by Buchthal and Schmalbruch.[2]

MOTOR UNIT

Major advances in identifying the properties and organization of motor units within muscles came from the histochemical staining for glycogen in cross-sections of muscle combined with isolation and repetitive stimulation of individual motoneurons.[3] A loss of glycogen identified those fibers (motor units) that had been active. A number of characteristics of the active fibers could then be identified from serial cross-sections stained by histochemical methods. Because of their invasive nature, these methods cannot be applied directly to the study of motor unit properties in human skeletal muscle.

However, some motor-unit mapping of human skeletal muscle has been done with electrophysiological methods.[4-6] Such studies have demonstrated a remarkable degree of similarity in the organizational pattern for human and animal muscle. The general characteristics of the motor unit are as follows. First, all fibers in a single motor unit are homogeneous with regard to histochemically identifiable contractile and metabolic properties.[4,7,8] Second, the fibers in a motor unit are distributed in a fairly large part of the cross-sectional area of the muscle.[9] Third, fibers belonging to a single motor unit are rarely positioned immediately proximal to each other. Fourth, a central locus for a motor unit exists, with the density of fibers in the unit declining as a function of the distance from the center.[3,10] In human muscle, there appear to be only 15 to 30 motor units contained in a 5- to 10-mm² cross-sectional area.[11-13] Motor units found in a given area can belong to all of the types represented in the muscle.

Fibers per Motor Unit

Data for human skeletal muscle are quite difficult to obtain. The must reliable estimates have come from counting the total number of motor nerves and muscle fibers.[14-16] Estimates based on electrophysiological measurements are less reliable.[5] The range of fibers per motor unit is from 110 for the lumbricals to 1,720 for the gastrocnemius medius muscles.[16] At present there are no exact determinations of the number of fibers in the different types of motor units found in human skeletal muscle.

Contractile Properties

The basic feature that differentiates motor units into types is their contractile properties. These are identified from the time to peak tension in a twitch and the closely related one-half relaxation time. Two general classes of motor units and, in some cases, of complete muscles can be identified from these contractile properties. One group of motor units possesses a relatively long time to peak tension (a slow twitch), and the other has a short time to peak tension (a fast twitch). Available data on the contractile properties of various motor units or muscle fibers within a single muscle illustrate the existence of a clear dichotomy of contractile speeds between fiber types.[7,8,17-24] However, a discrete dichotomy does not extend to the individual motor units, where there is a wide range of contractile speeds in spite of similar histochemical characteristics.

Biochemical Basis for Differences in Twitch Properties

A prime determinant of the twitch property of muscle is the rate at which myosin splits adenosine 5'-triphosphate (ATP), that is, its ATPase activity.[25-28] The relationship between the specific ATPase activity of myosin and the contractile speed for a variety of muscles with varying twitch times is presented in Figure 9–1.

The differences in the specific ATPase activity of myosin are attributable to the existence of multimolecular forms of the protein.[29-38] The

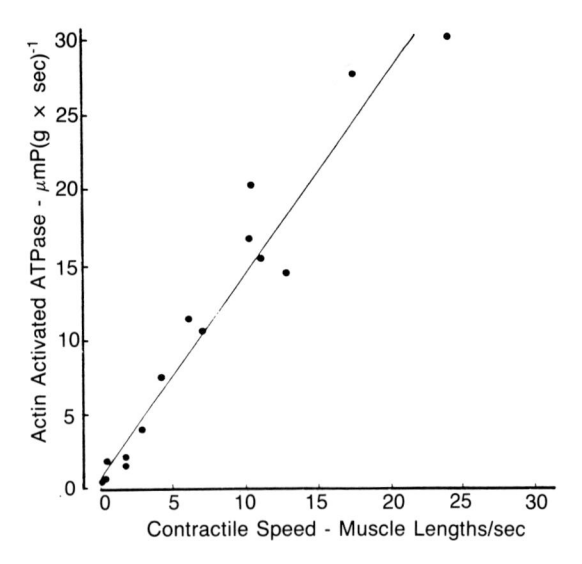

Figure 9–1 Relationship between maximal speed of shortening and actin-activated ATPase of myosin from a variety of animal species. Equation from the regression line is y = 0.34 + 1.37 x, and for the 2 variables, r = 0.97. (Plotted from original data published by Bárány M. J Gen Physiol 1967; 50 [Suppl pt 2]: 197–218.)

simplest method for identifying the myosin isozymes is based on their susceptibility to loss of ATPase activity in response to changes in pH.[30,31] Myosin from fast twitch (FT) muscles is alkaline stable but acid labile. The opposite is true for myosin from slow twitch (ST) muscles.

The multimolecular nature of myosin becomes a feature of all of the components that are assembled to form the functional protein complex.[39] This complex is composed of both a heavy- and a light-chain portion.[40-43] The heavy-chain portion can be divided into the structural subunits of the rod and the head. The ATPase activity is localized in the head subunit of myosin. Proteins of low molecular weight, the myosin light chains, are associated with the head portion of the heavy myosin. Identification of the components of myosin can be made through the use of immunological methods used in conjunction with histochemistry (Fig. 9–2). With these methods specific antibodies have been prepared against all subunits of the heavy chain and the individual light chains. Two classes of slow and three classes of fast ATP-splitting myosin have been identified with these techniques.[44-45] In general each muscle fiber contains only one class of myosin (that is slow or fast), but the relative proportion of the dif-

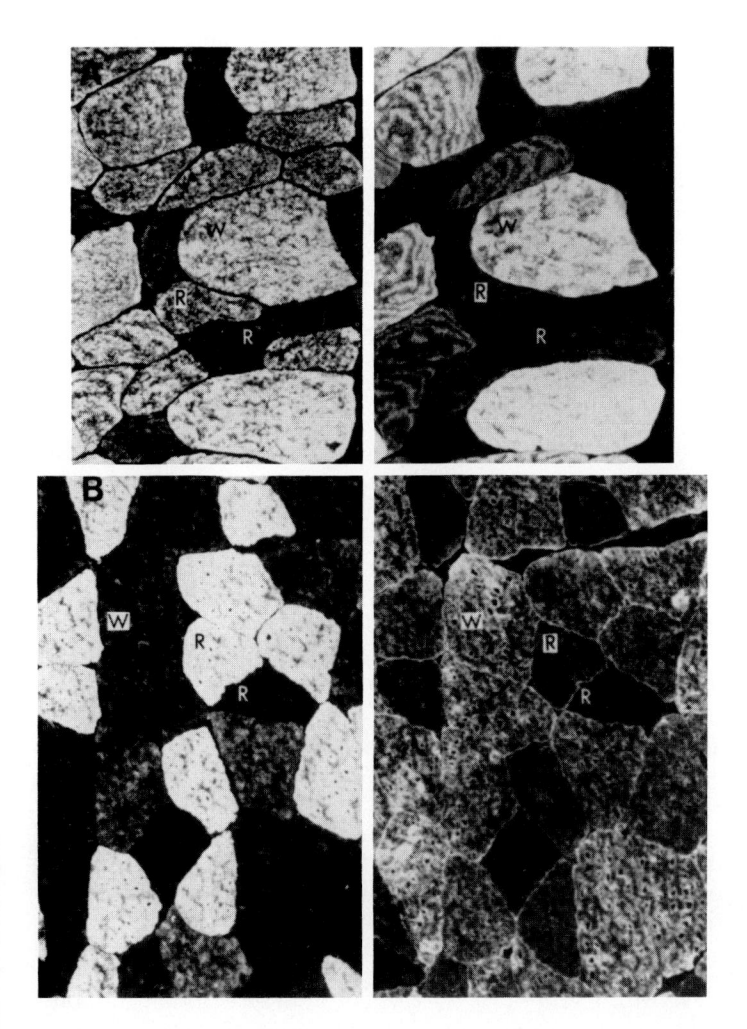

Figure 9–2 (A) Rat diaphragm, serial transverse sections. *Left* stained with antibody specific for alkali 1 light chain (anti-Δ1); *right* stained with antibody for alkali 2 light chain (anti-Δ2). Both antibodies react with same fibers (*W, I, black R*) that react with antibodies against whole white myosin. However, level of response to anti-Δ2 is lower in fast-twitch red fibers (*black R*) than in other fast-twitch fibers (*W, I*). (B) Cat flexor digitorum longus, serial sections. *Left*, anti-Δ1; *right*, anti-Δ2. Response of most fast-twitch fibers (*W*) is weak; compare with unreactive fibers (*white R*). However, level of response to anti-Δ1 (*left*) is more intense in one type of red fibers (*black R*) than in other fast-twitch fibers. Response to anti-Δ2 is less intense in this fiber (*black R*) than in other fast-twitch fibers. (From Gauthier GF. In: Pette D, ed. Plasticity of muscle. New York: de Gruyter, 1980: 83.)

ferent isozymes in this class can vary. However, there are instances in which fibers may contain a mixture of classes of myosin.[46–48] These immunologic methods hold great promise for positively establishing the existence of a specific type of myosin in a given fiber and the possible interconversion of fiber types in response to experimental perturbations such as chronic use or disuse.

Electrophoretic methods have also demonstrated the existence of different types of myosin in skeletal muscle.[35,36,47,48] In addition to isozymes of myosin, it has also been demonstrated that other proteins of the myofibrillar complex exist in polymorphic forms.[49–53] In summary, there are major differences between the proteins of the myofibrils of the FT and the ST muscles. On the basis of these differences, the fibers can be most reliably typed.

The general observation that only one class of contractile protein is found in a single muscle fiber does not preclude the existence of minor components of other types of proteins. Examples of this can be found in fetal and neonatal stages, during chronic electrical stimulation, and after cross-innervation and reinnervation.[7,23,32,44-48,54-58] The presence of more than one form of myosin in fetal and neonatal muscle is probably due to the existence of polyinnervation, which disappears with maturation.[59-63] Fast-twitch muscle fibers also possess a greater concentration of sarcoplasmic reticulum, and it changes with development, electrical stimulation, and cross-innervation.[64-68]

Histochemical Differentiation of Muscle Fibers

The difference in the sensitivity of myosin for retaining or losing ATPase activity after exposure to either high or low pH is a reliable method for the histochemical classification of muscle fibers.[38,69] It is a simple, rapid, and inexpensive method of determining the fiber composition of whole muscle or portions of muscles. This histochemical method for fiber identification is based on the ATPase activity remaining in myofibrils after preincubation of serial sections at pH 4.3, 4.6, and 10.3.[30] Immunologic methods have demonstrated that these histochemical staining patterns, produced by manipulation of the preincubation pH, are the result of the presence of different myosin isozymes.[32,33,70] This finding extends to the different classes of FT fibers, including those with either high or low oxidative capacities present in the limb muscle of most animals.[32] The staining pattern that exists in most mammalian muscles in response to variation in the pH of the preincubation is presented earlier in Figure 9-2. Although others have proposed that the fibers can be classified as type I and type II, in this chapter classification of skeletal muscle fibers is based on the histochemical differentiation of myofibrillar ATPase.[29-31,69,71-74] The assumption being made is that the acid stable and the alkaline stable myofibrillar ATPase correspond to slow and fast contractile characteristics, respectively. Hence the basic designation of the fibers is ST or FT. The FT fibers are further subdivided into FT_a, FT_b, and FT_c on the basis of differences in myofibrillar ATPase stability to low pH (Fig. 9-3). In the skeletal muscle of sedentary man, differences in metabolic potential can be identified from both histochemical (see Fig. 9-3) and biochemical (Tables 9-1 and 9-2) techniques when comparing subgroups of FT fibers, but these are small and an overlap is present. When subgrouping of the fiber types in human skeletal muscle is based on ATPase stains after both alkaline and acid preincubations rather than on stains for oxidative or glycolytic enzymes, fairly large differences are obtained, in which fibers can readily be assigned to the various groups.[29,30,75,76] Moreover this system eliminates the uncertainty that arises when changes in the oxidative potential occur in response to altered patterns of chronic physical activity. Thus, with extensive endurance training, all fiber types in the trained muscle may stain similarly for oxidative capacity, thereby making identification of fiber types based on this characteristic difficult if not impossible. Therefore it may be wrong to include abbreviations for the metabolic profile in the names to identify fibers, because these, at least for human muscle, can be misleading. The subscripts a, b, and c that we prefer to use indicate that there are certain differences in the populations of FT fibers. Whether they are related to differences in the myosin isozymes, energy metabolism, or other features of the muscle fiber cannot presently be ascertained.

Ultrastructural Basis for Skeletal Muscle Fiber Typing

Attempts have been made to identify the fiber types of skeletal muscle by ultrastructural features detectable by electron microscopy.[77-80] Sjöstrom and co-workers have examined the ultrastructural features of the Z and M bands of human skeletal muscle (Fig. 9-4).[81] The fibers were identified by histochemical staining for myofibrillar ATPase prior to electron microscopy. A higher degree of accuracy for fiber identification existed from examination of the M rather than the Z band (95 versus 70 percent). The identification of ultrastructural differences in skeletal muscle fibers supports the concept that the basic constitution of a fiber lies in the contractile proteins.

Other features commonly examined with electron microscopy are the size, shape, and concentration of the mitochondria. Examina-

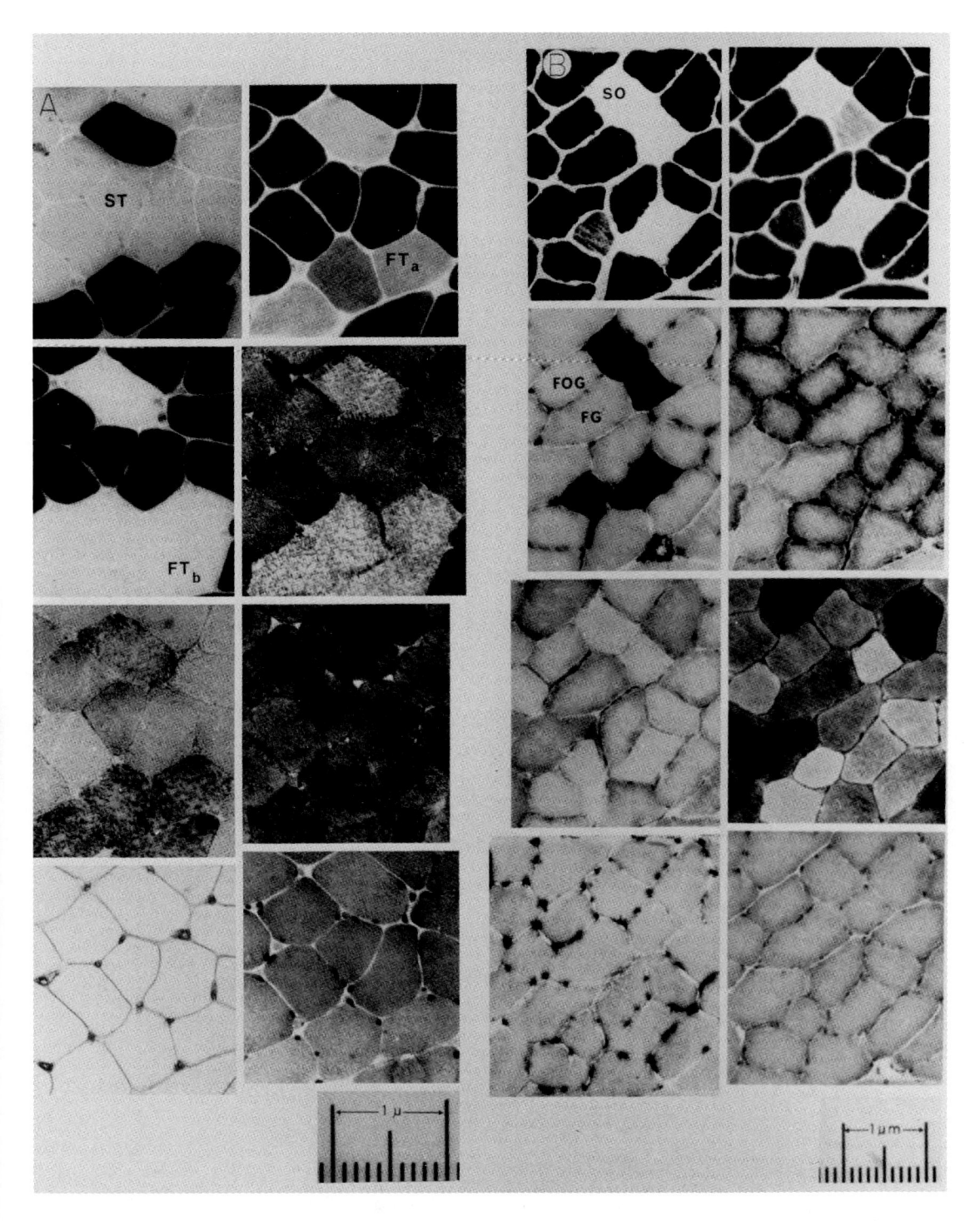

Figure 9–3 Serial transverse-sectioned frozen skeletal muscle from the lateral head of the gastrocnemius muscle of man (A) and the same muscle from rat (B). From *top* to *bottom* are the following stains (myofibrillar ATPase stained at pH 9.4 and preincubated at pH 10.3, 4.6, 4.3): nicotinamide adenine dinucleotide, reduced-tetrazolium reductase (NADH); α-GPDH, glycogen (periodic acid-Schiff, PAS); capillaries (man = amylase-treated sections stained with PAS; rat = alkaline phosphatase); and hematoxylin-eosin.

TABLE 9-1 Human Skeletal Muscle Substrate in Vastus Lateralis Muscle

Substrate	Mixed muscle, μmol/g wet wt	Fiber types, μmol/g wet wt ST	FT	FT_a	FT_b
Triglyceride	9.9 ± 0.6	7.1 ± 1.7	4.2 ± 1.2		
Glycogen (glucose units)	83.8 ± 18	77.8 ± 18	84.7 ± 19	83.1 ± 18	89.2 ± 21
ATP	5.0 ± 0.2	4.9 ± 0.1	5.1 ± 0.2	5.3 ± 0.2	4.9 ± 0.1
CP	10.7 ± 0.6	12.6 ± 0.2	14.7 ± 1.4	14.5 ± 1.1	14.8 ± 1.6

ST, slow twitch; FT, fast twitch; FT_a, fast twitch, a type; FT_b, fast twitch, b type; ATP, adenosine triphosphate; CP, creatine phosphate. Values are means ±1SD and are given for triglycerides in mixed muscles from refs. 118–120, 308, 405; glycogen from refs. 118, 119, 128, 178–180, 190; ATP and CP from refs. 135–137, 311. Corresponding values on fiber types are from refs. 124 (triglycerides); 121, 124, 130, 134 (glycogen); and 138, 139 (ATP and CP).

tion of mitochondria is based on the assumption that ST muscle possesses higher oxidative capacity and therefore a higher concentration of mitochondria than FT muscle. This relationship between mitochondrial concentration and contractile characteristics is not valid for FT muscles that possess high mitochondrial concentrations.[24,32,80] Moreover, the mitochondrial content of skeletal muscle is markedly influenced by the amount and type of activity of that muscle. Thus, an examination of mitochondrial features holds little promise as a reliable method for fiber identification.

Maximal Contractile Force

Considerable interest exists in identifying the factor or factors that contribute to the capacity of skeletal muscle to develop tension. A plethora of reports describe muscular strength increases in response to heavy-resistance exercise and decreases after inactivity. An interesting aspect of this topic is the question of whether any changes occur in the contractile properties of the fibers themselves in response to different patterns of physical activity. The central issue is whether changes occur at the level of the individual fiber. The capacity of a muscle or fiber to develop force is best related to the tension produced per unit of cross-sectional area.[81] Ikai and Fukunaga examined this relationship in humans by determining both the maximal voluntary contraction (MVC) and the cross-sectional area of the arm flexor muscle in children and adults.[82,83] Cross-sectional area of the muscles was estimated from ultrasound echoes; MVC was estimated to be 6.4 kg per square centimeter (64 newtons per cm²), with no differences between male and female subjects.

The maximal voluntary force as reported by Ikai and Fukunaga is an overestimate of the true capacity of human skeletal muscle.[82,83] The total muscle mass involved in elbow flexion includes the pronator teres, extensor carpi radi-

TABLE 9-2 Enzyme Activities in Human Skeletal Muscle (Vastus Lateralis) for Carbohydrate and Fat Metabolism Determined on Whole Muscle and on Fiber Types

Enzyme	Mixed muscle, $\mu mol \cdot g^{-1} \cdot min^{-1}$	Fiber types, $\mu mol \cdot g^{-1} \cdot min^{-1}$ ST	FT	FT_a	FT_b	Reference
Phosphorylase	6–7	2.8	7.3	5.8	8.8	124
Phosphofructokinase	20–25	7.5	15.4	13.7	17.5	121
		6.2	11.9			124
Lactate dehydrogenase	107–210	59	257	221	293	124
		94 ± 16	195 ± 12	179 ± 18	211 ± 3	141, 142, 145
Triosephosphate-dehydrogenase	134 ± 10	92 ± 3	175 ± 19	158 ± 9	191 ± 29	141, 142, 145
3-Hydroxyacyl-CoA dehydrogenase	6.2–12.0	14.8	9.3	11.6	7.1	124
		6.2 ± 0.2	3.4 ± 0.4	3.7 ± 0.2	3.1 ± 0.6	141, 142, 145
Succinate dehydrogenase	5.6–8.0	7.1	4.6	4.8	2.5	121, 124
Citrate synthase	6.0–11.5	10.8	7.5	8.6	6.5	121, 124

Activities are measured at 25°C.

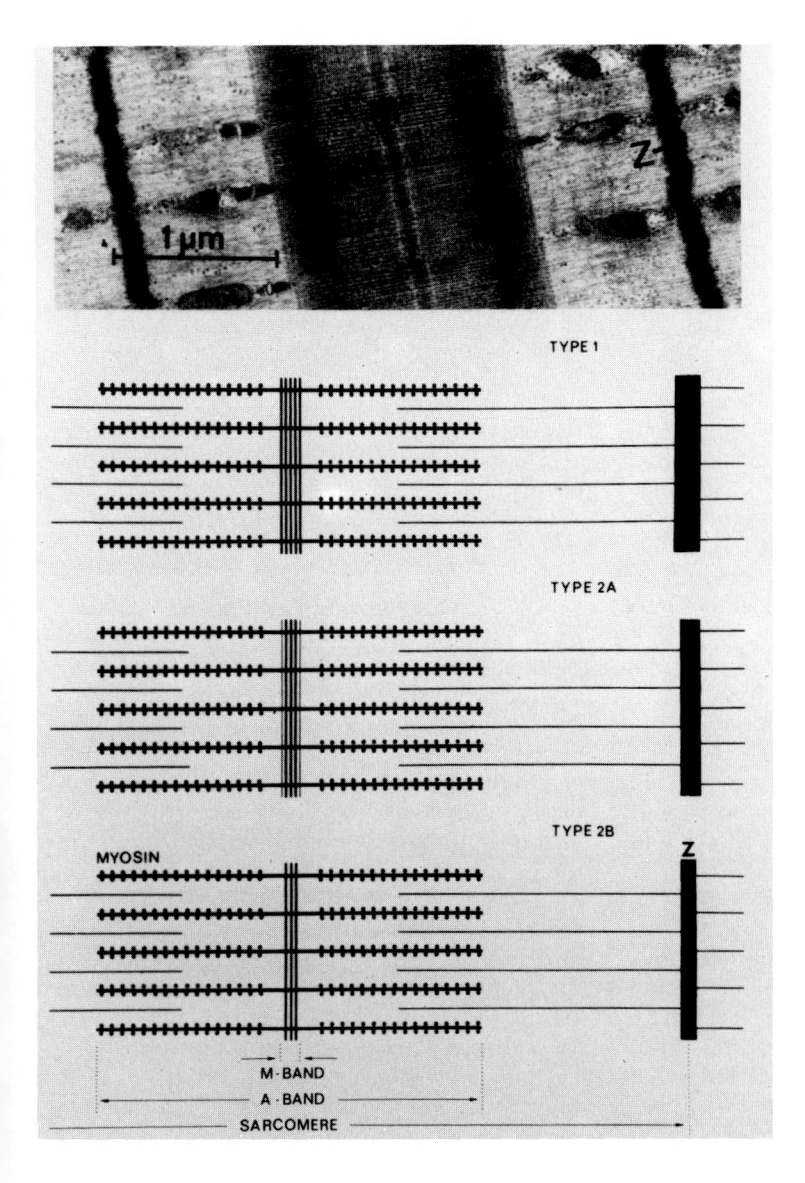

Figure 9-4 Part of a sarcomere from slow-twitch, ST (*micrograph* and *top panel*), fast-twitch, subtype a, FT$_a$ (*middle panel*), and fast-twitch, subtype b, FT$_b$ (*bottom panel*) fibers in combination with a schematic drawing of the respective fiber types. (From Angquist KA. Human skeletal muscle fibre structure. Effects of physical training and arterial insufficiency. Umeå, Sweden: Umeå University Medical Dissertations, New Series, No. 39, 1978.)

alis longus, and brachioradialis muscles.[84] Moreover, the placement of the origin and insertion of the biceps brachii muscle on the skeleton is such that in the position of elbow flexion used by Ikai and Fukunaga there is a 1 to 4.9 mechanical advantage.[85] On the basis of these factors the value given by Ikai and Fukunaga can be calculated to be about 47 newtons (N) per square centimeter. This is similar to a value of 40 N per square centimeter reported for the biceps brachii by Nygaard, and 39 N per square centimeter, as determined for the calf muscles by Haxton.[86,87]

The cross-sectional area of the upper arm flexors and knee extensors of man has also been estimated from x-ray computerized tomography (CT)[19,88,89] In two of these studies the fiber composition of the muscles was estimated from biopsy samples.[19,89] This revealed that the maximal voluntary strength of human skeletal muscle is related to fiber composition in only a minor way. Instead, total cross-sectional area appeared to be the decisive factor.

The ability of the different types of muscle and motor units to produce maximal tetanic tension has been examined in the mouse, rat, and cat. Conflict exists between those who found that the intrinsic capacity of the contractile elements to develop tension is similar for ST and FT muscle and those who found large differences in the maximal tetanic tension in ST versus FT motor units.[20,90–93] These differences could be due to the technical difficulties in assessing accurately the cross-sectional area of the motor units that were stimulated. If such large differences in force-developing capacity do exist between ST and FT motor units, their molecular basis is obscure. Differences could exist in excitation–contraction coupling, which ultimately involves the control of free calcium by the sarcoplasmic reticulum. Further studies into this problem are needed.

Speed of Contraction

The speed of contraction, that is, the time to peak isometric tension, of individual motor units has been studied most extensively in cat and rat skeletal muscle.[7,15,17,20,22,23,57,94–98] As described earlier, a close relationship exists between the contractile speed of a muscle and the specific activity of its myosin. Other elements in the excitation–contraction coupling system may also exert a regulatory influence on maximal speed of contraction of the individual motor units. Included are properties of the nerve and motor end-plate, interneuronal modulations, characteristics of the sarcolemma and transverse-tubular system for transmission of the neural impulse, the sarcoplasmic reticulum and its ability to release and sequester calcium, and finally, the role of the isozymes of troponin and tropomyosin in binding calcium and initiating contraction. Very little is known regarding these other regulatory factors.

Studies with man have lacked the precision for establishing contractile properties of the individual muscle or motor units of those from animals. In-situ stimluation of motor units has demonstrated the existence of FT and ST motor units.[4,5,99–110] Thus in the biceps muscle, bimodal distrubitions of contraction times with maximal values of 36 msec and 90 msec were observed, whereas in the midial head of the gastrocnemius muscle, the respective peak times were slightly longer. This does not necessarily signify that differences exist in contraction times between similar fiber types of these two muscles, because the methods for recording tensions were different in the two studies. There are also reports of contractile properties of biopsy samples of human skeletal muscle.[111–114] Although this type of study is open to question because the fibers had been cut and the integrity of the excitation-contraction coupling system was compromised, one-half relaxation times were also established and found to be approximately four times shorter in FT than in ST fibers.[114–116]

Fatigue Characteristics

In studies of human skeletal muscle motor units, a total of 57 single motor units of the medial gastrocnemius muscle were activated with a bipolar stimulating electrode (Fig. 9–5).[4] An electromyogram (EMG) of a single motor unit was recorded, and tension produced by activation of a motor unit was estimated from the torque measured in the ankle joint. Some motor units were more resistant to fatigue than others. The slowest contracting motor units demonstrated a small decline (2 to 20 percent) in twitch tension from the initial level after 3,000 stimuli were delivered over a 50-minute period. Two groups of FT fibers were discernible. One had fatigue-resistance properties similar to the ST fibers; the other had a reduction in tension from 50 to 75 percent during the same experiment period.

Metabolic Characteristics

Substrates

Human skeletal muscle contains stores of glycogen and lipids, in addition to the more immediate energy sources of ATP and creatine phosphate (CP). A summary of the average values for these stores, compiled from several studies in which they were estimated from bi-

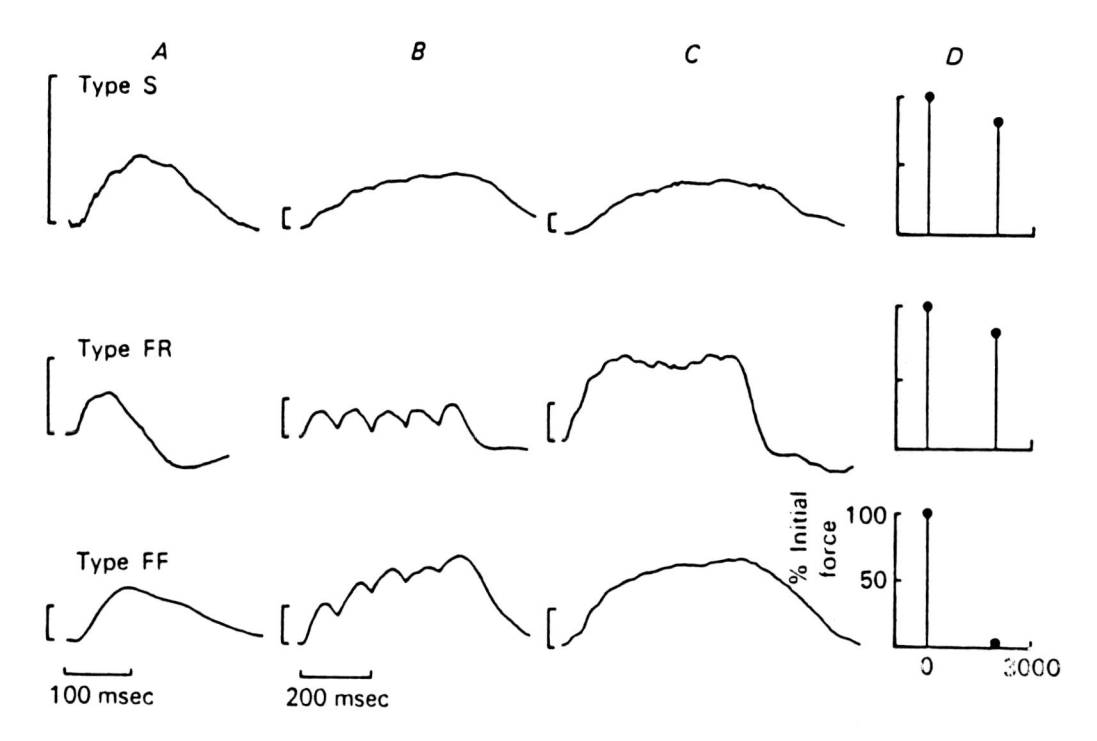

Figure 9–5 Examples of the three motor unit types found in human medial gastrocnemius. (A) Isometric twitch; (B) isometric tetanus 10 pulses/s; (C) isometric tetanus 20 pulses/s; and (D) fatique test, control and after 3,000 stimuli, expressed as a percentage of initial isometric tension. (From Garnett RAF, O'Donovan MJ, Stephens JA, Taylor A. J Physiol (Lond) 1978; 287:33–43.)

opsy samples of the extremity muscles, is presented in Table 9–1.[117]

Triglyceride Content. The triglyceride content of human skeletal muscle varies between 5 and 15 mmol per kilogram wet weight.[118–123] Although these values are from measurements made on samples of mixed-fiber muscle freed from visible fat, the possibility remains that part of this fat is localized in the extrafiber space. However, because bundles of fibers, carefully liberated from freeze-dried muscle samples, contain similar amounts of triglyceride as those given in Table 9–1, the extrafiber lipid store does not appear to have been appreciable.

The magnitude of the variation in the triglyceride stores between various muscles of the body is unknown. Measurements made on biopsy samples of muscles from the leg and arm suggest that the variation is small. The localization of fat within the muscle appears to be heterogeneous. Ultrastructural evaluations support the concept that fat is localized in small droplets at varying intervals in a fiber. An additional factor contributing to the variation of the triglyceride content in skeletal muscle is the distinct difference in the lipid content of the individual fibers, with the ST fibers containing three to five times higher concentrations than the FT fibers.[124] Therefore, differences in the lipid content must be expected when variation exists in the fiber composition of the tissue samples being analyzed.

Differences in the lipid content of the fiber types can be demonstrated when sections are stained with either Sudan black or oil red O.[125] With these treatments the ST fibers stain more intensely than the FT fibers.[90,91] Because mitochondrial membrane contains large amounts of lipid, which is also stained by Sudan black or oil red O, caution must be exercised in the interpretation of the histochemical staining method to estimate the triglyceride stores of the individual fibers. Consequently, this method seems to hold little promise for evaluating differences in lipid stores of the different fiber types or in estimating changes induced by exercise, diet, or training.

Glycogen Content. The average glycogen content (see Table 9–1) of human extremity muscle ranges from 50 to 90 mmol per kilogram of wet weight. (All glycogen concentrations are given as millimoles of glycosyl units.) Part of this rather wide variation appears to be related to the diet and state of physical activity of the subject.[126–128] Overall the glycogen granules are homogeneously distributed throughout the muscle fibers with only small differences existing in the glycogen content of ST and FT fibers or in the subgroups of FT fibers of humans.[121,124,129,130] Moreover, only minor variation in muscle glycogen is found when determinations are made on multiple samples from the same muscle or when assays performed on small samples are compared with those made on larger samples from the same muscle.[128]

The glycogen content of the gastrocnemius, the quadriceps femoris, the triceps brachii, and the biceps brachii muscles of humans all lie within the range of 50 to 90 mmol per kilogram wet weight.[128,131] Quantitative determinations of the glycogen content of the individual fiber types present in the vastus lateralis of the quadriceps muscle have revealed that at a glycogen concentration of about 75 mmol per kilogram wet weight ($\approx$300 mmol per kilogram dry weight) there is a 10 to 15 mmol per kilogram wet weight mean difference between the ST and FT fibers, with the latter fibers having the higher glycogen content.[121,124,130] It appears that for the subgroups of the FT fibers, the FT_b fibers may contain more glycogen than the FT_a fibers. These differences in glycogen content of the muscle fibers can be detected with periodic acid-Schiff (PAS) stain, but at a glycogen content of 80 to 100 mmol per kilogram wet weight or above, the staining intensity is homogeneous, and neither subjective ratings nor spectrophotometric methods can detect differences between fibers or fiber types.[132,133] The variation in the glycogen content within a single fiber type has been reported to be from about 50 to 650 mmol per kilogram dry weight for both the ST and FT fiber types.[121,124,130,134] The reason for this variation is unknown, but it may be due in part to the technical difficulties of separating the fiber from the support tissue and of weighing the small tissue fragments accurately. Thus, although a close relationship has been demonstrated between the histochemical evaluation of the glycogen content of muscle and the value determined biochemically, it is surprising that these differences are not more evident in tissue stained by standard histochemical methods.

Phosphagen. The phosphagen stores of skeletal muscle constitute 23 to 25 mmol per kilogram wet weight, with the CP concentration being 18 to 20 and the ATP being 4 to 5 mmol per kilogram wet weight (see Table 9–1).[135–137] Variations among muscles are small. The magnitude of the variation of these stores in the major fiber types of human muscle has been examined.[138,139] This has demonstrated a slightly higher ATP and CP concentration in ST fibers. However, these differences are so small (0.05 mmol per kilogram wet weight for ATP and 1 to 3 mmol per kilogram wet weight for CP) as to be physiologically unimportant. Measurements performed on samples with large differences in fiber composition also have failed to demonstrate any major differences in the concentrations of the high-energy phosphates.[139]

Enzyme Activities

The content or activities of enzymes for contraction and energy metabolism differ in the various fiber types of skeletal muscle.[140] For humans, in whom most muscles are homogeneous mixtures of the different types, quantitative data are difficult to obtain, and results at the individual fiber level are scarce. It has been possible, with the method developed by Essén and colleagues, to tease apart fragments of single fibers from freeze-dried muscle samples and to identify them histochemically according to type.[121] The remaining portion is then weighed on a quartz balance, and microchemical methods are applied.

The Ca^{2+}-activated myosin ATPase determined on pooled samples of a single fiber type was 2.5-fold higher in the FT than in ST fibers.[121] Major differences in creatine kinase activity of the fiber types also appear to exist in all skeletal muscle.

Histochemical staining of human skeletal muscle has demonstrated the existence of major differences in the metabolic profiles of the ST and FT fibers. The general pattern is for the

ST fibers to be well endowed with enzymes for end-terminal oxidation and a low anaerobic potential, and for the reverse to be true for the FT fibers. However, there is not a discrete relationship, and enzyme activities vary considerably within each of the fiber types. Some insight into this diversity within a given fiber type can be achieved from the varying staining intensities of the fibers. It has been further quantified from biochemical studies in which enzyme activities for carbohydrate and fat metabolism were determined at the level of the individual muscle fiber.[119,121,141-144] In some cases the fiber types were not histochemically identified. Instead, the activities of several enzymes were measured on each fiber and, of these, lactate dehydrogenase (LDH) activity was used to type the fibers.[141,142,145] The results of these studies are summarized, together with values for mixed-fiber muscles, in Table 9-2. Glycolytic and mitochondrial enzymes are quite consistent, that is, mitochondrial enzymes are higher in ST than in FT fibers, and the reverse is true for the glycolytic enzymes. An overlap is almost nonexistent. For all four glycolytic enzyme studies, there is a two-fold-higher mean value in the FT than in ST fibers. The subgroups of FT fibers also differ, with activities being 20 to 50 percent higher in the FT$_b$ than in FT$_a$ fibers.

The activities of 3-hydroxyacyl-CoA dehydrogenase (HAD), succinate dehydrogenase (SDH), and citrate synthase (CS) are 30 to 50 percent higher in the ST than in the FT fiber groups. However, when comparisons are made between FT$_a$ and ST fibers of the vastus lateralis muscle, the difference for CS is small or nonexistent. In contrast, HAD and SDH activities are 20 percent and 30 percent lower in the FT$_a$ than in ST fibers. In the study by Lowry and coworkers of the biceps brachii muscle, CS activity was about 20 percent lower in the FT$_a$ than in ST fibers.[142] The activity of these enzymes in the FT$_a$ fibers was approximately 50 percent of that found in the ST fibers, and 50 to 67 percent of that found in FT$_b$ fibers. Unfortunately, no data are available for human skeletal muscle for the activities of any respiratory chain enzymes at the individual fiber level.

In samples of muscle containing a mixture of fiber types, the activity of the mitochondrial enzymes appears to be about 6 to 10 μmol(mg^{-1}) (min^{-1}). In this case, little difference exists between activities for the three major oxidative pathways (fatty acid oxidation, citric acid cycle, or electron-transport system). A constant proportionality exists among mitochondrial enzymes.[146]

The activities of the glycolytic enzymes are generally higher than those for the end-terminal oxidation. In this pathway the enzymes also appear to be present in a constant proportion to one another.[147-150] No obvious deviation from this rule appears to exist when comparisons are made at the individual fiber level.

Ionic Composition of Skeletal Muscle

The various fiber types also contain different amounts of intracellular ions (Table 9–3). In human muscle, the sodium content of the fi-

TABLE 9–3 Muscle Electrolytes in Healthy Subjects

Muscle	Na$_m$	K$_m$	Mg$_m$	Reference
mmol/100 g FFW				
Vastus lateralis	11.6	44.7		117
	(2.7)	(2.0)		
Vastus lateralis	15.9	43.1		451
	(2.9)	(4.1)		
Different*	12.1	43.3	3.73	452
	(2.0)	(2.5)	(0.58)	
Vastus lateralis	9.3	46.7	4.48	453
	(1.5)	(0.9)	(0.08)	
mmol/100 g dry wt†				
Triceps brachii	12.7	45.0	3.86	131
	(5.0)	(2.0)	(0.33)	
Vastus lateralis	8.9	44.9	4.12	131
	(2.5)	(5.4)	(0.18)	
Soleus	12.5	43.3	4.07	131
	(3.3)	(4.7)	(0.45)	
Triceps brachii				
ST fibers	13.0	44.0	3.98	
FT fibers	11.6	46.2	4.15	131
Homogenate	11.7	44.5	3.79	
Vastus lateralis				
ST fibers	8.0	42.6	4.58	
FT fibers	8.9	43.0	4.76	131
Homogenate	8.3	44.2	4.12	
Soleus				
ST fibers	9.6	42.6	4.36	
FT fibers	9.6	43.2	4.52	131
Homogenate	10.7	41.8	4.09	

Values are means with 1 SD in parentheses. FFW, fat-free weight; ST, slow twitch; FT, fast twitch.
* In 6 subjects from sartorius or pectineus muscles and in 6 subjects from the internal oblique muscle
† Fat content averaged 8% (5%–14%) of dry weight. If expressed per 100 g FFW, value should be increased by this amount.

bers appears to be quite low, with no difference between fiber types. For intramuscular potassium concentrations in humans, no differences can be detected when comparing the different fiber types, the mean value for both ST and FT fibers being approximately 160 mM. Recently electron probe analysis has been used to study electrolyte concentration and intracellular distribution. Besides confirming that K^+ is of similar concentration in the ST and FT fibers in human skeletal muscle, with this method no differences between fiber types have been found for chlorine, sulfur, or phosphorus.[151,152] Magnesium, on the other hand, appeared to be slightly higher in the FT than in ST fibers.

Thus, fiber types in skeletal muscle can be distinguished by a number of characteristics. First is the time to peak isometric tension. For human skeletal muscle, few precise data are available, but indications are that the time to peak isometric tension is about 40 msec for FT units and 80 to 100 msec for ST units. It is unknown whether differences exist between the subgroups of FT units or what variation exists for the ST and FT units of different muscles.

Second, the ability of FT and ST units to develop force per unit of transectional area of muscle is a matter of controversy in various animal species. Although direct measurements of the force per unit area of ST or FT motor units are not available for human muscle, it appears that the force-developing capacity is similar for both FT and ST motor units.

Third are the fatigue characteristics of the motor units. In human skeletal muscle there is approximately a 25 percent decline in the force developed during a 60-minute period of stimulation. The FT_b fibers in human skeletal muscle retain up to 40 percent of the initial force developed after 50 minutes of stimulation and 3,000 contractions.

Fourth is the metabolic potential of the fiber types. The FT_a fiber has a rather low triglyceride content and a low concentration of enzymes for beta-oxidation. The enzymes for the citric acid cycle and electron-transport chain are usually present at lower concentrations than those found in the ST fibers in the muscle of sedentary humans.

MUSCLE FIBER COMPOSITION IN HUMAN SKELETAL MUSCLE

There is considerable interest in the percent composition and the size of the different fiber types in the skeletal muscle of normal humans and of athletes. Table 9-4 is a compilation of such data for normal sedentary subjects, as reported by a number of laboratories. Table 9-5 is a summary of the fiber composition and fiber area for several muscles from subjects who were either elite athletes or who had undergone specific training programs. These data are mostly from studies in which the muscle samples were obtained by the biopsy method (either needle or open). Data are available from entire muscles obtained at autopsy.[86,153-159] Comparisons have also been made between the open and the needle biopsy methods.[160]

Perhaps the most extensively studied human muscle is the lateral portion of the quadriceps femoris (vastus lateralis). In an early study, biopsy samples were obtained from 74 male subjects from 17 to 58 years of age, including sedentary men and highly trained athletes.[161] For this group the average fiber composition was 52.2 percent ST, with a range from 13 to 98 percent ST fibers. In an attempt to provide further information concerning the normal fiber composition of this muscle, 69 males and 48 females, all 16 years old and representing a random sample for this age group, were studied (Fig. 9-6). The mean fiber composition of the vastus lateralis muscle for this group was 54 and 52 percent ST fibers for the males and females, respectively. Within the FT fibers, the FT_a fibers were approximately twice as common as the FT_b fibers. Similar mean values for the percentages of ST, FT_a, and FT_b fibers were observed in studies of 26 men and 25 women around 25 years of age.[162] Thus, ample evidence is available to suggest that in the vastus lateralis muscle the ST and FT fibers are about equally common, and no differences exist between the sexes.

In the studies cited above, the relative percentage of fibers was estimated from small muscle samples obtained with the needle biopsy technique in which fragments of 200 to

TABLE 9–4 Summary of Some Published Values for Percent Distribution and Size of Fibers in Limb Muscles of Humans as Estimated From Biopsy Samples

					Slow-twitch fibers			Fast-twitch fibers			
Sex	Muscle	No.	Mean	Range	%	Range	X area, $\mu m^2 \times 10^2$	Range	%	X area, $\mu m^2 \times 10^2$	Range	Reference
	VM	11			42	26–63			58			454
	BB	7			49	39–61			51			454
M, F	VL	6			57	50–71	45.6	29.7–60.3	43	48.9	33.1–63.9	455
M, F	BB	7			48	37–61	40.6	27.2–54.3	52	61.4	34.2–87.1	455
M	G	2			64	55–69	33.7	33.0–34.4	36	46.0	39.8–50.2	455
M	S	2			72	65–78	53.3	47.8–58.7	28	94.3	71.1–117.5	455
M	VL	26	34	24–52	36	13–73	40.2	11.4–98.4	64	52.2	17.4–94.7	161
M	D	26	34	24–52	46	14–60			54			161
M	VL	8		23–32	48	29–65	45.6	33.0–60.3	52	50.7	37.0–71.7	241
M	VL	6		28–37	32	18–41	55.0	30.6–92.0	38	66.4	43.1–75.9	246
M	VL	4		16–18	41		50.6		59	55.0		446, 329
M	G	19	27		58		54.6		42	49.5		341
M	G	11	27	17–42	53	38–73	57.0	34.0–87.2	47	49.7	38.8–68.6	324
F	G	10	22	20–30	51	27–72	38.8	25.5–50.4	49	41.9	25.7–61.6	324
M	VL	4			36	20–48	33.0	22.6–41.8	64	37.6	22.3–51.9	348
F	VL	5			36	27–42	27.8	20.5–35.8	64	29.1	17.1–41.6	349
M	VL	19	27		58		54.6		42	49.5		457
M	VL	69		16–18	54		48.4		32[a] 13[b] 1[c]	52.7		344
M, F	VL	5		24–41	51	47–67			49			458
M, F	S	11		24–41	80	64–100			20			458
M, F	G	6		24–41	60	45–82			40			458
M	G	4	24	20–26	51	37–66	43.1	31.6–51.0	49	47.3	35.0–69.3	420
M	S	4	24	20–26	71	53–88	75.2	49.5–90.0	29	110.6	81.1–147.3	420
M	VL	8	24	20–31	53	45–62			47			459
M	VL	9	23		49	26–60	52.9		37[a] 18[b]	55.7 51.5		460
M	VL	5	24		47		55.9		29[a] 24[b]	68.0 62.7		242
M	G	19	32		53				23[a] 24[b]			461
F	VL	24	24		51				49			462
M	VL	6	6		43	42–72			57			463
F	VL	6	7		56	41–68			44			463
M	VL	11	26	20–29	60		29.4		40	36.6		464
M	VL	10	35	30–39	63		28.5		337	35.1		464
M	VL	8	43	40–49	52		31.3		48	33.6		464
M	VL	12	55	50–59			28.8		52	28.0		464
M	VL	10	62	60–69	45		22.6		55	21.2		464
M, F			59	21–83								153
					Autopsy Material							
	S	20			70	12–95			30			
	Med. gast.	24			50	14–84			50			
	Lat. bast.	9			48	37–62			52			
	Whole gast.	33			50	33–63			50			
	Vast. int.	14			47	30–71			53			
	VL deep	10			35	22–50			65			
	VL superf.	15			30	11–53			70			
	VL whole	25			32	19–48			68			
	BB autopsy			17–30	42	34–51			58			467
	D				53	43–63			47			467
	VL				38	27–48			62			467

M, male; F, female; G, gastrocnemius; S, soleus; BB, biceps brachialis; D, deltoid; VL, vastus lateralis; VM, vastus medialis; X, cross-sectional area. [a]Fast twitch, a type. [b]Fast twitch, b type. [c]Fast twitch, c type.

TABLE 9-5 Summary of Some Published Values for Percent Distribution and Size of Fibers in Limb Muscles of Humans in Training as Estimated From Biopsy Samples

Sex	Muscle	No.	Age Mean	Age Range	Slow-twitch fibers %	Slow-twitch fibers Range	Slow-twitch fibers X area, $\mu m^2 \times 10^2$	Slow-twitch fibers Range	Fast-twitch fibers %	Fast-twitch fibers X area, $\mu m^2 \times 10^2$	Fast-twitch fibers Range	Experiment	Reference
M	VL	6	33	29–40	32[a]	18–41	55.0	30.6– 92.0	68	66.4	36.8– 95.8	Endurance training on cycle ergometer, 6 mo	329
					36[b]	27–42	67.8	55.5– 89.0	64	61.4	43.1– 76.0		
M	VL	4	24	18–33	61	48–73	86.5[c]	58.0–127.6	39	99.5	75.4–147.9	Elite bicyclists	161
	D				51		54.7[c]	40.6– 72.5	49	73.4	46.4– 92.8		
M	VL	4	26	25–27	61	45–72	64.4[c]	36.6– 91.4	39	51.0	36.6– 65.8	Elite canoeists	161
	D				58	48–66	82.4[c]	58.5–131.6	42	83.9	54.8–109.8		
M	VL	4	25	23–29	46	25–60	60.4[c]	17.4–101.5	54	95.6	58.0–145.0	Weight lifters	161
	D				53	43–67	55.5[c]	29.0– 75.4	47	89.2	43.5–145.0		
M	VL	8	23	19–33	59	53–70			41			Distance runners	161
M	VL	11	52	47–58	69	47–96			31			Orienteers	161
	D				63	31–98			37				
F	G	2	20	18–21	27	27–28	37.5	35.4– 39.4	73	39.3	33.7– 45.0	Trained sprinters	324
M	G	2	20	17–22	24	21–27	58.8	39.8– 77.8	76	60.3	58.8– 61.9	Trained sprinters	324
F	G	7	20	16–25	61	44–73	60.7	30.8– 99.5	39	56.4	40.1– 75.0	Trained middle-distance runners	324
M	G	7	23	19–32	52	41–69	61.0	45.5– 84.5	48	71.2	48.9– 92.1	Trained middle-distance runners	324
M	G	5	24	20–32	69	63–74	66.1	36.4–101.1	31	76.3	47.3–113.3	Trained distance runners	324
F	G	3	22	21–23	49	37–61	41.6	35.0– 50.8	51	51.1	43.5– 66.2	Long and high jumpers	324
M	G	2	29	26–32	47	44–49	47.2	44.8– 49.6	53	65.2	63.0– 67.5	Long and high jumpers	324
F	G	3	21	17–26	42	41–42	48.6	42.6– 54.6	58	45.7	42.7– 48.7	Javelin throwers	324
M	G	3	25	23–30	50	46–56	55.9	25.7– 82.5	50	57.7	42.1– 76.1	Javelin throwers	324
F	G	2	24	21–26	51	48–54	51.9	32.9– 70.9	49	58.5	47.7– 69.4	Shot and discus throwers	324
M	G	4	27	21–32	38	13–52	77.0	50.4–103.5	62	94.8	91.3– 97.2	Shot and discus throwers	324
M	VL	4	21	17–28	69	60–83			20[d]		14 – 30	Distance runners after 18-wk aerobic training	240
									10[e]		1 – 20		
									1[f]		0 – 1		
M	VL	4	21	17–28	52	34–77			18[d]		7 – 28	Distance runners after 11-wk anaerobic training	240
									18[e]		4 – 29		
									12[f]		7 – 15		
M	G	13	35		55				43[d]			Trained distance runners	461
									2[e]				
		12	23		23				47[d]				
									2[e]				
F	G			18–26	39		32.5		61	35.0		Sprinters	468
F	G			18–26	54		37.5		46	30.0		Pentathletes	468
F	G			18–26	63		32.5		37	27.5		Middle-distance runners	468
F	G			18–26	73		36.0		27	21.0		Distance runners	468
M	G	26			56		54.3		44	54.2		Well-trained distance runners	465
M	VL	8			68				24[d]			Elite orienteers	344
									3[e]				
									4[f]				
M	G	7			67				29[d]			Elite orienteers	344
									2[e]				
									2[f]				

Table continues on following page

TABLE 9-5 (continued)

			Age			Slow-twitch fibers			Fast-twitch fibers				
Sex	Muscle	No.	Mean	Range	%	Range	X area, $\mu m^2 \times 10^2$	Range	%	X area, $\mu m^2 \times 10^2$	Range	Experiment	Reference
M	D	4			68				14[d] 17[e] 0[f]			Elite orienteers	344
M	VL	3	21	20–22	60	51–70			40			Elite skiers	459
M	VL	11	25		57		63.3		43	61.2		Elite cyclists	457
M	VL	11	25		53		60.6		47	57.6		Well-trained cyclists	457
F	VL	7	20		51		54.9		49	52.2		Well-trained cyclists	457
F	VL	5	23	20–32	48	24–82	43.1	31.1–71.7	52	38.2	15.2–76.9	Field hockey players	349
M	VL	3			45	30–60	44.3	31.6–58.9	55	67.7	58.1–76.6	Weight lifters	348
M	VL	3			44	29–54	46.1	33.9–69.0	56	43.1	25.1–69.0	Distance runners	348
M	VL	5	24		45		61.1		30[d] 25[e]	73.7 67.7		Leg 1 control	242
M	VL	5	24		42		58.9		35[d] 23[e]	73.8 71.2		Leg 1 after 7 wk of training 6 s, 4 times per wk	242
M	VL	5	24		48		48.7		28[d] 23[e]	62.3 57.7		Leg 2 control	242
M	VL	5	24		47		49.6		32[d] 21[e]	75.9 56.3		Leg 2 after 7 wk of training 30 s, 4 times per wk	242
M	D	6	23	18–28	53	41–74			47			Elite canoeists	318
M	G	14	26	21–32	79	50–98	83.42	48.5–151.4	21	64.9	31.8–115.2	Elite distance runners	341
M	VL	19	22		50	20–71	50.9		38[d] 12[e]	58.7 53.6		Elite ice hockey players	460
M	VL	8	20	16–29	44	24–55	45.5	35.7–65.8	56	74.3	59.5–92.4	Weight lifters	241
M	VL	4		16–18	41[a] 44[b]		50.6 51.9		59 56	55.0 57.4		Sprint training	456

M, male; F, female; VL, vastus lateralis; D, deltoid; G, gastrocnemius. [a]Before training. [b]After training. [c]Samples for single representative subjects. [d]Fast twitch, a type. [e]Fast twitch, b type. [f]Fast twitch, c type.

1,000 fibers are contained in each sample. The large variation observed in these samples could be a reflection of a heterogeneous mixture of fibers in the cross-section of the vastus lateralis muscle. The variability of the relative frequency and of the size of the various fiber types has been examined in whole cross-sections of muscles obtained at autopsy.[153,155,156,163]

The large range of the percentages of ST and FT fibers observed in the population in these studies implies that for a certain percent of the population of males and females, muscles are predominantly of one or the other fiber type. This interindividual variation appears to be genetically determined, because studies with mono- and dizygotic twins have shown almost identical fiber composition of the vastus lateralis muscle in the monozygotic but not in the dizygotic twins (Fig. 9–7).[164]

The various muscles of the human body differ in fiber composition. The extent of this variation is illustrated by data from an autopsy study in which the same muscles from several subjects were analyzed.[153,155–158,165] The results from six men and three women, who died suddenly without having a known muscle disease, are given in Figure 9–8B. It is apparent that some similarities exist among muscles from

MOTOR-UNIT RECRUITMENT

The contractile and metabolic properties that combine to produce the physiologic characteristics of the individual motor units in skeletal muscle enable them to engage in a wide variety of activities. The ST motor units, in all species, are well designed for prolonged activity, when ATP can be produced by directing substrate flux through the oxidative pathways of the mitochondria. The capacity of the ST fibers to develop force per unit of cross-sectional area does not appear to be significantly different from that of FT fibers.

The systematic use of the different motor units in response to distinct physiologic demands depends on the existence of an orderly procedure for their recruitment by the central nervous system. This system is based on the existence of motoneurons of varying size, threshold for activation, and conduction velocity. These properties of nerves were identified by Hursh and Rushton.[170,171] Their importance in the control of motor recruitment was elaborated by Henneman and co-workers.[172-176] In this scheme, now commonly referred to as the size principle, ST motor units are innervated by small, low-threshold, slowly conducting motor nerves; FT motor units are innervated by large, higher threshold, fast-conducting motor nerves. Rather than discrete differences in motoneurons, it appears that a continuum of thresholds for activation exists. In this manner a systematic procedure for mobilizing motor units exists, whereby the tension requirements for a specific muscular contraction pattern can be initiated by the central nervous system.

Evidence of an orderly recruitment of motor units in human muscle during a variety of physical activities has come from both histochemical (based on the depletion of glycogen from the fibers in biopsy samples) and electrophysiological data.[4,103-109,127,177-188] The method of biopsy and glycogen depletion is limited to exercise of sufficient duration and intensity to produce a discernible loss of PAS stain in the fibers. In some instances the metabolic profile of the fibers results in underestimating the involvement of ST units. Thus, during high-intensity exercise, the loss of glycogen from FT_b units would be greater than from ST units, simply because the ST units would also consume large amounts of oxygen, free fatty acids (FFA), and glucose, resulting in a smaller degradation of glycogen. Electrophysiological methods lack a definitive proof of the type of motor unit from which the electrical potential is recorded.

Histochemical studies (Fig. 9-9) have verified a primary involvement of ST motor units during low-intensity exercise in humans.[178,181] When such activity is prolonged or when its intensity is above a certain level, there is a progressive involvement of FT motor units, with the FT_a units being involved first, until, if the exercise extends to exhaustion, all motor units have been involved.[179] With high-intensity dynamic exercise, that is, above maximal oxygen uptake ($\dot{V}O_2$max) capacity, all types of motor units may be activated.[179,181] For some individuals, exhaustion does not result in complete depletion of glycogen from all FT fibers, regardless of whether the exercise has been of a moderate or high intensity.[178,181]

The exercise intensity required to activate FT motor units is debated. It has been suggested that activation may occur at intensities as low as 60 to 70 percent of the $\dot{V}O_2$max, and that this may be responsible for the elevation of lactate in the blood at these exercise intensities.[168,189] Definite proof for this concept is lacking in the published literature, and data are available to suggest that it is unlikely. The increase in the lactate concentration of blood that occurs during prolonged, moderately severe (60 to 70 percent $\dot{V}O_2$max) exercise usually peaks at about 10 to 20 minutes and then declines toward rest values as the exercise continues.[136,181,190] If the lactate production is a result of FT fiber use, its decline could be explained either by fatigue and inactivation of these fibers or by assuming that they have switched to terminal oxidation to support their energy requirements. If the FT fibers were exhausted, they could be expected to be depleted of glycogen as occurs during short, heavy exercise.[179] This is not the case. Because the power output is constant during such exercise, a loss of some motor units would necessitate the addition of others. Based on the concept of ST recruitment before FT units, this would imply addition of more FT units, but it would produce more lactate rather than less.[103-105] If the FT fibers had converted to oxidative metabolism, the total oxygen uptake would increase. This does not

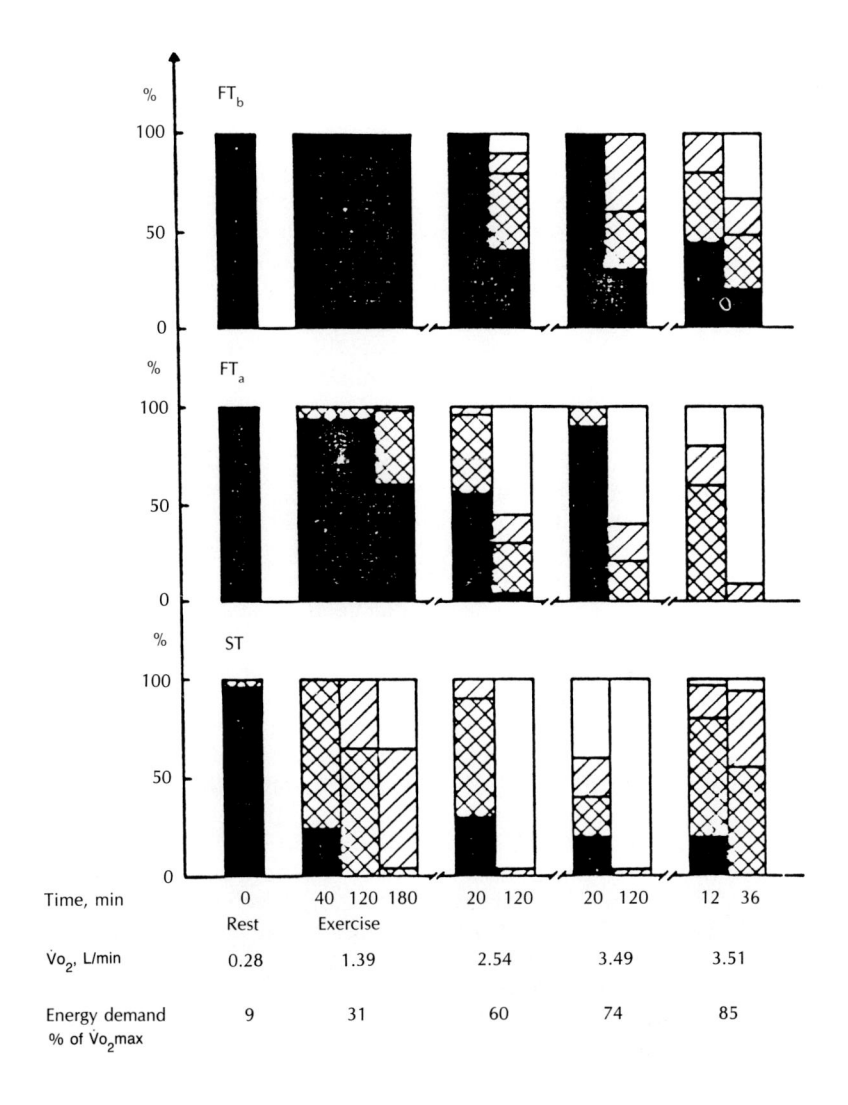

Figure 9–9 Schematic illustration of intensity of periodic acid-Schiff (PAS) stain (glycogen) in human skeletal muscle fibers at rest and after various times during prolonged exercise at relative work intensities ranging from 31% to 85% of the subject's maximal oxygen uptake. Graph is a summary of several studies. Findings at 74 percent $\dot{V}o_2$max show the PAS stain evaluated by microphotometry, whereas in the other studies results are based on a subjective rating (dark = *filled*; and white = *unfilled*, with various levels between as *crosshatched* and *hatched*). (Data from references 179, 181. Findings at 74 percent $\dot{V}o_2$max from Vøllestad K, unpublished material.)

occur.[178,181] However, as the exercise continues and ST fibers become glycogen depleted, there is evidence of a use of FT units.[178,181] This occurs without any rise in the lactate concentrations of the blood or in total-body oxygen uptake.[181] The latter circumstances suggest either that the FT fibers possess adequate mitochondrial enzymes and receive sufficient blood flow to support the terminal oxidation required for the levels of tension they produce during such exercise, or that the lactate produced is taken up and oxidized by other muscles. Such lactate could also be cleared by the liver.

Some of the discrepancies that exist in the

literature concerning the fiber type involvement at different exercise intensities may be attributable to the use of different modes of exercise. For example, cycle ergometers that are mechanically braked and have light flywheels often possess little inertial momentum. Thus for each pedal thrust a brisk contraction may be needed to keep a steady pace. From EMG studies it is known that the threshold for activation of a motor unit is reduced during brisk or ballistic type contractions.[103,106]

Clearly, recruitment order in humans may be related to the requirement for tension development, to the availability of oxygen, or to both. At exercise intensities that produce exhaustion in 4 minutes, less than one-half of the strength of the muscle is utilized.[191] In experiments in which static contractions were held with the knee extensors at tensions representing from 10 to 20 percent of the MVC, only ST units became glycogen depleted.[181] At higher tensions FT units also became depleted of glycogen. This suggests that with this type of muscular activity the availability of oxygen and the development of force influenced recruitment of FT units, because blood flow in the knee extensor group is restricted during sustained contraction above about 20 percent MVC.[192-194]

The EMG recordings from single fibers support the concept of an orderly recruitment of motor units in a progression from ST to FT units.[103-107,187,188,195,196] The observation that the individual motor unit is activated at specific levels of tension and ceases discharging when the tension falls below this set level points to the level of tension development as the primary factor in controlling motor unit recruitment.[197-199] Although there is evidence for an activation of FT motor units before or without ST units during high-intensity exercise, the data in support of this concept are equivocal.[108,109,200] There are also reports using either histochemical or electrophysiological techniques indicating exceptions to the orderly treatment of motor units as described above.[109,200,201]

The specific mechanism or sensing system to which the central nervous system responds with varying patterns of motor unit recruitment is unknown. It is easy to envisage a system centered upon the stretch receptors in muscle spindles or Golgi organs. Information from these receptors could signal the need for adding or subtracting motor units from the contraction. During prolonged submaximal exercise, when it appears that a progressive recruitment of motor units occurs starting with ST and finally using all units including FT units, this could occur as a result of failure of the ST units to produce the needed tension as their glycogen stores are depleted and their ability to produce the ATP needed to support contraction is diminished.

ADAPTIVE RESPONSE IN SKELETAL MUSCLE

Different types of motor units exist in skeletal muscles, and these are endowed with properties that uniquely qualify them for specific types of activity. In addition to the differences between major types of motor units, there are also differences between motor units that are histologically similar. Thus, there is a broad array of contractile speeds, fiber numbers, and metabolic potentials for the motor units in a single muscle. This section considers what effects growth and patterns of use (either overload or inactivity) have in establishing, maintaining, or changing the characteristics of skeletal muscle. Because activation of skeletal muscle by electrical stimulation or by voluntary means can produce very different mechanical and metabolic demands on the muscle depending on which fibers are engaged in generating the force, this must be considered when discussing muscle adaptation. To evaluate whether the mode of usage may elicit different adaptive responses, exercise is categorized as: high-resistance, few-repetition exercise (strength training); low-resistance, high-repetition exercise (endurance training); or varying intermediate combinations (for example, sprint training).

Clearly the changes in skeletal muscle that accompany either use or disuse as described in this chapter involve alterations in either the rate of protein synthesis or degradation. Recently attempts have been made to investigate these changes and to determine the mechanism by which they are induced and controlled.[202-216] This is an area for future investigation.

Muscle Size

In terms of its ability to adjust its size to physiologic demands, skeletal muscle is a very adaptable tissue. This is illustrated by the changes in weight that occur during normal growth and development and in the adult or growing animal in response to alterations in activity patterns. Because skeletal muscle consists (by weight) of about 85 percent fibers and 15 percent extrafiber material, a change in total weight is a simple, yet reliable, method for estimating changes in the fiber component of muscle.[217-221] Exceptions to this are instances in which experimental perturbations or pathologic changes produce modifications in the water and collagen content of muscle.[222,223] Human skeletal muscles possess a growth characteristic similar to that of other animals. This is illustrated by the increase in weight of the biceps brachii from about 2.0 g at birth to between 110 and 150 g in the adult (Saltin, Nygaard, and Colling-Saltin, unpublished observations). In addition, the absolute increase in the size of muscle depends on its function as determined by its location on the skeleton.

With changes in muscle size as a result of growth and maturity, there are also changes in the chemical composition of muscle of the fetus as compared to that of the adult. Fetal skeletal muscle is about 90 percent water.[224-227] At 4 to 7 months of age, this value is about 78.5 percent water; only minor changes occur thereafter, until attaining the adult value of about 76 percent water. There are also major changes in the protein fractions of muscle (Fig. 9-10). This is exemplified by a 2.8-fold increase in total protein from the 14th week of gestation to the adult human being. Of the various protein fractions, the biggest increase occurs in the fibrillar fraction, which increases 3.5-fold. There are also changes in the intracellular ion concentration from fetal life to maturity (Fig. 9-11).

Postnatal Development

Aherne and associates examined changes in the fibers of the deltoid, biceps brachii, rectus femoris, and gastrocnemius muscle of man in the age range from 37 weeks of gestation to 18 years of age.[228] This material was from 22 individuals, 14 males. Only rarely was there more than one sample for a given age, and not all years were represented. In this sample the fibers in the muscles at 37 weeks of gestation ranged from 36.5 to 48.2 μm^2, with the smallest fibers in the rectus femoris and the largest in the gastrocnemius muscles. Over the entire age range examined, there was a nearly linear increase in the cross-sectional area of the muscle fibers as a function of body dimension (Fig. 9-12). Unfortunately, the fibers were not subdivided into the different types. In mature individuals, the average fiber areas were approximately 2,000 μm^2, with those in the leg muscles being larger than those of the arm muscles. Nevertheless, during skeletal growth the longitudinal growth of the muscle fibers is such that the average sarcomere length in the mature muscle fibers is not markedly different from that of the young animal.[1,229]

Colling-Saltin has examined muscular growth in the lateral portion of the quadriceps, rectus abdominis, deltoid, biceps brachii, soleus, and gastrocnemius muscle of 86 fetuses and 50 infants and children to age 7.[224-226,230] The fetal samples included material from as early as 12 to 14 weeks of gestation. The majority of the samples were from males. The samples were fresh frozen and stained with histochemical methods to identify the different fiber types. These data illustrated that early in fetal life the muscle fibers had not developed to a stage at which they could be typed. Some differentiation of fibers into types appeared at about the 21st week of gestation and thereafter continued, with differentiation being nearly complete at approximately 1 year of age (Fig. 9-13). These studies revealed that at about 12 weeks of gestation the average cross-sectional area was 36.3 μm^2. This remained relatively constant until about 21 weeks of gestation, when ST fibers with an average area of about 128 μm^2 appeared in cross-sections. These ST fibers constituted about 3 percent of the total fiber population, with the remainder still being small, undifferentiated fibers. During the subsequent period of gestation, the percent of fibers that could be identified as a specific type increased, as did the average cross-sectional area of the fibers. At the time interval from 38 to 42 weeks of fetal life, approximately 80 percent of the fibers could be typed. These fibers averaged about 200 μm^2 in cross-sectional

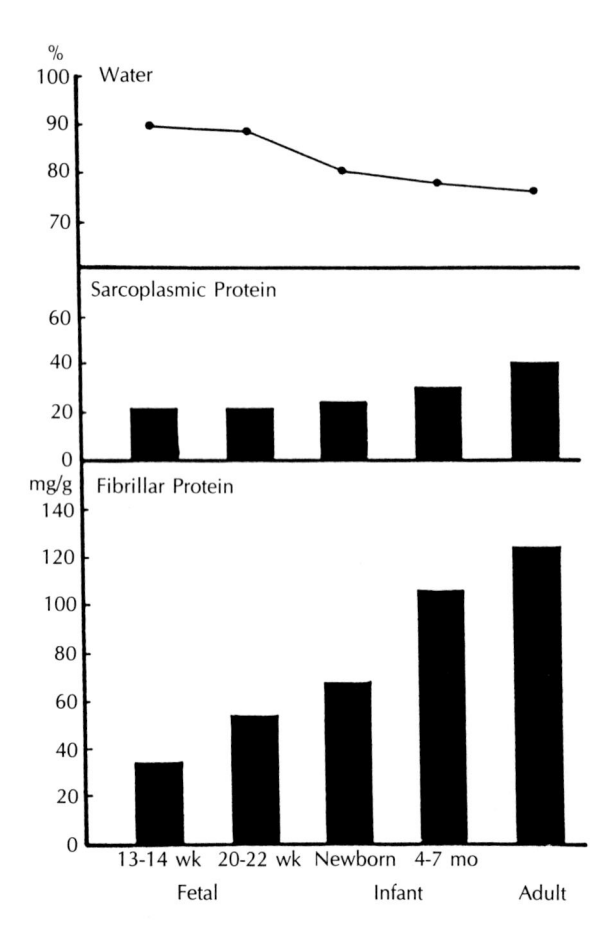

Figure 9-10 Changes in the percent of water and concentration of protein in the sarcoplasmic and fibrillar fractions of human skeletal muscle as a result of growth and development. (Adapted from Dickerson JWT, Widdowson EM. Biochem J 1960; 74:247–257.)

area. At the age of 1 year the cross-sections of the fibers ranged from 500 to 600 μm^2. The cross-sectional areas reported by Colling-Saltin are larger than those observed by Aherne and associates.[228] This difference can probably be attributed to the different methods used to prepare the tissue. Cross-sectional areas ranging from about 2,500 to 10,000 μm^2 have been observed in cryostat sections of fresh-frozen adult human limb skeletal muscle (see Table 9-5). There are a number of other studies in which fiber size was determined in muscle of children and adults.[75,76]

In addition to problems associated with methods of fixation (paraffin versus fresh frozen), there are difficulties associated with the assessment of the cross-sectional area of skeletal muscle fibers.[9,231-232] First is that the fibers, once removed from the intact muscle usually shorten.[233] Moreover, several methods can be applied in the actual determination of the area, which can also influence the results.[234,235]

Postnatal increases in muscle size are closely associated with hypertrophy of the preexisting fibers. Data on the number of fibers in human skeletal muscle come primarily from studies of the sartorius muscle as reported by MacCallum and Montgomery.[236,237] MacCallum made fiber counts from cross-sections of five fetuses and one full-term infant and concluded that fiber number was established before birth. Montgomery employed similar methods to estimate the total number of fibers in the sartorius muscle from samples including three stillborn (two fetal and one full-term) infants, two well-nourished infants (4 and 13 months old), and two adults (64 and 74 years old) of unspecified sex. The number of fibers

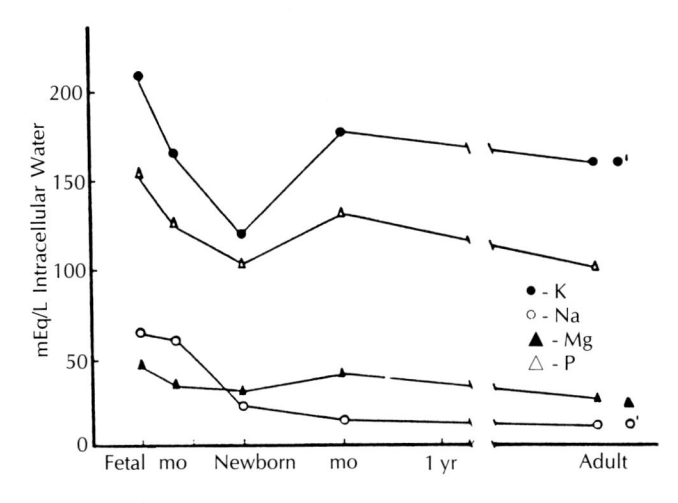

Figure 9-11 Intracellular ion concentrations for human skeletal muscle from fetal life to adulthood. The data points marked (') are averages of samples collected from the triceps brachii, vastus lateralis, and soleus of 6 male and 6 female adults. (Data from Dickerson JWT, Widdowson EM. Biochem J 1960; 74:247–257; except those marked ['] from Sjøgaard G. Water spaces and electrolyte combinations in human skeletal muscle. Thesis. Copenhagen: University of Copenhagen, 1979.)

appearing in the cross-section of the 4-month old infant was about twice that observed for the 32-week old fetus. There were no major differences in total fiber number with advanced age. Histologic examination of the muscle sections in the late stages of fetal life did not reveal any evidence of mitotic activity or of fibers undergoing "longitudinal splitting." On this basis Montgomery concluded that the apparent increase in fiber number of the sartorius muscle of humans during later fetal and early postnatal life was the result of a longitudinal fiber growth, such that more fibers appeared in the histologic cross-section. The lack of increase in fiber number in the sartorius muscle is in agreement with the observation that there is no evidence of fiber division in the biceps brachialis muscle of humans after midgestation. Moreover, no myoblasts have been observed in the muscle of human beings after birth, and the number of fibers in the biceps of infants is similar to that of adults.[14,86,238]

Use and Disuse

Muscular Strength. Heavy-resistance exercise results in increases in muscle bulk in excess of that which occurs during normal growth and development. This is exemplified by the conspicuous musculature of persons who engage in heavy physical labor or in athletic events in which heavy-resistance exercise is practiced (body building). The importance of the increase in size in response to functional overloads lies in the fact that the strength of a muscle is closely related to its cross-sectional area.[82,83,86] This principle is based on the concept that all motor units are maximally activated during MVC.[81,113] Moreover, there was little difference in the strength per square centimeter among boys, sedentary males, and highly trained judo athletes.[82,83] This supports the general contention that the capacity of muscle to develop force per unit of cross-sectional area is constant. If one accepts the concept that all individuals can maximally activate all motor units in a muscle, it is difficult to explain both the increases in force-developing capacity that occur in the nontrained limbs of individuals who train a contralateral limb and the instances in which training does not produce increases in the cross-sectional area of muscle.[142,199,239] Such changes in the force-developing capacity may be a function of the central nervous system rather than of the muscle.[187] Further, isometric training, consisting of three maximal contractions sustained for 10 seconds and separated by 1 minute of rest continued for 100 days, has been reported to produce a near doubling of the volitional strength of the forearm flexor muscles.[240] This increase occurs with only a 23 percent increase in the cross-sectional area of the muscles. The nontrained arms of these subjects increased in strength by 30 percent without any change in cross-sectional area of the muscles.

Fiber Cross-Sectional Area. There are several reports in which the cross-sectional area of the fibers in skeletal muscle of weight lifters

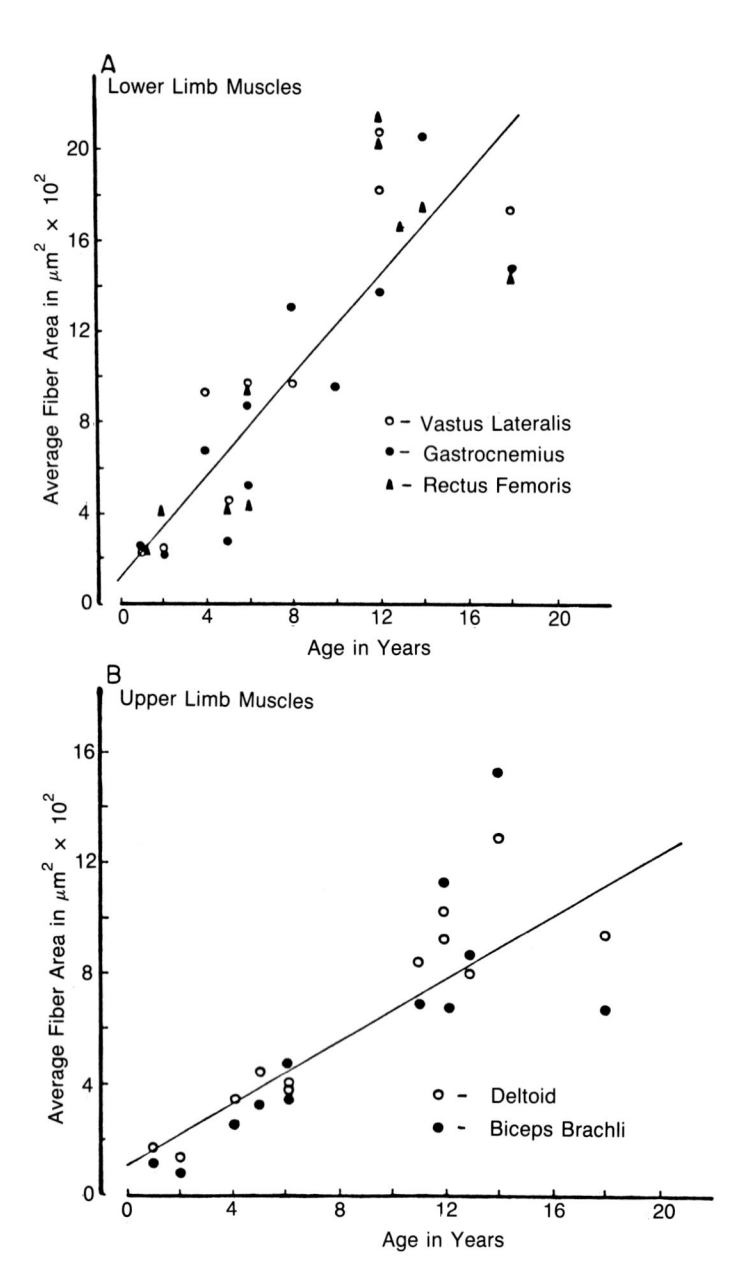

Figure 9–12 Data are for muscle from human subjects ranging in age from 2 mo to 18 yr. Fiber areas for infants less than 1 yr are not plotted. (A) Relationship between age and muscle fiber cross-sectional area in the lower limb muscles of humans. Equation of the regression line y = 115 + 111x. Between age and fiber area r = 0.92; between age and body height r = 0.98. (B) Relationship between age and muscle fiber cross-sectional area in the upper limb muscles of humans. Equation of the regression line is y = 112 + 56x. Between age and fiber area r = 0.85 (Data from Aherne W, et al. J Neurol Sci 1971; 14:17–182.)

or those who have engaged in a variety of sports events have been examined (see Table 9–5). The general conclusion from such studies has been that weight lifters generally have larger fiber areas than sedentary individuals or those who engage in endurance-type activities.[161] Edström and Ekblom, Costill and co-workers, and MacDougall and co-workers have reported that a period of strength training results in increases in the cross-sectional area of the FT fibers.[241-244] However, Thorstensson and associates did not observe a similar finding in subjects who had participated in 8 weeks of strength training.[245] In the latter study this was true in spite of an increased muscle mass and total body potassium. Muscle mass increased by only 1 kg (2.5 percent), which is probably too little to detect in fiber size if the increase

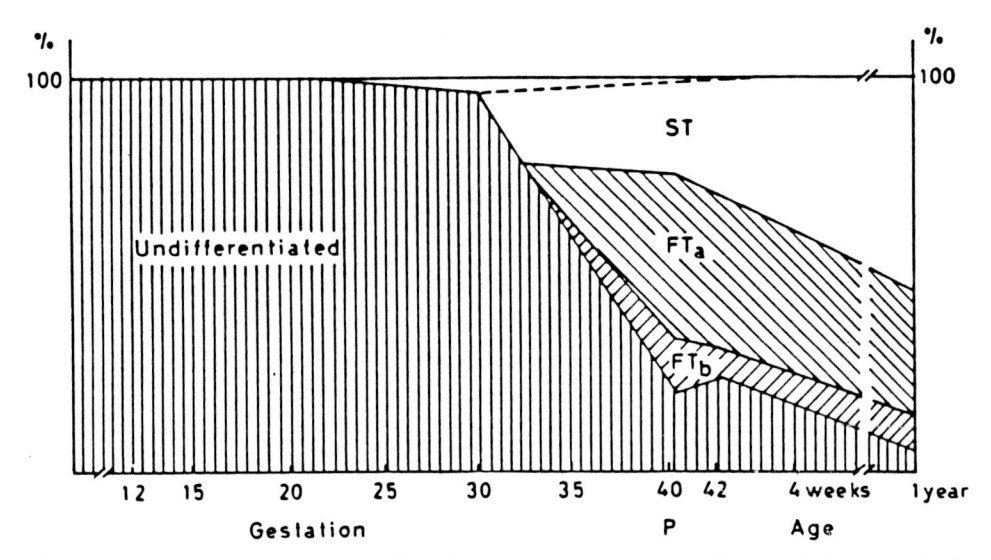

Figure 9–13 A summary description of the relative occurrence of various fiber types in human skeletal muscle during gestation and 1st year of life. The slow-twitch (ST) fibers are divided by size with the small fraction of Wohlfart's B fiber above the *dashed line*. (Data from Wohlfart G. Acta Psychiatry Neurol Scand (Suppl) 1937; 12:1–119.)

is not confined to only a few muscle groups. Gollnick and associates did not observe a selective enlargement of ST fibers after a 6-month endurance-training program.[246] MacDougall and co-workers have also examined the effect of weight-lifting activities on the cross-sectional area of the fibers in the triceps muscle of humans and found muscle-fiber hypertrophy.[243,244]

Forced inactivity, such as after injury, reduces the cross-sectional area of the fibers in skeletal muscle.[89,243,247] Subjects whose legs are immobilized in fixed casts as a result of radical knee surgery readily demonstrate this phenomenon.[185] In these subjects the cross-sectional area of the fibers was similar in the normal and the injured leg prior to surgery. After a 5-week immobilization there was a 27 percent decline in the cross-sectional area of the ST fibers of the vastus lateralis muscle. However, there was no change in the area of the FT fibers. Data are also available from subjects whose one leg had been immobilized for 15 weeks as a result of fracture.[248] Such immobilizations did not alter the composition of the muscle in terms of the percentages of the different fiber types. However, the cross-sectional area of both ST and FT fibers was lower by an average of 47 percent and 38 percent, respectively. The reduced FT fiber area after a 15-week immobilization, as opposed to no change after a 5-week immobilization, is probably attributable to the fact that in the latter study the patients were encouraged to perform intensive isometric contractions of the thigh. With such contractions FT fibers are recruited, and this may be an adequate stimulus for maintaining normal size of the FT fibers. This was evident from the relatively large FT fibers in these patients. When such exercise is not performed, the FT fibers also become smaller after a 4- to 6-week period of inactivity induced by putting a cast on the leg.[185]

The effect of physical conditioning on the fiber size of a normal leg and a leg after 6 to 8 weeks of immobilization has also been examined.[247] In these experiments CT was used to establish the total cross-section of the thigh muscles. These experiments have firmly established an atrophy of the thigh muscles as a result of chronic immobilization. This atrophy was almost exclusively restricted to the knee extensors, whereas the hamstring muscles were almost unchanged.[247] Moreover, the relative changes in the knee extensor cross-section and fiber size were closely correlated. A similar conclusion was reached by Renstrom in his study of the knee extensors in below-the-knee amputees.[89] In these investigations the total cross-sectional area was reduced by 30 percent and that of the fibers, by 26 percent.

Hypertrophy Versus Hyperplasia

There has been considerable interest over the years in the mechanism(s) by which skeletal muscles increase in size in response to heavy-resistance exercise. The early studies of Morpurgo, in which increases in muscle weight produced by training did not alter the number of fibers contained in the cross-section of the sartorius muscle of the dog (one muscle having been removed before and the other after training), have been the cornerstone of evidence that muscular growth in response to functional overloads occurs by hypertrophy of the fibers and not by hyperplasia.[249,250] Subsequent studies support this general concept.[42,251,252] There is also general agreement with the concept that normal growth of muscle occurs by hypertrophy of the fibers present in the muscle at birth.

The concept of a postnatal growth of muscle occurring by a combination of longitudinal and circumferential hypertrophy of the preexisting fibers has recently been challenged by reports of larger numbers of fibers in enlarged muscle than in control muscle.[213,253-261] In some cases the suggestion has been made that the increase in fiber number was the result of new fibers formed by a longitudinal division of preexisting fibers.[256,258-268] This suggestion is based in part on the observation that fibers with points of branching or with central cleavages exist in skeletal muscle.[254,258,266,267,269-272] The existence of such fibers in skeletal muscle was reported in 1866 by VonEulenberg and Cohnheim and in 1891 by Erb.[273,274] The major impetus for espousing the concept that increases in fiber number occur as a result of fiber division (a so-called fiber splitting) during muscular enlargement produced by functional overload comes from the studies of Van Linge and Reitsma.[266,268] These investigators produced muscular enlargement in the hindlimb muscles of the rat by either denervation or surgical ablation of synergistic muscles. In some cases exercise was used in combination with inactivation of a synergist to produce further muscular enlargement. Van Linge observed what were considered to be new fibers in histologic sections of the overloaded, enlarged muscles.[268] These "new fibers" were described as small fibers interspersed among normal-sized fibers. It was suggested that these represented "young muscle fibers, the growth of which was stimulated by strenuous training." Technical difficulties were cited by Van Linge as making it impossible to count all of the fibers in the muscle from histologic cross-sections. Subsequently Reitsma reported the existence of similar small fibers in histologic cross-section of experimentally enlarged muscle.[266] Moreover, when enlarged muscles were digested in nitric acid and fibers were teased free, some fibers with branches and appendages of varying length were isolated. The presence of such fibers was interpreted as evidence that a longitudinal splitting of the fibers was occurring. Unfortunately the total number of fibers in the muscles was not determined, nor was the frequency of the branched fibers established.

Little is known about the number of fibers in human skeletal muscle. Etemadi and Hosseini reported that the number of fibers in the human biceps brachii muscle was larger in an athletic subject (316,243 fibers) than in two sedentary individuals (227,233 and 199,240 fibers).[275] Of these subjects, the one with well-developed musculature also had the greater fiber diameter (45.25 µm as compared to about 23 µm for the sedentary individuals).[276]

Because there has been a rather wide acceptance of the concept that the total number of fibers in skeletal muscle can increase with work-induced growth, it seems appropriate to comment on the methodology that was used to arrive at this conclusion. Basically three methods are used to determine total fiber number in skeletal muscle. These are: counting all fibers that appear in a cross-sectional cut of the muscle; counting the fibers in a given cross-sectional area cut, and then estimating total fiber number by an extrapolation to the total area of the section; and making a cross-sectional cut, dispersing the fibers in saline, and counting the fragments with an electronic device.[277] All methods appear valid for estimating the total number of fibers in the cross section of muscle. However, these methods assume either that all of the fibers in a muscle are contained in the cross-section or that changes in the number of fibers contained in the single section are representative of any change in the entire muscle. These assumptions appear to be tenable only when the fibers lie parallel to the long axis of the muscle and traverse the point where the cross-section is made. However, this is not the case for muscles in which the fiber arrangement is penniform. In addition, the angle that the fibers form with the longitudinal axis of the muscle is known to change during muscular enlargement.[85,278,279] A change in fiber angle in the mature animal is necessary to accommodate the large fiber diameter without any change in the total length of the muscle. The difficulty in determining the fiber number in a muscle with a multipennate fiber arrangement is illustrated from the studies of Gollnick and associates and of Gonyea and co-workers.[253,254,280]

The total number of fibers in the human biceps has been estimated from measurements of the total cross-sectional area of muscle determined by CT and of the area of the individual fibers determined from biopsy samples, assuming that the majority of the fibers extend through the whole muscle.[162,281,282] In sedentary male and female subjects, the cross-sectional area of the muscle averaged 11.6 cm^2 (range: 9.8 to 16.1) and 8.7 cm^2 (6.8 to 10.6), respectively. These values were 12.3 cm^2 (11.9 to 12.9) and 9.0 cm^2 (7.7 to 9.7) for trained male and female swimmers. The total number of fibers in the biceps averaged 280,000 (280,000 to 290,000) and 420,000 (340,000 to 500,000) for the sedentary female and male subjects. This was in contrast to 320,000 (240,000 to 380,000) and 350,000 (280,000 to 400,000) for the trained female and male subjects. These data demonstrate the existence of considerable variation in the fiber number of subjects and considerable overlap between the sexes and between the sedentary and trained groups. There is no evidence of a systematic difference between the sedentary and trained groups, the greater total cross-sectional area of the muscle being attributable to the larger cross-sectional area of the individual fibers.

The tedious process of isolating all of the fibers of a muscle has deterred researchers from applying this method to the study of normal growth and development and of hypertrophy versus hyperplasia during work-induced muscular enlargement. Gollnick and co-workers dissected, counted, and examined each fiber over its entire length for bifurcations.[280] In these studies there was no change in fiber number in enlarged as compared to control skeletal muscle in the rat. The appearance of branched fibers in all muscles was interpreted as an indication that these abnormal fibers are normally present in small percentages and do not represent an active process of a longitudinal division of fibers.

The finding of Gollnick and associates supports the older concept that the number of fibers in skeletal muscle is established early in life, and that the exceptional enlargement that occurs in response to a variety of overloads is a true hypertrophy.[236,237,251,280,283,284] This supports the conclusion of Hall-Craggs and co-workers and of James that if a splitting of fibers in skeletal muscle does occur during enlargement, it is of minimal importance in the overall increase in muscular size.[263–265,285]

There are reports of increases in the DNA content of skeletal muscle during normal growth and work-induced hypertrophy.[286–288] This could be interpreted as an indication of the addition of new fibers. However, the bulk of the increase in DNA arises from the addition of connective tissue to support enlarged fibers.[211,289] Part of the increase in DNA is associated with a proliferation of the satellite cells of muscle.[213,290–296] Some of these are apparently incorporated into the existing muscle fibers. This has been proposed as a mechanism whereby the ratio of nuclear material to other cellular components is maintained at a constant level within the cell. Of some interest is the observation that blocking DNA synthesis does not stop the hypertrophy of muscle fibers in the rat soleus muscle after tenotomy of the synergists.[297] Such blocking did completely inhibit connective tissue proliferation; an almost complete lack of new nuclei was observed in histologic sections.

In summary from birth to full maturity there is an increase in muscle weight from 100- to 200-fold in the skeletal muscle of most mammals. This increased muscle size is the result of a longitudinal growth produced by the addition of sarcomeres to the ends of the existing muscle fibers and by circumferential growth produced by the addition of myofibrils. During the growth process the total number of nuclei increases, so that the ratio between cellular material and nuclei remains rather constant. With added physical demands, such as heavy manual labor or weight lifting, there is an additional increase in muscle mass. This increased muscle mass is produced by further increases in total cross-sectional area of the individual fibers and not by the addition of more muscle fibers. With disuse or with inadequate nutrition there is a loss of muscle mass as a result of a decrease in cross-sectional area.

Metabolic Capacity

Postnatal Development

The skeletal muscle of the newborn contains substrate concentrations and enzyme activities, expressed per unit of dry weight, that are only slightly below those found in later life.[225] This could be interpreted as indicating that parallel increases occur in all muscular components with postnatal maturation. However, with growth there is a continued differentiation of the fiber types that necessitates a preferential synthesis of either mitochondrial, cytoplasmic, or myofibrillar proteins, depending on the type of fiber that develops. How this differential growth is regulated is unknown. Because it is the rule rather than the exception, different stimuli and regulatory mechanisms must be present for the increases in contractile proteins and metabolic enzymes. Evidence suggests that this is regulated, at least in part, by the motor nerve.[61-63,65,298-303]

Use and Disuse

Phosphagen Stores. There are reports of increases and of no change in the ATP and CP concentrations of human skeletal muscle with either endurance or strength training.[136,244,304,305] Increases in both ATP and CP concentrations have been reported in the limb muscles of adolescent and adult males after programs of endurance training.[136,304,305] However, when the training was extended from 3 to 6 months in the adult group, the ATP and CP concentrations returned to the pretraining level. Only a few studies are available dealing with the effects of immobilization or termination of training on the phosphagen stores of muscle. Studies with animals suggest that, although there may be increases in the phosphagen stores after training, these modifications are small and probably biologically unimportant.[306,307] Further proof that changes in the immediately available energy stores of ATP and CP are not important features of adaptation to training comes from observations of elite athletes. In these individuals, whether they have trained for strength development or for endurance, the ATP and CP concentrations in the muscles do not differ more than a few moles per kilogram of wet weight (approximately 100 percent) from those of sedentary individuals. Attempts have been made to determine whether differences exist between the ST and FT fibers.[139] In these studies the ATP and CP concentrations were found to be slightly higher in the ST than in the FT fibers in the muscle of female athletes competing in endurance events.[138]

Glycogen. In the first studies on the glycogen stores of human skeletal muscle in which the influence of exercise was examined, it was noted that higher values existed in trained than in sedentary individuals.[190] Thereafter several studies, both longitudinal and cross-sectional, demonstrated that subjects undergoing strength-, sprint-, or endurance-training programs possessed larger muscle glycogen stores, although in some instances the difference between the trained and sedentary state was small.[128,136,244,246] Conversely immobilization or detraining results in a reduction in the glycogen concentration of skeletal muscle.[185] However, the changes observed with activity and inactivity are well within the more dramatic variation in the glycogen concentration of skeletal muscle that can be induced with dietary manipulations with or without exercise.[126,127,308-310] The one-leg model, in which one leg is trained and the other is left untrained, has been useful to assess objectively the quantitative effect of exercise on muscle glycogen stores, divorced from either dietary or hormonal influences. At least three such studies are available in which the vastus lateralis muscles of a control and of an endurance-trained leg were examined.[133,311,312] In these studies the glycogen concentration of the trained leg was from 6 to 60 mmol per kilogram of wet weight higher than that of the untrained leg. An alternative approach to this problem has been to examine the glycogen content in the arm and leg muscles of individuals whose training is primarily with either the arms or the legs, such as bicyclists, canoeists, and swimmers. Such studies have revealed that the muscle glycogen content is higher in the trained than in the control muscles, with differences varying from 20 to 101 mmol per kilogram of wet weight. Training increases glycogen synthase activity.[133,251,313-318] When activities of hexokinase and glycogen synthase were also compared in the two legs of which only one leg was trained, both enzymes were found to be increased in the trained leg, with the relative increments being about 30 percent to 50 percent.[133] The muscle glycogen concentrations in these studies were also increased from 38 to 50 mmol per kilogram of wet weight. These differences represented relative increases of 47 percent to 100 percent.

Triglyceride Stores. Few studies have measured the triglyceride concentration in human skeletal muscle, and of these, only three were longitudinal with measurements made on the same subjects before and after training.[311,319,320] Quantitative morphometric techniques applied to electron micrographs have demonstrated that the lipid content in muscles of sedentary humans varies between 0.1 and 0.6 vol%, depending on the muscle examined.[321-323] In muscle from trained subjects, the range for the same muscles was from 0.2 to 0.8 vol%. Strength and endurance training altered the triglyceride content of muscle. Morgan and co-workers, and Bylund-Fellenius and associates observed elevation in the triglyceride content of the quadriceps muscle after endurance training.[316,319,320] The increase was about 50 percent from an initial value of approximately 10 µmol per gram of wet weight. Of special interest are results from a study in which subjects trained only one leg, thereby permitting comparison with the nontrained leg to obviate the effects of diet. In this instance there was no difference in triglyceride content of the muscles of the two legs.[311] There are also reports of a decline in the triglyceride content of skeletal muscle of humans with exercise.[123] Thus, factors other than physical activity, such as percent of lipid in the diet, may dominate in determining the triglyceride content of skeletal muscle.

Glycolytic Enzymes. The number of longitudinal training studies focusing on changes in the activities of glycolytic enzymes in human skeletal muscle is limited. When these studies are divided into reports concentrating on improving strength, speed (sprinting), or endurance capacity, only one, or at the most two, reports are available in each area. Although this is the case, the adaptive response of the glycolytic enzymes in skeletal muscle to varying patterns of increased use is rather clear. Training regimens designed to increase maximal strength have not produced alterations in the activities of phosphorylase (PHOS), phosphofructokinase (PFK), or lactate dehydrogenase (LDH).[239,242] This is true for both dynamic and static exercise. The response of muscle appears to be related to the total duration of the exercise. Thus, no changes were noted in muscle when the resistance was so high that the total number of repetitions to exhaustion was completed in 6 seconds.[242] However, when the resistance was lowered and the exercise extended to 30 seconds, there was a 10 to 20 percent elevation in PHOS and PFK activities, but LDH was unchanged. A high-intensity endurance training did produce an increase in PFK activity.[246,304] Hexokinase also has been reported to be elevated with training.[316]

Further information concerning the adaptive response of the glycolytic system comes from cross-sectional studies of athletes competing in typical strength and sprint-type events. Shot-putters, weight lifters, and discus throwers have PHOS, PFK, and LDH activities well within the range of sedentary subjects, whereas sprinters, jumpers, and runners (400 to 800 m) usually have elevated levels of these enzymes.[161,324]

The influence of sprint and endurance training on total LDH activity and on the isozymes of LDH has been examined.[325,326] Cross-sectional comparisons were also made between weight lifters and endurance athletes.[245,325,327-329] Total LDH activity was not altered by sprint training. These results, and also the report of high values in the muscles of weight lifters, contrast with some mentioned above.[325,327] It has been found that the muscle of sprint-trained individuals contains a relatively high percent of LDH4-5, whereas muscle from endurance-trained individuals is especially high in LDH1-2.[325] Part of the explanation for the differences between athletic groups may lie in the fiber composition of the muscle. Thus, it is known that ST fibers not only show lower LDH activities but also have high percentages of LDH1-2.[325,328] The type and cellular location of the LDH is also different for the fiber types and could be an important factor in their function.[330-335] Clearly in future studies in which adaptations of LDH are investigated, close attention must be given to the nature of the muscle sample that is analyzed.

Mitochondrial Enzymes. Although it has been known for a long time that the capacity of muscle to consume oxygen was related to the level of activity of the citric acid cycle and electron-transport system, studies of adaptations in the mitochondrial enzymes of human skeletal muscle were not undertaken until the late 1960s and early 1970s. Over a period of time results from cross-sectional studies of men and women performing physical activity of an endurance type were published.[73,133,161,241,246,304,312,319,321-324,326,327,336-353] Cytochrome oxidase (CYTOX) and succinate dehydrogenase (SDH) activities were found to be elevated in the trained skeletal muscle.

Exercise designed to develop strength does not alter the activities of the mitochondrial enzymes.[161,242,243] When this type of exercise is practiced over a long time, it leads to a disproportionate proliferation of the contractile proteins, resulting in a dilution of the mitochondrial concentration in the muscle fiber, and the activities of the enzymes expressed per unit of muscle become lower than those of muscle from sedentary individuals.[161,243]

Sprint training, in contrast to high-resistance training, causes a definite adaptive response with significant elevation of the mitochondrial enzymes.[312] Intermittently performed isometric strength training places a severe stress on oxygen utilization and also induces increases in mitochondrial enzymes.[354] Thus, it appears that the concentration of mitochondrial enzymes is increased whenever there is a chronic demand for a high-oxygen consumption by the muscle. In line with this is the finding that the largest increases in these enzymes occur after typical endurance-training programs.[246,312] It appears to make little difference whether the exercise is performed intermittently or continuously, although changes at the level of the individual fiber may be affected.[355] Other evidence of differences in the concentration of oxidative enzymes based on the relative use of a muscle can be obtained from sedentary individuals in whom the activities of the oxidative enzymes for end-terminal oxidation are higher in the leg than the arm muscles, in spite of a similar fiber-type distribution.[161] The muscles of the legs are presumably used more in endurance activity than those of the arms.

The time course for the change in oxidative enzyme activities and the concomitant change in whole-body $\dot{V}O_2max$ (Fig 9–14) suggest that there is a close relationship of these variables over the first 3 to 4 weeks of training.[336] Thereafter the increase in $\dot{V}O_2max$ levels off, but the activity of the mitochondrial enzymes continues to rise. This disparity in the response of the $\dot{V}O_2max$ and mitochondrial enzyme activity is further illustrated by comparisons of endurance athletes and sedentary individuals. The $\dot{V}O_2max$ of the athletes may be twice that of the control subjects, whereas the activity of the mitochondrial enzymes of the muscle is three- to four-fold higher than those of the sedentary individuals.[356] As pointed out earlier, the adaptive response in enzyme activity is local in nature. Competitive cyclists and endurance runners have higher activity levels for the mitochondrial enzymes in their legs that do sedentary individuals. Canoeists resemble sedentary people in their leg muscles but have elevated enzyme concentrations in arm muscle.[161] Moreover, training one limb induces changes in the muscle of that limb but not in the muscle of the contralateral untrained limb (Fig. 9–15).

The enzymes in the various metabolic pathways of the muscle cell are found in a rather constant ratio to one another.[146-150] The question arises whether this constant proportionality is retained when adaptations occur in response to increased muscle use. For human skeletal muscle, almost all existing data support the concept of a constant proportionality of enzymes. Thus, increase in SDH and CYTOX activities occur in concert.[357,358] The capacities of the citric acid cycle and the electron-transport chain change in parallel. Whether enzymes in the β-oxidation pathway adapt in similar proportion is unknown. In one of the few studies in which marker enzymes for all of the major mitochondrial pathways were followed citrate synthase (CS) and CYTOX increased similarly, although with a slightly different time course, but HAD was unchanged.[319] In fact a small decline was noted after 6 months of training. These data are in contrast to those from a study with middle-aged men, in whom a similar type of training (jog-

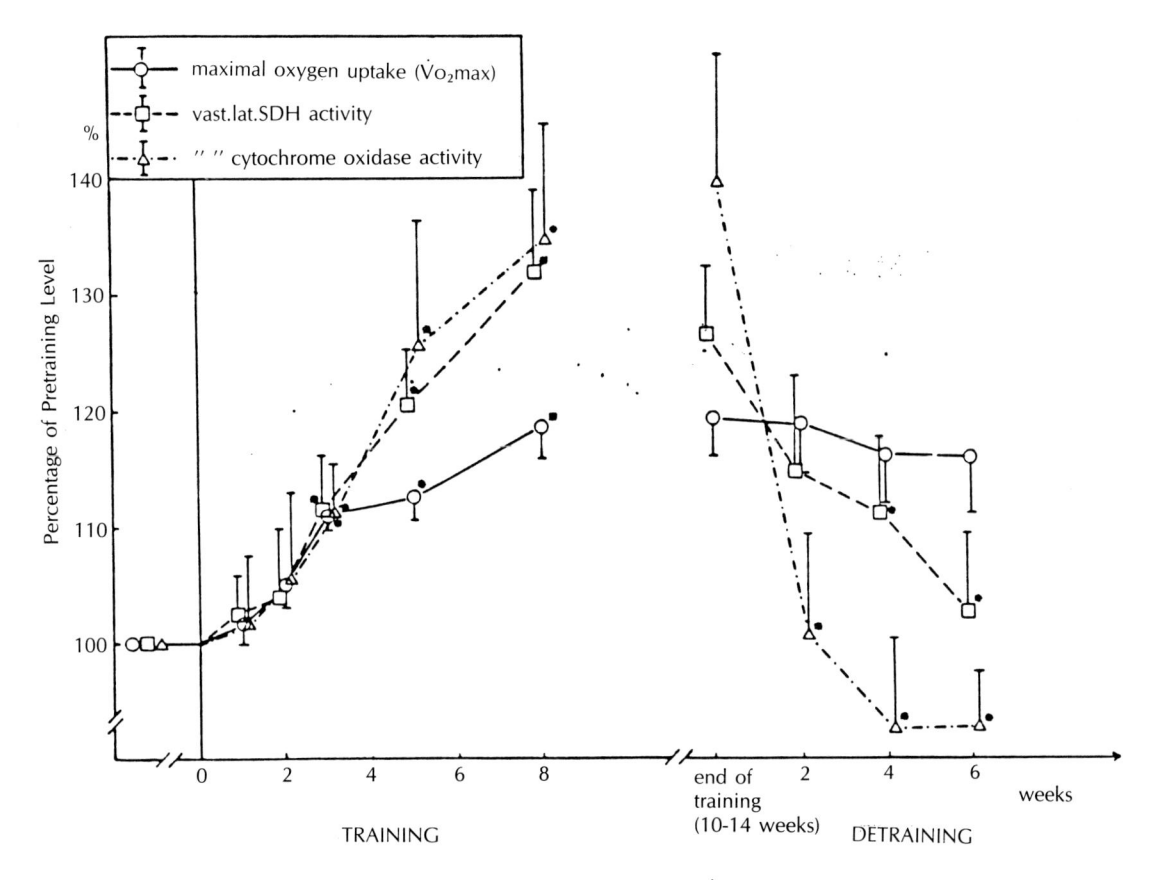

Figure 9-14 Time courses for changes in two mitochondrial enzymes and $\dot{V}O_2$max during physical conditioning and deconditioning. *Significant changes in time (paired t test) for the selected variables. (Adapted from Henriksson J, Reitman JS. Acta Physiol Scand 1977; 99:91-97.)

ging, playing basketball, etc.) produced parallel increases in SDH, CS, and HAD activities.[359] The activity of HAD was observed to be present in a constant proportion to SDH, CS, or CYTOX in cross-sectional studies of endurance-trained subjects, with the ratio being close to 1.0 (0.8 to 1.4).[321,344] However, it is conceivable that training could produce differential responses in enzymes of β-oxidation as compared to the citric acid cycle or the electron-transport chain as a function of the type or intensity of the exercise regimen. With intense interval training, which is as effective in producing increases in $\dot{V}O_2$max as continuous exercise, FFA utilization may be less and thereby may fail to elicit any adaptive response in the enzymes of the β-oxidation pathway. An indication of this possibility is found in a study of eight long-distance runners, all having $\dot{V}O_2$max above 70 ml (kg^{-1})(min^{-1}).[344] Those who trained with continuous exercise possessed higher HAD activities in the leg muscles than those who trained with intermittent exercise, despite the fact that SDH activities were identical. Additional support for this possibility comes from sprint-training studies in which CS, SDH, and CYTOX were elevated but HAD was unchanged.[319] In concert with this are the results from a study of sedentary subjects and individuals involved in a variety of sports activities.[359] Those persons who participated in game-type activities had lower ratios of HAD to CS than did the sedentary or endurance-trained individuals.

Histochemical staining for NADH-nitrotetrazolium reductase or SDH clearly demonstrates that the elevation of oxidative enzymes can occur in all fiber types. Morphometric

rectly to the actual use of the fiber. This suggests that the inducers of these modifications are local in nature and depend on the internal conditions within the muscle fibers. Because similar adaptations can be induced by continuous or interval exercise, there are obviously many methods for inducing these local changes. Presently there is no indication about the nature of the inducer for the synthesis-specific proteins or how it is related to physical activity. The adaptations preclude the existence of a general inducing factor, such as a change in the level of an unknown factor in the blood.

It is known that synthesis of enzymes can be induced by elevation in substrate concentrations.[404] There are a number of substrates that become elevated during exercise including citrate, lactate, malate, and glucose 6-PO_4.[119,120,405] None of these has been demonstrated to be an inducer for the synthesis of components of the metabolic pathways. The fact that all components of the oxidative system increase in concert appears to suggest that the general flux of substrates through the system may be the inducer. Fitch and Chaikoff suggested the involvement of a concept of "throughput," because the enzyme content of tissue appears to be directly related to the amount of substrate conversion that occurs in a given tissue. With the elevated metabolic rates associated with exercise and the total substrate conversion during prolonged endurance-type exercise, it is entirely possible that a substrate flux through the system could be involved in the induction of the increased oxidative capacities of the different fiber types. This may be important from the standpoint of the stability of enzymes. Enzymes are known to be more stable in the presence of their substrates.[406]

In recent years a great deal of information has been generated about the adaptability of skeletal muscle to a variety of patterns of use and disuse. It would appear that there is little need for further experiments to explore additional types and intensities of exercise that can influence some of these well-documented changes. Therefore more attention should be directed toward furthering the understanding of the processes that induce the specific synthesis of proteins and control the genetic apparatus of the cells involved.

CONNECTIVE TISSUE

Limited data are available that show the effects of training on the connective tissue of skeletal muscle and of differences between the types of skeletal muscle. However, it has been demonstrated that with a work-induced growth of muscle there is an increased synthesis of both deoxyribonucleic acid (DNA) and RNA in skeletal muscle.[211,297] The bulk of this DNA has been shown to be localized in the connective tissue.[211,297,407] When DNA synthesis was inhibited, chronic overload still produced an increase in the cross-sectional area of the muscle fibers but without a concomitant proliferation of the interfiber support structures.[297] Only limited data are available that concern the effect of training on the connective tissue of human skeletal muscle. In one study it was reported that an 8-week training program increased the activity of propyl hydroxylase in the vastus lateralis muscle of 69-year-old female but not male subjects.[408] In a population of men ranging in age from 33 to 70 years, Suominen and Heikkinen observed higher activities of propyl hydroxylase in the vastus lateralis muscle of those who were habitually active than in sedentary individuals.[351] Clearly this is an area in which additional data are needed.

CAPILLARIES

The capillary is the interface between the skeletal muscle and the vascular supply that makes the exchange of bloodborne materials possible. Many of the features of this exchange were described by Krogh in his now-classic studies.[409,410] Since these pioneering studies there has been considerable effort directed towards furthering the understanding of this system. Because the functioning of skeletal muscle during exercise depends to a large extent on the perfusion of the muscle with blood, attention is focused here on some of the factors that contribute to this process. This includes a description of the number, length, and diameter of the capillaries as they are related to and surround the muscle fibers. Although such measures do not give any indication of the number of open capillaries, of blood flow either at rest or during exercise, or of the permeability characteristics of the exchange process—all of which are essential in determining the transport rate for specific substances—they do give estimates of the upper capacity for blood flow in the muscle. This situation is similar to the use of maximal activity (V_{max}) for enzymes as an indicator of the potential substrate flux through a specific metabolic pathway.

There has been some attention paid to the effect of varying patterns of physical activity on the capillary supply to muscles and of the differences in capillary supply that may exist among the different types of muscle fibers. The results of such studies depend on the methodology used. Basically three methods have been used to visualize capillaries in skeletal muscle: injection of a dye into the capillary lumen, staining of the capillary wall, and vital microscopy. There are problems associated with all three methods.[336,411,412]

Anatomy

The arrangement of the capillaries in skeletal muscle was the focus of many of the early studies.[411,413,414] In summary, in white muscle the majority of capillaries run parallel to the muscle fibers, but there are also capillaries that encircle the fibers. In red muscle the capillaries have a more tortuous arrangement. They also seem to form parallel loops.

Capillary Density

Capillary number in a cross-section of a muscle fiber bundle can give information on several subjects of importance for the understanding of skeletal muscle capillary physiology.

Growth and Development

Because postnatal growth of skeletal muscle is due to enlargement in both diameter and length of existing muscle fibers, the capillaries surrounding the fibers are pushed apart, and the number of capillaries per square millimeter (density) decreases. However, in animal studies the reduction in capillary density is less than could be anticipated from the growth of fiber size. This is due then, to an increase in capillaries per fiber found with development.[415,416]

Muscle Fiber Types and Potential for Oxidative Metabolism

Ranvier was the first to demonstrate a difference in red and white muscles in degree of capillarization.[413] Since then quite a few studies have presented evidence in support of this early finding, but systematic studies on the subject are scarce. The explanation is that with injection techniques it is difficult to identify fiber types and their metabolic potential. Romanul, combining a stain for alkaline phosphatase to visualize capillaries in muscles from the rat, rabbit, and man with stains for mitochondrial enzymes, has made a plea for a very close coupling between the oxidative metabolic capacity of a fiber and the number of capillaries surrounding the fiber.[417] Further, in studies with cross-innervation of muscles, the capillary count did change in relation to alteration in the oxidative capacity of the muscle fibers.[418] He supports his contention with excellent micrographs, but no detailed mathematical treatment of the results is presented. However, ample evidence is available to demonstrate differences in capillaries of ST and FT fibers (see Fig. 9–3).

The size of the various fiber types also has to be taken into account, because ST fibers usually are smaller than FT fibers. Many of the studies of capillaries in human muscle have used serial frozen sections in which staining of the capillary basement membranes was done concurrently with evaluation of metabolic profile and muscle fiber type.[73,86,207,230,234,419–421] In mixed muscles such as the gastrocnemius, the number of capillaries surrounding a specific fiber type is between three and four for ST fibers, 2.5 to three for FT_a, and two to three for FT_b fibers. Not until the fiber size is taken into account can a significant difference in capillarization of the various fiber types be established. In the untrained muscles studied, the average area a capillary supplies is 20 to 30 percent more for FT_b and 10 to 20 percent more for FT_a than for ST fibers. The absolute values may vary markedly among individuals and also among muscles, but the overall pattern is remarkably stable. What contributes to this rather small difference is the fact that in large parts of mixed muscle, FT fibers share capillaries with adjacent ST fibers. In locally homogeneous areas of mixed muscle where an individual muscle fiber is surrounded only by those of similar type, it was found that there are one to four capillaries per FT fiber, but four to 11 capillaries per ST fiber (G. Sjøgaard, personal communication). Accounting for differences in fiber size, the ratio for the fiber-type area each capillary had to supply could be estimated to be in the order of 3 to 1 for ST to FT fibers.

From among variables used to quantitate capillarization, the question of which serves as the best indicator of diffusing conditions is still unsettled. Although it appears essential to include an estimate of diffusing distance, it is not immediately apparent whether the critical distance is to the center of the muscle fiber or to the most distant point between capillaries along the periphery of a fiber in cross-section; the point being that mitochondrial density is largest underneath the sarcolemma and smaller, centrally.[321,322] What adds to the importance of this question is that, although it is commonly believed that the diffusion of oxygen is the key factor, there may be situations during exercise when substrate uptake, release of a metabolite, or heat dissipation is just as essential.

Use and Disuse

Capillary Density

Recent studies using both electron microscopy and histochemistry have demonstrated that human skeletal muscle adapts to use by increasing the number of capillaries.[155,162,336,421-424] In fact, all variables (capillaries per fiber, capillaries per square millimeter, and number of capillaries found around a fiber) are increased. Because the last two variables also are a function of muscle fiber size, the variable most frequently used is capillaries per fiber. This indicator of capillarization in trained muscle is closely linked to whole-body maximal oxygen uptake of a subject, and alteration in activity level causing a change in maximal oxygen uptake results in a parallel change in the number of capillaries per fiber. A doubling of maximal oxygen uptake corresponds approximately to a doubling of the number of capillaries per fiber. In untrained muscles FT (FT_b) fibers have the largest fiber area per capillary and the lowest level of oxidative capacity, but with use these fibers adapt and become almost indistinguishable from ST fibers for these variables. This supports the concept of Romanul and others that there is a close coupling between the number of capillaries and the capacity for oxidative metabolism of the fibers they supply.[417,418] Further, in animal experiments it appears as though the capillaries begin to proliferate before changes can be noted in the oxidative enzymes. Just as importantly, it proves that the FT fibers have the ability to adapt to aerobic metabolism, which is similar to the metabolism of ST fibers.

In well-trained endurance swimmers, mean muscle fiber area was the smallest in the most trained muscles, and in marathon runners the areas of muscle fibers in the gastrocnemius muscle were also small.[421] Further, 2 weeks of no training caused the muscle fibers of the gastrocnemius to become slightly larger.[425] These findings may support the notion that the distance to the center of the muscle cell is a critical factor. Whether it is the transport of gas or substrate that is crucial is still obscure. Because myoglobin markedly enhances the oxygen transport within the cell and is elevated with enhanced oxidative capacity, the reduction in diffusing distances of substrates other than oxygen may be the crucial limiting factor.[426]

The effect of inactivity on muscle capillarization is less well studied in man (Fig. 9-16). The picture that emerges from available detraining studies or studies in which a limb is placed in a cast is that the number of capillaries per fiber is reduced. Notably, it appears as if early in the time course the reduction in the number of capillaries is slightly slower than a possible change in fiber size, resulting in slightly shorter diffusing distances the first week of inactivity.[356] After some weeks both variables approach a new level of adaptation.[362] With tenotomy, reduction in capillary density has also been observed.[427,428]

Regulation

Little is known about the factors involved in capillary proliferation. Myrhage and Hudlická cite Ashton as saying that "endothelial cells them-

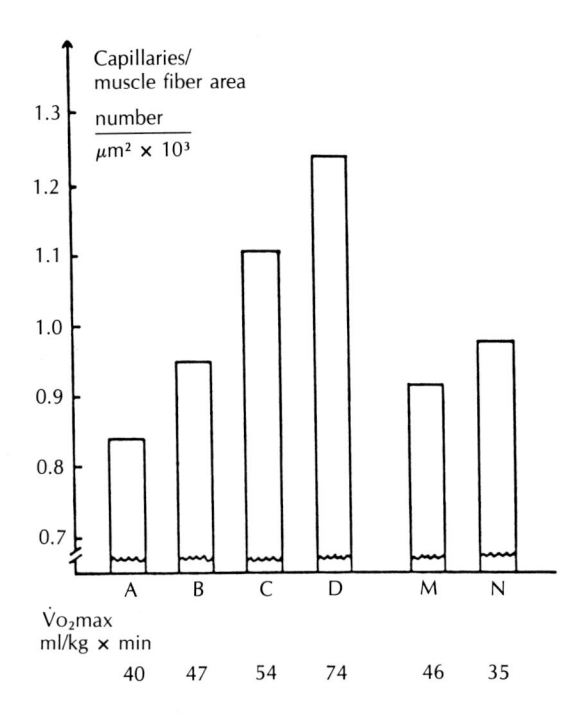

Figure 9–16 Mean values for number of capillaries per 1,000 μm² of muscle fiber area. (*Bar A*) Results from a group of sedentary subjects (73). (*Bars B* and *C*) Values before and after 8 wk of conditioning (336,362). (*Bar D*) Values from well-trained men (425, 344, 421, 73). (*Bar M* and *N*)) Values from subjects deconditioned for 7–14 days (362; Saltin B, unpublished observations). V̇o₂max below *bars M* and *N* was estimated from heart rate response to submaximal exercise (subjects were recovering from minor knee injury).

selves are in some way directly sensitive to oxygen—multiplying at low O_2 levels, resting at normal O_2 levels, and dying at high O_2 concentrations."[412,429] They base this belief, that tissue partial pressure of O_2 (P_{O_2}) is the crucial variable, on the same reports of high capillary counts in skeletal muscle of animals living at or exposed to high altitude.[430–432] In man, when sea-level residents stay at high altitude (elevation 3,700 m) for months, the muscle fibers become slightly smaller but the number of capillaries per fiber is unchanged (Fig. 9–17). Further, permanent residents at this altitude do not have a high number of capillaries per fiber, but they have small muscle fibers resulting in high values for capillaries per square millimeter. When the high-altitude residents are divided into physically inactive and physically active groups, the latter group has the higher number of capillaries per fiber, similar to the results found in sea-level residents. Thus, it appears likely that tissue oxygen tension is not the key factor for capillary proliferation.

Unfortunately, no other obvious alternative for a stimulus and regulatory factor has been suggested. In tissue injury some substance is thought to be released, serving as a stimulus for capillary proliferation, but with increased use of muscle, no signs of tissue damage or inflammation are observed.[412,433] Because sprouting capillaries are most frequently found branching off where the capillary is bent and its diameter widens, the pressure in the capillaries at both arteriolar and venular ends may serve as stimulus for proliferation.[412] However, this hypothesis has not been experimentally tested.

SIGNIFICANCE OF ADAPTATION

In this section we analyze what the specific role may be for the adaptations that occur in skeletal muscle as a result of changes in patterns of use and disuse. More specifically, the focus is on how these may alter metabolism and performance. A schematic overview of the varying systems and the interactions among them is given in Figure 9–18. We briefly sum up the possibilities that exist for each of the essential adaptations under study and discuss their contribution to a change in the metabolic response to exercise. Further, we evaluate whether such a change would aid in explaining a change in performance capacity. Finally, we discuss why certain adaptations do not occur in spite of the fact that they would appear likely and beneficial.

Muscular Size

The capacity of skeletal muscle to develop tension per unit of cross-sectional area is not altered by training. At the molecular level, this implies that the tension developed per cross-bridge interaction is constant. This is what could be anticipated. A large variation does exist in the number of fibers contained in the same muscle of humans and rats. This is probably a function of genetic endowment and a likely factor in limiting the maximal growth potential of a muscle. Because fiber number is not influ-

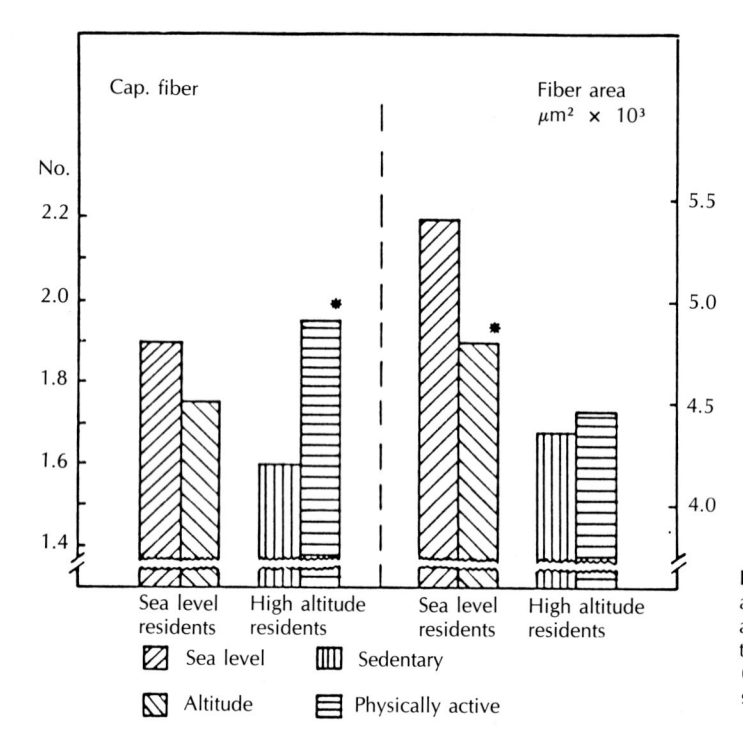

Figure 9-17 Capillaries per fiber and fiber area in sea-level residents at sea level and after an average 32 wk (6–52 wk) at elevation 3,500 m and in high-altitude residents. (Adapted from Saltin B, Nygaard E, Rasmussen B. Acta Physiol Scand 1980; 109:31A.)

enced by the activity level, the only resource available for increasing total muscular strength is for the muscles to increase in cross-sectional area.[81] This is accomplished by a hypertrophy of the existing muscle fibers. It might seem just as logical to have mechanisms for increasing the number of fibers in a muscle rather than restricting the number of those present either at or shortly after birth. However, there are a number of arguments against the efficacy of adding fibers to preexisting muscles. First it could disturb the existing architecture in the muscle by having to provide new attachments on the bone or tendons that serve as origin and insertions. If the fibers arose within the muscle without appropriate attachments, they would be ineffective.[434] Second, and perhaps of greater importance, is the problem of how they would be innervated and incorporated into preexisting motor units. A lateral sprouting of the existing motor units might also result in reducing the capacity for neuromuscular coordination.

Although the capacity for skeletal muscle to enlarge appears to be great, there may not always be a direct relationship between the degree of enlargement and the torque that a muscle can develop around a joint. This is because, for muscles with pennate fiber arrangements, the angle of attachment to the tendon becomes greater as they are enlarged.[278,279] Because the force developed along the long axis of the muscle depends on the angle of attachment, this change in angle results in a diminution in the tension transferred to the tendon. Although increases in strength can be closely related to changes in the total cross-sectional area of a muscle, there are many reports of increases in muscular strength without changes in muscle bulk. This can be explained on the basis of an increased capacity for motor unit recruitment and activation.

Substrate Stores

Stores of phosphagen (ATP, CP) and glycogen are influenced by the state of training only to a very minor extent. With short, intense exercise there is a rapid depletion of glycogen from the FT fibers in skeletal muscle. A failure to sustain multiple bouts of such exercise may be re-

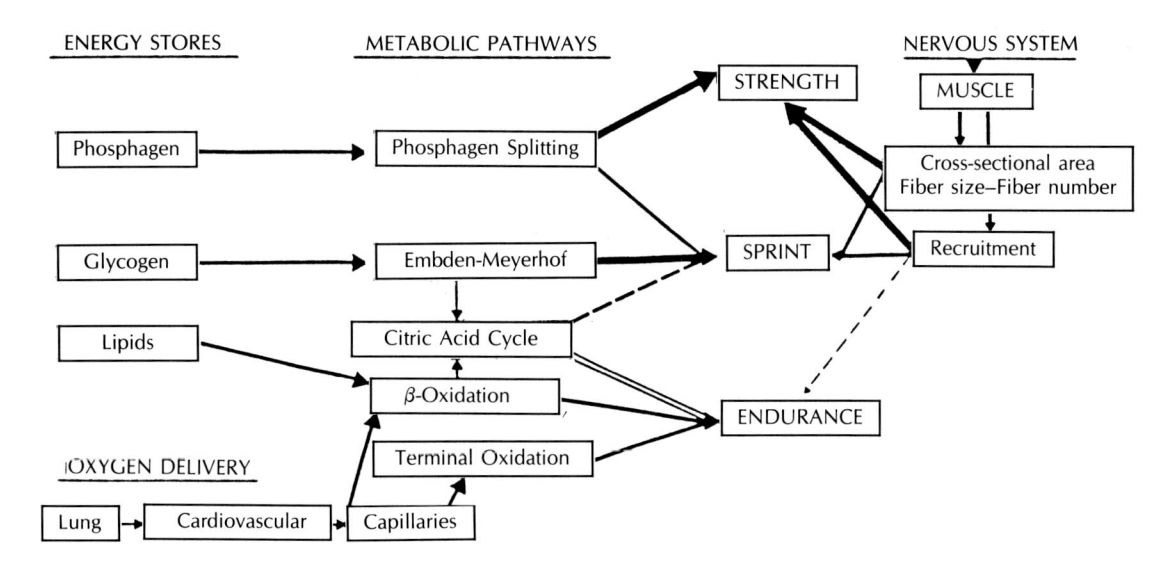

Figure 9–18 A schematic summary with indication of relative importance of various energy stores and metabolic pathways for performance in strength, sprint, and endurance events. Also included in the scheme are indications of how oxygen delivery and the nervous system are interacting.

lated to an exhaustion of the local glycogen in the FT fibers. An elevation in the glycogen stores could forestall exhaustion in such activities.

The immediate energy stores of muscle are sufficient for up to 200 minutes of submaximal exercise. Thus, it is obvious that extramuscular substrates also are important. This has been demonstrated in experiments in which mobilization of fats has been inhibited. At exhaustion the carbohydrate stores of the body were nearly depleted, and the importance of this energy store as a determinant of exercise capacity has been demonstrated.[126,190,246,435-438] Consumption of a fat and protein diet decreases exercise tolerance by about 25 percent, whereas exercise capacity is doubled following consumption of a high-carbohydrate diet.[126,127] Subsequent experiments have established that these dietary manipulations alter the glycogen store of the muscle and that a linear relationship exists between exercise capacity and the muscle glycogen concentration.[126] The role of stored triglyceride is unknown. However, it is well known that increases in the local glycogen stores can increase exercise capacity. This is even more important when coupled with the increased oxidation of fat that occurs with training.

Enzyme Activities

Anaerobic Metabolism

There are reports of increases in the activities of some enzymes in the glycolytic pathway. In some instances these changes are small and appear to exist in only select enzymes of the system. Moreover, in some cases the enzymes that have been reported to increase are not those whose activity is known to be regulated (PHOS, PFK) and which thus exert control over the flux of substrate through the system. Overall, the data available concerning adaptations in the glycolytic system are less certain than those for the enzymes for end-terminal oxidation.

Aerobic Metabolism

In addition to substrate levels and mitochondrial enzymes, the role of oxygen delivery is important for a discussion of the aerobic energy yield in muscle. To discuss this subject thoroughly, we need to summarize some of the adaptations that occur within the cardiovascular system as a response to varied levels of physical activity. From the results in Figure 9–19

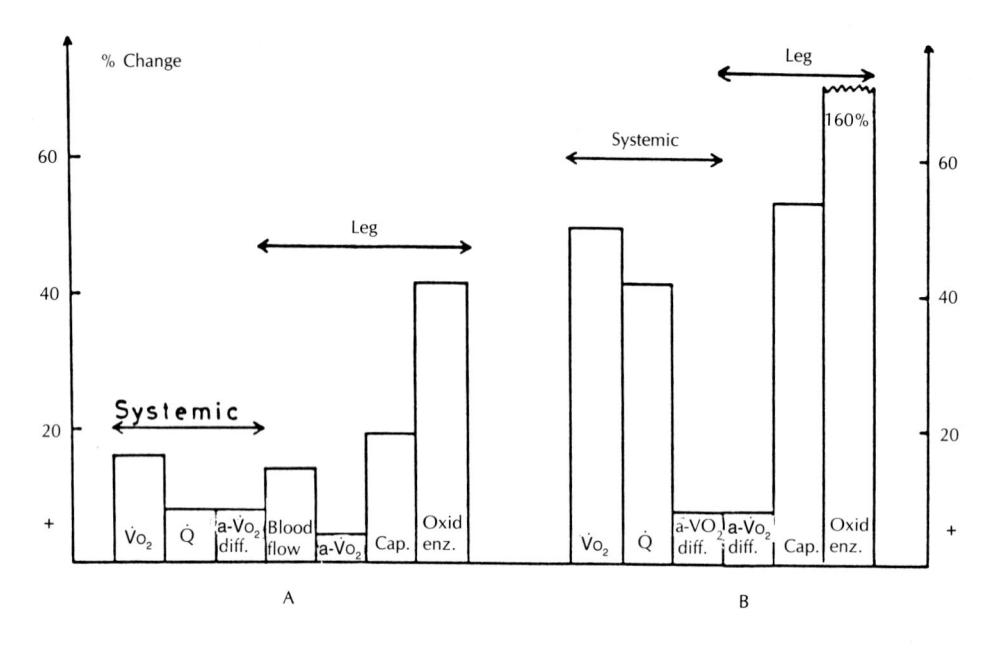

Figure 9-19 Summary of changes associated with a moderate (*panel A*) and a large (*panel B*) increase in Vo₂max in response to physical conditioning. (A) From longitudinal studies in which sedentary subjects were conditioned for 2–3 mo. (B) (Also longitudinal studies) subjects participated either in a conditioning program for 2–3 yr starting from a sedentary level (Vo₂max 45 ml · kg⁻¹ · min⁻¹ [see ref. 445]) or in an intense conditioning program for some months starting from very low Vo₂max (34 ml O₂ · kg⁻¹ · min⁻¹ [see ref. 466]). (A: circulatory data, refs. 445–447. Leg blood flow and arteriovenous O₂ differences are collected from refs. 338, 448, 449 and from Saltin B, unpublished observations. Muscle data, ref. 358 for enzymes, 420 for capillaries. B: central circulatory data, refs. 445, 446. Leg arteriovenous O₂ differences, ref. 446. Muscle capillarization and enzyme data are from unpublished studies by Saltin B, Halkyaer-Kristensen J, and Ingemann-Hansen T.)

it is apparent that at maximal exercise (running or bicycling) eliciting maximal oxygen uptake, both systemic cardiac output and a widening of arteriovenous difference contribute to the improved maximal oxygen uptake. After a short period of adaptation to endurance training, these two factors increase to the same extent. After a long period of training, enlargement of the cardiac output contributes the most to the increased maximal oxygen uptake. Muscle capillary density and mitochondrial enzyme activities are enhanced after both shorter and longer periods of adaptation. The percentage increase in capillarization occurs in parallel with maximal oxygen uptake, whereas the increase in mitochondrial enzyme potential is far in excess of maximal oxygen uptake. The question, then, is whether these changes in the muscle are necessary to increase maximal oxygen uptake. Because close relationships exist among the degrees of capillarization, the activity of a marker enzyme for oxidative capacity, and maximal oxygen uptake in experimental material with large variations in training studies, many researchers use the degree of capillarization as a criterion to illustrate the importance of these variables in attaining maximal oxygen uptake.

It is true that many links in the transport of oxygen to the tissues are closely related, but this does not mean that they are limiting.[438,439] Exercise with a single muscle group, such as the knee extensor muscles, illustrates this problem. In a sedentary person blood flow to these muscles at maximal exercise may average 2,000 to 3,000 ml (kg⁻¹) of muscle (min⁻¹), $\dot{V}o_2$ may attain values of 400 to 500 ml O₂ (kg⁻¹) of muscle (min⁻¹), and the femoral arteriovenous oxygen difference is maintained at around 160 to 180 ml per liter.[440] Thus, when the capacity of the cardiovascular system can be diverted to a small, maximally activated muscle mass, considerably larger blood flow and oxygen uptake (milliliter per kilogram of active muscle) are observed than in ordinary whole-body exercise when systemic cardiac output is shared by a much larger muscle mass. Although blood flow through the knee extensors is tremendous, an extremely wide femoral arteriovenous oxygen difference is maintained. Taken in total, we conclude from these results that neither the capillarization of the muscle nor the concentration of mitochondrial enzymes limits whole-body aerobic power in healthy human subjects.

If we cannot ascribe any significant role to the adaptation in capillarization or mitochondrial enzyme concentrations for attainment of maximal oxygen uptake, why do these variables change so dramatically in response to physical training? An obvious effect of increasing the number of capillaries, and also of the observed small decrease in the size of the muscle fibers with extreme endurance training, would be to reduce the diffusion distances within the muscle. This may be crucial for gas and substrate transport, especially FFA, from the blood to the muscle cell.

In the trained state the number and volume of mitochondria increase, which increases the surface area for the exchange of metabolites, cofactors, and end products between the cytosol and the mitochondrial matrix. Of particular interest here might be an increasing capacity for the transport of fatty acids into the mitochondria and the ATP out into the cytosol. This could in part be responsible for the increased use of FFA, the decreased rate of glycogen depletion, and the lower lactate levels that occur in response to a standard exercise test after training. These differences occur despite lack of change in oxygen uptake and cardiac output at standard work loads before and after training.

A possible effect of increasing the activities of oxidative enzyme in muscle would be to elevate the capacity of the low oxidative fibers for terminal oxidation. Thus the FT fibers, and particularly the FT_b fibers, could more effectively utilize the intracellular glycogen stores and perhaps rely to a greater extent on the oxidation of FFA during prolonged exercise. This would be important when such fibers ultimately are recruited during prolonged exercise, as well as during more intense exercise in which these motor units may be engaged from onset of exercise. Fine tuning of the control of oxidative metabolism could be responsible for the lower respiratory exchange ratio and lactate levels in muscle and blood that occur during exercise after training. Conversely a decrease in physical activity with a resulting loss of oxidative capacity would have an opposite effect on metabolic control.

In summary, then, the stage is set. In submaximal exercise with limited amounts of glycogen (and after dietary manipulation) and with the predominant fraction of the lipids stored outside the muscle cell, the ultimate factor that determines the intensity and duration of work is the body's capacity to utilize extramuscular fat stores. At least five steps are required for the transport of FFA from the adipocytes to the skeletal muscles, where the lipids are finally oxidized in the mitochondria. These are: the release from the fat cell, transport to the muscle by the blood, transport from the capillary across the interstitial space to the muscle cell, transport into the muscle and mitochondria, and oxidation by the mitochondria. In both the untrained and the trained state, the mobilization of lipids appears to be sufficient, and the exercising muscles are offered ample amounts of FFA. Only a very small percentage (3 to 5 percent) of the FFA that is offered by the blood is taken up by the muscle.[405,441,450] This is also true in situations lacking all other substrates, which indicates that the limitations in the utilization of FFA lie either within the muscle or in the transport of the FFA from the blood into the muscle cell.[442-444] There may be a larger FFA uptake by trained muscle, but if this is so, it is within the methodologic variation and thus has not been substantiated.[208,311] It is not known which of the three remaining possibilities for limiting the uptake of FFA by skeletal muscle is the most important. Presently, it appears that the transport of FFA through the interstitial space with its low protein concentration may constitute the major hindrance. For obvious reasons (colloid osmotic pressure and hydrostatic pressure balance over the capillary wall), interstitial protein concentration cannot be elevated. With training, adaptations take place on both sides of this hindrance, by increasing the number of capillaries and by elevations in mitochondrial volume and the capacity for β-oxidation. The importance of these adaptations is illustrated in Figure 9–20, which shows that when subjects, who have trained one leg, exercise using both, the utilization of FFA is greater and the produc-

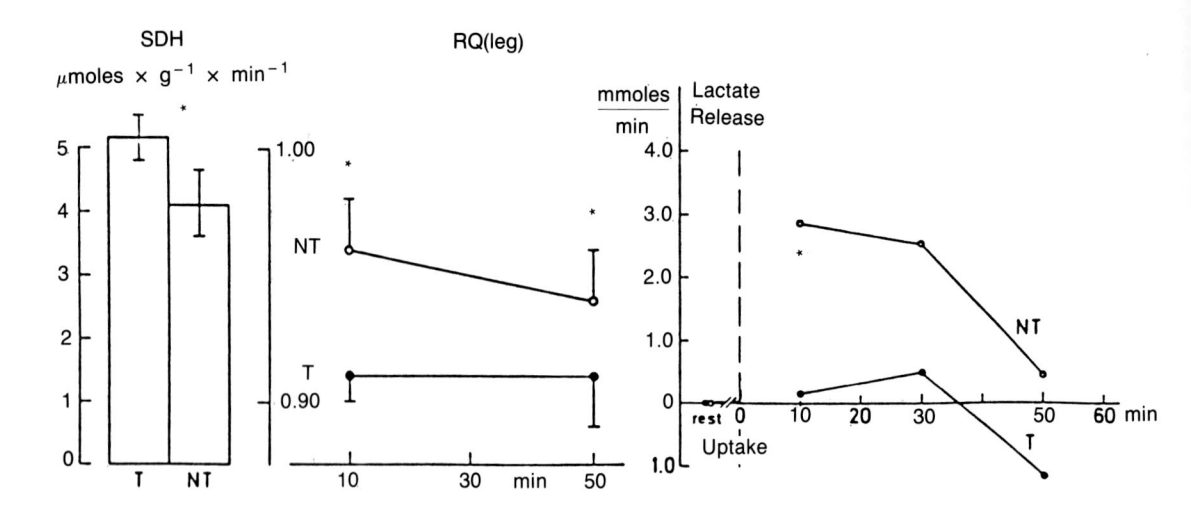

Figure 9–20 Succinate dehydrogenase activity (μmol · g^{-1} wet wt · min^{-1}) in trained (T) and nontrained (NT) leg (*left*), respiratory quotient (RQ) values (*middle*), and release/uptake of lactate (*right*) for both legs during a posttraining metabolic study. Means ± SE are given.* Significant difference between trained and nontrained leg (p<0.05). (Adapted from Henriksson J. Human skeletal muscle adaptation to physical activity. PhD thesis. Copenhagen: University of Copenhagen, 1976.)

tion of lactate is less by the trained leg, in spite of the fact that both legs were offered similar amounts of oxygen and FFA. Of note is that the increase in mitochondrial protein is maintained as long as the training stimulus persists. After termination of training the "excessive" metabolic apparatus is rapidly disassembled, and the muscle returns to the nontrained state.

Part of the answer to why increases occur in total oxidative capacity rather than in substrate storage with training may lie in the fact that the total protein needed to produce a doubling of mitochondria and the oxidative enzymes is relatively small, amounting to only a few milligrams per gram of fresh weight. Such an increase appears to add very little to the overall bulk of the muscle and to produce no measurable disturbance of the ionic and osmotic balance.

This chapter is based on information previously published by the American Physiological Society. Saltin B, Gollnick PD. Skeletal muscle adaptability: significance for metabolism and performance. In: Peachey LD, ed. Handbook of physiology. Skeletal muscle. Bethesda, MD: American Physiological Society, 1983: 555.

REFERENCES

1. Close RI. Dynamic properties of mammalian skeletal muscles. Physiol Rev 1972; 52:129–197.
2. Buchthal F, Schmalbruch H. Motor unit of mammalian muscle. Physiol Rev 1980; 60:90–142.
3. Edström L, Kugelberg E. Histochemical composition, distribution of fibers, and fatiguability of single motor units. J Neurol Neurosurg Psychiatry 1968; 31:424–433.
4. Garnett RAF, O'Donovan MJ, Stephens JA, Taylor A. Motor unit organization of human medical gastrocnemius. J Physiol (Lond) 1978; 287:33–43.
5. McComas AJ, Fawcett PRW, Campbell MJ, Sica REP. Electrophysiological estimation of the number of motor units within human muscle. J Neurol Neurosurg Psychiatry 1971; 34:121–131.
6. McComas AJ, Thomas HC. Fast and slow twitch muscles in man J Neurol Sci 1968; 7:301–307.
7. Kugelberg E. Histochemical composition, contraction speed, and fatiguability of rat soleus motor units. J Neurol Sci 1973; 20:177–198.
8. Kugelberg E, Lindegren B. Transmission and contraction fatigue of rat motor units in relation to succinate dehydrogenase activity of motor unit fibres. J Physiol (Lond) 1979; 288:285–300.
9. Eisen A, Karpati G, Carpenter S, Danton J. The motor unit profile of the rat soleus in experimental myopathy and reinnervation. Neurology 1974; 24:878–884.
10. Kugelberg E, Edström L, Abruzzese M. Mapping of motor units in experimentally reinnervated rat muscle. J Neurol Neurosurg Psychiatry 1970; 33:319–329.
11. Buchthal F, Ermino F, Rosenfalck P. Motor unit territory in different human muscles. Acta Physiol Scand 1959; 45:72–87.
12. Buchthal F, Guld C, Rosenfalck P. Multielectrode study of the territory of a motor unit. Acta Physiol Scand 1957; 39:83–104.
13. Buchthal F, Kamieniecka Z, Schmalbruch H. Fibre types in normal and diseased human muscles and their physiological correlates. In: Exploratory concepts in muscular dystrophy II. Amsterdam: Excerpta Medica 1974:526.

14. Christensen E. Topography of terminal motor innervation in striated muscles from stillborn infants. Am J Phys Med 1959; 38:65–78.
15. Close RI. Dynamic properties of fast and slow skeletal muscle of the rat after nerve cross-section. J Physiol (Lond) 1969; 204:331–346.
16. Feinstein B, Lindegård B, Nyman E, Wohlfart G. Morphologic studies of motor units in normal human muscles. Acta Anat 1955; 23:127–142.
17. Burke RE, Levine DN, Salcman M, Tsairis P. Motor units in cat soleus muscle: physiological, histochemical, and morphological characteristics. J Physiol (Lond) 1974; 238:503–514.
18. Burke RE, Levine DN, Tsairis P, Zajac FE III. Physiological types and histochemical profiles in motor units of the cat gastrocnemius. J Physiol (Lond) 1973; 234:723–748.
19. Burke RE, Levine DN, Zajac FE III, et al. Mammalian motor units: physiological-histological correlation in three types in cat gastrocnemius. Science 1971; 174:709–712.
20. Burke RE, Tsairis P. Anatomy and innervation ratios in motor units of cat gastrocnemius. J Physiol (Lond) 1973; 234:749–765.
21. Burke RE, Tsairis P. The correlation of physiological properties with histochemical characteristics in single muscle units. Ann NY Acad Sci 1977; 301:144–159.
22. Fitts RH, Holloszy JO. Contractile properties of rat soleus muscle: effects of training and fatigue. Am J Physiol 1977; 233 (Cell Physiol 2): C86–C91.
23. Kugelberg E. Adaptive transformation of rat soleus motor units during growth. Histochemistry and contraction speed. J Neurol Sci 1976; 27:269–289.
24. Peter JB, Barnard RJ, Edgerton VR, et al. Metabolic profiles of three fiber types of skeletal muscle in guinea pigs and rabbits. Biochemistry 1972; 11:2627–2633.
25. Bárány M. ATPase activity of myosin correlated with speed of muscle shortening. J Gen Physiol 1967; 50 (Suppl pt 2):197–218.
26. Bárány M, Close RI. The transformation of myosin in cross-innervated rat muscles. J Physiol (Lond) 1971; 213:455–474.
27. Samaha FJ, Guth L, Albers RW. Differences between slow and fast muscle myosin. Adenosine triphosphatase activity and release of associated proteins by p-chloromercuriphenylsulfonate. J Biol Chem 1970; 245:219–224.
28. Sréter FA, Seidel JC, Gergely J. Studies on myosin from red and white skeletal muscles of the rabbit. I. Adenosine triphosphatase activity. J Biol Chem 1966; 241:5772–5776.
29. Brooke MH, Kaiser K. Muscle fiber types: how many and what kind? Arch Neurol 1970; 23:369–379.
30. Brooke MH, Kaiser K. Three "myosin adenosine triphosphatase" systems: the nature of their pH lability and sulfhydryl dependence. J Histochem Cytochem 1970; 18:670–672.
31. Brooke MH, Kaiser K. The use and abuse of muscle histochemistry. Ann NY Acad Sci 1974; 228:121–144.
32. Gauthier GF. Distribution of myosin isoenzymes in adult and developing muscles fibers. In: Pette D, ed. Plasticity of muscle. New York: de Gruyter, 1980:83.
33. Gauthier GF, Lowey S. Polymorphism of myosin among skeletal muscle fiber types. J Cell Biol 1977; 74:760–779.
34. Gauthier GF, Lowey S. Distribution of myosin isoenzymes among skeletal muscle fiber types. J Cell Biol 1979; 81:10–25.
35. Hoh JFY. Neural regulation of mammalian fast and slow muscle myosins: an electrophoretic analysis. Biochemistry 1975; 14:742–747.
36. Hoh JFY, McGrath PA, White RI. Electrophoretic analysis of multiple forms of myosin in fast-twitch and slow-twitch muscles of the chick. Biochem J 1976; 157:87–95.
37. Lowey S. An immunological approach to the isolation of myosin isoenzymes. In: Pette D, ed. Plasticity of muscle. New York: de Gruyter, 1980:69.
38. Padykula HA, Herman E. The specificity of the histochemical method for adenosine triphophatase. J Histochem Cytochem 1955; 3:170–183.
39. Bormioli SP, Sartore S, Vitadello M, Schiaffino S. "Slow" myosins in vertebrate skeletal muscle. An immunofluorescence study. J Cell Biol 1980; 85:672–681.
40. Locker RH, Hagyard CJ. The myosin of rabbit red muscles. Arch Biochem Biophys 1968; 127:370–375.
41. Lowey S, Risby D. Light chains from fast and slow muscle myosin. Nature (Lond) 1971; 234:81–85.
42. Sréter FA, Sarkar S, Gergely J. Myosin light chains of slow twitch muscle. Nature (Lond) 1972; 239:124–125.
43. Weeds AG, Pope B. Chemical studies on light chains from cardiac and skeletal muscle. Nature (Lond) 1971; 234:85–88.
44. Rubinstein NA, Kelly AM. The sequential appearance of fast and slow myosins during myogenesis. In: Pette D, ed. Plasticity of muscle. New York: de Gruyter, 1980:147.
45. Rubinstein N, Mabuchi K, Pepe F, et al. Use of type-specific antimyosins to demonstrate the transformation of individual fibers in chronically stimulated rabbit fast muscles. J Cell Biol 1978; 79:252–261.
46. Kelly AM, Rubinstein NA. Patterns of myosin synthesis in regenerating normal and denervated muscles of the rat. In: Pette D, ed. Plasticity of muscle. New York: de Gruyter, 1980:161.
47. Pette D, Schnez U. Coexistence of fast and slow type myosin light chains in single muscle fibers during transformation as induced by long-term stimulation. FEBS Lett 1977; 83:128–130.
48. Weeds A. Myosin: polymorphism and promiscuity. Nature (Lond) 1978; 274:417–418.
49. Dhoot G, Fearson N, Perry SV. Polymorphic forms of troponin T and troponin C and their localization in striated muscle types. Exp Cell Res 1979; 122:339–350.
50. Dhoot GK, Gell PGH, Perry SV. The localization of the different forms of troponin I in skeletal muscle and cardiac muscle cells. Exp Cell Res 1978; 117:357–370.
51. Dhoot GK, Perry SV. Distribution of polymorphic forms of troponin components and tropomyosin in skeletal muscle. Nature (Lond) 1979; 278:714–718.
52. Dhoot GK, Perry SV. Factors determining the expression of the genes controlling the synthesis of the regulatory proteins in striated muscle. In: Pette D, ed. Plasticity in muscle. New York: de Gruyter 1980:256.
53. Syska H, Perry SV, Trayer IP. A new method for preparation of troponin I (inhibitory protein) using affinity

chromatography. Evidence for three different forms of troponin I in striated muscle. FEBS Lett 1974; 40:253–257.
54. Margreth A, Salvati G, Libera LD, et al. Transition in membrane macromolecular composition and in myosin isoenzymes during development of fast-twitch and slow-twitch muscles. In: Pette D, ed. Plasticity of muscle. New York: de Gruyter, 1980:193.
55. Weeds A. Myosin light chains, polymorphism and fibre types in skeletal muscles. In: Pette D, ed. Plasticity of muscle. New York: de Gruyter, 1980:55.
56. Whalen RG. Contractile protein isoenzymes in muscle development, the embryonic phenotype. In: Pette D, ed. Plasticity of muscle. New York: de Gruyter, 1980:177.
57. Bárány M, Close RI. The transformation of myosin in cross-innervated rat muscles. J Physiol (Lond) 1971; 213:455–474.
58. Margreth A, Libera LD, Salviati G. Postnatal changes in myosin composition of slow muscle in relation to the differentiation of the motoneurons (Abstr). Muscle Nerve 1980; 3:273.
59. Brown MC, Jansen JKS, Van Essen D. Polyneuronal innervation of skeletal muscle in new-born rats and its elimination during maturation. J Physiol (Lond) 1976; 261:387–422.
60. Brown MD. Role of activity in the differentiation of slow and fast muscle. Nature (Lond) 1973; 244:178–179.
61. O'Brien RAD, Österberg AJC, Vrbová G. Observations on the elimination of polyneuronal innervation in developing mammalian skeletal muscle. J Physiol (Lond) 1978; 282:571–582.
62. O'Brien RAD, Purves RD, Vrbová G. Effect of activity on the elimination of multiple innervation in soleus muscles of rats (Abstr). J. Physiol (Lond) 1977; 271:54P.
63. O'Brien RAD, Vrbová G. Nerve muscle interactions during early development. In: Pette D, ed. Plasticity of muscle. New York: de Gruyter, 1980:271.
64. Dickerson JWT, McAnulty PA. The response of hindlimb muscles of the weanling rat to undernutrition and subsequent rehabilitation. Br J Nutr 1975; 33:171–180.
65. Heilig A, Pette D. Changes induced in the enzyme activity pattern by electrical stimulation of fast-twitch muscle. In: Pette D, ed. Plasticity of muscle. New York: de Gruyter, 1980:409.
66. Heilmann C, Pette D. Molecular transformation of sarcoplasmic reticulum in chronically stimulated fast-twitch muscle. In: Pette D, ed. Plasticity of muscle. New York: de Gruyter, 1980:421.
67. Drachman DB, Johnston DM. Development of mammalian fast muscle: dynamic and biochemical properties correlated. J Physiol (Lond) 1973; 234:29–42.
68. Sréter FA, Luft AR, Gergely J. Effect of cross-reinnervation on physiological parameters and on properties of myosin and sarcoplasmic reticulum of fast and slow muscles of the rabbit. J Gen Physiol 1975; 66:811–821.
69. Engel WK. The essentiality of histo- and cytochemical studies of skeletal muscle in the investigation of neuromuscular disease. Neurology 1962; 12:778–794.
70. Gauthier GF. Ultrastructural identification of muscle fiber types by immunochemistry. J Cell Biol 1979; 82:391–400.
71. Engel WK. Fiber type nomenclature of human skeletal muscle for histochemical purposes. Neurology 1974; 24:344–348.
72. Brooke MH, Williamson E, Kaiser K. The behavior of four fiber types in developing and reinnervated muscle. Arch Neurol 1971; 25:360–366.
73. Saltin B, Henriksson J, Nygaard E, et al. Fiber types and metabolic potentials of skeletal muscle in sedentary man and endurance runners. Ann NY Acad Sci 1977; 301:3–29.
74. Sjøgaard G, Houston ME, Nygaard E, Saltin B. Subgrouping of fast twitch fibres in skeletal muscles of man. Histochemistry 1978; 58:79–87.
75. Brooke MH, Engel WK. The histographic analysis of human muscle biopsies with regard to fiber types. 1. Adult male and female. Neurology 1969; 19:221–223.
76. Brooke MH, Engel WK. The histographic analysis of human muscle biopsies with regard to fiber types. 4. Children's biopsies. Neurology 1969; 19:591–605.
77. Gauthier GF. On the relationship of ultrastructural and cytochemical features to color in mammalian skeletal muscle. Z Zellforsch Mikroskop Anat 1969; 96:462–482.
78. Gauthier GF, Dunn RA. Ultrastructural and cytochemical features of mammalian skeletal muscle fibres following denervation. J Cell Sci 1973; 12:525–547.
79. Payne CM, Stern LZ, Curless RG, Hannapel LK. Ultrastructural fiber typing in normal and diseased human muscle. J Neurol Sci 1975; 25:99–108.
80. Tomanek RJ. Ultrastructural differentiation of skeletal muscle fibers and their diversity. J Ultrastruct Res 1976; 55:212–227.
81. Sjöström M, Kidman S, Larsen-Henriksson K, Angquist KA. Z- and M-band appearance in different histochemically defined types of human skeletal muscle fibers. J Histochem Cytochem 1982; 30:1–11.
82. Ikai M, Fukunaga T. Calculation of muscle strength per unit cross-sectional area of human muscle by means of ultrasonic measurement. Int Z Angew Physiol Einschl Arbeitsphysiol 1968; 26:26–32.
83. Ikai M, Fukunaga T. A study on training effect on strength per unit cross-sectional area of human muscle by means of ultrasonic measurement. Int Z Angew Physiol Einschl Arbeitsphysiol 1970; 28:173–180.
84. Bouisset S, Lestienne F, Maton B. Relative work of main agonists in elbow flexion. In: Komi PV, ed. Biomechanics. Baltimore: University Park Press, 1969:272.
85. Hansen TE, Lindhard J. On the maximum work of human muscles, especially the flexors of the elbow. J Physiol (Lond) 1923; 57:287–300.
86. Nygaard E. Morfologi og funktion im biceps brachii. Thesis. Copenhagen: University of Copenhagen, 1981.
87. Haxton HA. Absolute muscle force in the ankle flexors of man. J Physiol (Lond) 1944; 103:267–273.
88. Ingemann-Hansen T, Halkjaer-Kristensen J. Computerized tomographic determinations of human thigh components. Scand J Rehabil Med 1980; 12:27–31.
89. Renstrom P. The below-knee amputee. Thigh muscle

atrophy in below-knee amputees. Thesis. Goteborg, Sweden: University of Goteborg, 1981:72.
90. Sexton AW. Isometric tension of glycerinated muscle fibers following adrenalectomy. Am J Physiol 1967; 212:313–316.
91. Sexton AW, Gersten JW. Isometric tension differences in fibers of red and white muscles. Science 1967; 157:199.
92. Faulkner JA, Niemeyer JH, Maxwell LC, White TP. Contractile properties of transplanted extensor digitorum longus muscles of cats. Am J Physiol 1980; 238 (Cell Physiol 7): C120–C126.
93. Burke RE, Edgerton VR. Motor unit properties and selective involvement in movement. Exercise Sport Sci Rev 1975; 3:31–81.
94. Barnard RJ, Edgerton VR, Furukawa T, Peter JB. Histochemical, biochemical, and contractile properties of red, white, and intermediate fibers. Am J Physiol 1971; 220:410–414.
95. Brust M, Cosla HW. Contractility of isolated abdominal skeletal muscle. Arch Phys Med Rehabil 1967; 48:534–555.
96. Close R. Properties of motor units in fast and slow skeletal muscles of the rat. J Physiol (Lond) 1967; 193:45–55.
97. Fidler MW, Jowett RL, Troup JDG. Myosin ATPase activity in multifidus muscle from cases of lumbar spinal derangement. J Bone Joint Surg (Am) 1975; 57:220–227.
98. McPhedran AM, Wuerker RB, Henneman E. Properties of motor units in a homogeneous red muscle (soleus) of the cat. J Neurophysiol 1965; 28:71–84.
99. Buchtal F, Dahl K, Rosenfalck P. Rise time of the spike potential in fast and slowly contracting muscle of man. Acta Physiol Scand 1970; 79:435–452.
100. Buchtal F, Schmalbruch H. Spectrum of contraction times of different fibre bundles in the brachial biceps and triceps muscles of man. Nature (Lond) 1969; 22:89.
101. Buchtal F, Schmalbruch H. Contraction times and fibre types in intact human muscle. Acta Physiol Scand 1970; 79:435–452.
102. Buller NP, Ismail HM, Ranatunga KW. Recording of isometric contractions of human biceps brachii muscle (proceedings). J Physiol (Lond) 1978; 277:11P–12P.
103. Desmedt JE, Godaux E. Ballistic contractions in man: characteristic recruitment pattern of single motor units of the tibialis anterior muscle. J Physiol (Lond) 1977; 264:673–693.
104. Desmedt JE, Godaux E. Fast motor units are not preferentially activated in rapid voluntary contractions in man. Nature (Lond) 1977; 267:717–207.
105. Desmedt JE, Godaux E. Mechanism of the vibration paradox: excitatory and inhibitory effects of tendon vibration on single soleus muscle motor units in man. J Physiol (Lond) 1978; 285:197–207.
106. Desmedt JE, Godaux E. Recruitment patterns of single motor units in the human masseter muscle during brisk jaw clenching. Arch Oral Biol 1979; 24:171–178.
107. Desmedt JE, Godaux E. Voluntary motor commands in human ballistic movements. Ann Neurol 1979; 5:415–421.
108. Grimby L, Hannerz J. Recruitment order of motor units on voluntary contraction: changes induced by proprioceptive afferent activity. J Neurol Neurosurg Psychiatry 1968; 31:565–573.
109. Grimby L, Hannerz J. Firing rate and recruitment order of toe extensor motor units in different modes of voluntary contraction. J Physiol (Lond) 1977; 264:865–879.
110. Salmons S, Vrbová G. The influence of activity on some contractile characteristics of mammalian fast and slow muscles. J Physiol (Lond) 1969; 20:535–549.
111. Eberstein A, Goodgold J. The use of biopsies in the study of human skeletal muscle. Life Sci 1967; 6:655–661.
112. Eberstein A, Goodgold J. Slow and fast twitch fibers in human skeletal muscle. Am J Physiol 1968; 215:535–541.
113. Edwards RHT, Young A, Hosking GP, Jones DA. Human skeletal muscle function: description of tests and normal values. Clin Sci Mol Med 1977; 52:283–290.
114. Moulds RFW, Young A, Jones DA, Edwards RHT. A study of the contractility, biochemistry, and morphology of an isolated preparation of human skeletal muscle. Clin Sci Mol Med 1977; 52:291–297.
115. Edwards RHT. Physiological analysis of skeletal muscle weakness and fatigue. Clin Sci Mol Med 1978; 54:463–470.
116. Wiles CM, Young A, Jones DA, Edwards RHT. Relaxation rate of constituent muscle-fibre types in human quadriceps. Clin Sci 1979; 56:47–52.
117. Bergström J. Muscle electrolytes in man. Scand J Clin Lab Invest (Suppl) 1962; 68:1–110.
118. Essén B. Intramuscular substrate utilization during prolonged exercise. Ann NY Acad Sci 1977; 301:30–44.
119. Essén B. Studies on the regulation of metabolism in human skeletal muscle using intermittent exercise as an experimental model. Acta Physiol Scand (Suppl) 1978:454.
120. Essén B, Hagenfeldt, Kaijser L. Utilization of blood-borne and intramuscular substrates during continuous and intermittent exercise in man. J Physiol (Lond) 1977; 265:489–506.
121. Essén B, Jansson E, Henrikson J, et al. Metabolic characteristics of fibre in human skeletal muscle. Acta Physiol Scand 1975; 95:153–165.
122. Fröberg SO, Hultman E, Nilsson LH. Effect of noradrenaline on triglyceride and glycogen concentrations in liver and muscle from man. Metabolism 1975; 24:119–126.
123. Fröberg SO, Mossfeldt F. Effect of prolonged strenuous exercise on the concentration of triglycerides, phospholipids, and glycogen in muscle of man. Acta Physiol Scand 1971; 82:167–171.
124. Essén B, Henriksson J. Metabolic characteristics of human type 2 skeletal muscle fibers (Abstr). Muscle Nerve 1980; 3:263.
125. Lillie RD. Various oil soluble dyes as fat stains in the supersaturated isopropanol technic. Stain Technol 1944; 19:55–58.
126. Bergström J, Hermansen L, Hultman E, Saltin B. Diet, muscle glycogen, and physical performance. Acta Physiol Scand 1967; 71:140–150.
127. Gollnick PD, Piehl K, Saubert CW IV, et al. Diet, ex-

ter Muskelhypertrophie. Verh Ber Med Ges 1866; 1:191–210.
274. Erb WH. Dystrophia muscularis progressiva. Klinische und pathologische Studien. Dtsch Z Nervenheilk 1891; 1:173–261.
275. Etemadi AA, Hosseini F. Frequency and size of muscle fibers in athletic body build. Anat Rec 1968; 162:269–274.
276. Julian LM, Cardinett GH III. Fiber sizes of the biceps brachii muscle of dogs which differ greatly in body size. Anat Rec 1961; 139:243.
277. Thompson EH, Levine AS, Hegarty PVJ, Allen CE. An automated technique for simultaneous determinations of muscle fiber number and diameter. J Anim Sci 1979; 48:328–337.
278. Binkhorst RA, Van't Hof MA. Force-velocity relationship and contraction time of the rat fast plantaris muscle due to compensatory hypertrophy. Pflügers Arch 1973; 342:145–158.
279. Meara PJ. Postnatal growth and development of muscle, as exemplified by the gastrocnemius and psoas muscles of the rabbit. Onderstepoort J Vet Sci Anim Ind 1947; 21:329–482.
280. Gollnick PD, Timson BF, Moore RL, Riedy M. Muscular enlargement and the number of fibers in the skeletal muscles of rats. J Appl Physiol: Respirat Environ Exerc Physiol 1981; 50:936–943.
281. Nygaard E. Number of fibers in skeletal muscle of man (Abstr). Muscle Nerve 1980; 3:268.
282. Schwarzacher HG. Über die Länge und Anordnung der Muskelfasern in menschlichen Skelettmuskeln. Acta Anat 1959; 37:217–231.
283. Eliot TS, Wigginton RC, Corbin KB. The number and size of muscle fibres in the rat soleus in relation to age, sex, and exercise. Anat Rec 1943; 85:307–308.
284. Walker MG. The effect of exercise on skeletal muscle fibers. Comp Biochem Physiol 1966; 19:791–797.
285. James NT. Compensatory hypertrophy in the extensor digitorum longus muscle of the rat. J Anat 1973; 116:57–65.
286. Hamosh M, Lesch M, Baron J, Kaufman S. Enhanced protein synthesis in a cell-free system from hypertrophied skeletal muscle. Science 1967; 157:935–937.
287. Hubbard RW, Ianuzzo CD, Matthew WT, Linduska JD. Compensatory adaptation of skeletal muscle composition to a long-term functional overload. Growth 1975; 39:85–93.
288. Morkin E, Ashford TP. Myocardial DNA synthesis in experimental cardiac hypertrophy. Am J Physiol 1968; 215:1409–1413.
289. Armstrong RB, Marum P, Tullson P, Saubert CW IV. Acute hypertrophic response of skeletal muscle to removal of synergists. J Appl Physiol: Respirat Environ Exerc Physiol 1979; 46:835–842.
290. Allbrook DB, Han MF, Hellmuth AE. Population of muscle satellite cells in relation to age and mitotic activity. Pathology 1971; 3:233–243.
291. Moss FP. The relationship between the dimensions of the fibers and the number of nuclei during normal growth of skeletal muscle in the domestic fowl. Am J Anat 1968; 122:555–564.
292. Moss FP, Leblond CP. Nature of dividing nuclei in skeletal muscle of growing rats. J Cell Biol 1970; 44:459–462.

293. Schiaffino S, Bormioli SP, Aloisi M. The fate of newly formed satellite cells during compensatory muscle hypertrophy. Virchows Arch B 1976; 21:113–118.
294. Schmalbruch H. Satellite cells of rat muscles as studied by freeze-fracturing. Anat Rec 1978; 191:371–376.
295. Schmalbruch H, Hellhammer H. The number of satellite cells in normal human muscle. Anat Rec 1976; 185:279–282.
296. Shafiq SA, Gorycki MA, Mauro A. Mitosis during postnatal growth in skeletal and cardiac muscle of the rat. J Anat 1968; 103:135–141.
297. Fleckman P, Bailyn RS, Kaufman S. Effects of the inhibition of DNA synthesis on hypertrophying skeletal muscle. J Biol Chem 1978; 253:3320–3327.
298. Henriksson J, Galbo H. Blomstrand E. The importance of the motor nerve for the stimulation-induced oxidative enzymatic adaptation in cat skeletal muscle (Abstract). Muscle Nerve 1980; 3:274.
299. Hudlická O, Brown M, Cotter M, et al. The effect of long-term stimulation of fast muscles on their blood flow, metabolism, and ability to withstand fatigue. Pflügers Arch 1977; 369:141–149.
300. Lømo T, Westgaard RH, Engebretsen L. Different stimulation patterns affect contractile properties of denervated rat soleus muscle. In: Pette D, ed. Plasticity of muscle. New York: de Gruyter, 1980:297.
301. Pette D, Dolken G. Some aspects of regulation of enzyme levels in muscle energy-supplying metabolism. Adv Enzyme Regul 1975; 13:355–377.
302. Pette D, Ramirez BA, Müller W, et al. Influence of intermittent long-term stimulation of contractile, histochemical, and metabolic properties of fibre populations in fast and slow rabbit muscles. Pflügers Arch 1975; 361:1–7.
303. Purves D. Long-term regulation in the vertebrate peripheral nervous system, In: Porter R, ed. Neurophysiology II. Balitmore University Park Press, 1976:125.
304. Eriksson BO, Gollnick PD, Saltin B. Muscle metabolism and enzyme activities after training in boys 11–13 years old. Acta Physiol Scand 1973; 87:485–497.
305. Karlsson J, Diamant B, Saltin B. Muscle metabolities during submaximal and maximal exercise in man. Scand J Clin Lab Invest 1971; 26:358–394.
306. Fredman D, Feinschmidt O. Über Einfluss des Trainierens des Muskels auf seinen Gehalt and Phosphorverbindungen. Hoppe-Seyler's Z Physiol Chem 1929; 183:216–268.
307. Palladin A, Ferdmann D. Über den Einfluss der Trainings der Muskeln auf ihren kreatingehalt. Hoppe-Seyler's Z Physiol Chem 1928; 174:284–294.
308. Jansson E. Diet and muscle metabolism in man. Acta Physiol Scand (Suppl) 1980;487.
309. Jansson E. Acid soluble and insoluble glycogen in human skeletal muscle. Acta Physiol Scand 1981; 113:337–340.
310. Piehl K. Time course for refilling of glycogen stores in human fibres following exercise-induced glycogen depletion. Acta Physiol Scand 1974; 90:297–302.
311. Henriksson J. Training-induced adaptation of skeletal muscle and metabolism during submaximal exercise. J Physiol (Lond) 1977; 270:677–690.
312. Saltin B, Nazar K, Costill DL, et al. The nature of the

training response; peripheral and central adaptations to one-legged exercise. Acta Physiol Scand 1976; 96:289–305.
313. Burke RE, Cerny F, Costill D, Fink W. Characteristics of skeletal muscle in competitive cyclists. Med Sci Sports 1977; 9:109–112.
314. Houston ME. The use of histochemistry in muscle adaptation: a critical assessment. Can J Appl Sport Sci 1978; 3:109–118.
315. Houston ME. Metabolic responses to exercise, with special reference to training and competition in swimming. In: Eriksson B, Furberg B, eds. Swimming medicine IV. Baltimore: University Park Press, 1978:207.
316. Morgan TE, Cobb LA, Short FA, et al. Effects of long-term exercise on human muscle mitochondria. In: Pernow B, Saltin B, eds. Muscle metabolism during exercise. New York: Plenum, 1971:87.
317. Taylor AW, Thayer R, Rao S. Human skeletal muscle glycogen synthase activities with exercise and training. Can J Physio Pharmacol 1972; 50:411–415.
318. Tesch P, Piehl K, Wilson G, Karlsson J. Physiological investigations of Swedish elite canoe competitors. Med Sci Sports 1976; 8:214–218.
319. Bylund-Fellenius AC, Bjurö T, Cederblad G, et al. Physical training in man. Skeletal muscle metabolism in relation to muscle morphology and running ability. Eur J Appl Physiol Occup Physiol 1977; 36:151–169.
320. Morgan TE, Short FA, Cobb LA. Effect of long-term exercise on skeletal muscle lipid composition. Am J Physiol 1969; 216:82–86.
321. Hoppeler H, Lüthi P, Claassen H, et al. The ultrasturcture of the normal human skeletal muscle: a morphometric analysis on untrained men, women, and well-trained orienteers. Pflügers Arch 1973; 344:217–232.
322. Kiessling K-H, Pilström L, Bylund A-C, et al. Enzyme activities and morphometry in skeletal muscle of middle-aged men after training. Scand J Clin Lab Invest 1974; 33:63–69.
323. Kiessling K-H, Pilström L, Bylund A-C, et al. Morphometry and enzyme activities in skeletal muscle from middle-aged men after training and from alcoholics. In: Howald H, Poortman JR, eds. Metabolic adaptation to prolonged physical exercise. Basel: Birkhäuser, 1975:384.
324. Costill DL, Daniels J, Evans W, et al. Skeletal muscle enzymes and fiber composition in male and female track athletes. J Appl Physiol 1976; 40:149–154.
325. Sjödin B. Lactate dehydrogenase in human skeletal muscle. Acta Physiol Scand (Suppl) 1976; 436:5–32.
326. Sjödin B, Thorstensson A, Frith K, Karlson J. Effect of physical training on LDH activity and LDH isozyme pattern in human skeletal muscle. Acta Physiol Scand 1976; 97:150–157.
327. Karlsson J, Sjödin B, Thorstensson A, et al. LDH isoenzymes in skeletal muscles of endurance and strength trained athletes. Acta Physiol Scand 1975; 93:150–156.
328. Tesch P, Sjödin B, Karlsson J. Relationship between lactate accumulation, LDH activity, LDH isozyme, and fibre type distribution in human skeletal muscle. Acta Physiol Scand 1978; 103:40–46.
329. Thorstensson A, Sjödin B, Karlsson J. Enzyme activities and muscle strength after "sprint training" in man. Acta Physiol Scand 1975; 94:313–318.

330. Fahimi HD, Amarasingham CR. Cytochemical localization of lactic dehydrogenase in white skeletal muscle. J Cell Biol 1964; 22:29–48.
331. Fahimi HD, Karnovsky MJ. Cytochemical localization of two glycolytic dehydrogenases in white skeletal muscle. J Cell Biol 1966; 29:113–128.
332. Gollnick PD, Armstrong RB. Histochemical localization of lactate dehydrogenase isozymes in human skeletal muscle fibers. Life Sci 1976; 18:27–32.
333. Karlsson I, Frith K, Sjödin B, et al. Distribution of LDH isozymes in human skeletal muscle. Scand J Clin Lab Invest 1974; 33:307–312.
334. Peter JB, Sawaki S, Barnard RJ, et al. Lactate dehydrogenase isoenzymes: distribution in fast-twitch red, fast-twitch white, and slow-twitch intermediate fibers of guinea pig skeletal muscle. Arch Biochem Biophys 1971; 144:304–307.
335. Van Wijhe M, Blanchaer MC, St. George-Stubbs S. The distribution of lactate dehydrogenase isozymes in human skeletal muscle fibres. J Histochem Cytochem 1964; 12:608–614.
336. Andersen P, Henriksson J. Capillary supply of the quadriceps femoris muscle of man: adaptive response to exercise. J Physiol (Lond) 1977; 270:677–690.
337. Andersen P, Henriksson J. Training induced changes in the subgroups of human type II skeletal muscle fibres. Acta Physiol Scand 1977; 99:123–125.
338. Ångquist KA, Bylund AC, Bjurö T, et al. Physical training in man. Skeletal muscle metabolism in relation to muscle morphology and running ability. Eur J Appl Physiol Occup Physiol 1977; 36:151–169.
339. Bergman H, Björntorp P, Conradson T-B, et al. Enzymatic and circulatory adjustments to physical training in middle-aged men. Eur J Clin Invest 1973; 3:414–418.
340. Bylund AC. Skeletal muscle metabolism in man. Studies with special reference to methodology and effects of physical training. Thesis. Goteborg, Sweden: University of Goteborg, 1977.
341. Costill DL, Fink WJ, Pollock ML. Muscle fiber composition and enzyme activities of elite distance runners. Med Sci Sports 1976; 8:96–100.
342. Holm J, Björntorp P, Scherstén T. Metabolic activity in human skeletal muscle. Eur J Clin Invest 1972; 2:321–325.
343. Ingwall JS, Weiner CD, Morales MF, et al. Specificity of creatine in the control of protein synthesis. J Cell Biol 1974; 63:145–151.
344. Jansson E, Kaijser L. Muscle adaptation to extreme endurance training in man. Acta Physiol Scand 1977; 100:315–324.
345. Örlander J, Aniansson A. Effects of physical training on skeletal muscle metabolism and ultrastructure in 70- to 75-year old men. Acta Physiol Scand 1980; 109:149–154.
346. Örlander J, Kiessling K-H, Ekblom B. Time course of adaptation to low intensity training in sedentary men: dissociation of central and local effects. Acta Physiol Scand 1980; 108:85–90.
347. Örlander J, Kiessling K-H, Karlsson J, Ekblom B. Low intensity training, inactivity, and resumed training in sedentary men. Acta Physiol Scand 1977; 101:351–362.
348. Prince FP, Hikida RS, Hagerman FC. Human muscle fiber types in power lifters, distance runners, and un-

ization with extreme endurance training in man. In: Eriksson B, Furberg B, eds. Swimming medicine IV. Baltimore: University Park Press, 1978:282.
422. Brodal P, Ingjer F, Hermansen L. Capillary supply of skeletal muscle fibers in untrained and endurance-trained men. Am J Physiol 1977; 232 (Heart Circ Physiol 1):H705–H712.
423. Ingjer F. Maximal aerobic power related to the capillary supply of the quadriceps femoris muscle in man. Acta Physiol Scand 1978; 104:238–240.
424. Ingjer F, Brodal P. Capillary supply of skeletal muscle fibers in untrained and endurance-trained women. Eur J Appl Physiol Occup Physiol 1978; 38:291–299.
425. Houston ME, Bentzen H, Larsen H. Interrelationships between skeletal muscle adaptations and performance as studied by detraining and retraining. Acta Physiol Scand 1979; 105:163–170.
426. Wittenberg B, Wittenberg JB. Role of myoglobin in the oxygen supply to red skeletal muscle. J Biol Chem 1975; 250:9038–9043.
427. Józsa L, Bálint J, Réffy A, et al. Capillary density of tenotomized skeletal muscles. II. Observations on human muscles after spontaneous rupture of the tendon. Eur J Appl Physiol Occup Physiol 1980; 44:183–188.
428. Józsa L, Järvinen M, Kvist M, et al. Capillary density of tenotomized skeletal muscles. I. Experimental study in the rat. Eur J Appl Physiol Occup Physiol 1980; 44:175–181.
429. Ashton W. Neovascularization in ocular disease. Trans Ophthalmol Soc UK 1961; 81:145–161.
430. Appell H-J. Morphological studies on skeletal muscle capillaries under conditions of high-altitude training. Int J Sport Med 1980; 1:103–109.
431. Cassin S, Gilbert RD, Bunnell CE, Johnson EM. Capillary development during exposure to chronic hypoxia. Am J Physiol 1971; 220:448–451.
432. Valdiva E. Total capillary bed in striated muscle of guinea pigs native to the Peruvian mountains. Am J Physiol 1958; 194:585–589.
433. Brånemark P-I. Capillary form and function—the microcirculation of granulation tissue. Bibl Anat 1965; 7:9–28.
434. Muscle fibre splitting—a reappraisal. Lancet 1978; 1:646.
435. Fitts RH, Booth FW, Winder WW, Holloszy JO. Skeletal muscle respiratory capacity, endurance, and glycogen utilization. Am J Physiol 1975; 228:1029–1033.
436. Rennie MJ, Winder WW, Holloszy JO. A sparing effect of increased plasma fatty acids on muscle and liver glycogen content in the exercising rat. Biochem J 1976; 156:647–655.
437. Wohlfart G. Über das Vorkommen verscheidener Arten von Muskelfasern in der Skelettmuskulatur des Menschen und einiger Säugetiere. Acta Psychiatry Neurol Scand (Supp) 1937; 12:1–119.
438. Booth FW, Narahara KA. Vastus lateralis cytochrome oxidase activity and its relationship to maximal oxygen consumption in man. Pflügers Arch 1975; 349:319–324.
439. Simon LM, Robin ED. Relationship of cytochrome oxidase activity to vertebrate total and organ oxygen consumption. Int J Biochem 1971; 2:569–573.
440. Adams RP, Andersen P, Sjøgaard G, et al. Knee-extension as a model for the study of isolated exercising muscle in man (Abstr). Med Sci Sports Exerc 1981; 13:99.
441. Gollnick PD. Free fatty acid turnover and the availability of substrates as a limiting factor in prolonged exercise. Ann NY Acad Sci 1977; 301:64–71.
442. Neely JR, Rovetto MJ, Oram JF. Myocardial utilization of carbohydrates and lipids. Progr Cardiovasc Dis 1972; 15:389–396.
443. Rose CP, Goresky CA. Constraints on the uptake of labeled palmitate by the heart. Circ Res 1977; 41:534–545.
444. Gollnick PD, Saltin B. Fuel for muscular exercise: role of fat. In: Horton ES, Terjung RL, eds. Exercise, nutrition, and energy metabolism. New York: MacMillan, 1988:72.
445. Ekblom B. The effect of physical training on oxygen transport system in man. Acta Physiol Scand (Supp) 1969; 328:1–45.
446. Saltin B, Blomqvist G, Mitchell JH, et al. Response to exercise after bed rest and after training. Circulation 1968; 38 (Suppl 7):1–78.
447. Rowell LB. Factors affecting the prediction of the maximal oxygen intake from measurements made during submaximal work with observations related to factors which may limit maximal oxygen intake. Thesis. Minneapolis: University of Minnesota, 1962.
448. Jorfeldt L, Wahren J. Leg blood flow during exercise in man. Clin Sci Mol Med 1971; 41:459–473.
449. Wahren J, Saltin B, Jorfeldt L, Pernow B. Influence of age on the local circulatory adaptation to leg exercise. Scand J Clin Lab Invest 1974; 33:79–86.
450. Gollnick PD, Pernow B, Essén B, et al. Availability of glycogen and plasma FFA for substrate utilization in leg muscle of man during exercise. Clin Physiol 1981; 1:27–42.
451. Graham JA, Lamb JF, Linton AL. Measurements of body water and intracellular electrolytes by means of muscle biopsy. Lancet 1967; 2:1172–1176.
452. Valentin N, Olesen KH. Measurements of muscle tissue water and electrolytes. Scand J Clin Lab Invest 1973; 32:155–160.
453. Bergström J, Alvestrand A, Fürst P, et al. Influence of severe potassium depletion and subsequent repletion with potassium on muscle electrolytes, metabolites, and amino acids in man. Clin Sci Mol Med 1976; 51:589–599.
454. Edström L. Histochemical changes in upper motor lesions, parkinsonism and disuse. Differential effect on white and red muscle fibers. Experientia 1968; 24:916–918.
455. Edström L, Nyström B. Histochemical types and sizes of fibres in normal human muscles. Acta Neurol Scand 1969; 45:257–269.
456. Thorstensson A, Larsson L, Tesch P, Karlsson J. Muscle strength and fiber composition in athletes and sedentary men. Med Sci Sports 1977; 9:26–30.
457. Burke RE. Motor unit types of cat triceps surae muscle. J Physiol (Lond) 1967; 193:141–160.
458. Gollnick PD, Sjödin B, Karlsson J, et al. Human soleus muscle: a comparison of fiber composition and enzyme activities with other leg muscles. Pfluegers Arch 1974; 348:247–255.
459. Tesch P, Larsson L, Eriksson A, Karlsson J. Muscle glycogen depletion and lactate concentration during downhill skiing. Med Sci Sports Exerc 1978; 10:85–90.
460. Green HJ, Thomson JA, Daub WD, et al. Fiber composition, fiber size, and enzyme activities in vastus lateralis of elite athletes involved in high intensity ex-

ercise. Eur J Appl Physiol Occup Physiol 1979; 41:109–117.
461. Costill DL, Fink WJ, Getchell LH, et al. Lipid metabolism in skeletal muscle of endurance-trained males and females. J Appl Physiol: Respirat Environ Exerc Physiol 1979; 47:787–791.
462. Campbell CJ, Bonen A, Kirby RL, Belcastro AN. Muscle fiber composition and performance capacities of women. Med Sci Sports 1979; 11:260–265.
463. Bell RD, MacDougal JD, Billeter R, Howald H. Muscle fiber types and morphometric analysis of skeletal muscle in six-year-old children. Med Sci Sports Exerc 1980; 12:28–31.
464. Larsson L, Grimby G, Karlsson J. Muscle strength and speed of movement in relation to age and muscle morphology. J Appl Physiol: Respirat Environ Exerc Physiol 1979; 46:451–456.
465. Foster C, Costill DL, Daniels JT, Fink WJ. Skeletal muscle enzyme activity, fiber composition and $\dot{V}O_2$max in relation to distance running performance. Eur J Appl Physiol 1978; 39(2):73–80.
466. Hedberg G, Jansson E. Skelettmuskelfiberkomposition. Kapacitet och in tresse för olika fysiska aktiviteter bland elever i gymnasieskolan. Umeå, Sweden: Pedagogiska Institute, 1976 (Rep. 54).
467. Jorfeldt L, Wahren J. Leg blood flow during exercise in man. Clin Sci Mol Med 1971; 41:459–473.
468. Gregor RJ, Edgerton VR, Perrine JJ, et al. Torque-velocity relationships and muscle fiber composition in elite female athletes. J Appl Physiol: Respirat Environ Exerc Physiol 1979; 47:388–392.

Chapter 10
Muscle Strength and Local Endurance Training

BARBARA J. de LATEUR

RESPONSE OF MUSCLE TO EXERCISE

Muscle responds to exercise by hypertrophy, by improvement in motor control, and by an adaptive response of enzymes that decrease the fatigue with sustained effort concurrently with an increase in strength and an increase in absolute muscle endurance. Increase in relative endurance that involves a change in shape of the intensity duration curve is also possible, although the results are less dramatic than the increase in absolute muscle endurance.

Hypertrophy

It has long been established that larger muscles are, other things being equal, stronger muscles. Although reported figures vary, there is general agreement that the *absolute strength* of a muscle is 3.6 kg per square centimeter of physiologic cross-sectional area. For a long parallel muscle, the physiologic cross-sectional area is the same as the cross-sectional area at the widest portion of the muscle. Pennate muscles with the same overall volume have a much larger physiologic cross-sectional area than do parallel muscles; thus, they can develop far more force. In order to obtain the physiologic cross-sectional area of a pennate muscle, one takes multiple sections at right angles to the muscle until all fibers are included (Figs. 10–1 and 10–2). Thus, a parallel muscle is said to be built for speed, and a pennate muscle is built for "power" (actually force). A typical pennate muscle would be the vastus medialis, which is responsible for the last 15 degrees of *forceful* extension at the knee, especially when the hip is flexed. Hip flexion shortens the distance over which the rectus femoris contracts; this muscle must use its excursion to "take up the slack" and is not effective in extending the knee.

Muscle responds to at least some types of exercise by hypertrophy. The surest way to produce hypertrophy of muscle is to use a weight that is at or near the one-repetition maximum (1RM), to do as many repetitions as possible (usually one to three), and, after a short rest, to do repeated sets at this high weight. In order to be sure of muscle hypertrophy, some lengthening contractions should be included in the regimen. There is some evidence that hypertrophy does not occur with isokinetic exercise that is purely concentric (shortening only; see the section on isokinetic exercise).[1]

Improvement of Motor Control

Moritani and deVries have devised a clever system for sorting out, with isometric strength, the

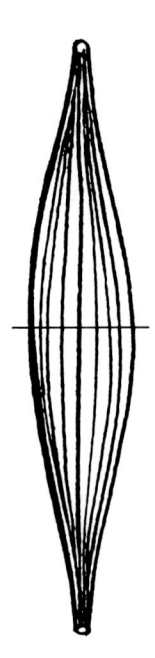

Figure 10-1 Parallel arrangement of muscle fibers. "Physiologic" cross-section is equal to cross-section of muscle belly. (From Brunnstrom S. Clinical kinesiology. 2nd ed. Philadelphia: FA Davis, 1966.)

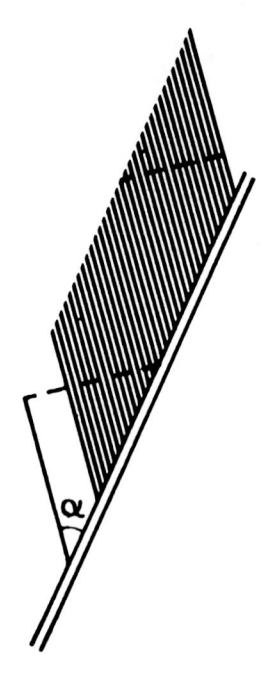

Figure 10-2 In pennate muscle, the physiologic cross-section is determined by multiple sections at right angles to the fibers until all are included. (From Brunnstrom S. Clinical kinesiology. 2nd ed. Philadelphia: FA Davis, 1966.)

amount of improvement of muscle performance that is due to hypertrophy and that which is due to "neural" or other learning factors.[2] The relationship of integrated electrical myographic (IEMG) activity of the muscle to the force generated by that muscle is a linear one, provided that the exercise is purely an isometric one and that the surface electrode is kept over the same portion of the same muscle with the joint(s) held in the same position from session to session. There are two ways that a muscle could, in theory, improve its performance, as demonstrated by this technique. Figure 10-3 shows a theoretical possibility in which the slope of the line relating force to IEMG activity remains the same, but the line is extended, indicating that the subject has somehow generated more electrical activity. This could be described as learning or, using Moritani and deVries' term, improved performance because of neural factors. Figure 10-4 shows another theoretical possibility in which the line is not extended but, with training, the line shifts or slopes to the right; this indicates that, for any given amount of neural or motor unit action potential activity, the amount of force generated is greater. This would be caused by a change of the muscle itself, i.e., hypertrophy. Figure 10-5 shows how one could sort out the relative contribution of learning and of hypertrophy. Figure 10-6A shows the trained side of an actual subject. It should be noted that, in response to the first 2 weeks of training, the main improvement is caused by neural factors, i.e., learning. This provides a good explanation of the remarkable increases in strength often seen at the beginning of a strength training program. Following week 2, there is slight further extension of the line, but the main changes come from a slope of the subsequent lines downward to the right, i.e., for any given amount of IEMG or electrical effort, the amount of force generated is greater. This is caused by muscle hypertrophy. This technique of Moritani and deVries can also be used to document and to explain the phenomenon of cross-training (crossed limb training) that sometimes occurs. One can see in Figure 10-6B that in the opposite, untrained limb there is some improvement in muscle strength, but this is all caused by an increased electrical activation, without any change in the slope of the line. It is not surprising that some

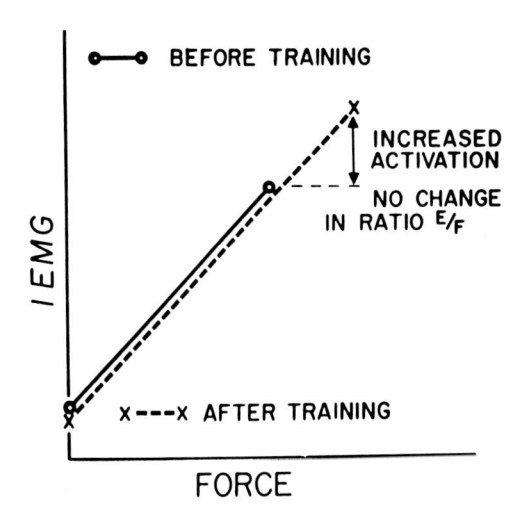

Figure 10-3 Increase of integrated electromyographic activity (IEMG) plotted against force of contractions, as an index of strength due to neural factors gained during training. (Redrawn from Moritani T, deVries HK. Neural factors versus hypertrophy in the time course of muscle strength gain. Am J Phys Med 1979; 58:115–130.)

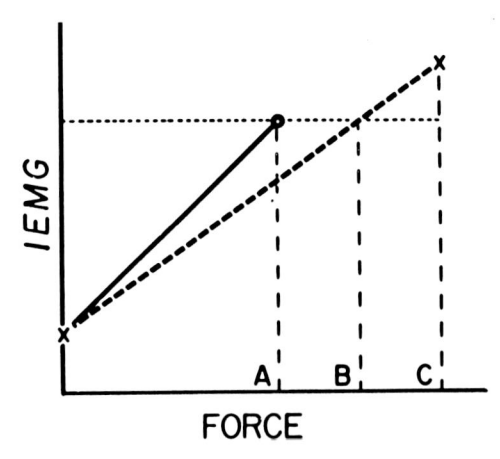

Figure 10-5 Schema for evaluation of percent of contribution of neural factors (NF) versus muscular hypertrophy (MH) to the gain of strength through progressive resistance exercise based upon efficiency of electrical activity (EEA). Strength increase percent MH = (B-A)/(C-A) × 100. Strength increase percent NF = (C-B)/(C-A) × 100. (Redrawn from Moritani T, deVries HK. Neural factors versus hypertrophy in the time course of muscle strength gain. Am J Phys Med 1979; 58:115–130.)

learning would take place on both sides. It is equally unsurprising that no hypertrophy occurs on the untrained side.

Milner-Brown and associates have shed some light on what may be happening to improve the "neural factors" for brief, high-force contractions.[3] For such contractions, it is important that motor units be activated as synchronously as possible. Milner-Brown studied synchronization ratios in weight lifters and in those who use their muscles in brief, high-force contractions in their occupations. As shown in Figure 10-7, these persons have higher synchronization ratios than controls. Control subjects who are then put on a weight training program increase their ability to activate motor units synchronously. Milner-Brown and colleagues showed that a 20 percent increase in maximal isometric force (maximum voluntary contraction [MVC]) was associated with a doubling of the synchronization ratio.

In addition, the experienced weight lifter observes that improvements in technique enable him to keep lifting higher weights in some competitive activities even after hypertrophy would have been expected to level off. This may represent greater synchronization and/or accelerating the weight in certain favorable portions of the range and allowing momentum to assist during more difficult portions of the range of motion.

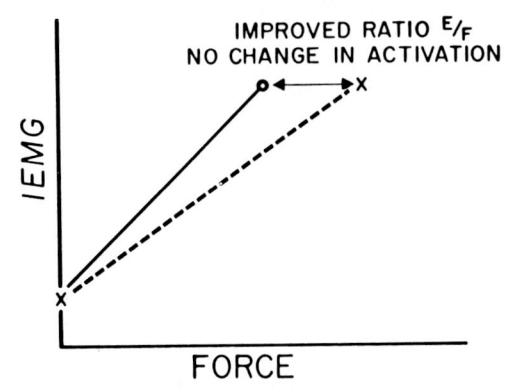

Figure 10-4 Strength gained because of hypertrophy when neural activity is constant. (Redrawn from Moritani T, deVries HK. Neural factors versus hypertrophy in the time course of muscle strength gain. Am J Phys Med 1979; 58:115–130.)

Adaptive Response of Enzymes

Although it is possible that athletes may choose their sport, and therefore their preferred form of exercise, according to their native endow-

Isokinetic Exercise

Isokinetic exercise is defined by the measurement system. In an isokinetic system, one can preset the maximal rotational velocity, and the equipment accommodates any torque produced in the attempt to accelerate beyond this preset maximal contraction velocity. Thus isokinetic exercise is also referred to as *accommodated resistance exercise*. This permits the subject to vary his torque maximally (or, for that matter, minimally) throughout the range of motion. Motivational factors are of great importance in this type of exercise.

Cam-Varied Load Exercise

The Nautilus system (Fig. 10–8) utilizes a cam to vary the resistance produced by a constant load. It does this according to the formula: force equals mass times acceleration (F = ma). The cam, which is thought by some to resemble the cross-section of a Nautilus sea creature, makes a longer distance for the load to travel in certain parts of the range of motion in which the muscle is ordinarily able to produce more torque. Thus, although the mass is kept the same, the acceleration of the load (at a constant joint rotational velocity) is greater in this part of the range, and the force demanded to produce this acceleration is greater.

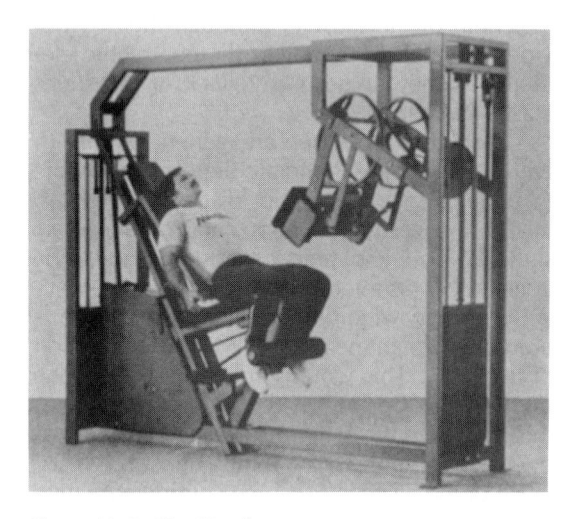

Figure 10–8 The Nautilus system.

Typical Exercise Training Programs

DeLorme Technique

The DeLorme program requires the initial and weekly determination of the 10-repetition maximum (10RM), i.e., the highest weight that the subject can lift through the full range of motion 10 times only.[6] Although the actual program has gone through a number of variations, a typical DeLorme program would involve daily performance of 10 repetitions at 50 percent of the 10RM value, 10 at 75 percent, and 10 at 100 percent of the 10RM. Except for the inconvenience of having to determine the 10RM weekly on each group of muscles trained, this program has much to recommend it. It utilizes an initial warm-up, i.e., the 10 repetitions each at 50 percent and 75 percent of the 10RM, and it generally pushes the muscle to fatigue or near fatigue, which is desirable as shown below.

Figures 10–9 through 10–12 show three types of relatively simple equipment that can be used for quadriceps strengthening. They could be used not only with the DeLorme technique but also with the Oxford, Hellebrandt, and University of Washington techniques.

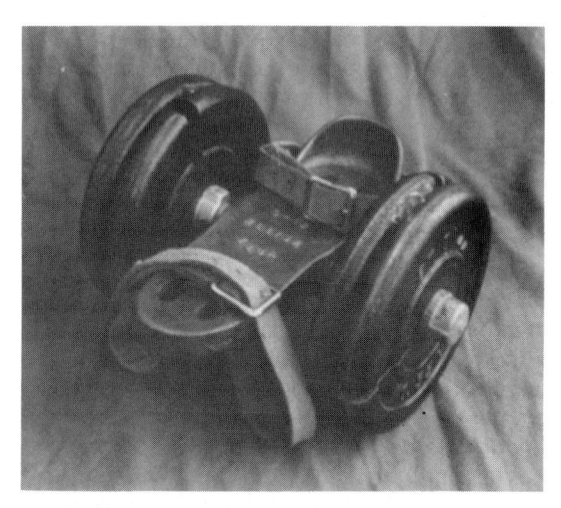

Figure 10–9 Quadriceps boot with crossbar and weights. (From de Lateur BJ. In: Kottke FJ, Stillwell GK, Lehmann JF, eds. Krusen's Handbook of Physical Medicine and Rehabilitation. 3rd ed. Philadelphia: WB Saunders, 1982.)

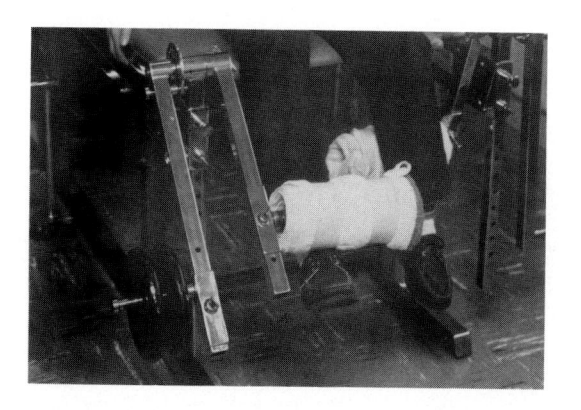

Figure 10–10 Exercise table with the angle between the load and lever arm set at 0 degrees. (From de Lateur BJ. In: Kottke FJ, Stillwell GK, Lehmann JF, eds. Krusen's handbook of physical medicine and rehabilitation. 3rd ed. Philadelphia: WB Saunders, 1982.)

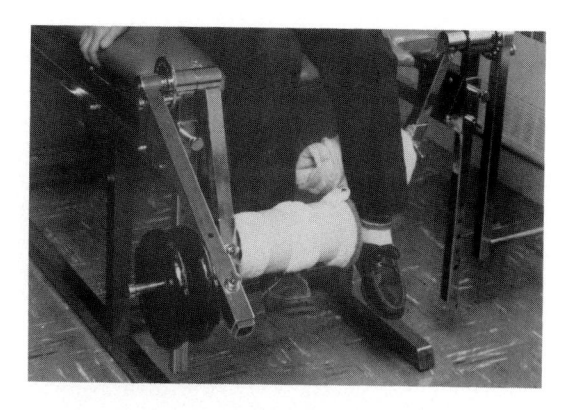

Figure 10–11 Exercise table with the angle between load and lever arm set at 45 degrees. (From de Lateur BJ. In: Kottke FJ, Stillwell GK, Lehmann JF, eds. Krusen's handbook of physical medicine and rehabilitation. 3rd ed. Philadelphia: WB Saunders, 1982.)

Oxford Technique

The so-called Oxford program is, or can be, in all respects similar to the DeLorme program including equipment, except that one begins with 10 repetitions of the 10RM and follows this with 10 repetitions at 75 percent and 50 percent of the 10RM.[7] Although the definitive study comparing these two programs has not yet been done, one would expect that the DeLorme program would obtain superior results.

Hellebrandt Technique

Hellebrandt and Houtz demonstrated that one may progressively "overload" and thereby improve the performance capacity of muscle not only by progressively increasing the load but also by keeping the load constant for a relatively long period of training time and gradually increasing the contraction velocity.[8] The principle that underlies this is the torque–velocity relationship. Figure 10–13 illustrates that if one fully recruits the available motor units, i.e., gives full effort and motivation, one is able to produce less tension in the muscle and less net torque with a faster shortening contraction than with a slow shortening contraction or an isometric contraction. Thus, if one begins with a high weight and slow contraction, and on an every-other-day basis increases the metronome setting, the progressively taxed muscle adapts by an improvement in work capacity, including strength. One begins setting the metronome at 40 beats per minute, elevating the weight on "tic" and lowering it *smoothly* to strike the floor on "toc" (allowing it to drop to the floor would defeat the purpose of the program). One then proceeds to accomplish a fixed number of repetitions, such as 20. (If it is possible to go much beyond this, the weight is too low.) The metronome setting is increased every other day. This program has the advantage of taking a slightly shorter length of time each day. A metronome

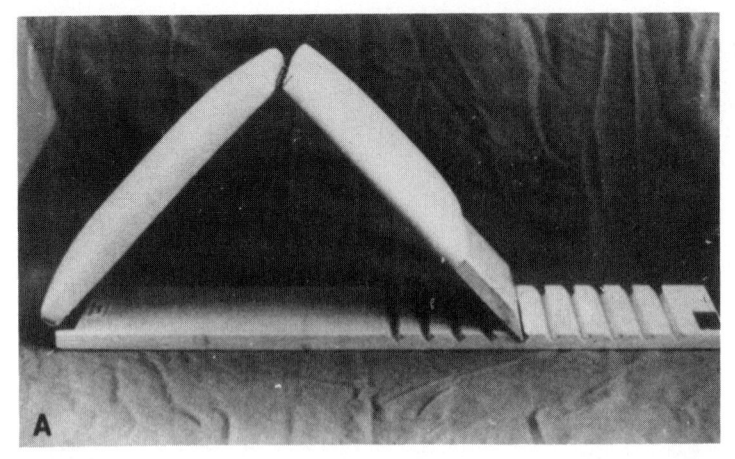

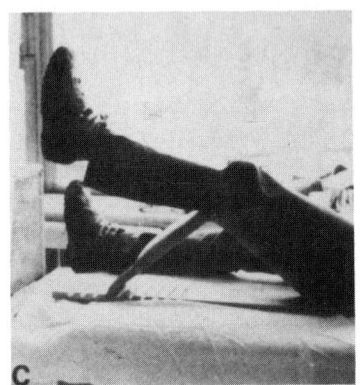

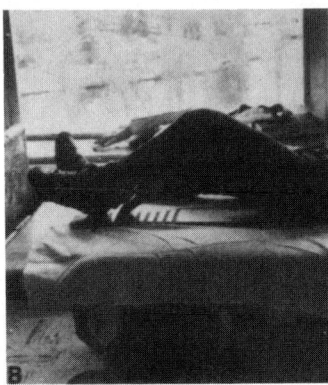

Figure 10–12 The quadriceps board or fracture board. (A) The angle of the knee is determined by the slot in which the distal portion of the board is placed. (B) Subject using fracture board, knee flexed. (C) Subject using fracture board, knee extended. (From de Lateur BJ, Lehmann JF. In: Leek JC, Gershwin ME, Fowler WM Jr, eds. Principles of physical medicine and rehabilitation in musculoskeletal disease. Orlando: Grune & Stratton, 1986.)

is required, and some find the sound annoying, although there are electronic metronomes that can be made only to flash and to produce no sound.

University of Washington Technique

A system developed at the University of Washington involves taking a relatively high weight, i.e., one that the subject could lift three to seven or eight times, and having the subject continue lifting the weight through the full range of motion until muscle fatigue is achieved, counting the number of repetitions. When a fixed number of repetitions is reached, such as 20, the weight is increased a small amount. This is very efficient; it obviates the need for determining a weekly 10RM but still gives a quantifiable measure of progress to follow. When possible repetitions are relatively few, it is more likely that genuine muscle fatigue is achieved rather than boredom, joint pain, or other overuse problems. A metronome is desirable, but not absolutely essential.

Nautilus System

The Nautilus system applies several physiologic and biomechanical principles: the well-known torque–velocity curve (Fig. 10–13); the fact that the torque which can be developed varies throughout the range of motion (and that this variation is, in turn, dependent upon changes in the length–tension relationship and changes in the angle of insertion of the muscle tendon throughout the range); and, finally, the

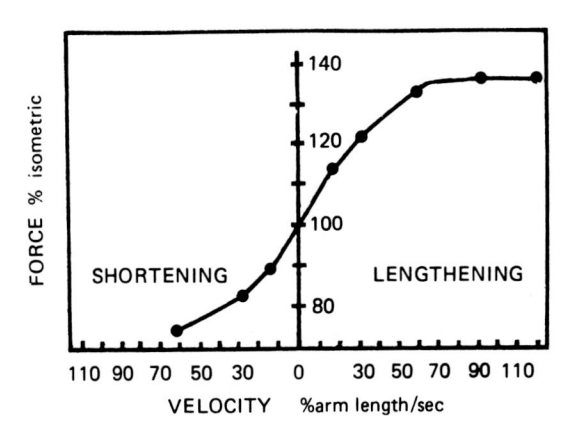

Figure 10-13 Relationship of maximal force of human elbow flexor muscles to velocity of contraction. Velocity on abscissa is designated as percent of arm length per second. (From Knuttgen HG, ed. Neuromuscular mechanisms for therapeutic and conditioning exercises. Baltimore: University Park Press, 1976).

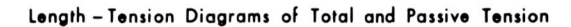

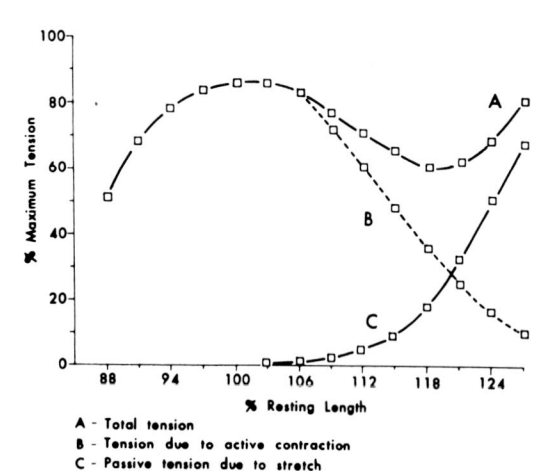

Figure 10-14 Length–tension diagram for passive stretch of an unstimulated muscle is shown in lower curve C. Curve A, showing total isometric tension when the muscle is stimulated at various lengths, from maximal stretch through moderate shortening, represents the sum of active contraction and passive tension caused by the stretch. Active tension caused solely by muscular contraction is obtained by subtracting passive tension (C) from total tension (A) and is represented by curve B. Normal resting length is 100 percent. (Redrawn from Schottelius BA, Senay LC. Effect of stimulation-length sequence on shape of length–tension diagram. Am J Physiol 1956; 186:127–130.)

fact that some component of eccentric or lengthening muscle exercise appears to be essential in order to train the muscle optimally. Pure concentric isokinetic protocols might not lead to muscle hypertrophy. In addition, muscle is called upon to perform some loaded eccentric contractions during sport activities. Figure 10-14 illustrates an idealized length–tension diagram or Blix diagram. If, for example, in an anesthetized animal, one detaches the Achilles tendon from its insertion and allows the muscle tendon unit of the triceps surae to be put in a very short or slack position, no tension would be measured in this unit. If one draws the muscle tendon unit out to progressively greater lengths, that length at which tension just begins to register is called the *resting length* of the muscle. As one draws the muscle tendon unit out to progressively greater lengths, progressively greater tensions are recorded, until such time as this unit ruptures. If one stops before rupture and goes back to a short length (for example 88 percent of resting length) and sends a tetanizing volley of electrical stimuli down the motor nerve, a certain tension develops. This total tension is seen in curve A as equal to the active plus the passive tensions. Because the passive tension is, by definition, zero until the resting length is achieved, the total tension is equal to the active tension alone at all lengths below the resting length. As can be seen, the greatest active and total tension is achieved a or slightly beyond the resting length, as so defined. If one then goes to the intact human subject and uses the biceps brachii as an example, one would expect the greatest torque to be developed when the muscle is in a relatively long position, as when the elbow is near full extension. However, the length–tension relationship is not the only consideration. Figure 10-15 shows two ways of computing torque that take into consideration the angle of insertion of the muscle tendon into the bone. Here, F is the total muscle force or resultant force vector which is a function of the length–tension relationship (and also of the force–velocity curve). The rotatory force or torque is equal to the resultant force times the perpendicular distance from this resultant force vector to the joint axis. A somewhat easier way of computing this would be to multiply the resultant force by the sine of alpha. Thus, when the elbow is almost fully extended, the angle of application of the tendon, alpha, is very small, and the sine of alpha is therefore small. Figure 10-16 shows how the

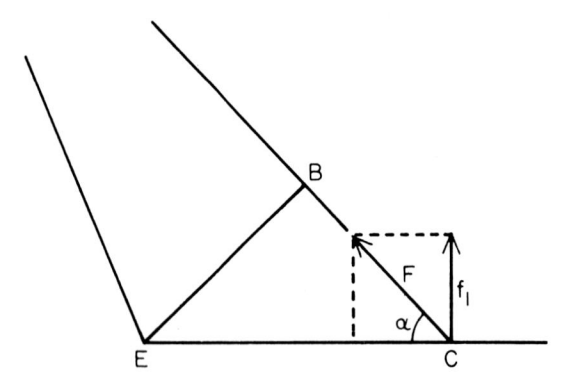

Figure 10–15 Two methods of computing torque. Torque equals $f_1 \times EC$ or $F \times EB$. (From Brunnstrom S. Clinical kinesiology. 2nd ed. Philadelphia: FA Davis, 1966.)

leverage resulting from this angle of application can be considered apart from the muscle size. In this respect, the brachioradialis has the greatest leverage, but the leverage of all of the elbow flexors is greatest at or beyond (slightly more flexed than) 90 degrees. If leverage were the only consideration, then the brachioradialis would be the most powerful elbow flexor, but, as was previously shown, the muscle force itself is in proportion to the physiologic cross-section of the muscle, and the biceps is a much larger muscle. Figures 10–17 through 10–19 show the net interaction between the physiologic (length–tension relationship) and mechanical (leverage, angle of insertion) factors for isometrically measured torque for elbow flexors and extensors, forearm pronators and supinators, and shoulder flexors and extensors, respectively. The interaction of the physiologic and mechanical factors is somewhat different for each muscle group. The relationships among the physiologic factors of length–tension, speed of contraction, and the mechanical factor of leverage are shown as measured isokinetically for the quadriceps and hamstrings at three different speeds.

As described in a previous section (cam-varied load), the Nautilus system uses a cam to attempt to force the muscle tendon joint unit to exert the maximum torque of which the muscle is capable throughout the range of motion. Because the weight is lowered by the same muscle group, an eccentric component is present.

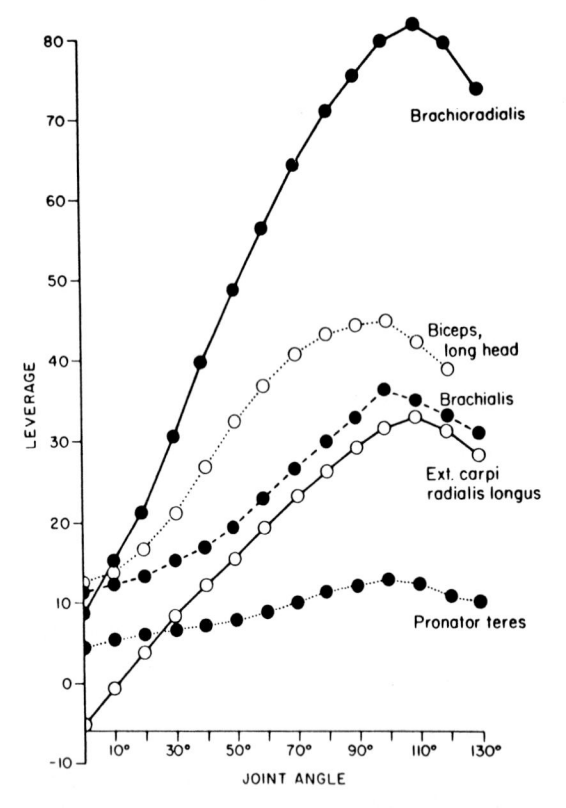

Figure 10–16 Leverage curves of elbow flexors. Zero degrees = elbow extended. (From Brunnstrom S. Clinical kinesiology. 2nd ed. Philadelphia: FA Davis, 1966.)

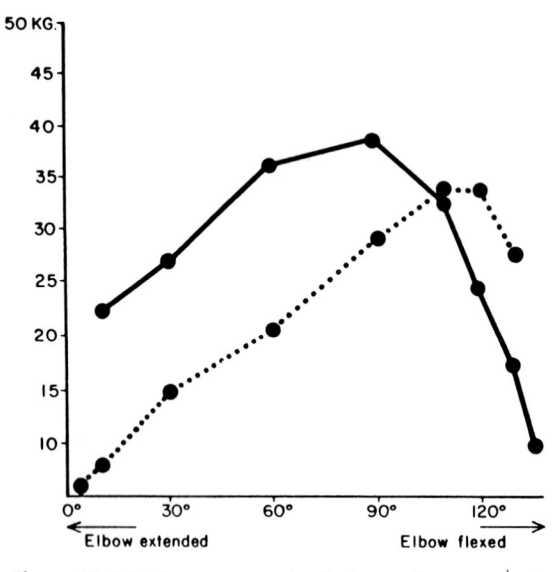

Figure 10–17 Torque curves for flexion and extension of right elbow, from determinations on four male subjects (*solid curve*, elbow flexion; *dotted curve*, elbow extension). (From Brunnstrom S. Clinical kinesiology. 2nd ed. Philadelphia: FA Davis, 1966).

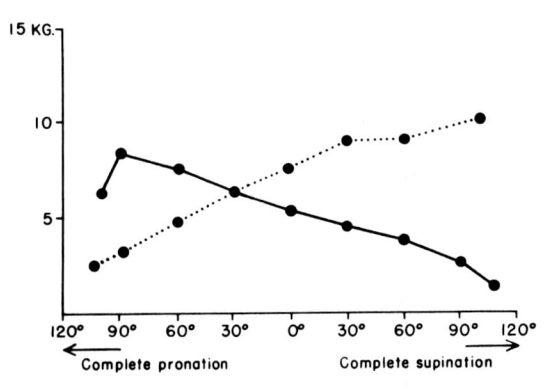

Muscle Strength and Local Endurance Training / 253

Figure 10–18 Torque curves for pronation and supination of right elbow, derived from determinations on four male subjects. Elbow at 90 degrees of flexion (*solid curve*, supination; *dotted curve*, pronation, zero, thumb upward). (From Brunnstrom S. Clinical kinesiology. 2nd ed. Philadelphia: FA Davis, 1966).

However, because muscles can develop more tension with a lengthening contraction than with any type of shortening contraction, this lengthening portion of the exercise is relatively untaxing to the muscle. Some subjects increase the vigor of the lengthening component by having a companion apply an additional force during the lengthening portion of the exercise. The Nautilus program bears some similarity to the University of Washington system in that a relatively low number of contractions is performed (10 to 15 for the lower body, eight to 12 for the upper body) prior to adding a small amount of weight. This is a routine used for general conditioning. If a body building program is desired, the weight is increased so that fewer repetitions can be done, and, after a brief rest, the set is repeated.

Cybex System

The Cybex (Fig. 10–20) or other pure isokinetic system is different from the Nautilus system in at least two ways. One is that it permits but does not force the subject to exert the maximum torque throughout the range. The Cybex system allows one to preset a maximum rate of contraction and then accommodates any torque the subject develops in attempting to accelerate the lever arm beyond this preset limiting rate. If one does not attempt to accelerate beyond the preset limit, one could push the lever arm throughout the range of motion with very little

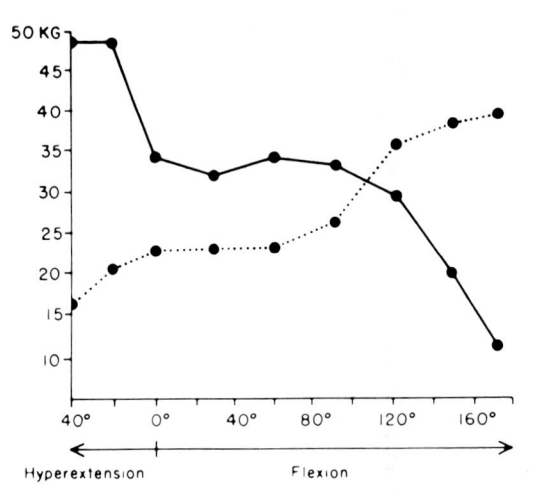

Figure 10–19 Torque curves for flexion and extension of right shoulder, derived from determinations on four male subjects (*solid curve*, flexion, *dotted curve*, extension). (From Brunnstrom S. Clinical kinesiology. 2nd ed. Philadelphia: FA Davis, 1966.)

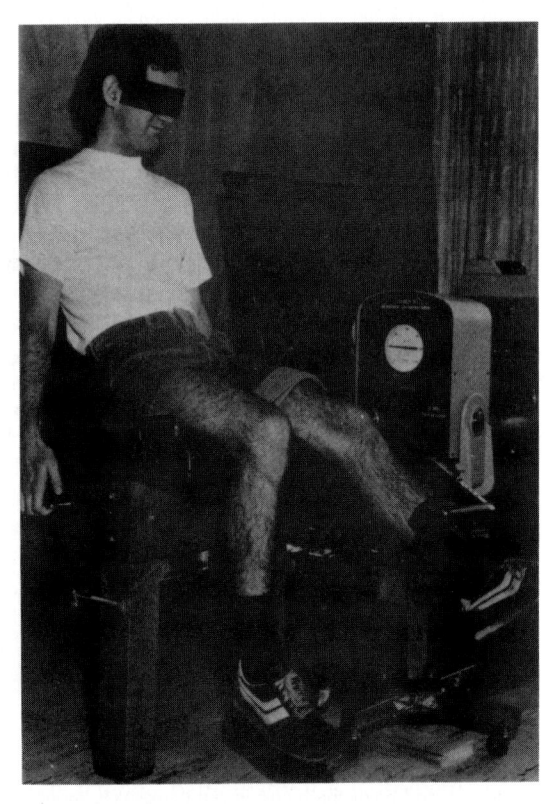

Figure 10–20 The Cybex isokinetic exerciser.

ARTICULAR CARTILAGE COLLAGEN ALIGNMENT

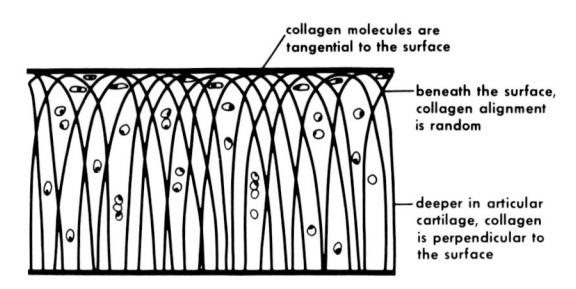

Figure 11-1 Beninghoff arcade of collagen alignment in articular cartilage.

cate this magnificent structure, there are many more sugar side chains attached to the protein core. These *glycosaminoglycans* (GAG) are replete with negatively charged (anionic) sulfate and carboxyl groups on the chondroitin and keratan sulfate components of glycosaminoglycan (Fig. 11-2).

Mechanically, this multiplicity of anionic groups creates considerable resiliency in the proteoglycan matrix, with like charges repelling each other diffusely throughout articular cartilage. This creates a cushion effect; when compression of articular cartilage pushes these negative charges closer together, the anions push away from each other to provide some degree of cartilage resilience. In articular cartilage, one may conceive of a balance of like charges on sulfated proteoglycans, repelling each other within a collagen "retaining wall." This simplified view of articular cartilage provides an attractive illustration of how cartilage responds to compression in athletics, as well as in normal day-to-day activities.

Water is attracted osmotically to proteoglycan and provides an important structural component of articular cartilage, particularly because it is the main constituent of normal articular cartilage.[1] Normal cartilage function depends on water extrusion through articular cartilage "pores," which are large enough to allow water to flow freely in and out, but small enough to restrain macromolecules within the articular cartilage matrix. The normal function of articular cartilage is probably best understood, then, as a complex interrelationship between static alignment forces (including collagen support and electronegative charge balance) and hydrodynamic factors, in which water is extruded from articular cartilage in front of an advancing load on the cartilage but is "imbibed" back into the cartilage with removal of the load. This mechanism of stress resistance is certainly extremely important for the normal ability of articular cartilage to resist athletic stress. As the amount of stress increases with running, jumping, and vigorous activity, the health of articular cartilage is particularly critical. Normal fluid flow in articular cartilage is important also for flow of nutrients from synovial fluid to chondrocytes in the matrix, because articular cartilage has no blood supply.

Chondroitin - 4 - Sulfate

Chondroitin - 6 - Sulfate

Keratan Sulfate

Figure 11-2 Negatively charged sulfate and carboxyl groups on chondroitin and keratan sulfate glycosaminoglycans (GAG) repel each other when placed in proximity in articular cartilage matrix. This helps produce cartilage resiliency.

Any structural defect in articular cartilage that weakens the collagen-restrained polyanionic proteoglycan and water complex makes articular cartilage prone to breakdown. The sequence of events that can follow is described in the section on pathologic joint function. Likewise, the presence of excessive water (in effusion), degradative enzymes (collagenases, proteoglycanases, etc.), or destructive chemicals (prostaglandins and bradykinins) produced by an inflammatory response can cause alteration of this complex matrix and impairment of normal articular cartilage function.

The entire structure of articular cartilage as outlined thus far might be regarded as incredibly well adapted to resist stress. Subchondral bone may also help articular surfaces to resist impact and stress. In the diaphysis (midportion) of long bones, there is a peripheral rim of cortical bone supporting most of the longitudinal stress. In the subchondral area, this cortical rim, particularly in weightbearing bones, flares out and thins, thus providing a broader weight-bearing surface under the articulating surfaces. Clearly, then, this distributes impact over a broader area at the joint. The spongy, cancellous layer of bone under articular cartilage provides a somewhat more resilient base of support for articular cartilage than would a thick cortical bone layer. The bony structure supporting joints, then, is also well suited to providing resiliency and withstanding loads.[4] Damage to subchondral bone, from a fracture or excessive impact, can lead to thickening of this subchondral layer in some regions and can result in loss of resiliency with reduced resistance to normal impact loading.[5]

Both cartilage and bone are *viscoelastic*.[6] Viscoelastic structures respond differently to impact, depending on the rate at which a load is applied. If a load is applied quickly, as is often the case in sports, the cartilage and bone supporting a joint surface may be less able to resist the load than if the same stress is applied over a longer period of time. This is the reason why good cushion in an athletic shoe is important to protect articular surfaces. The cushion delivers an impact load more slowly to musculoskeletal structures. As the impact stress is delivered more slowly (lower strain rate), bone and cartilage adapt to the load better, the stress–strain relationships change, and there is less chance of bone or cartilage fracture (Fig. 11–3). The cartilage (or bone underlying it) can provide more cushion when an impact is delivered more slowly.

Finally, it is important to recognize that articular cartilage, like bone, actually becomes thicker in response to stress.[7] It is likely that this occurs as a result of direct chondrocyte stimulation and not because of any neurologic factors, because cartilage is aneural as well as avascular. An immobilized or unloaded joint actually loses articular cartilage mass, making it less able to withstand stress.[3] It is very important, therefore, to provide enough time for joint cartilage restoration after immobilization and to avoid vigorous athletic involvement until there has been adequate reconstitution of a joint that was immobilized following injury.

Synovial fluid normally protects articular cartilage by providing both lubrication and nutrition. Because there is no blood supply to articular cartilage, the availability of normal synovial fluid nutrients to articular cartilage is imperative for cartilage survival. It is not surprising, then, that effusions eventually cause articular cartilage attenuation. Enzymes and prostaglandins in an effusion cause articular cartilage matrix depletion, while depriving chondrocytes of normal synovial fluid nutrition. The normal hyaluronic acid concentration of synovial fluid diminishes as effusion increases; consequently there is less protection against shear stress. Normal synovial fluid, then, is important for healthy articular cartilage function.

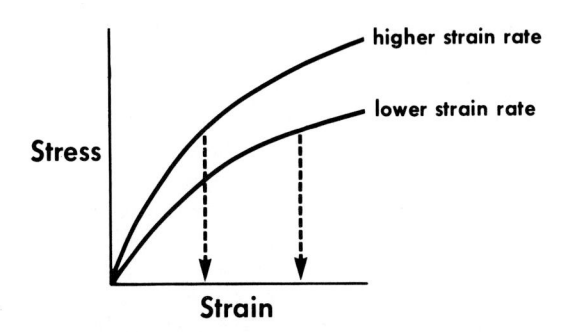

Figure 11–3 Stress–strain curves for a viscoelastic material. At a higher strain rate, a given load is applied more rapidly and less strain (deformation) occurs. By applying the same load more gradually (lower strain rate), the stressed material (cartilage, bone, etc.) can adapt and behave more as a cushion.

The synovial membrane normally produces synovial fluid, but it also releases degradative enzymes and prostaglandins when it is inflamed. Galasko and colleagues showed elevated levels of prostaglandins in the synovium of knees with injured menisci.[8] However, under normal circumstances synovial membrane functions simply to provide synovial fluid for normal articular lubrication and nutrition.

In arthroscopic or conventional joint surgery, there is some risk to articular cartilage. Aside from the obvious risk of mechanical injury to articular cartilage, solutions irrigating a joint (including normal saline, bupivacaine, and even lactated Ringer's solution) cause some transient inhibition of proteoglycan synthesis.[9] Corticosteroids can cause considerable inhibition and attenuation of articular cartilage.[10] Therefore, prompt, accurate articular surgery (arthroscopic or conventional) and minimal use of exogenous agents (particularly corticosteroids) permit more rapid return of an athlete to vigorous activity.

MENISCUS

The menisci of the knee (also known as semilunar cartilages) are extremely important. Although historically the menisci were not considered very important for knee function, it is now well recognized that menisci help in absorbing impact and controlling motion of the knee. Meniscus injury is fairly common in athletics. In the past, injury to a meniscus would usually result in complete removal of the torn meniscus. Degeneration of the meniscus-deficient compartment has since proven predictable.[11] Recently, arthroscopic surgery has permitted removal of only the damaged portion of a meniscus. Although not yet proven, knee degeneration should be less if only a small piece of a meniscus is removed, particularly if the main weightbearing portion of the meniscus can be preserved and if basic meniscus stability is retained. To understand the adverse effects of meniscus removal on a knee, one must first understand the normal structure and function of the menisci.

The medial and lateral menisci of the knee joint minimize shear stress on articular cartilage. They do this by moving with the femoral condyles as they flex, extend, rotate, and slide on the tibia.[12] The lateral meniscus is somewhat loosely attached at its posterior aspect and therefore moves considerably; the medial meniscus is more firmly attached at its periphery. The medial meniscus is also attached to the collateral ligament, whereas the lateral meniscus is not. This helps to explain why the posterior medial meniscus is more prone to tearing.

Normally, the menisci move posteriorly with flexion and anteriorly with knee extension. The femoral condyles roll posteriorly with knee flexion, placing particular pressure on the posterior aspects of the menisci in flexion (explaining why flexion causes pain in many people with posterior horn meniscus tears). In fact, this is why McMurray's test (rotation of the knee with flexion beyond 90 degrees) can elicit a click in some people with posterior horn meniscus derangement.

Motion of the knee joint is particularly complex including rotation, sliding, and rolling, in addition to pure flexion and extension. The medial and lateral condyles move at different rates across the tibial surface with knee flexion and extension. At terminal extension, the medial femoral condyle rolls posteriorly at a rapid rate, pushing the medial meniscus slightly posteriorly. This process is reversed as knee flexion begins from a position of full extension, with contraction of the popliteus muscle laterally. The popliteus pulls the lateral condyle into external rotation and thereby pulls the medial femoral condyle slightly forward on initiation of knee flexion. This "unlocks" the knee from its most stable position in extension. The menisci are important in maintaining this knee stability in extension, but they also "buttress" the femoral condyles, thereby adding to knee stability throughout flexion and extension.

The predominant collagen orientation within the menisci is circumferential, with radial strands of collagen presumably helping to prevent separation of the circumferential collagen.[13,14] Towards the meniscal surface, collagen is oriented tangentially, as in articular cartilage. The wedgelike shape of the menisci and the solid fixation of the peripheral meniscus help control motion of the femoral condyles.[15]

The menisci, like articular cartilage, also contain proteoglycan. However, the concentration of proteoglycan is only about one-eighth that of hyaline cartilage.[16] Nevertheless, from a mechanical point of view, the shear stiffness of meniscal tissue is very similar to that of articular cartilage.[6] Stress across the knee joint, then, can be spread out over a larger surface area and shared by the menisci.[13] As previously noted, subchondral bone also provides a cushion, under normal circumstances, for articular cartilage. Consequently, the menisci and subchondral bone can modify substantially the impact loads delivered to the knee. The lateral meniscus absorbs most of the weight applied to the lateral knee, while the medial meniscus and exposed cartilage share the medial load equally (up to 150 kg). Without a meniscus, there would be considerable loss of articular load transmission and energy-absorbing functions, as well as a diminished buttress effect.[16]

Arnoczky and Warren have shown that the menisci receive their blood supply from the inferior and superior geniculate arteries.[17] The end capillaries of these vessels form a plexus in the synovium and capsule. These vessels lie around the periphery of the menisci (Fig. 11–4), and they project in a radial fashion into the menisci, thus providing a blood supply to the peripheral portions of the meniscus. This blood supply permits healing of peripheral meniscal tissue following fixation by sutures or other materials (adhesives or staples may eventually replace sutures for meniscus repair). Consequently, restoration of the meniscal loadbearing function is possible following repair of a torn meniscus. However, generally only more peripheral meniscal tears are repaired because the blood supply and healing capacity of meniscal tissue diminishes toward the free edge of the meniscus. When possible, therefore, it is desirable to restore a torn meniscus rather than to remove it, particularly in an athlete who places high demands on his or her knees.

LIGAMENT STRUCTURE AND HEALING

Ligaments and *retinacula* can be defined as fixed connective tissue structures that connect and restrain joints or other moving structures in the body. These functions are extremely important to the athlete. A *capsule,* on the other hand, encloses a joint; it limits motion to some extent, but its primary function is not so much restraint as enclosure.

A thin connective tissue capsule runs in continuity with the synovium surrounding each joint. On the other hand, each joint has specific ligaments (such as the anterior cruciate, posterior cruciate, medial collateral, and lateral collateral ligaments in the knee) that restrain motion in certain planes of motion. In the shoulder, the superior, middle, and inferior glenohumeral ligaments prevent excessive anterior shoulder mobility. There are other retinacular restraints that function in a manner similar to ligaments, but they are generally more sheetlike and multifaceted in their restraint function. The best example in the knee joint is the lateral peripatellar retinaculum.[18] This structure runs mostly from the iliotibial band to the patella. It controls medial displacement of the patella while modulating movement of the patella in the femoral trochlea. Similar retinacular structures provide restraining, as opposed to enclosing, functions. Chronic trauma to such structures, caused by joint imbalance (as in the patellofemoral joint), may lead to neuromatous degeneration of retinacular small nerves and pain around the joint.[19]

Ligaments and retinacula are well adapted to resist tensile stresses. Specifically, fibers in ligaments and retinaculum run in the direction

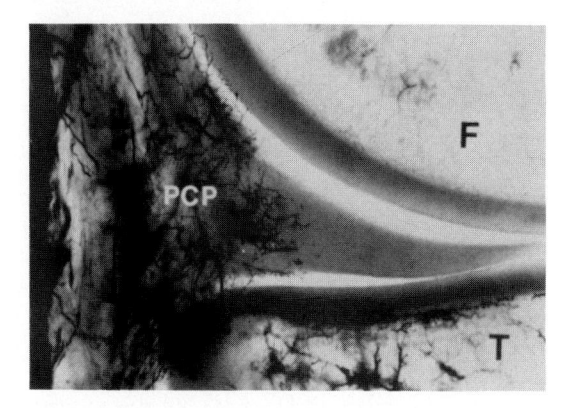

Figure 11–4 The vascular supply enters the menisci peripherally through the perimeniscal capillary plexus (PCP). (From Arnoczky S, Warren R. Am J Sports Med 1982; 10:91; with permission.)

necessary to control tensile loading. In the ankle joint, the anterior talofibular ligament is tight as the talus is drawn forward on the tibia. In contrast, the posterior talofibular ligament becomes taut as the talus is pushed posteriorly on the tibia. The fibulocalcaneal ligament helps to prevent dislocation of the talus but is more suited to block inversion of the ankle. Consequently, each of these ligaments functions to control motion of the ankle joint in specific planes. Histologically, the fibers of these ligaments and of other ligaments in the body run parallel to one other, with bundles of collagen also running parallel to the direction of function. In addition, there are condensations of connective tissue at the edges of some joints to block excessive motion. Such *labral* condensations are particularly notable in the hip and shoulder. Other joints, such as the elbow and ankle, rely more on bony contours of the joint. This adds to stability and minimizes, but does not eliminate, risk of joint dislocation.

Fibroblasts in ligaments and retinacula produce collagen, replacing damaged collagen and adapting to the loads applied. New collagen, as in an injured or reconstructed ligament, is more fragile than mature collagen. Cross-linking and linear orientation occur in more mature collagen and add considerably to the tensile strength of the linearly oriented ligament fibers.[20] Immature collagen, on the other hand, resists tensile loading poorly, largely because there is less cross-linking. This is particularly important to note with regard to surgical repair or reconstruction of deficient ligaments. Early collagen formation in a tendon graft used for ligament reconstruction is immature, with less cross-linking, so it cannot resist tensile stresses as well as it would following a normal process of collagen maturation and cross-linking. It is important to recognize also that the collagen formed even in a normal healing ligament (such as the talofibular ligament injured in an ankle sprain) is weak for months. Adequate rehabilitation and taping or bracing of injured ligaments help prevent inadvertent reinjury to healing ligaments that have too little strength to resist even a modest amount of stress. Furthermore, techniques such as deep friction massage should generally be avoided in the first few months after sprain, because repeated pressure on a healing ligament may prevent clot fibrosis and optimal healing.

Ligament Reconstruction

Unfortunately, some torn ligaments never heal adequately, and a surgical procedure may be necessary to restore adequate stability. When a tendon graft must be used to build a new ligament, autogenous tendon graft is probably best, because it can revascularize and form autogenous connective tissue most readily, with minimal risk to the patient (Fig. 11–5).

The anterior cruciate ligament in the knee is particularly important in resisting excessive knee rotation in athletics and is commonly reconstructed when torn. Its reconstruction was first described in the early 1900s.[21] However, until recently there has not been much understanding of the behavior of tendon grafts placed into the knee for replacement of a deficient intra-articular ligament. Lundborg and Rank have shown that tendons remain viable when placed in the intra-articular environment.[22] It was not until Amiel that these tendon grafts were shown to synthesize biochemically appropriate collagen.[23] In fact, Amiel and colleagues suggested that "there may be ligamentization of the tendon graft used inside a joint to reconstruct a

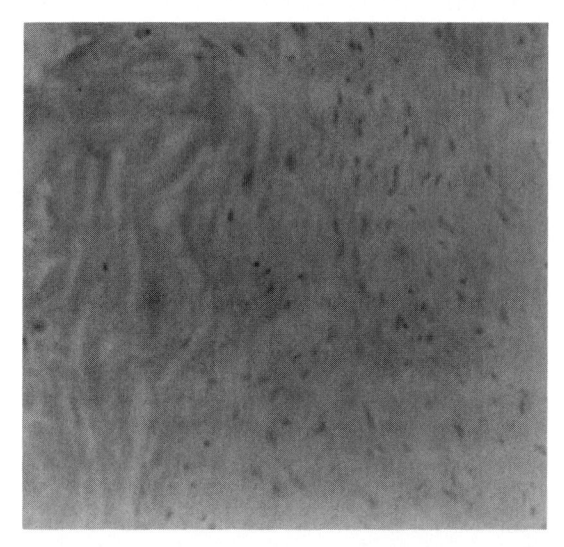

Figure 11–5 Collagen degeneration and disorientation are readily apparent in a tendon graft transplant at 6 weeks from the time of surgery. Adjacent immature new collagen is also apparent.

deficient intra-articular ligament." Other studies, such as that by Van Rens and associates, have questioned the ultimate mechanical integrity of tendon grafts placed in the knee joint to replace the anterior cruciate ligament.[24] Clancy found that there was good return of tensile strength in tendon grafts used to reconstruct monkey anterior cruciate ligaments.[25] It is important to recognize that there is a gradual reformation of healthy connective tissue over a long period of time (probably years) following tendon graft reconstruction. We have further shown in our laboratory that intra-articular tendon grafts survive and form abundant new collagen following vascularization.[26] However, the ultimate strength of the new ligament may not be adequate for a long time after surgery.

Usually, an athlete is restricted from returning to vigorous sports for at least 9 months from the time of tendon graft reconstruction of a deficient cruciate ligament, because tendon remodeling is slow and possibly even somewhat inadequate.[24,25,27] In addition to the time required for remodeling, factors that affect the function of a reconstructed anterior cruciate ligament include initial selection of an adequately strong tendon for grafting and appropriate placement of the graft in the knee joint. Although our work, along with that of Amiel and colleagues and Clancy and colleagues, is encouraging with regard to reformation and quality of reconstructed ligaments, van Rens has raised serious questions about the actual amount of strength ultimately achieved by reconstructed ligaments.[23-26] It is also important to consider how reconstructed ligaments provide joint protection. Is the strength of the reconstruction most important, or is appropriate reinnervation of the graft at its ends important to provide sensory input to modulate knee motion? Kennedy showed that there are neural elements innervating the anterior cruciate ligament, predominantly in multiple clefts at the tibial origin.[28] Perhaps reinnervation of a reconstructed ligament is important to its ultimate ability to withstand stress.

Adding to the complexity of ligament reconstruction is the multicentric flexion and rotation of most joints. Replacement of an anterior cruciate ligament, for instance, cannot really restore the fan-shaped complex orientation of a *normal* anterior cruciate ligament. So, in reality, most reconstructions provide limitation of joint motion in certain extremes of motion, but do not permit completely normal joint function. High-level, precise athletic performance requires a joint that functions well; consequently treatment must provide precise reconstruction and vigorous, appropriate rehabilitation, realizing that absolute normality is rarely achieved following severe ligamentous injury.

There is interest now in synthetic material and allograft replacement of defective ligaments. Any "matrix" may permit fibroblast infiltration and connective tissue formation within its structure, assuming that the replacement ligament is accessible to cells. However, fatigability of synthetic materials is a problem, and there is no secure evidence yet that artificial ligaments can stand the test of time.

Allografts offer human tissue that may provide tensile strength while permitting autogenous fibroblast infiltration. Although there may be some merit in using allograft ligaments, primarily the ability to avoid using autogenous structures for ligament reconstruction, there have been concerns about introducing occult viruses or infection into the recipient. There is currently no evidence that allograft reconstruction of a deficient ligament is better than, or even equal to, autograft reconstruction. However, with further experience it is possible that synthetic or allograft ligament replacement will be suitable for selected patients, particularly those who have already lost autogenous support structures around the knee.

Fortunately, some joint injuries, such as detachment of the anterior labrum genoidale in the shoulder, permit virtual anatomic restoration of the injured structure without need for ligament reconstruction. Using arthroscopic technique, anatomic fixation of a detached labrum glenoidale is possible.[29] This sort of restoration is particularly desirable for the athlete who wishes to return to competitive athletics, but return to high-performance throwing sports after shoulder reconstruction is uncommon.

PATHOLOGIC JOINT FUNCTION

With joint instability and excessive loading, attenuation of articular cartilage can occur for purely mechanical reasons. Simply explained, there is a limit to the amount of impact and stress that normal articular cartilage can tolerate. Cartilage begins to deteriorate if loading involves recurrent impact.[30] Such loading causes subchondral microfractures, subsequent stiffness, and eventual cartilage degeneration.[30] Although superficial injury to articular cartilage may remain stable, deep articular cartilage injury does not result in replacement of the injured cartilage by normal articular cartilage.[31]

With excessive articular loading and mechanical joint deterioration, fragments of articular cartilage are released into a joint and the concentration of free proteoglycan in the joint increases. George and Chrisman have shown that the excessive proteoglycan in a joint eventually causes chemical as well as mechanical articular damage.[32] An inflammatory response results from free intra-articular proteoglycan. Increased levels of prostaglandins, catheptic enzymes, and inflammatory by-products can lead, then, to chemical deterioration of a joint.[33-35] Prostaglandins cause accelerated loss of articular cartilage proteoglycan by the cascade phenomenon described by Chrisman and associates.[35] Cathepsins cause further destruction of articular cartilage macromolecules. Both proteoglycanases and collagenases appear during the inflammatory response, causing destruction of articular cartilage proteoglycan and collagen. It is possible that acute articular cartilage injury causes considerable arachidonate release and subsequent production of prostaglandins and enzymes by Chrisman's cascade.[35,36] With loss of normal articular cartimacromolecules, the joint is more susceptible to high loads and breaks down mechanically at some point with even normal loading. The result is progressive joint deterioration.

This unfortunate scenario occurs also, although slowly, after total removal of a meniscus from the knee.[11] Although there are many who seem to control excessive joint motion after cruciate injury and who have limited joint degeneration, anterior cruciate ligament (ACL) insufficiency may lead to progressive joint deterioration in many people.[37] Vigorous athletes are likely to injure an ACL-deficient knee further, and progressive deterioration is more likely in them.

Patellar malalignment, particularly abnormal tilt, can lead to articular degeneration in a similar way. Chronic patellar malalignment particularly limits athletes, often because of pain in the peripatellar lateral retinaculum, but joint degeneration may occur later because of excessive shear stress, concentration of stresses on the lateral patellar facet, and cartilage breakdown, as previously described.[19,38]

Other joints are also known to deteriorate because of chronic imbalance or instability. Small joints in the hand, injured early in life during athletics or other activity, can degenerate and stiffen by the same process described in larger joints. The trapeziometacarpal joint, as well as other carpal joints, may deteriorate later in life after early injury. Elbow joint deterioration is common in baseball pitchers, with excessive medial elbow stretching and lateral joint compression (Little League elbow in youngsters). This can lead to bony changes, osteochondral injury, articular cartilage damage, and eventual joint degeneration. The shoulder can degenerate as a result of chronic instability, but all the upper extremity joints are less prone to rapid degeneration because they do not bear body weight. Consequently, mild upper extremity articular instability can be tolerated by some athletes if adequate strengthening and activity modification can control symptoms. Ultimately, the fate of an unstable joint is determined by the amount of shear stress and overload. Athletes often put extreme stress on injured joints, the result being articular overload, excessive articular cartilage wear, and substantial impact loading of already weakened (by prostaglandins, enzymes, and mechanical injury) articular cartilage. This can cause or hasten the appearance of degenerative arthritis.

Therefore, treatment of athletes with unstable joints should be designed primarily to limit or prevent later joint degeneration. If an athlete can control excessive joint mobility with adequate bracing, strengthening of supporting muscles, and modification of activities, there is no reason to stabilize every unstable joint surgically. On the other hand, a knee, shoulder, ankle, or other joint that swells recurrently because of chronic irritation (causing prostaglandin and enzyme production), that subluxes or dislocates causing gross joint damage, or that in any way demonstrates signs of uncontrollable instability (resulting in extreme amounts of shear stress and eccentric loading) may require surgical stabilization *early,* before arthrosis and an irreversible pattern of progressive joint destruction occur.

JOINT MOBILITY AND INSTABILITY

Synchronous joint motion with appropriate intermittent loading is necessary for joint homeostasis and preservation. Joint instability caused by genetic deficiency, structural malalignment, or damage to the normal supporting (retinacular) structures can lead to progressive, and often irreversible, changes in a joint, as described in the previous section.

There is a spectrum of connective tissue tightness related predominantly to heredity. At one end of this spectrum are people with collagen defects and extreme hyperelasticity of their joints. A genetic deficiency of one enzyme, such as lysyl oxidase, can result in defective collagen structure and excessive connective tissue laxity, as in the Ehlers-Danlos patient. At the other end of this spectrum are people with excessive joint stiffness. Conditions such as arthrogryposis, another congenital deficiency, cause excessive joint stiffness and loss of motion. There are also people who can hyperextend their joints and can maneuver joints into positions that are impossible for most normal people. This can be beneficial in activities such as gymnastics and dance, which require unusual joint mobility. On the other hand, unstable joints can limit some types of athletic activity. Sometimes there is a fine line between joint laxity that permits excellent gymnastic or dance performance, and joint laxity that causes problems.

Pathologic joint laxity can lead to recurrent joint subluxation and dislocation. Shoulders and knees are particularly susceptible to excessive joint laxity. If a joint dislocates recurrently because of excessive laxity, the trauma from this recurrent injury eventually leads to permanent articular damage and arthrosis.

Inborn structural defects in joint alignment, such as a congenitally dislocated hip, can be particularly destructive, because they can involve extreme concentration of loads to limited areas of an articular surface, unusually great amounts of shear stress, and resulting loss of articular cartilage early in life. Such conditions are uncommon and usually preclude normal athletic participation.

Joint injuries, on the other hand, are common in athletes. Disruption of joint capsule and ligaments can lead to a similar pattern of concentrated loading and excessive shear stress. Injury to the shoulder joint, resulting in recurrent dislocation, injury to the acromioclavicular joint with instability and excessive motion, unstable finger joints, recurrent ankle sprains, knee laxity related to ligament injury, and recurrent patellar dislocation or subluxation can lead to joint arthrosis in the area afflicted by recurrent excessive loading and shear stress. It may be that this process starts because of arachidonic acid production by injured chondrocytes after impact.[36] If there is inflammation also, enzymes, prostaglandins, and excessive fluid in the joint may hasten joint deterioration.

It is difficult to define the precise line between tolerable and intolerable joint laxity. However, as a general principle, one may accept some degree of inherent or induced joint laxity if rehabilitation and bracing permit adequate function without mechanical and biochemical evidence of progressive joint deterioration. Once a pattern of chemical and mechanical joint degeneration becomes predictable because of recurrent instability, consideration should be given to correcting this process before it becomes irreversible.

REFERENCES

1. Mankin H, Thrasher A. Water content and binding in normal and osteoarthritic human cartilage. J Bone Joint Surg (Am) 1975; 57:76–80.
2. Weiss C. Light and electron microscopic studies of normal articular cartilage. In: Simon WH, ed. The human joint in health and disease. Philadelphia: University of Pennsylvania Press, 1978.
3. Fulkerson J, Edwards C, Chrisman OD. Articular cartilage. In: Albright J, Brand P, eds. The scientific basis of orthopaedics. East Norwalk, CT: Appleton and Lange, 1987:347.
4. Radin EL, Paul IL. Importance of bone in sparing articular cartilage from impact. Clin Orthop 1971; 78:342–344.
5. Radin EL, Paul IL, Lowy M. A comparison of the dynamic force-transmitting properties of subchondral bone and articular cartilage. J Bone Joint Surg (Br) 1974; 56:381.
6. Hayes WC, Bodine AJ. Flow-independent viscoelastic properties of articular cartilage matrix. J Biomech 1978; 11:407–419.

7. Palmoski MJ, Colyer R, Brandt K. Joint motion in the absence of normal loading does not maintain normal articular cartilage. Arth Rheum 1980; 23:325–334.
8. Galasko C, Rushton S, Lacey E. Prostaglandins and the synovitis associated with meniscal lesions. Trans Orthop Res Soc 1980; 5:61.
9. Fulkerson J, Winters T. Articular cartilage response to arthroscopic surgery: a review of current knowledge. Arthroscopy 1986; 2:184–189.
10. Behrens F, Shepard N, Mitchell N. Alteration of rabbit articular cartilage by intra-articular injections of glucocorticoids. J Bone Joint Surg (Am) 1975; 57:70–76.
11. Fairbank T. Knee joint changes after meniscectomy. J Bone Joint Surg (Br) 948; 30:664–670.
12. Hollinshead WH. Anatomy for surgeons. Vol. 3. The back and limbs. Hagerstown, MD: Harper & Row, 1969.
13. Bullough P, Vosburgh F, Arnoczky S, Levy IM. The menisci of the knee. In: Insall J, eds. Surgery of the knee. New York: Churchill-Livingstone, 1984:135.
14. Bullough PG, Munuera L, Murphy J, Weinstein AM. The strength of the menisci of the knee as it relates to their fine structure. J Bone Joint Surg (Br) 1970; 52:564–570.
15. Beaupre A, Choukroun R, Guidouin R, et al. Knee menisci: correlation between microstructure and biomechanics. Clin Orthop Rel Res 1986; 208:72–75.
16. Krause WR, Pope MH, Johnson RJ, Wilder DG. Mechanical changes in the knee after meniscectomy. J Bone Joint Surg (Am) 1976; 58:599–604.
17. Arnoczky SP, Warren RF. Microvasculature of the human meniscus. Am J Sports Med 1982; 10:90–95.
18. Fulkerson J, Gossling H. Anatomy of the knee joint lateral retinaculum. Clin Orthop 1980; 153:183–188.
19. Fulkerson J, Tennant R, Jaivin J, Grunnet M. Histologic evidence of retinacular nerve injury associated with patellofemoral malalignment. Clin Orthop 1985; 197:196–205.
20. Tanzer M. Cross-linking of collagen. Science 1973; 180:561.
21. Hey-Groves EW. The cruciate ligaments of the knee joint: their function, rupture, and operative treatment. Br J Surg 1920; 7:505.
22. Lundborg G, Rank F. Experimental intrinsic healing of flexor tendons based upon synovial fluid nutrition. J Hand Surg 1978; 3:21.
23. Amiel D, Kleiner J, et al. The phenomenon of ligamentization: ACL reconstruction with autogenous patellar tendon. J Orthop Res 1986; 4:162.
24. Van Rens T, van den Berg A, Huiskas R, Kuypers W. Substitution of the anterior cruciate ligament: a long-term histologic and biomechanical study with autogenous pedicled grafts of the iliotibial band in dogs. Arthroscopy 1986; 2:139.
25. Clancy W, Narenchania R, et al. Anterior and posterior cruciate ligament reconstruction in rhesus monkeys. J Bone Joint Surg (Am) 1981; 63:1270.
26. Fulkerson J, Gossling H, Waite J. Collagen synthesis in vascularized and nonvascularized patellar tendon transplants in rabbit knees. Trans Orthop Res Soc 1983; 8:111.
27. Noyes F, Butler D, Paulos L, Grood E. Intra-articular cruciate reconstruction: perspectives on graft strength, vascularization, and immediate motion after replacement. Clin Orthop 1983; 172:71–77.
28. Kennedy J, Alexander I, Hayes K. Nerve supply of the human knee and its functional importance. Am J Sports Med 1982; 10:329–335.
29. Morgan C, Bodenstab A. Arthroscopic bankart suture technique and early results. Arthroscopy 1987; 3:111–122.
30. Radin E, Parker H, Pugh J, et al. Response of joints to impact loading III. J Biomechanics 1973; 6:51–57.
31. Mankin HJ. The response of articular cartilage to mechanical injury. J Bone Joint Surg (Am) 1982; 64:460–466.
32. George R, Chrisman OD. The role of cartilage polysaccharides in osteoarthritis. Clin Orthop 1968; 57:259.
33. Teitz C, Chrisman OD. The effect of salicylate and chloroquine on prostaglandin-induced articular damage in rabbit knees. Clin Orthop 1975; 108:264.
34. Fulkerson JP, Damiano P. Effect of prostaglandin E2 on adult pig articular cartilage slices in culture. Clin Orthop 1983; 179:266.
35. Chrisman OD, Ladenbauer-Bellis I-M, Fulkerson J. The osteoarthritic cascade and associated drug actions. Osteoarthritis Symp Semin Arthritis Rheum 1981; 11(Suppl I):145.
36. Chrisman, OD, Ladenbauer-Bellis I-M, Panjabi M. The relationship of mechanical trauma and the early biochemical reactions of osteoarthritic cartilage. Clin Orthop 1981; 161:275.
37. Feagin J. The syndrome of the torn anterior cruciate ligament. Orthop Clin North Am 1979; 10:81–90.
38. Fulkerson J. Awareness of the retinaculum in evaluating patellofemoral pain. Am J Sports Med 1982; 10:147–149.

Chapter 12
Biomechanics

GIDEON B. ARIEL

Biomechanics is an integration of the two disciplines of biology ("bio") and physics ("mechanics"). It recognizes that all bodies on earth, whether animate or inanimate, are affected in the same way by gravity, and it provides a better understanding of performance. In other words, a bridge, a car, a baseball player, and a horse must all adhere to the laws of mechanics. The additional factors that must be included to assess motion for the biological entities more accurately include such things as bone capacity, neuromuscular coordination, and physiologic attributes. From the understanding of each component comes a greater appreciation of the integrated result, which is called biomechanics.

Da Vinci once observed that, although drops of rain are in fact independent of one another, they appear to the human eye as "continuous threads descending" from the clouds, and that therein lies the truth of how the eye "preserves the impression of moving things which it sees."[1] Therein also lies the visual distortion that allows us to see motion pictures. Because of the properties of the human eye and the visual system, a series of separate images on film becomes a smoothly flowing image when projected onto a screen at a certain speed—a movie.

Movement of the human body is also a series of separate, individual actions. These actions begin with minute electrochemical processes that are infinitely swifter and more complicated than any set of film images traveling at 24 frames, or 1.5 feet, per second. Our muscles are thin strands of fibers which, when inactive, have all the strength of jelly. But when they contract or relax because of these electrochemical reactions, the result is movement of the body with a fluidity that prevents even the sharpest eyes from distinguishing the separate actions. For instance, the simplest of human movements, such as crooking a finger or raising an eyebrow, involves a complex of neuromuscular happenings that cannot be duplicated by artificial means. In fact, the best robot still moves in jerks and stops when compared with the subtle, flowing pace of a human.[2]

People fathom the nature of things by tracking their motion. All motion follows mechanical principles. Like the machines they make, people are a set of levers whose movements copy the geometry of classical mechanics. These levers are powered by muscles, whose actions can be as simple as their characters are complex. Each of the more than 600 muscles is abundantly supplied with nerves that link the muscles to the brain and spinal cord and that often follow labyrinthian circuits, humming with signals, to control the ebb and flow of muscular energy. Many muscles must work harmoniously together in order to perform even the simplest task.[3]

The study of biomechanics is an attempt to understand how these neuromuscular events occur and to analyze a series that the naked eye sees only dimly and the mind often fails to comprehend. Biomechanics is a science that depends on the known facts of biology, physics, and, to a lesser extent, chemistry. To reap the rich rewards of the more satisfying, fulfilling life this science can offer, a thorough understanding of both the "bio" and the "mechanics" of biomechanics must be gained.

NEUROMUSCULAR INTEGRATION

The "bio" part of biomechanics deals with the functioning living organisms or their parts. The smallest elements of the body, which maintain all the functions of life, are the cells. Furthermore, in the 500 million years that the human species has been on earth, the basic nature of the cells has remained relatively unchanged. Therefore, what was true for the cells of cave people continues to apply to modern human beings. Activities that produced fitness in the cells of prehistoric humans do the same today, because the human body has remained essentially unchanged over the eons. What has changed, and quite dramatically in Western civilizations, is the environment in which the body functions. Our cells have been forced to adapt to this fast-changing world.

The building or structural units of the human body are the bones, which are connected by ligaments. At the joints, cartilage cushions the shock of bone on bone, and the joint is lubricated by synovial fluid that can be pumped in and out of articular cartilage.

However, bones have no power to move. Like the frame of an automobile, they provide the basic structure on which the body rests. The engine that supplies the power to move comes from the muscles. It is the 600 muscles of the body, which account for about 40 percent of body weight, that do the work.[4]

Biomechanical engineers are principally concerned with the voluntary muscles. These are controlled by conscious and rather programmable routines that enable the skeletal system to move in a prescribed manner. The control programs are generated by the brain and can be modified by training. Muscles are caused to contract by signals from the central nervous system. The actions of the body can be likened to a link system in which those reciprocating engines, the muscles, move the bones of the foot, ankle, shank, thigh, and so on, under the controlled stimulation of the central nervous system.

Consider some of the complexities of the simple act of walking. There must be a neurologic program and control of the nervous system pattern of firings and relaxations, chemical processes must be appropriately regulated, and muscular actions must be generated so that the activity is consistent with the laws of physics. Thus, muscle action is used to adjust the position of the body, keeping that center of gravity in line with the base. Each time this line of gravity is displaced out of the base, the body is in the act of falling. Muscles, in effect, act as cables pulling on bones. The tug of the cable makes motion possible, but it should be remembered that a muscle can only contract. Because muscles are paired, one contracting muscle pulls a bone forward, while the paired muscle can contract to pull the bone back in the opposite direction.

In all cases, the number of muscles involved in an action of the body is more than the eye observes.[5] The arms, hands, and fingers contain 52 pairs of muscles. The typesetting of this page employs all 52, although only the fingers and hands appear to shift positions significantly. The thighs, legs, and feet have 62 pairs of muscles. The back is composed of 112 pairs. Even when standing motionless, the muscles that are used in walking must be constantly at work to prevent falling. It is not possible for a corpse or skeleton to stand up, because there are no muscles to work at maintaining the proper distribution of body segments.

The three basic elements of the musculoskeletal system—bone, muscle, and connective tissue—normally perform with perfect teamwork. Their mission is to support the body, shield its delicate internal organs, and make it mobile. The coordination and interactions of these individual components is the responsibility of the nervous system.

In the 1700s, Galvani studied the movements of frog muscles and saw that they contracted when electrically stimulated. He deduced that electrical current must be involved in the normal muscle contraction process. Both chemical and mechanical interactions affect muscular contractions, but any understanding of biomechanics requires an appreciation of biocybernetics, the study of control and communication in humans. The central nervous system consists of the brain and both the sensory and motor pathways that innervate the musculature. In the brain, 10 billion cells, about the same number as stars in our galaxy, engage in an electrochemical operation that, in conjunction with other body parts, permits us to see, hear, reason, imagine, create, love, hate, move, and be aware of exactly which process we are involved in, through the capacity to incorporate feedback.[6]

The building block of the system is a specialized nerve cell known as a *neuron*. Bundles of neurons are organized into larger entities, the *nerves*. Nerves serve as pathways for constant streams of information from eyes, ears, nose, and other areas, to the neurons of the brain. The brain evaluates the data in light of evolution and individual experience. In addition, nerves with receptor cells monitor such stimuli as pain, cold, touch, pressure, and even blood and body chemistry. Motor neurons within the brain and at the target sites control the movement of muscles. They not only trigger the chemicomechanical process of working muscles but also try to govern the actions.

The input for one neuron comes from other neurons and receptors by means of a synapse. Pathways for signals of motor neurons lie along the spinal column, which is why severe spinal injury can lead to paralysis of limbs. Motor neurons cause muscle fibers to contract. But the action in which a muscle fiber ceases to contract, in which it relaxes or lengthens, does not occur because of some signal to the motor neuron. Rather, it is the absence of a signal ordering the fiber to contract that allows the tissue to relax.

The intricate programming that coordinates this choreography of balance resides in the brain and central nervous system. This network relies on continuous feedback in much the same way as control of today's modern automobile. No matter how frail he or she might be, the modern driver can control a vehicle with the flick of a wrist or ankle, because sophisticated mechanisms assist in steering, braking, and shifting. These mechanisms have sensors that measure some physical variable and use the "feedback" information to control the devices. In our bodies, there are numerous automatic feedback mechanisms of this kind controlling physiologic functions without any mental effort on our part. For example, blood pressure, respiratory rate, and levels of insulin are regulated by feedback control between the brain and the receptor targets. Certain body sensors control muscle tension while others measure responses to changes in muscle length (Fig. 12–1).

These receptor, feedback, control center programs are actually extremely complicated and require continuous activity when smooth, normal, coordinated behavior is desired. For example, suppose a person is asked to flex an elbow steadily against a load. If there were a sudden unexpected increase in the weight, his elbow would have to extend, and a larger contraction of the biceps muscle would be needed to sustain the load. Conversely, a decrease in load brings a relaxation of the biceps. The control of muscular contraction is very sophisticated and highly programmed.

Consider another example, a person's signature. Whenever John Smith signs his name, it always looks the same (or enough so to be recognizable) and different from what any other person can write, even one who was trying to sign the name of John Smith. If Mr. Smith uses chalk and signs his name on a blackboard, the signature still appears the same, even though he used different muscles than those employed when writing on paper. The individuality remains. In this complex handwriting movement, there is a preprogrammed control mechanism. Optimum performance depends on the control efficiency, not on the strength of the muscles or the efficiency of the metabolism. The control of these processes is the most important factor. Most people believe the brain is primarily used for thinking, yet research shows it to be first and foremost a control system.

Some think that the brain is like a computer. However, the single computer element in the brain is the cell. Each cell acts like a computer, and we have 10 billion of them. Posture sensors detect the position of joints, tension in tendons, and the length and velocity of muscle contraction. Inertial sensors control rolling, twisting, turning, acceleration, and the position of the head with respect to gravitational attraction. Hormonal sensors, thermosensors, and blood chemistry analyzers report on the internal biological condition of the whole organism. All of this information is analyzed and processed in innumerable computing centers that detect patterns, compare incoming data with

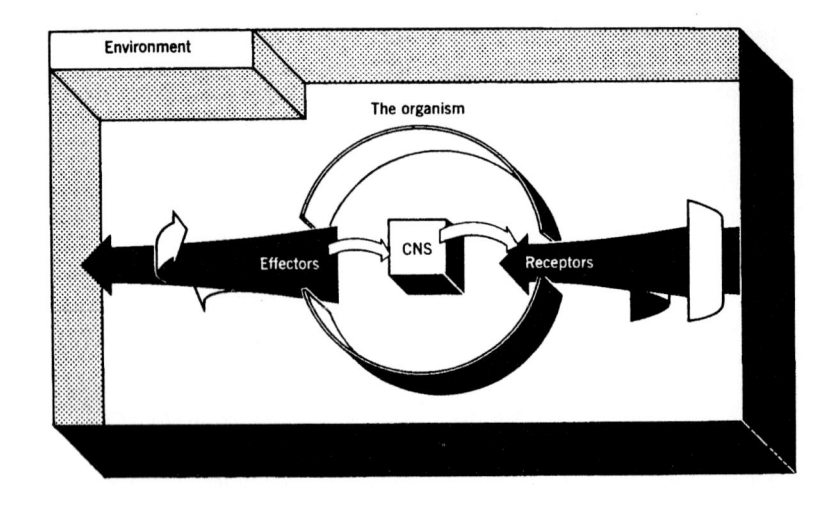

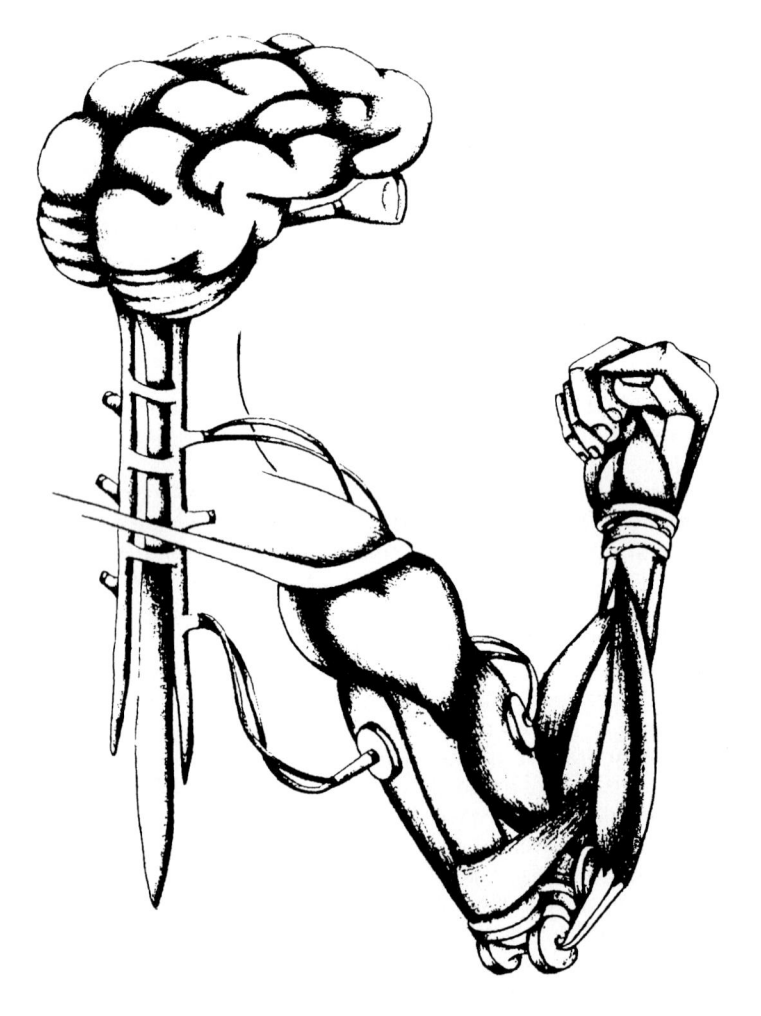

274 / Scientific Foundations of Sports Medicine

Figure 12-1 Feedback control of muscular contraction.

stored expectations, and evaluate the results. Perhaps one of the more significant features of the brain is that many computations proceed simultaneously in many different places. The brain does not execute sequential programs of instructions like a computer; rather, it executes many parallel processes simultaneously.

The fineness of control depends upon the number of motor nerve units per muscle fiber.[7] The more neurons, the finer the ability to maneuver, as in the case of the muscles that operate the eye. When there are fewer motor nerve units involved, the action becomes less fine or precise. The individual muscle fibers that make up a muscle contract and relax in an elaborate synchronization. The arrangement permits all of them to arrive at a peak of action simultaneously. But certain diseases, such as polio or cerebral palsy, destroy the normal recruitment pattern of the muscle fibers. This causes weak or spasmodic muscle action.[8] In the absence of other symptoms, some diseases may therefore be diagnosed by analyzing the form of the aberrations in the sequence of muscle fiber firing.

Synchronization of muscle firing is critical for optimizing athletic performance. In the power events, such as throwing the discus or the high jump, it is extremely important that the muscle action be simultaneously activated to optimize the force. The central nervous system does this by sending signals to the individual muscle fibers. Lack of synchronization in power events results in less force and poorer performance. On the other hand, in events of endurance such as long distance running, asynchronization is important, because fewer fibers are needed to maintain the action, thus permitting other fibers to "rest." It is a fact that the long distance runner who "over recruits" muscle fibers feels fatigue sooner.

Technique is important in achieving optimal performance. How does the brain adapt to the requirements? The answer relies on the great number of approximations that seem to add up to the correct signal. The brain achieves its incredible precision and reliability through redundancy and statistical techniques.[9] Many axons carry information about the value of the same variable, each encoded slightly differently. The statistical summation of these many imprecise and noisy information channels results in the reliable transmission of precise messages over long distances. In a similar way, a multiplicity of neurons may compute on roughly the same input variables. Clusters of such computing devices provide statistical precision and reliability in orders of magnitude greater than that achievable by any single neuron. The outputs of such clusters are transmitted and become inputs to other clusters, which perform additional analog computations. These computations result in fantastic numbers of signals terminating on the motor neurons that stimulate the muscles for movement.[10]

Movement, then, could be used to differentiate between a dead thing and a live thing, and by this definition, human beings are obviously different from stones. But are they different from machines? Machines are often in restless movement; wheels spin, levers thrash, pistons pump, but clearly they are not "alive." What are two basic constituents of movement for a, biologically speaking, living thing? The first is muscle and the second, a signaling system that makes muscles contract in an orderly manner.

To begin with, although the molecular or cellular processes of each nerve or muscle cell may be similar, tasks and innervation ratios differ; because tasks differ, not all muscles work in the same way. Consider the operations required of the human eye and arm. Eye muscles must operate with great speed and precision in orienting the eyeball quickly to close or distant points of focus, as well as in tracking movement. At the same time, the eye muscle does not have to contend with such external demands as lifting weight. The fine control needed in eye movement calls for a high innervation ratio (the ratio of the number of neurons with axons terminating on the outer membrane of muscle cells to the number of cells in the muscle). For eye muscle, the innervation ratio is about 1 to 3, which means that the axon terminals of a single motor neuron release their chemical transmitter to no more than three individual muscle cells.

In contrast to this high innervation ratio, the axon terminals of a single motor neuron innervating a limb muscle, such as the biceps of the arm, may deliver a chemical transmitter to hundreds of muscle fibers. The muscle may, therefore, have a low ratio, one motor neuron to many hundreds of muscle cells. As a result, the output of the motor unit in limb muscle is correspondingly coarse.

One of the most elementary movements for humans is walking.[11-13] All mammals and other land animals are born with the ability to walk and run. In experiments with babies between 4 and 6 weeks of age, infants started to walk when supported, raised to a standing position, and placed on a treadmill. It seems that a baby at this early age possesses and can utilize the built-in walking mechanism with which it was endowed by its genes. The nerve cells controlling the mechanism come from the spinal cord.

In order to understand complicated movement such as that of an athlete jumping or throwing or of a musician playing the violin, it is necessary to understand the brain, one of the few remaining frontiers to be explored. Humans' control of their movements comes from a system that is capable of novel and creative solutions to problems of movement.

Our movements are generated in different ways depending on the level of skill we are able to use. Athletes recruit their muscles in different ways depending on their level of acquired skill. The motor program is constantly changing in order to produce efficient movement. As mentioned above, each individual has a unique signature that appears approximately the same regardless of whether it was written with a pen on paper, chalk on a blackboard, or a stick in the sand. Yet for each of these signatures, a different set of muscles is utilized. Instructions to the muscles must come from the nervous system, but because the combinations of different muscles result in the same signature, the internal model is not simply a series of directives to a specific set of muscles. Somewhere in the nervous system a model of movement is formed that is not related to its muscular means of achievement. In other words, the optimal motor control of skilled movement is generated by a program controlled in our central nervous system.

In addition to the control by the nervous system, the human body is composed of linked segments, and rotation of these segments about their anatomical axes is caused by force. Both muscle and gravitational forces are important in producing these turning actions, which are fundamental in bodily motions in all sports and in daily life. Pushing, pulling, lifting, kicking, running, walking, and other human activities are results of rotational motion of the links, which consist of bones.

In motor skills, muscular forces interact to move the body parts through an activity. The displacement of the body parts and their speed of motion are important in the coordination of the activity and are also directly related to the forces produced. However, it is only because of the control provided by the brain that the muscular forces follow any particular displacement pattern. Without these brain controls, there would be no skilled athletic performance. In every planned human motion, the intricate timing of the varying forces is a critical factor for successful performance.[6]

The accurate coordination of the body parts and their velocities is essential for maximizing athletic performance. Muscular forces generated by the individual fibers must occur at the right time for optimum results. The strongest weight lifter cannot put the shot as far as an experienced shotputter, because although the weight lifter may possess greater muscular force, he has not trained his neuromuscular system to produce the correct forces at the appropriate time or speed.

Different athletic performances can be likened to a spectrum. On one side of the spectrum are the explosive activities, such as throwing, jumping, sprinting, and weight lifting. At the other end of the spectrum are the esthetic events, such as gymnastics, diving, and figure skating, in which success depends on the ability of the athlete to create movements that are pleasing to the judges. In the middle of the spectrum are the endurance activities, for which the athlete tries to maintain muscular contractions for long periods of time at submaximal intensity levels. Within this spectrum are events that demand that the athlete repeatedly shoot at a target with a high level of consistency and accuracy. Other activities, such as team sports, incorporate many overlapping characteristics. For example, football players need explosiveness, endurance, and accuracy.

In characterizing the movements of a person, we specify the particular activity, not the independent contraction of hundreds of thousands of muscle fibers. Walking, running, throwing, and jumping are movements that result from contractions of muscles and their synergists in relatively standard patterns of coordinated activity.

The combination of muscle and bone forms a lever system that is one of the most basic mechanical systems for performing work. A lever is a machine by which force applied at one point does work at another.[14,15] Each joint in the human body is a fulcrum of a particular lever. There are different types of lever systems, and the human body uses all types. The forces on the different levers are applied by the muscular system. Muscles do all their work by contraction, or shortening. That means that they can only pull, never push. Although it may appear that the legs, arms, and body are used to push an object, nevertheless the mechanism that produces force is still muscles that are pulling. The explanation lies in the fine symmetry that characterizes so much of the human organism. Muscles, like so many other features of our anatomy, operate in pairs, agonists and antagonists. When a limb is flexed, the agonist muscle contracts while the antagonist lengthens. The two work together in a coordinated movement, with one assisting the other for desired optimal action.

For the body to regulate movement and muscular contraction, it must receive information about what it controls. In order to accomplish this, a servomechanism must be introduced. Many current concepts about the mechanisms of movement have evolved from the work of the British physiologist, Charles Scott Sherrington.[16] Early in this century, Sherrington studied the function of the motor neuron in certain reflexive forms of motor activity, such as scratching and walking. Signals from many different areas of the brain impinge on the spinal cord motor neurons, and Sherrington characterized motor neurons as the "final common pathway" linking the brain with muscle action. He studied muscle movements in animals whose spinal cords were severed, effectively separating the motor neurons from the brain. He found that within a few months after a dog's spinal cord was severed, a scratch reflex could be elicited by such mechanical stimuli as tickling the animal's skin or lightly pulling on its hair anywhere within a large, saddle-shaped region of the upper body. In describing these responses, he stated that the movements were "executed without obvious impairment of direction or rhythm."

Sherrington's work led to today's concept of the "triggered movement" based on a "central program" involving a spinal rhythm generator. Not long after Sherrington, another British physiologist, Graham Brown, showed that rhythmic limb movements similar to those involved in walking were also possible in dogs deprived of connections between the brain and spinal cord. Evidently, spinal rhythm generators existed for walking as well as for scratching.[17,18]

Many current investigations of the neurophysiology of locomotion are aimed at clarifying the interaction between what may be termed central programs from the brain and sensory feedback from outside the nervous system. Indeed, Sherrington's work was particularly concerned with the ways motor neuron activity could be regulated by sensory feedback. Sherrington introduced the term "proprioception" to describe sensory inputs arising in the course of centrally driven movements when "the stimuli to the receptors were delivered by the organism itself." Sherrington chose the prefix "proprio" (from the Latin, *one's own*) because he believed the major function of the proprioceptors was to provide feedback information on the organism's own movements.

These control mechanisms in the muscles and tendons themselves are governed by higher level mechanisms in the brain. In fact, the control of movement relies on a hierarchical structure. The sensory information in the muscle itself processes local information and transmits net results to higher centers. Feedback enters the hierarchy at every level.[6] At the lowest levels, the feedback is unprocessed; hence, it is fast-acting with very short delay. Thus, a simple patellar tendon reflex is executed more rapidly and with a shorter "program" than a complex task like hitting a golf ball off the tee 150 yards down the center of the fairway.

In more complicated tasks necessitating higher-level control, feedback data pass through more and more stages of an ascending sensory processing hierarchy. Thus, feedback closes a real time control loop at each level in the hierarchy. The lower-level loops are simple and fast acting. The higher-level loops are more sophisticated and slower. The combination gen-

284 / Scientific Foundations of Sports Medicine

rotational speed is related to the fact that both performers are affected by the conservation of angular momentum.

The product of a turning body's moment of inertia and its angular velocity is called its *angular momentum*. According to the law of conservation of angular momentum, a turning body, isolated from external forces, has a constant angular momentum; that is to say, the product of moment of inertia and angular velocity about the axis of rotation is constant. If, for example, a man is standing on a revolving turntable without friction, he may increase his resistance to turning three-fold by stretching his arms sideways (Fig. 12–4). By the same token, if a man rotating on the same frictionless turntable pulls his hands toward his body, the rotational velocity increases three-fold, because the moment of inertia has decreased.

A figure skater makes use of these laws on ice. At first, as rapid a spin as possible is produced with arms extended. The arms are then brought down, and the body spins on the point of one skate with remarkable velocity. The same principle allows discus throwers or shotputters to generate higher speed across the circle of throwing.

These laws of motion are critical when applied to the muscles and bones of the body. To understand the application of motion, we must first understand the use of a basic tool, the lever.

The lever is one of the most basic mechanical systems for performing work. Each joint in the human body is the fulcrum of a particular lever. There are different types of lever systems and the human body uses all types. The forces on the different levers are applied by the

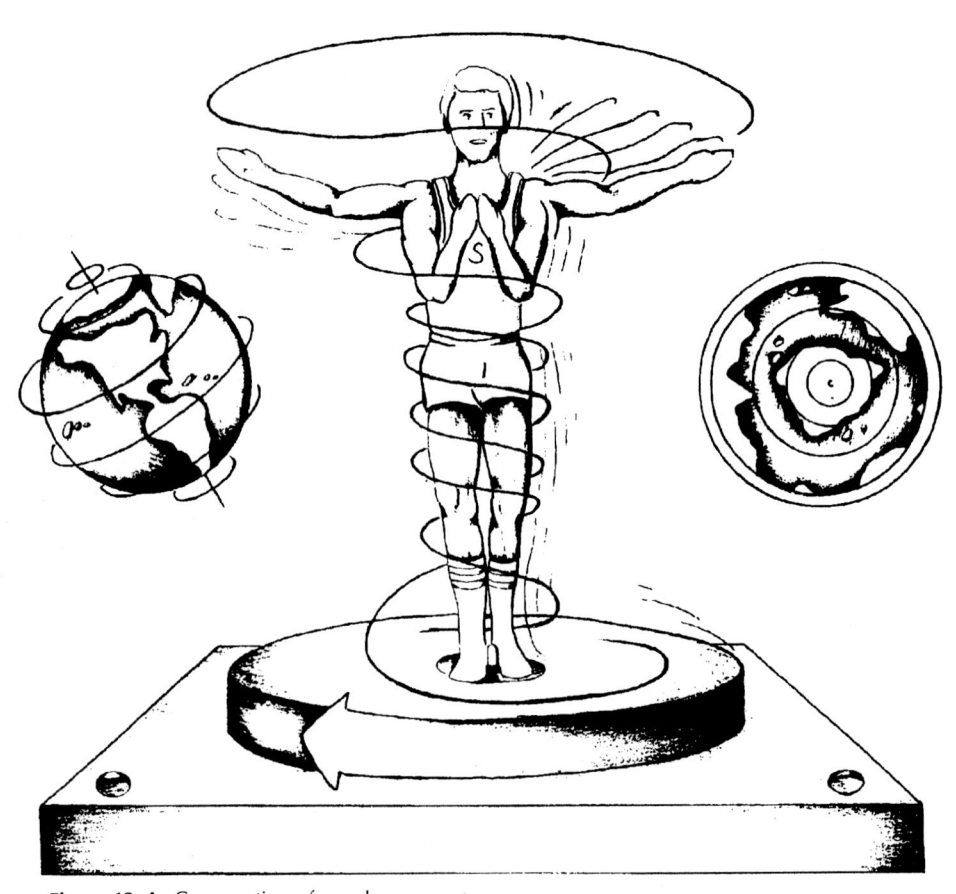

Figure 12–4 Conservation of angular momentum.

muscular system. Activity occurs because the muscles contract or pull the various bones, which constitute the levers employed in the mechanical properties of motion.

As mentioned above, muscles operate in pairs known as agonists and antagonists. Bending the arm at the elbow, for example, requires the biceps to contract while the extensors, the triceps, relax. In order to stop this bending motion, the biceps must stop contracting at the appropriate time and the triceps must begin to contract in order to slow and subsequently stop the action. The neural coordination of this system was previously discussed in the "bio" section.

Physics divides levers into three classes.[14] In the first of these, force is applied at one end of the lever and the resistance to be overcome or the work to be done lies at the other end. The fulcrum, or pivotal point, lies between. Two children bouncing up and down on a playground teeter-totter exemplify a class one lever.

In the second class, the force is applied at one end but the resistance is located above the pivot or fulcrum. A crow bar underneath a tree stump is an example of class two leverage.

In the third type, force is exerted between the pivot point and the resistance, and this is the common lever system within the human body. When you lift a weight with your arm, the pivot is the elbow joint, the force is exerted between your elbow and your hand by your biceps muscle, and the weight in your hand is the resistance (Fig. 12–5).

A lever may either increase the amount of work that can be done with a given input of force or it may cause the work to be done at a faster rate than the application of the force. Archimedes once bragged that he could move the world if given a long enough lever.[21] To perform the feat, Archimedes would have used a second class lever, with his fulcrum very close to earth; he himself would have dangled on his elongated lever somewhere deep in outer space.

A mechanical advantage is gained with use of a lever. The amount of force is multiplied many times over to produce greater output at the other end. Note that this is true if the fulcrum is situated closer to where the force is applied than to where it is executed. If the reverse is true, and the fulcrum is nearer to the point where the force is executed than to the point of force application (a class three lever), the result is a mechanical disadvantage.

For humans, the fulcrum usually falls closer to the point where the force is executed or initiated than to where it is applied, or where the k is done. The biceps attaches to the radius bone quite close to the elbow. Therefore, to lift a 1-lb weight with your hand, your biceps operates at a mechanical disadvantage of approximately seven to one: To lift 1 lb requires a force of 7 lb.

However, the same principle that governs mechanical advantage and disadvantage has its compensations. The hand at the end of the lever of the arm moves seven times faster than the point at which the biceps attaches to the radius. It is easily seen that only a slight movement upward of the forearm near the elbow causes the hand to move several inches during the same time interval. Obviously, the hand travels considerably faster than the elbow.

For most human joints, the length of the lever does not produce a mechanical advantage. Nonetheless, there is still more potential for production of speed if the human levers are longer. The knees are particularly vulnerable to injury, not only because of their limited range but also because, in some instances, the whole body becomes one long lever applying its force at the knees. A sport that illustrates this point is skiing. If the boot does not release when the shear forces are excessive, the long skis and the body can create an exaggerated and destructive lever, ultimately resulting in injury.

While Archimedes would have required a very long lever to move a very large ball (the earth), Hannibal needed a shorter lever to throw large balls from his catapult. Individuals concerned with much smaller spheres, such as golf and baseball, can apply still more force to the object of their intentions with a longer lever. Golfers should play with the longest clubs they can comfortably manage, as should batters in baseball.

However, the longer the lever, the less fine the control, and the greater the requirement for muscular force. Thus, the putter, the club used for a deft, accurate stroke, is the shortest in the bag. Many good golfers further reduce the potential margin for error by shortening up on the putter and holding it lower on the shaft.

In addition to some of the important com-

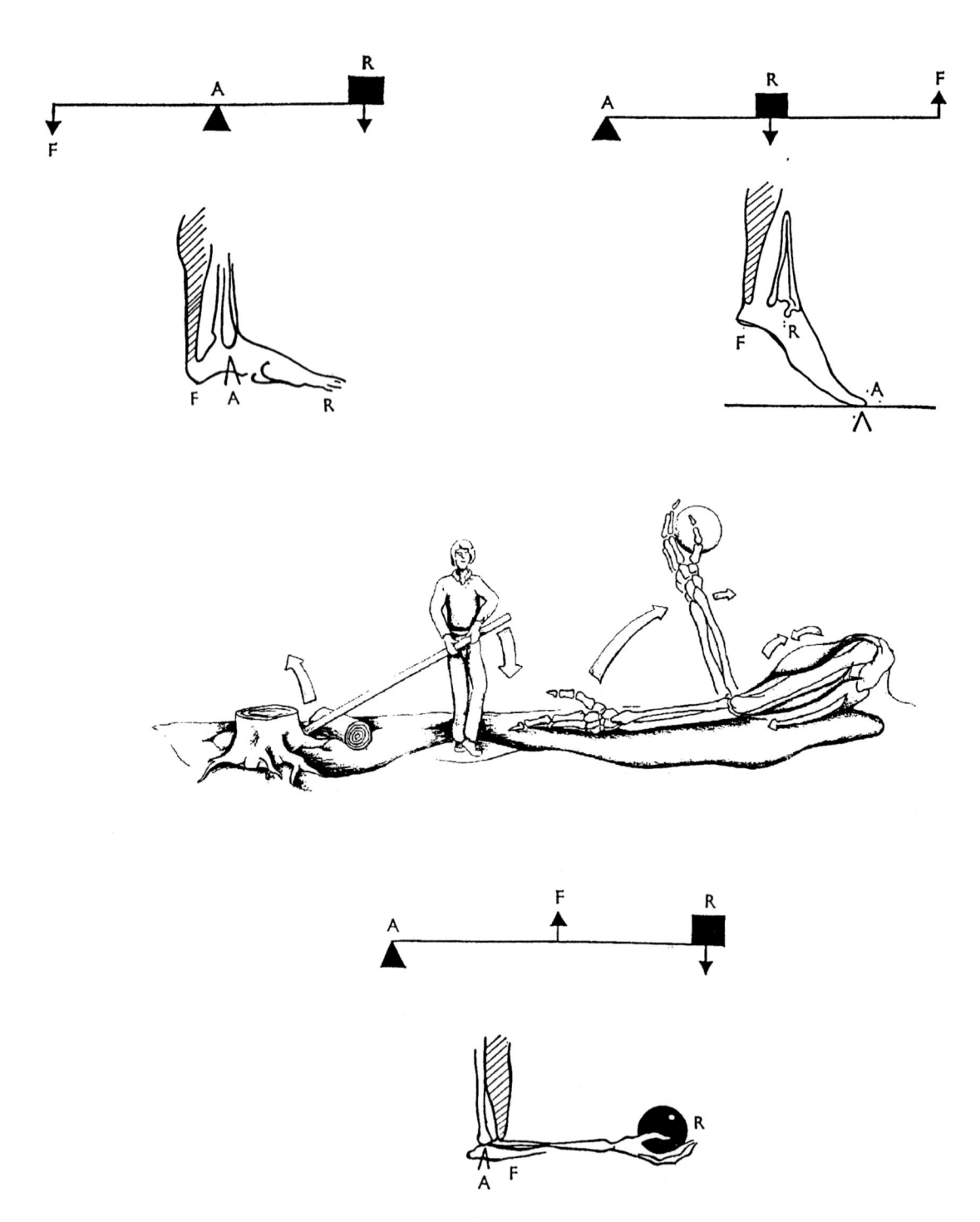

286 / Scientific Foundations of Sports Medicine

Figure 12-5 Levers: F = applied force, R = resistance, A = fulcrum.

ponents of mechanics, it is also essential to understand the other laws of motion. Newton neatly encapsulated these laws into three principles. The first states that an object remains at rest until some force acts upon it. If the object is already in motion, it continues at a constant speed unless some outside force is brought to bear. In other words, until the levers of foot and leg are applied to a soccer ball, it remains at rest on the ground. However, once it is kicked, the ball continues to roll at a constant rate until it is acted on by the outside force of friction from ground or air, or by contact from another system of levers in the form of an opposing soccer player.

When two or more forces act on an object, the subsequent force is known by physicists as the resultant force. If player A kicks a soccer ball due north simultaneously with player B's kick of the same ball due west, the ball will travel northwest along a path determined by which athlete delivered the most force. The route taken by the ball and its velocity are the resultant force supplied by players A and B.

Newton declared that the main task of mechanics was to learn about forces from observed motions. The physics behind movement is related to the law of momentum, which is part of Newton's second law. Momentum is a concept that consists of velocity multiplied by the mass of the moving object. *Momentum,* in terms of physics, is distinguished from force, which is defined as mass multiplied by acceleration, or the rate of change in velocity. Alteration of momentum, or a change in motion, declared Newton, is governed by the force brought to bear upon the object, which then follows the straight line in which the force acts.

Consider the problem of a man leaping over a small puddle. He runs toward the puddle, creating many forces including horizontal ones. As he nears the water, the central nervous system, the movement coordinator, orders the muscles of the feet and legs to contract, generating a vertical force for the jump. The height depends on the man's ability to generate enough force to exceed gravitational force temporarily. If the man weighs 150 pounds and produces only 140 pounds of vertical force, he will have wet feet. Once airborne, he can no longer add any force to the jump. The force of momentum, the velocity at take-off multiplied by the man's weight, must be enough to overcome the demands of gravity in order to jump over, not into, the puddle. The vertical force combines with the horizontal force for the leap. That is to say, the body does not travel in either a purely vertical direction or a solely horizontal one. Rather the path becomes a combination of horizontal and vertical forces, a direction that physicists call a *resultant.*

Newton's third law is that for every force that acts upon an object, the object itself exerts an equal and opposite amount of force. When you kick a ball with your bare foot, the painful sensation in your big toe confirms Sir Isaac's third law. The recoil of a fired rifle is also an example of equal and opposite reactions. A car striking a bridge abutment at 60 miles per hour is demolished, while one that nudges the wall at 5 miles per hour remains intact. The wreck is an example of a much greater degree of equal and opposite force.

Another principle affecting the body is derived partly from theories of Einstein. An old bedroom farce joke uses the punch line, "Everybody's got to be someplace," and Albert Einstein said that energy can be neither created nor destroyed. In other words, energy or a visible manifestation of it in the form of force also always must "be someplace."

This means that when one generates a force by swiveling the back and then suddenly tries to stop the movement of the back, the force developed in the trunk of the body does not simply disappear. It must go someplace. The secret to efficient use of a body for work or sport, for fitness or injury prevention, depends to a great extent on where these forces go or how well they are exploited.

In the human body, the bones, or levers, move in a rotational manner. These angular movements create linear movement for the total body. The same laws that govern linear motion also govern angular motion. The only difference is that the length of the lever also plays an important part. If the body begins a rotation, it continues to turn on its axis until the movement is altered either by a change in body position or by the application of some other force. Imagine that the ice skater mentioned above begins a spin with the arms abducted or outstretched, building up angular momentum by the maneuver. If this athlete suddenly drops the arms to the side, the velocity of the spin increases, because the momentum that was ini-

body and its segments without reference to the forces that cause the motion, and *kinetics,* which describes the forces that cause the movement. The kinematic parameters include linear and angular displacement, velocity, and acceleration. The kinetic parameters include the external and internal forces that act on the body segments.

In order to measure the kinematic and kinetic parameters, it is necessary to make a few assumptions. If it were possible to disassemble and reassemble the human body like other machines, measurements could be taken more accurately. However, this is obviously impossible. Therefore, some of the measurements are derived from cadavers, and additional assumptions are made based upon the linkages of the human body. This is not different from any other field involved with living bodies. In the field of physiology, for example, many assumptions are made about the ability of the body to consume oxygen. In the conversion of energy measurements from external measurements to internal measurements, many reasonable assumptions are made. In determining the composition of different muscles and their classification into fast and slow twitch muscles, many assumptions are made about the chemical staining methods and the counting methods. Of course all statistical methods, which are the basis for most behavioral research, utilize assumptions about the normality of the populations and the distribution of the data samples.

Therefore, to view the human as a machine made of links is an oversimplification, but it is possible to create a representation of the body in a humanoid model made of rigid segments. This model facilitates quantitative analysis of movement. The links that represent the body's limbs are a series of interconnected rigid segments that demonstrate independent motion.

This system can be applied more accurately if we realize that there are different body types. It is clear that body differences in shape occur between ages and sexes, and within individuals. The field which deals with the measurement of size, weight, and proportions of the human body is anthropometry.[23]

Anthropometric data are fundamental to biomechanics, because some of the assumptions made in the calculation of movement parameters are based on them. When a scientist performs a biomechanical analysis of any movement, the human body is considered to be a system of mechanical links, with each link of known physical size and shape according to anthropometric measurement (Fig. 12–7).

After adapting the anthropometric measurements to the different body segments, the next assumption is that this link system is connected at identifiable joints. Because the body landmarks or the body segments are covered by muscle, fat, and skin, it is sometimes difficult to identify joints such as the hips and shoulders. However, with the aid of statistical and numerical methods, some of the errors can be filtered out.

Some of the pioneers in the field of anthropometry are Braune and Fischer, Dempster, and Snyder, Chaffin, and Schulz.[24–26] They have made tremendous contributions by dissecting cadavers and measuring the location of joint centers. Using cinematographic techniques, it is possible to trace the intersections of the long axes of the segments during movement. Some of the landmarks used in the field of biomechanics are illustrated in Figures 12–7 and 12–8.

In addition to landmarks required for biomechanical tracing, it is important to predict

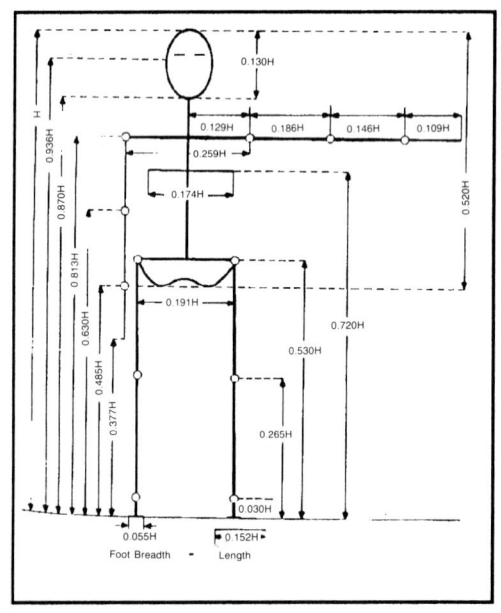

Figure 12–7 Anthropometric measurements of the human body.

the segment mass and location of the center of the mass (see Fig. 12–8). The National Aeronautics and Space Administration has made detailed measurements of human body composition and the relative mass for segments such as arms, legs, and hands, given the overall height and weight of the individual. The specifications may not be exactly accurate for each individual, but they are close enough to humans in general for the purposes of even the most exacting scientists. Body segment mass and volume are related to the density of the segment. Density can be determined by immersing cadaver body segments in water and measuring the volume of water displaced. The equation used is $D = M/v$, where D equals average density, M equals the mass of the segment, and v equals the volume of water displaced. The values thus obtained for the different body segments are available in various biomechanics textbooks.

In addition to the segment mass and volume, the distribution of the mass within the segment is necessary in order to compute the kinetic information. From this distribution of the mass, it is possible to calculate the mass center or the center of gravity of the segment. There are a few methods to calculate the segment center of gravity. One method determines the distribution of forces when a person is suspended between two force platforms by calculating the change in vertical forces created by moving various segments to different angles. Another method involves submersion of the segment in water. Regardless of the method used, a sufficient data base exists from various investigations that have calculated the center of mass for different segments and for different populations, so that these parameters need not be recalculated for each analysis.

Knowledge of the center of gravity of each segment and its weight and length allows the calculation of the static force and torque at each body joint for a given posture as described in the mechanics section of this chapter. However, in athletic performances and in normal human life, we are seldom concerned with static posture. More realistic are the dynamic performances in which the forces caused by motion plus the forces caused by gravity act upon the body.

For these dynamic analyses of the human body, it is necessary to know the inertial property of the segment. This property is referred to

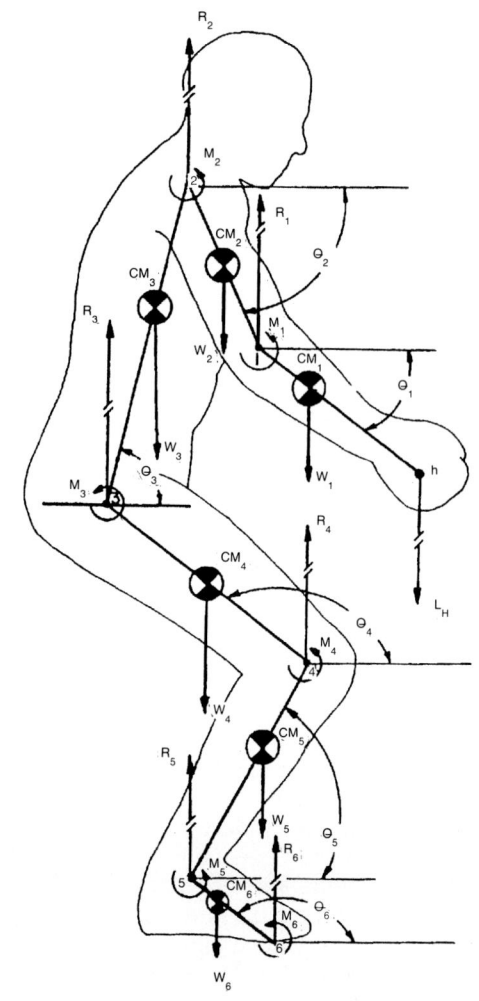

Figure 12–8 Coplanar link system: R = reaction force, M = moment, CM = center of mass, W = weight.

as the *moment of inertia*. The formula that describes the moment of inertia follows:

$$I = M \times R \times R$$

That is, the moment of inertia of the segment is equal to the mass of the segment times the square of the perpendicular distance from a given axis. There are different methods for calculating the moment of inertia of the individual body segments. These are described in various biomechanics textbooks.

It is also important to calculate the place on the body segment at which the moment of inertia affects the segment. This point can be derived by knowing the *radius of gyration*. The radius of gyration is equal to the square root of the moment of inertia divided by the mass of the segment.

According to Drillis and Contini, the radius of gyration is "the distance from the axis of rotation to an assumed point where the concentrated total mass of the body would have the same moment of inertia as it does in its original distributed state."[27] This information is necessary to quantify the dynamics of human motion in conjunction with other parameters.

It should be remembered that all of these estimated parameters are used in calculating the dynamic forces rather than merely in describing movement in qualitative terms. These parameters are available in numerous sources, and the normal analysis of human movement does not require the individual calculation of all of these parameters. The information resides in tables and charts that can be accessed at will. The normal analysis of movement relies on this information, in the same way that physiologists depend on the tables presenting characteristics of different gases and their coefficients at various temperatures and pressures.

Quantification of an action, whether to evaluate it or to attempt to improve it, can be accomplished through biomechanical analysis. Biomechanical assessments normally begin with quantification of the kinematic portion. This is usually accomplished by utilizing high-speed cinematography or videography, which allows careful scrutiny of even the fastest movements of humans or animals. The films or videos are traced, and the resulting data are stored in a computer that calculates the results by applying the principles of physics and mechanical engineering. Tables and graphs can then be generated, giving a precise profile of what actually occurred during the execution of the movement. The researcher then carefully examines this output in order to understanding the motion and, in the case of an athlete, to determine which patterns are most important in distinguishing championship from average performances.

Biomechanics is a science still in its adolescence with many discoveries yet to be made. Hand analysis of high-speed films is a slow and tedious process, and it is only recently that the computer has been harnessed to make the process more efficient. Development of this technology in the United States has meant that many complex analyses can now be executed in a relatively short time.

In the past, athletic achievement depended mainly on the individual's talent, although skill was often enhanced or ruined by existing facilities, equipment, and, undeniably, coaches. Athletes with superior genetic compositions who successfully interacted with the available facilities dominated the list of world records. Continual improvement of equipment and techniques has complemented raw talent.

However, with the advent of new measurement tools and knowledge in the field of sport science, athletic achievement has attained a new dimension. The athletic teams of the United States, which for years dominated amateur sports, are no longer the leaders. Countries such as those of Eastern Europe and Cuba, which have relatively small populations, have achieved a spectacular level of success in athletic events. Current evidence suggests this trend may continue through the remainder of the 1980s and 1990s. Such domination stems from the application of science to the realm of athletic performance.

Modern coaches can use biomechanical means to optimize the human body in each event. Because the human body obeys the same physical laws as all other earthly objects, the laws of motion govern its performance. In order to throw, run, or jump, physical laws must be obeyed. It is impossible to throw the shot 20 meters if the shot velocity and angle of release do not attain certain values. These values do not differ for different athletes, because for each particular shot velocity, there is one specific optimal angle.

For the jumper to leap 8 meters, it is necessary to produce certain forces on the ground to propel the body with a specific reaction force at a particular angle. This force is unique, and it is impossible to cover the same distance with only a fraction of the force because gravitational pull acts uniformly regardless of the jumper.

The concept to be reemphasized here is that all bodies, athletes, implements, or machines are affected by and must adhere to the laws of motion. The science of biomechanics deals specifically with motion of the body and the resultant forces. A number of scientists have long recognized these facts of force and motion and their relationship to humans, but the kind of equipment that could measure and analyze the motion and forces involved was lacking. Thus, further research was impeded.

Without a computer to store information, retrieve it, and perform the myriad computations, such calculations can place the scientist in an impossible position. But before a computer can perform its job, whether it is to guide a robot, print a check, or retrieve a space vehicle, it needs a program, a sequence of instructions that tell it how and what to do.

Programming a computer involves hundreds and, at times, thousands of hours of work. But once the instructions have been fed into the computer, it can automatically execute the hundreds of steps without any need for further instructions, and the execution may only take a few seconds. The beauty of a computer is that it can play the great game of "what if?" In sports, one could ask, "What if I hold the shot down here and then whirl in this fashion?" The computer can calculate the distance the shot would travel, applying the amount of force developed in previous analysis. Through use of the computer, then, biomechanics can write equations and construct models to obtain optimal performances.

Another critical element is the camera, either a high-speed movie or sufficiently fast video system. It provides sequences of the body in motion. Knowing the speed with which film or video tape travels through the camera allows calculation of the velocity and acceleration of body segments using the joints as points of reference. For example, if the shutter speed on the camera is 200 frames per second, one can identify the location of the right knee at the start of a sprint, compare the position of the right knee in frame 20 of the film, and learn how far the right knee has moved in one-tenth of a second. The data can be further utilized to determine velocity, acceleration, and, with some additional information, even the forces involved. The forces can be calculated by measuring the length of the leg, for example from knee to ankle, and, by using the NASA specifications, determining the mass of that segment and the center of gravity. Using these values, quite reasonable estimates of the exact forces and torques around the joint center can be calculated (Fig. 12-9).

Along with analyses based on films taken during actual events, highly sensitive force plates have been developed for precise impact measurements. These allow controlled laboratory testing of forces, such as when an object like the human foot strikes the plate during a sprint, or when a monkey leaps from the plate onto a table. The plate is capable of recording three different components of forces—vertical, horizontal, and sideways or lateral—as well as the moment or torque.

Any kind of athletic movement or work action that can be photographed with a high-speed motion picture or video camera can be fed into the computer. Forces can be plotted for each segment of the body as the accelerations and lengths of the segments are measured. The maximum amount of force that can be generated using a particular approach in an activity can be calculated.[28] For instance, it is feasible to calculate how high a jumper might go if he changed from his customary form of the roll to the flop style, assuming he was able to generate the amount of force for the flop as he did for the roll. Analyses have shown that the flop happens to be a more efficient use of forces for athletes who do not possess extremely powerful legs.

It is important to remember that because of both gross and subtle variations in the neuromuscular system of each human, the biomechanical actions of individuals are as unique as their fingerprints. The shades of difference from one person to another are, in fact, great enough to permit the development of a foolproof method for guaranteeing a signature. A person could file his or her signature in a computer bank. The information in the computer would contain not only the shapes of the letters, but the amount of force the individual applied to every loop, line, and curve. With this device, a buyer in a store need only sign the chit on a force plate or use a pen with a force-sensitive transducer that transmitted the information directly to the computer. The patterns of force would be compared instantly and, if not the same, the new one would be rejected.

Similarly, detection of variations or errors in human movement has always been one of the most difficult problems facing coaches,

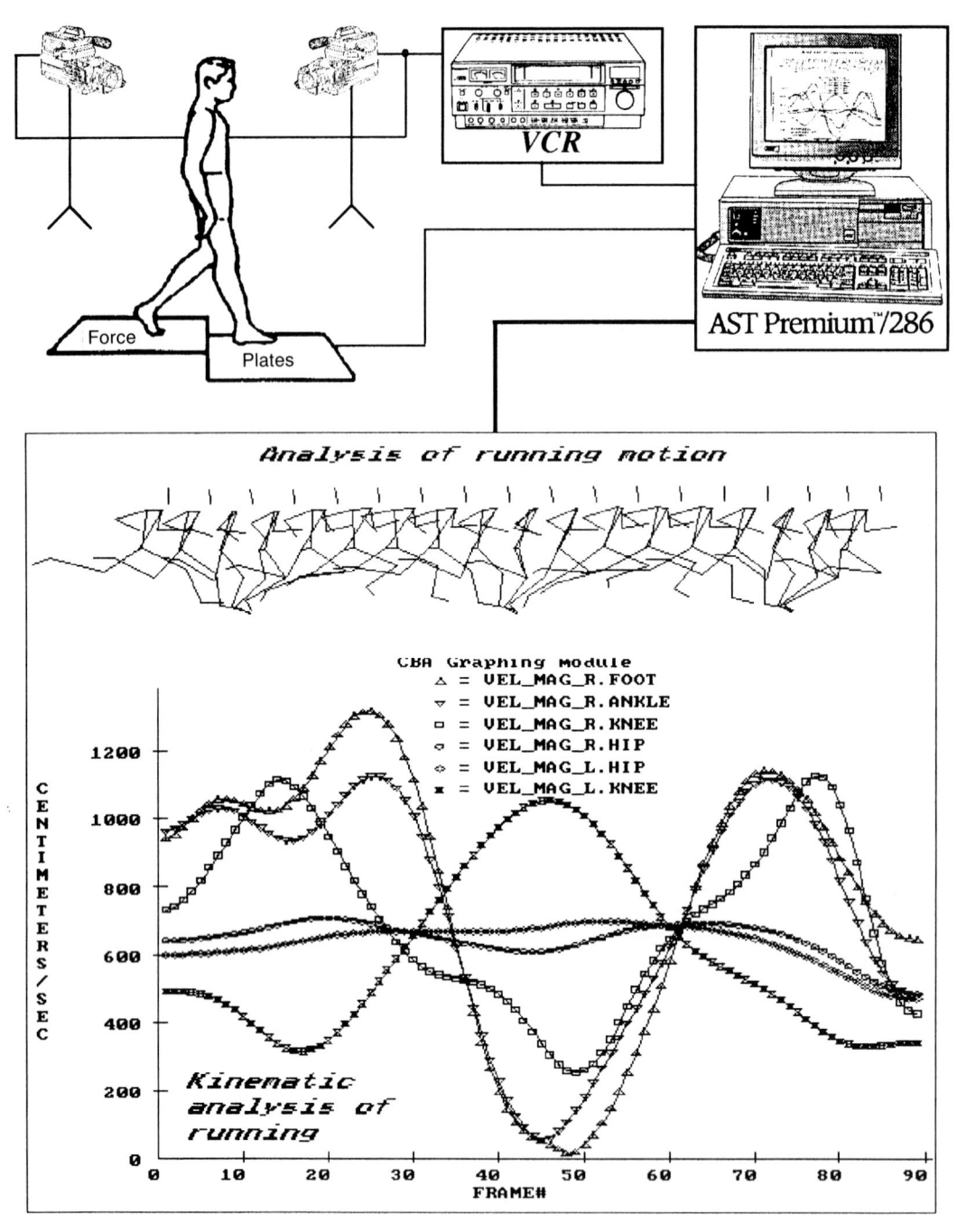

Figure 12-9 Computed performance analysis.

trainers, and physicians in athletic situations. If the error detection is inaccurate or nonspecific, the quality of correction is poor. Failure to recognize the causes of error stems from an inadequate understanding of the mechanisms of human motion. Impact in sports, automobile accidents, falls, and other movements involving forces can be acccurately quantified through biomechanical applications.

The designer of protective equipment for sports such as hockey and football must have an understanding of biomechanics, because it is necessary to comprehend before the equipment is designed how the human head reacts to impact forces or how a skier's leg reacts to twisting forces. The forces produced by the human body cause a change in acceleration or speed. The change might involve the entire body, as in sprint starting, skating, or volleyball (in a vertical jump to block). It may also be a body segment or combination of segments, as with a boxer's upper arm and forearm, a golfer's arms, or a soccer player's thighs and lower legs. Through use of biomechanical analysis, it is now possible to detect errors scientifically that are beyond the visual capabilities of the human eye.

To enhance the understanding of biomechanics, we should now consider a few physical terms that refer to muscular activity. When a muscle contracts, it produces *force*. This force moves the limb and may move an external object to perform *work*. This work is executed in a certain time to produce *power*.

A muscle may contract in various ways. If the movement involved is of a constant speed, the movement and the contraction are called *isokinetic*. When muscular force development results in no change in length for the muscles and in no skeletal movement, the contraction is termed *isometric*. If the force generated by the muscles results in a shortening contraction, the contraction is called *concentric*. If the force generated by the muscles results in an elongation of the muscle, the contraction is called *eccentric*.

When the muscle contracts and there is a change in limb position, work is performed. When time is required to perform the physical work, then units of power measurement are employed, because the rate of work is power. In human performance, striving for excellence on the athletic field or in recreation, it is important to be able to sum the forces exerted on the various joints. This principle is called the *summation of joint forces.*

For example, in swinging the golf club in the drive, the amount of force exerted by the club on the golf ball depends on how much of the total force exerted by the body actually reaches the club. If there is any loss of force due to bad timing, the golf club head will not move at the same velocity. Any violation of the principle of summation of joint forces can result in too small a force being exerted by the golf club.

Another important biomechanical principle is that of continuity of joint forces. This is illustrated by the fact that the golfer not only must use all body joints efficiently, but also must time their use so that the motion begins at the larger segment (such as the thigh) and then continues and is overlapped by motion of the hip and trunk. There must be no pauses in the flow of motion from the legs to the trunk and to the club. It must be continuous. A violation of this principle results not only in too small a force but also in bad timing and a poor "feel" on the golf club.

Because club speed is determined by the force applied and the length of time of force application, the best combination of force application should be determined—a large force in a short time or a small force for a longer time.

There is an optimal combination for each activity. The size of the force multiplied by its time of application is called "impulse" and it is actually this force–time combination that produces the golf club velocity. Therefore, the impulse in any activity should be determined to result in optimum efficiency. Although compromises in the size of force and duration of application often have to be made in sports to achieve an optimal combination, one such combination to be avoided is a small force applied for a short time.

The size of the force an athlete can produce is determined by his or her ability to comply with the principles of summation and continuity of joint forces. In the absence of measuring devices, assessing whether the force application time is as great as possible presents yet another problem. In general, if each joint has gone through a complete range of motion, one can be assured that the maximum time available has been used.

It was previously pointed out that not only must the range of motion of the joint be complete, but the joint must straighten fast and the combined joint motion must be continuous. The concept of the combined effect of force and duration of application in producing speed changes is called the *principle of impulse*. Violation of this principle causes further errors in performance.

Direction of force application is another important principle. The direction of the application of force to the golf club is vital, but, so is the direction from the club head to the golf ball. In an optimal situation, the force is exactly 90 degrees to the club, and the club head hits the ball exactly at its center. However, some deviation is at times necessary if the flight of the ball has to be changed in a predetermined pattern. Incorrect direction of force can be disastrous in events such as gymnastics and diving. A good technique implies that the principle of direction of force has been followed.

A final principle is the *summation of body segment speeds*. Especially in any throwing, kicking, and striking events, it is important to obtain as high a hand, foot, stick blade, racket head, or club head speed as possible at the instant of impact or release. The speed of the last segment in the chain is built by adding the individual speeds of all the preceding segments with appropriate timing. If any of the segments contributes low or negative values, the resultant measured for the last segment is less than optimum. This principle is similar to summation of joint forces and is closely related to it.

In summary, any motion should obey the principles of summation of joint forces, continuity of joint forces, impulse, and the direction of joint forces. Through the use of biomechanics, all of these principles can be quantified and optimized so that better and safer results can be obtained.

REFERENCES

1. Plantanida S, Baroni C, eds. Leonardo da Vinci New York: Reynal and Company, 1956.
2. Granit R. The basis of motor control. New York: Academic Press, 1970.
3. Crosby EC, Humphrey T, Lauer EW. Correlative anatomy of the nervous system. New York: Macmillan, 1962.
4. Guyton AC. Textbook of medical physiology. 3rd ed. Philadelphia: WB Saunders, 1966.
5. Travell JG, Simons, DG. Myofascial pain and dysfunction. Baltimore: Williams & Wilkins, 1983.
6. Arbib MA. The metaphorical brain. New York: Wiley-Interscience, 1972.
7. Granit R. Demand and accomplishment in voluntary movements. In: Stein RB, Pearson KG, Smith RS, Redford JB, eds. Control of posture and locomotion. New York: Plenum Press, 1973:3.
8. Stein RB, Milner-Brown HS. Contractile and electrical properties of normal and modified human motor units. In: Stein RB, Pearson KG, Smith RS, Redford JB, eds. Control of posture and locomotion. New York: Plenum Press, 1973:73.
9. Bizzi E. Coordination of movements. In: Herman R, Grillner S, Stein RB, Stuart, eds. Neural control of locomotion. New York: Plenum Press, 1976:798.
10. Davis J. Central activation of movements. In: Herman R, Grillner S, Stein RB, Stuart, eds. Neural control of locomotion. New York: Plenum Press, 1976:804.
11. Eberhart HD. Physical principles of locomotion. In: Herman R, Grillner S, Stein RB, Stuart, eds. Neural control of locomotion. New York: Plenum Press, 1976:1.
12. Herman R, Wirta R, Bampton S, Finley FR. Human solutions for locomotion: single limb analysis. In: Herman R, Grillner S, Stein RB, Stuarts eds. Neural Control of locomotion. New York: Plenum Press, 1976:13.
13. Craik R, Herman R, Finley FR. Human solutions for locomotion: interlimb coordination. In: Herman R, Grillner S, Stein RB, Stuart, eds. Neural control of locomotion. New York: Plenum Press, 1976:51.
14. Meriam JL. Statics. New York: John Wiley & Sons, 1966.
15. Meriam JL. Dynamics. New York: John Wiley & Sons, 1966.
16. Sherrington CS. The integrative action of the nervous system. New Haven: Yale University Press, 1906.
17. Grillner S. Some aspects of the descending control of the spinal circuits generating locomotor movements. In: Herman R, Grillner S, Stein RB, Stuart, eds. Neural control of locomotion. New York: Plenum Press, 1976:351.
18. Arshavsky YI, Kots YM, Orlovsky GN, et al. Investigation of the biomechanics of running by the dog. Biophysics 1965; 10:737–746.
19. Severin FV, Orlovsky GN, Shik ML. Work of the muscle receptors during controlled locomotion. Biofizika 1967; 12:575–586.
20. Basmajian JV. Muscles alive. Baltimore: Williams & Wilkins, 1978.
21. Asimov I. Understanding physics: motion, sound, and heat. New York: New American Library, 1966.
22. Shames IH. Engineering mechanics—statics and dynamics. 2nd ed. Englewood Cliffs, NJ: Prentice Hall, 1967.
23. Chaffin DB, Andersson GBJ. Occupational biomechanics. New York: John Wiley & Sons, 1984.
24. Braune W, Fischer O. The center of gravity of the human body as related to the German infantryman. Cited in: Chaffin DB, Andersson GB. Occupational biomechanics. New York: John Wiley & Sons, 1984.
25. Dempster WT. Space requirements of the seated operator. WADC-TR-55-159, Ohio: Aerospace Medical Research Laboratories, 1955.

26. Snyder RG, Chaffin DB, Schulz RK. Link system of the human torso. HSRI Report 71-112, Highway Safety Research Institute, University of Michigan, Ann Arbor, MI and AMRL-RT-71-88, Ohio: Aerospace Medical Research Laboratories, 1972.
27. Drillis R, Contini R. Body segment parameters. BP174-945, Tech. Rep. No. 1166.03, New York: School of Engineering and Science, New York University, 1966.
28. Ariel G. Computerized biomechanical analysis of human performance. Mechanics and Sport. 1973; 4:267–275.

Chapter 13
Overuse Injuries

CAROL C. TEITZ

Overuse injuries, by definition, are injuries that occur from trying to do too much too quickly, i.e., from being poorly conditioned. They imply that the musculoskeletal tissues involved may not be strong enough, warm enough, or, in the case of soft tissues, flexible enough to withstand the stresses imposed. Generally the tissues of the musculoskeletal system are capable of adapting to loads, if these loads are gradually increased. Traumatic injuries usually occur when loads beyond the ultimate load-bearing capacity of the tissues are applied suddenly. Overuse injuries, in contrast, are caused by relatively low loads, which are applied so frequently that normal adaptive processes cannot occur. Overuse injuries in sports are probable, for example, when the casual runner decides to attempt a marathon and increases her training markedly 1 month prior to the marathon. Similarly, someone who ordinarily plays tennis 1$\frac{1}{2}$ hours twice per week and then goes to tennis camp, where he practices tennis skills and plays 6 to 8 hours per day, is likely to suffer an overuse injury. In addition, a rather sedentary person who begins an athletic activity in a sudden desire to become instantly fit is likely to suffer an overuse injury unless he or she introduces the new physical activity gradually.

Causes of Overuse Injury

Recognized causes of overuse injury include poor training, technique, anatomical alignment, equipment, and environment. Poor training is probably the most common cause of overuse injuries. Training considerations include frequency of athletic participation, intensity of participation, and duration of each burst of activity. Obviously, the more intense the activity, the shorter the duration needs to be to stress the musculoskeletal system. High-intensity activity produces the type of loads seen in traumatic injuries. Duration of activity is limited by the vascular supply to the involved tissues. Previous conditioning affects the utilization of glucose and glycogen by these tissues. Frequency of participation is often the critical factor producing an overuse injury.

Many have had the experience of having sore muscles 48 hours after undertaking more activity than usual. The muscle ache is a sign that the metabolic and load-bearing capacities of the involved muscles have been exceeded.[1] By 72 hours, recovery generally occurs, and return to activity is possible. Trying to return to the same activity within the first 48 hours, often prior to the appearance of clinical symptoms of overuse, is likely to potentiate the inflammatory response to the initial stress and thereby produce a clinically significant overuse injury. A training-related overuse injury is likely in a runner who decides to increase his or her frequency of training from 3 miles three times per week to alternate days of running 3 miles and 2 miles. In the process, the total mileage to which the limbs are exposed goes from 9 miles to 17 miles per week, almost a 100 percent increase. The frequency of training simultaneously increases, not allowing the musculoskeletal tissues time to recover from the stresses to which they are exposed. Similar examples include a runner who increases the speed at which he runs, or one who continues to run 3 days per week but increases the mileage from 3 miles to 5 miles per run, again almost doubling the weekly mileage.

Technique is often a factor in overuse injuries as well. Although there are "natural" athletes, one of the important aspects of coaching is that of developing efficient technique. In the recreational athlete in particular or the athlete or dancer who has been poorly coached and trained, various musculotendinous units can be used unnecessarily and inefficiently, thereby suffering greater stress. A dancer, for example, who uses the rectus femoris muscle to raise her leg to the front, is using a muscle that does not have much mechanical advantage across the hip joint. She will ultimately develop rectus femoris tendinitis. In contrast, if she can be taught to use her iliopsoas muscle, a much stronger hip flexor, she can achieve this particular movement much more efficiently. The movement will be less likely to produce tendinitis and will be aesthetically more desirable because there will not be an obvious contraction of the thigh muscle. In addition, a dancer can often raise the leg higher using the iliopsoas, because the rectus femoris tendon at the hip joint is more relaxed and therefore can fold into the groin crease without blocking the ability to fold the leg up onto the torso.

Variations in anatomical alignment also can produce abnormal biomechanical stresses on the musculoskeletal system, overstressing certain parts of the body that otherwise might not be loaded. A common example is the athlete with flat feet who engages in an impact-loading activity of the lower extremities such as running or aerobic dancing. Every time contact is made between the foot and the impacting surface, the foot flattens and the posterior tibial tendon is drawn around the ankle posterior to the medial malleolus and stretched around the medial aspect of the foot prior to inserting into the navicular bone. Because of this constant stretching of the posterior tibial tendon from either static or dynamic pronation of the foot, more strain is put on the tendon than is necessary or desirable. The strains, in turn, are more likely to produce microtears in the tendon.

Equipment often plays a role in overuse injuries. In general, equipment is designed to enable the athlete to function more efficiently and often with more power. For example, if a tennis racket is made of nonshock-absorbent material, is strung very tightly, or does not fit the player's hand properly, more shock from the contact of the racket and the ball is transferred to the tennis player's arm. The absorption of this shock by the musculotendinous tissues in the upper extremity leads to overuse injuries, usually tendinitis.

The environment in which an athlete practices or performs also may contribute to overuse injuries in a number of ways. (See chap. 1.) The first is shock absorption. Most runners know that running on asphalt is more likely to lead to lower extremity injuries than is running on soft dirt or a composite surface. Dancers and gymnasts like to perform on sprung wood floors, which also are very shock absorbent. Second, the grade of the terrain on which one exercises is also important, in that if one leg is functionally longer than the other, the soft tissue structures on the outer side of that limb are likely to be stretched more. Third, particularly cold or hot environments may influence the metabolic rates and vascular supply of the soft tissues thereby limiting their ability to work efficiently for any length of time.

The most common overuse injuries include tendinitis, stress fractures, and chronic compartmental syndromes. These particular overuse injuries are discussed below from a basic science perspective. In each case, the normal physiology is reviewed, followed by the pathophysiology and some highlights of the clinical presentation. Finally, principles for treating these injuries are described.

TENDON

Normal Physiology

Function

Tendon functions to transmit force from muscle to bone and is therefore subject to great tensile stresses. In order to carry out this function successfully, tendon must be capable of deforming and returning to its original shape; accepting loads of various magnitude, direction, and speed; and responding to changes induced by exercise, aging, and hormonal changes (e.g., pregnancy). In fact, tendons are remarkable structures that do have all of the characteristics mentioned above. These are due to the biochemical constituents and the macrostructure and microstructure of tendon.

Structure

Tendon is made up of dense, regularly arranged collagen fibrils. Most of the collagen in tendon is genetic type I, although lesser amounts of types III and V are present. Collagen is a protein of unique conformation made by fibroblasts. The molecule consists of three polypeptide chains wound together to form a ropelike triple helix. In the polypeptide chain, glycine occurs at every third residue, and proline is common at the other two positions of a repeating tripeptide pattern. Within the fibroblast, about half of the proline residues and some lysines are hydroxylated (mediated by enzymes that require iron and vitamin C as cofactors) just before the chains twist into a triple helix to form the procollagen molecule. At both ends of the procollagen are nonhelical peptides (domains). After procollagen is extruded from the fibroblast, these extra domains are enzymatically cleaved to form the collagen molecule sometimes called tropocollagen.[2] These collagen molecules pack together in a head-to-tail overlapping array ("quarter stagger") to form collagen fibrils (Fig. 13-1). Intermolecular cross-linking between specific amino acids on adjacent chains is essential for aggregation at the fibril level and provides the strength necessary for collagen to be a structural protein that functions under mechanical loads. Adjacent molecules within fibrils are staggered by 0, 1, 2, 3, or 4 times 670 angstroms, which creates the cross-striated appearance seen in electron micrographs of collagen. Gellike ground substance decreases friction between fibrils and fibril bundles (fibers). Finally, fibers are organized into fascicles, which are wavy when they are not under tension. Endotenon binds fascicles of collagen within tendon and permits longitudinal movement of bundles while supporting blood vessels, lymphatics, and nerves. A group of fascicles surrounded by *epitenon* makes up a tendon. The epitenon continues within the attached muscle as the *epimysium*.

Tendons that move in a straight line are surrounded by *paratenon*, a loose areolar tissue containing blood vessels that are coiled and can stretch along with the tendon fibers. Tendons that go around corners are enclosed by a tendon sheath that is a bifoliate mesotenon. An example of this type of tendon is the tibialis posterior tendon, which travels around the corner posterior to the medial malleolus and is subject to excessive strain when the hindfoot pronates. Gliding is assisted by synovial fluid produced by both the parietal and the visceral synovial membranes of the epitenon. At the bone tendon interface, the tendon fibers become incorporated into a fibrocartilage that is relatively avascular and that decreases the stress riser of going from a soft tissue to a hard tissue.

Vasculature of tendon is variable. Blood supply originates at both the musculotendinous and bone-tendon junctions and comes from the perimysium, periosteum, and surrounding soft tissues by way of the paratenon and mesotenon. Vascular tendons are surrounded by paratenon and receive vessels all along their borders. Avascular tendons are in sheaths and receive vessels through vascularized conduits called vincula. The blood vessels within the tendon are fed by vessels in the epitenon that branch and enter the tendon radially through the endotenon. In the endotenon the vessels are aligned in the tendon's long axis. These arterioles are flanked by two venules. Capillaries loop from the arterioles to the venules but do not penetrate the collagen bundles. The paratenon also is largely responsible for blood supply to the middle third of the tendon. "Small branches from vessels in the paratenon run transversely toward the tendon and branch several times before assuming a course parallel to the tendon's long axis."[3] A number of longitudinal vessels can be seen traversing the musculotendinous junction, but they are found only in the perimysium. The capillary circulations of muscle and tendon are separate. Tendon vasculature is compromised at sites of friction, torsion, or compression. Spontaneous degenerative rupture of the tibialis posterior and Achilles tendons is extremely common. Although the Achilles tendon does not actually have to go around a corner, its fibers twist during their

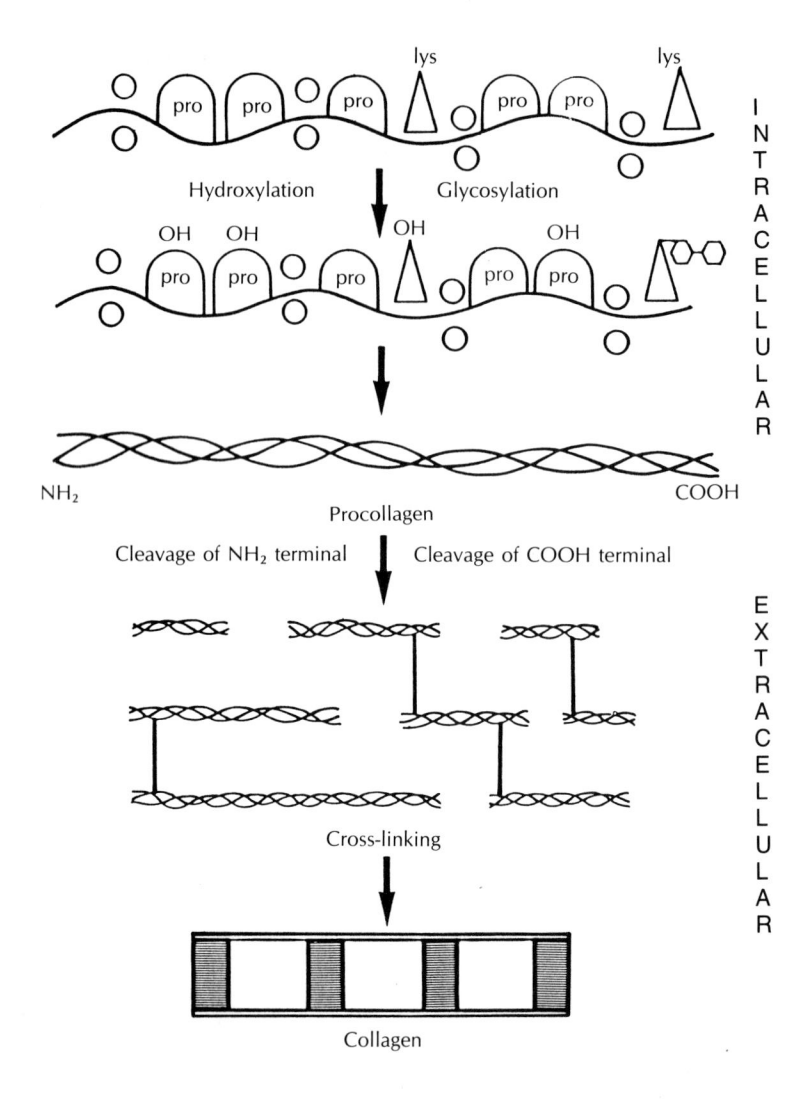

Figure 13–1 Production of collagen.

passage from the gastrocnemius and soleus muscles into the calcaneus, thus subjecting them to similar types of torsional strain. In addition, the Achilles tendon does not have a true tendon sheath, so it is slightly less vascular than other tendons and is more subject to degenerative tears.[4]

Proprioceptive information is obtained through nerve endings near the musculotendinous junction. In addition, Golgi tendon organs and lamellated corpuscles act as mechanical receptors in the tendon. The Golgi tendon organs respond to tension in the tendon by producing contraction and shortening of the tendon, whereas the lamellated corpuscles seem to respond to pressure transmitted by way of the surrounding tissue.[5]

In addition to collagen, which accounts for 30 percent of the wet weight of tendon, tendon contains 2 percent elastin, and 58 to 70 percent water. Whereas collagen is predominantly responsible for the structural integrity of tendon and for resisting deformation, elastin contributes to the "flexibility" of tendon. Although fibroblasts make elastin as well as collagen, chemically elastin does not contain much hydroxyproline or lysine and no hydroxylysine, in contrast to collagen. Thus, elastin does not form helices and is a hydrophobic molecule. Elastin can, under appropriate conditions, elongate up to 70 percent of length without rupture, as compared with collagen, which generally elongates only 4 percent of its original length prior to failure. Amorphous elastin fibers appear to elongate, rather than slipping on each other as do collagen fibrils.[6] In healing wounds, very little elastin is produced, resulting in rigid scar tissue. In summary, the behavior of soft tissues under load is a function of the structural orientation of the fibers, the properties of collagen and elastin, and the proportions of collagen and elastin.

Biomechanics

Collagen is responsible for resisting tensile force applied to tendon. "Because the collagen fibrils are crimped, the initial response to tensile force is straightening of the fibers so that these waves, or crimps, disappear. Greater loads stress the fibrils themselves."[3] The elongation of tendon fibers in response to load is shown in a stress–strain curve (Fig. 13–2). *Stress* is the force divided by the unit area, whereas *strain* is the change in length divided by the original length (Table 13–1). The stress–strain curve is thus independent of physical dimensions and tells us more about the elastic property of the material under study. In the toe region of the curve (see Fig. 13–2), the tissue elongates with only a small increase in load, because the wavy fibers are straightening and matrix may be shearing. In the second part of the curve, tissue deformation begins and responds linearly to load. In region three, some fibers begin to fail. In the fourth region, both tensile failure of fibers and shear failure between fibers occurs producing macroscopic tendon failure.[7] There is a large gap between the stresses that cause tendon failure and those that are experienced during physiologic loading. Tensile strength of tendon is estimated at 49 to 98 N per square meter.[8] Physiologic loading produces strain and is found in the safe zone of the stress–strain curve (less than 4 percent) representing straightening of the crimped collagen fibers. Elliott, and also Walker, Harris, and Benedict have suggested that tendon is probably never stressed to more than one-quarter of its ultimate tensile strength during normal activities.[8,9] On the other hand, force during kicking has been estimated by Wahrenberg, Lindbeck, and Ekholm at 5,200 N, larger than the values cited by Elliott.[10,11] Zernicke,

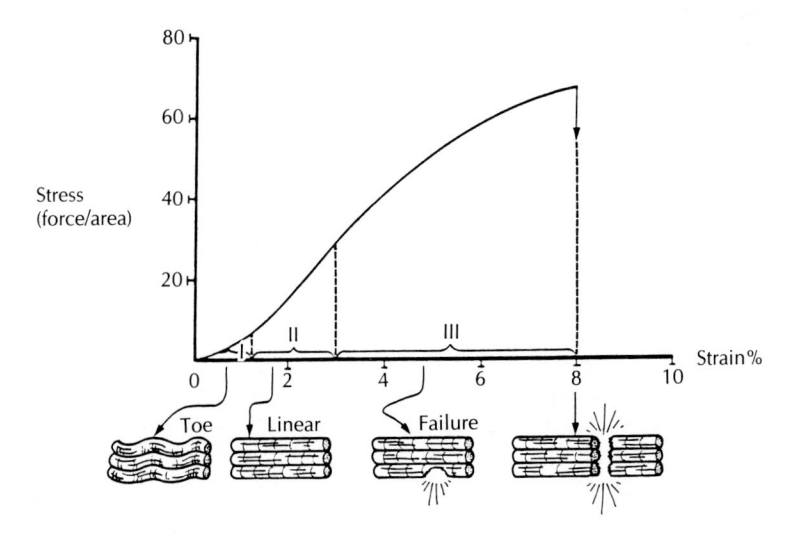

Figure 13–2 A stress-strain curve for tendon. (From Curwin S. Stanish WD. Tendinitis; its etiology and treatment. Lexington, DC Heath and Company, 1984. Reprinted with permission.)

TABLE 13–1 Terms

Term	Definition
Load	Any mechanical force applied to a structure from without. The load deforms or strains it, and the resistance of the structure's intermolecular bonds to that deformation represents its internal stress. A unit load constitutes the load-per-unit cross-sectional area of the structure material.
Modeling	The collection of bone surface motions in tissue space that determines a bone's architecture, including its shape and outside cortical diameters. The term has the same meaning as in sculpting or modeling with clay.
Remodeling	A quantized, package form of bone turnover in multicellular units, called BMU, that need not alter a bone's architecture.
Strain	Deformation of a structure by an externally applied load, which, for bones, can represent muscle forces, body weight, and accelerations of the body and its parts against the inertial force of its mass. It can be measured directly, e.g., by strain gauges of various types. *Unit strain* is the relative change in a unit length of the structure under load. Thus, a unit compression strain of 0.0008 is equivalent to a shortening of 0.08% and also to 800 microstrain.
Stress	The resistance of intermolecular bonds of matter to the deformation or strain induced by an applied load. It is usually inferred from measurements of strain and load.

(Adapted with permission from Frost HM. A determinant of bone architecture. Clin Orthop 1983; 175:286–292.)

Garhammer, and Jobe estimated patellar tendon tensile force as equal to approximately 17 times the body weight of a skilled weight lifter at the moment he ruptured his patellar tendon.[12] Unfortunately, tendons are usually tested in a laboratory as isolated specimens loaded in tension. This simplistic form of stress rarely occurs in athletics "where maximum effort is made, movement is uncertain or unexpected, or gravity or an opposing muscle stretches a contracting muscle."[13] According to Barfred, tendon is most vulnerable in six situations when: tension is applied quickly, tension is applied obliquely, the tendon is tense before the trauma, the attached muscle is maximally innervated, the muscle group is stretched by exterior stimuli, or the tendon is weak in comparison with the muscle.[14] Eccentric muscle contraction is associated with a higher incidence of tendinitis than is concentric contraction.[15] *Concentric contraction* occurs when the muscle shortens while producing tension. In an *eccentric contraction*, the muscle lengthens while producing force. Figure 13–3 shows that the force production during eccentric contraction appears to be greater than that during concentric exercise, thereby subjecting the tendon to larger loads.

The ability of tendon to deform without suffering structural damage is due in part to its viscoelastic properties. A viscoelastic material exhibits both solid and fluid properties, and its mechanical behavior is rate dependent. The rate at which forces are applied determines the amount of force that the tendon can withstand prior to rupture. Generally, tendon can withstand larger forces when these forces are applied rapidly. Viscoelasticity is also a feature in the rate of relaxation of tendon. "If a load is applied rapidly and maintained while the length is allowed to vary, the tissue lengthens with time."[3]

Both the range of motion of a musculotendinous unit and the force applied to the tendon are functions, in part, of the orientation of the muscle fibers relative to the axis of the tendon. The greater the longitudinal array of muscle fibers, the greater is the range of motion of the

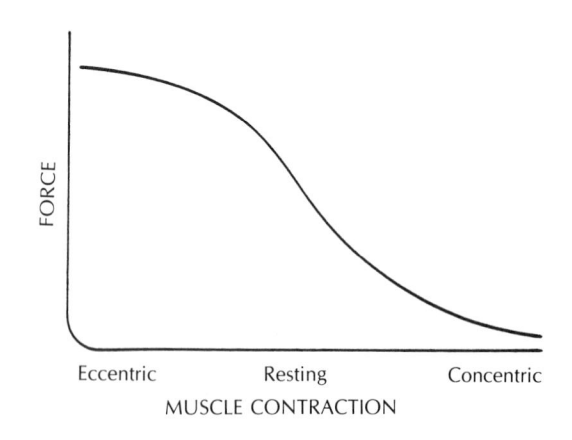

Figure 13–3 Forces produced during different types of muscle contraction.

muscle and tendon. A fusiform muscle also exerts greater tensile force on its tendon than does a pennate muscle, because all of the force in a fusiform muscle is applied in series with the longitudinal axis of the tendon. The greater the obliquity of the muscle fibers, the more force is dissipated laterally relative to the axis of the tendon. The greater the cross-sectional area of tendon, the greater the applied load it can withstand prior to deformation. Longer fibers also elongate more at the same load. Tendons that course around corners are subject not only to interference with vascularity, as mentioned above, but also are subject to greater than usual strain. This has been shown nicely in the supraspinatus tendon, in which studies of vascularity reveal that the area within 1 cm of the insertion, i.e., that part of the tendon tensed over the humeral head, is relatively avascular, particularly when the arm is hanging at the side.[16] In addition, where tendons wrap around articular surfaces, compressive forces may be experienced, in contrast to the usual tensile forces seen in tendon. These compressive forces can alter the histologic structure of tendon to make it more like cartilage.[17]

Metabolism

Tendon is metabolically active, although its rate of metabolism is relatively slow compared to that of liver, for example. Normal collagen metabolism involves a balance between synthesis and degradation. During growth or following injury, the synthesis of collagen increases. By 10 days after a tendon laceration, the collagen production has increased to 15 times normal, peaking at 22 times normal by 14 to 28 days after injury. There is a slow decline in this injury-induced collagen production, so that 84 days after tendon laceration, the collagen production rate is still 15 times normal.[18] Collagen metabolism can be affected by heredity and systemic problems. Inborn errors of metabolism and nutritional deficiencies can lead to abnormalities in amino acid content, hydroxylation, and cross-linking. Vitamin C is vital for collagen synthesis; it is required for the hydroxylation of the procollagen molecule. Vitamin-C deficiency results in decreased extrusion of procollagen molecules from the fibroblast cell. The molecules that are extruded are usually defective. Under the influence of certain hormones such as corticosteroids, the rate of collagen degradation exceeds that of synthesis. Corticosteroids also inhibit the production of new collagen. Insulin and the sex hormones, testosterone and estrogen, may actually increase the production of new collagen.

Landi and associates found in rabbits that the enzymes required for collagen synthesis decreased with age, thereby potentially slowing or lessening repair of soft tissue injury with age.[19] The ultrastructure of tendon, i.e., the collagen microfibrils, changes in response to aging and temperature. With aging, cross-linking between tropocollagen molecules increases. This, in turn, stiffens the tendon and may make it more likely to tear when it is subjected to strain. At approximately 104°F, a change in the microstructure of collagen occurs. It is thought that the intermolecular physical bonding becomes partially destabilized.[20] Therefore, when collagenous tissue is stretched at an elevated temperature rather than when body temperature is normal, these microstructural changes allow greater relaxation of the tissue and increase the relative proportion of plastic deformation following cooling. "Plastic or permanent lengthening is most favored by lower force, longer-duration stretching at elevated temperatures, but allowing the tissue to cool before releasing the tension."[21]

Exercise improves both the mechanical and structural properties of tendon. Exercise increases weight: length ratios of tendon, ultimate tendon strength and stiffness, and junctional strength of tendon–bone interface.[22-24] Three mechanisms implicated in these improvements include: changes in the synthesis of proteoglycans and collagen, changes in collagen cross-links on intramolecular and intermolecular levels, and changes in the deposition and arrangement of collagen fibers.[25] Inactivity or immobilization, in contrast, results in increased collagen degradation, decreased weight, decreased junctional strength, and decreased concentration of oxidative enzymes.[26] Although when nerve supply to tendon and muscle is interrupted, atrophy occurs and collagen content decreases, it is unclear whether loss of neural input or mechanical causes are responsible for these findings in inactive tendon.

Pathophysiology

What, then, is the process by which overuse of a musculotendinous unit produces a clinically apparent overuse injury such as tendinitis? As noted above, no damage is thought to occur when the tendon is not stretched more than 4 percent of its resting length. However, if larger loads are applied, microfailure occurs. The amount of applied force that can cause structural damage is a function of the size and number of the collagen fibrils present. Because all of the fibrils are in parallel alignment, the force is shared among linked fibrils. As fibrils slip on one another, the weakest fibers rupture, increasing the load on the remaining fibers. Continued load under these circumstances ultimately leads to failure and macroscopic rupture of the tendon. Extensive elongation of the fibrils and tendon may also interfere with the vascular supply to the tendon, thereby adding to the insult. Once microtears have occurred, an inflammatory response ensues, and it is this inflammatory process that produces the clinical signs and symptoms of tendinitis.

The inflammatory response is characterized on the microscopic level by increased vessel permeability leading to swelling around the tendon. Damaged cells release prostaglandins and enzymes that cause a further increase in vessel wall permeability and that attract scavenger polymorphonuclear leukocytes to the area to phagocytize and digest the damaged tissue. These neutrophilic cells also contribute to tissue destruction by release of lysosomal enzymes. Lysosomal enzymes have the capability of destroying vascular basement membrane, elastin, collagen, and cell membranes.[27,28] Complement, which is chemotactic for neutrophils, can also be activated by neutral proteases from lysosomal granules.[29] In addition, lysosomal phospholipases can transform membrane phospholipids to arachidonic acid, generating substrate for prostaglandin synthetase. Prostaglandins can reproduce all of the manifestations of inflammation. Prostaglandin E_1 (PGE_1) is nociceptive and can produce erythema, polymorphonuclear leukocyte chemotaxis, and increased vascular permeability, leading to swelling. PGE_1 also may increase collagen biosynthesis. It is apparent, then, that the inflammatory response, once initiated, can easily be self-sustaining through regulation of various cellular processes. This regulation may occur by cyclic nucleotides.[30] Both cyclic AMP (cAMP) and cyclic GMP (cGMP) have been shown to be capable of inhibiting antigen-induced release of histamine from basophils. Agents that increase cAMP levels increase proportionately with the level of inhibition of many of the cellular components of the inflammatory process.[31] "It seems likely that the chronic regulation of inflammation is mediated by intracellular concentration of these two cyclic nucleotides in dynamic tension, with cyclic AMP depressing and cyclic GMP stimulating inflammation."[32] It may also be the balance between PGE and prostaglandin F (PGF) that determines the outcome, so that the inflammatory response does not lead to massive tissue destruction.

The inflammatory response generally lasts about 48 hours. Continued excessive physical activity during this period of time with further microscopic damage to the tendon in its already weakened state is likely to prolong the inflammatory phase and to cause more damage owing to the relative hypoxia, excessive extracellular fluid, and acidic environment caused by the proteolytic enzymes released from polymorphonuclear leukocytes. Ordinarily on the third or fourth day following the initiation of the inflammatory response, fibroblasts from the surrounding connective tissue begin to lay down a gellike substance composed of proteins, carbohydrates, and water, all of which are necessary for the aggregation of collagenous protein into collagen fibrils. During these first 4 days the collagen is predominantly immature, because mature cross-links have not yet formed between tropocollagen molecules. Therefore, a significant proportion of the collagen tends to be soluble and may be liable to further breakdown if the inflammatory response continues. During the second week following the initiation of the inflammatory response, solubility data suggest that mature cross-links are forming.[33] The first 2 weeks following the injury are called the *proliferative phase* of connective tissue healing.

The second phase of connective tissue healing is the *formative phase*, during which time the new collagenous tissue is organized. Initially collagen fibrils are laid down in random directions. Obviously the tensile force that can be resisted by multidirectional fibers is limited, thus making newly forming scar more subject to tearing under load. The collagen fibers subsequently reorient themselves in line with the tensile force applied to the tissue.[34] Tension may be applied through contraction of the attached muscle but may be markedly reduced if the nearby joints have been immobilized. Akeson, Amiel, and LaViolette have shown that tendons lose from 20 to 40 percent of their ground substance during joint immobilization and that less elastin may be formed in the new connective tissue if immobility is prolonged.[35] Early mobilization has been found to produce greater tensile strength and greater gliding function in tendons. These findings are also associated with an accelerated change in the peritendinous vessel density and configuration as well as with increased DNA at the repair site.[36] Early motion not only produces stresses that are important in collagen alignment but also may help pump synovial fluid and nutrients into the interstices of the tendon.[37] How the magnitude and duration of controlled passive motion might affect tendon healing is unknown. Mason and Allen found that healing tendon tensile strength in rabbits initially decreased, then rapidly increased with a plateau between 14 and 16 days. If the neighboring joint was immobilized, there was a slight rise in strength at 19 days and a subsequent plateau over the next 2 weeks. If activity was allowed earlier than the third week following injury, tensile strength was much greater than in the immobilized animals, suggesting that function seems to accelerate maturation.[38] Similarly, Woo and co-workers, in a study of lacerated dog flexor tendons, found that controlled passive mobilization after 3 weeks of immobilization accelerated the tendon repair strength and increased tendon excursion, compared to tendons around joints that had been immobilized longer. In this study there was no increase in strength seen during the first 3 weeks of immobilization, suggesting that perhaps mobilization could begin even sooner than 3 weeks.[39] Early mobilization also improves tendon excursion by preventing adhesions of tendon to surrounding connective tissue.[40] Tendon excursion is critical, so that the tendon is capable of going around corners or under pulleys.

The third phase of connective tissue healing is called the *remodeling phase*. It begins in the third to fourth week after injury and may continue for a year or more. During the early remodeling phase, the fibrils reorganize themselves parallel to the long axis of the tendon, i.e., along lines of stress, into functional tendon fibers that are capable of withstanding the loads normally applied. This reorientation along the lines of stress may be due to piezoelectric charges in the collagen fibrils, produced by tension from contraction of the muscle.[34,41] During the remodeling phase, tensile strength increases at the same time as the mass of scar tissue decreases. Because tendon strength is a direct function of the number, size, and orientation of the collagen fibers, it is important that protected motion be encouraged in the third week after the injury. By the twentieth week, only minimal histologic differences exist between the scar and normal tendon. These differences are in the form of increased vascularity and cells in the scar. Although there is still a small amount of remodeling that occurs until 1 year after the time of injury, most tendons are able to withstand normal stresses 6 weeks after injury.

Clinical Correlation

The clinical hallmarks of tendinitis include tenderness to palpation of the involved tendon and pain during use of the musculotendinous unit, especially against resistance. Stretching the tendon may produce pain. When the inflammation is particularly acute, there is redness, swelling, and crepitus around the tendon. Local application of ice and deep heat is often recommended for treating tendinitis. Ice is especially useful in the first few days after injury, because it decreases the swelling that follows increased vascular permeability. Also, it reduces the rate of chemical activity and therefore potentially minimizes the inflammatory response. In addition, cold is an effective analgesic. Heat, particularly in the form of ultrasound or diathermy, may be used later in the healing process to try to produce mechanical waves that affect the scar tissue being formed and make it more susceptible to remodeling. Curwin and Stanish recommended that ultrasound be followed by exercise, so that the tendon is subjected to appropriate tensile stresses to tell the collagen fibrils how to align.[13] Application of these forms of heat therapy prior to formation of scar would be fruitless because there would be nothing to remodel.

It should be obvious that controlled motion is helpful, particularly during the second week following injury when tension is important for the orientation of newly forming collagen fibrils. The amount of motion must be one that would load the tendon without exceeding a 4 percent strain. Generally, normal use of the involved extremity and musculotendinous unit, without the addition of extraneous weights or excessive loading caused by impact activities, provides appropriate amounts of load and strain.

Because eccentric loading elicits greater force production, greater stress on the tendon occurs during this type of activity, and it is often associated with tendinitis. A program designed theoretically to train the tendon to withstand eccentric loads was devised by Curwin and Stanish. This training regimen focused on three areas:

1. Length: stretching was an integral part of the program based on the theory that by increasing resting length of the muscle tendon unit, the strain taken for any given range of motion during activity might be lessened.
2. Load: progressive resistive exercise, i.e., increasing the load, is the basis for many strengthening programs; however, in this particular program the load was often applied in an eccentric manner.
3. Speed of contraction: because the force on the tendon was related to the speed of muscle contraction, increasing the speed could also gradually increase the load on the tendon. Curwin and Stanish also recommended that ice be applied immediately after each exercise session to minimize any inflammatory response to the exercise.[42]

Another method of strengthening, transcutaneous electrical muscle stimulation, is becoming more popular for two reasons. First, it often provides pain relief. Second, it has been shown that the loads applied to the musculotendinous unit by electrical stimulation are often less than those applied during actual use of the musculotendinous unit, thereby providing the benefit of loading without the risk of overloading.[43]

The two most commonly discussed medications in the treatment of tendinitis are nonsteroidal anti-inflammatory drugs (NSAIDs) and corticosteroids. The NSAIDs generally inhibit the synthesis of prostaglandins and thereby lessen the increased vascular permeability, some of the nociceptive input, and the attraction of cells to the injured area. It would be detrimental to use these drugs during the first 2 days after injury, because cell migration and phagocytosis of detritus are required for healing to take place. The use of anti-inflammatory agents in the treatment of experimental muscle strains in rabbits decreased the inflammatory reaction seen in the early postinjury period but also decreased the muscle regeneration; hence, it is felt that a certain amount of inflammation early in the process is necessary for a normal healing response to occur.[44] However, if symptoms of inflammation persist, these drugs may be quite useful in decreasing the inflammatory response so that the fibroblast can get on with the job of making new collagen fibers. Injection of corticosteroids into inflamed tendons is frowned upon because evidence indicates that corticosteroid injection decreases the tensile strength of tendon and inhibits the production of collagen and ground substance, potentially leading to tendon rupture.[45,46]

In summary, overuse injuries occur when the amount of stress applied to the tendon exceeds its ability to elongate without disrupting structural integrity. The amount of stress on the tendon is related to the magnitude of the force generated by the muscle, the direction of the force applied, the physical dimensions of the tendon, its relative vascularity, and its course, i.e., any angles it must take to its insertion. Persistent excessive strain in the first few days following microscopic injury tends to produce a chronic inflammatory state. Hence, rest is often recommended in the first few days after an injury during the proliferative stage of soft tissue healing. Ice is also useful during the initial 48 hours after injury, because it keeps the inflammatory response to a minimum without totally inhibiting it. During the formative stage, limited amounts of tensile stress should be applied to encourage functional tissue remodeling.

Various forms of heat and limited exercise may be useful during this stage of soft tissue healing and remodeling (see chap. 15).

BONE

Normal Physiology

Function

Bone serves as a storehouse of calcium and, early in life, as a producer of blood cells. Bone functions predominantly to transmit loads in association with muscles and gravity. Bone must resist muscle pull and support body weight. "A relatively consistent relationship seems to exist between muscle mass and bone mass, with each adapting to changes in the other."[47] During growth from newborn to adult, bone mass increases 20 times, whereas muscle mass increases 40 times. Although the proximal segments of both the upper and lower limbs contain twice as much muscle as the distal segments, and the lower limbs contain more muscle and bone than the upper limbs, the proportion of bone to muscle mass remains relatively constant in both.[47]

Structure

"Despite obvious differences in configuration, all bones have certain structural features in common. These include a cortical shell of varying thickness that encompasses all external surfaces, thus forming a closed container; loose-meshed spongy (cancellous) bone within the cortical shell; and myeloid or fatty marrow in the cavities between the trabeculae."[48] Bone can be classified as *cortical* (also known as dense or compact bone), or *trabecular* (also known as spongy or cancellous). Cortical bone is found both in cuboid bones and in long bones subject to bending, torsion, and compression. Haversian bone is a type of cortical bone made up of vascular channels surrounded by circumferential bony lamellae producing a structure known as the osteon (Fig. 13–4). These cylinders are usually oriented along the long axis of the bone and are the major structural units of cortical bone. Trabecular bone is generally found in metaphyseal areas of long bones and in cuboid bones such as the vertebrae. The spicules in trabecular bone form a three-dimensional lattice that is in general alignment with applied stresses. This type of bone is subject mainly to compression.

The relative quantity of cortical and trabecular bone varies among bones and in different parts of the same bone and is determined by the load requirements of each area. Usually the diaphysis has the thickest cortical shell in long bones. It is also cylindrical. The most efficient shape for a structure that must resist torsional and bending forces is a cylinder, because it provides an equivalent moment about any transverse axis. The farther mass is distributed away from the center of an object, the greater the moment of inertia and therefore the greater the strength of the object in torsion and bending. At the ends of a long bone where the forces are predominantly compressive, the bone becomes wider. This broader supporting surface containing trabecular bone makes the metaphysis more resilient and aids in the transfer of forces through the joint.

All bone is composed predominantly of mineralized organic matrix laid down on a collagen framework. A longitudinal orientation of collagen fibers increases the tensile strength of bone, and a transverse orientation increases the compressive strength. One can distinguish two types of bone tissue microscopically—*woven bone* and *lamellar bone*. The collagen fibers are randomly distributed in woven bone and are highly ordered in lamellar bone. Both trabecular bone and cortical bone can be woven or lamellar. Woven bone is usually found in areas of endochondral ossification, at sites of tendinous or ligamentous attachments, in fracture callus, osteogenic sarcoma, or metastases. Lamellar bone can be found in trabecular lamellae, outer and inner circumferential lamellae, interstitial lamellae, and osteons with concentric lamellae. Lamellar bone, whether compact or cancellous, is highly organized. The collagen is stress oriented in lamellar bone; therefore, the mechanical behavior differs as a function of the orientation of the force applied. Woven bone has more cells per unit volume than lamellar bone. The mineral content varies, and cells and fibers are randomly arranged. Mechanical behavior is similar regardless of the

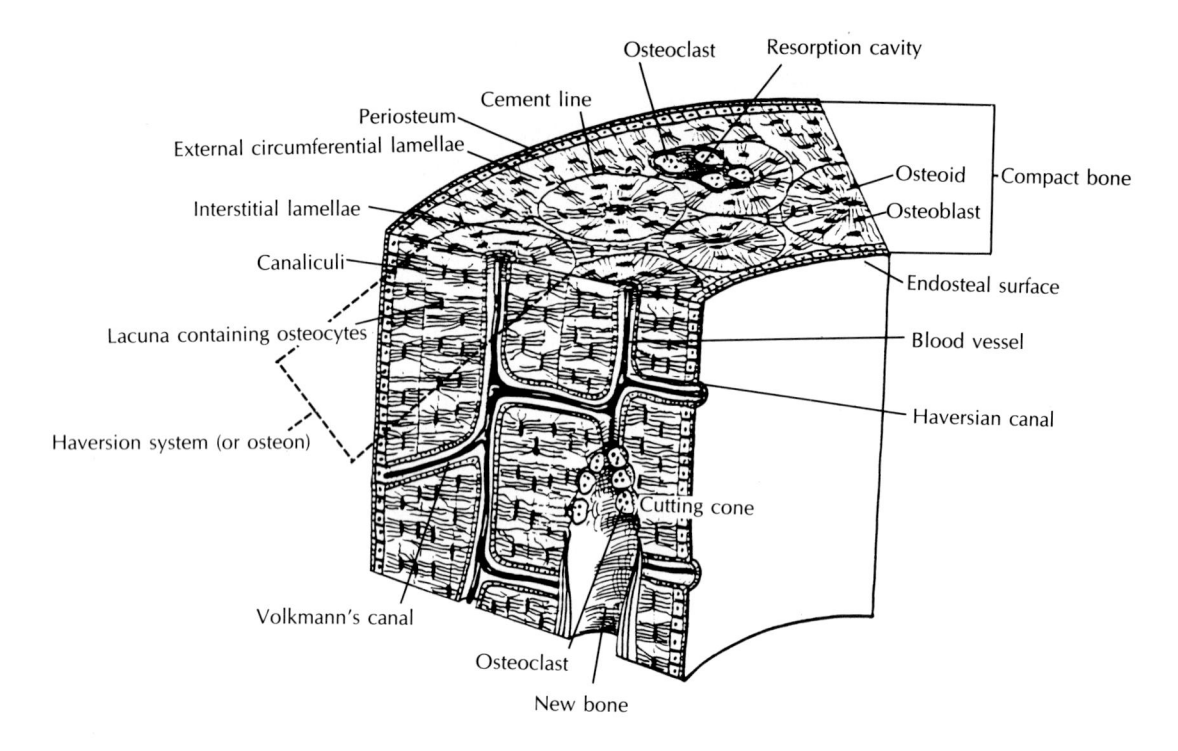

Figure 13-4 Three-dimensional representation of the diaphyseal cortex in a long bone. (From Harris WH, Heaney RP. Skeletal renewal and metabolic bone disease. N Engl J Med 1969; 280:193–203. Reprinted with permission.)

orientation of the applied forces. It is thought that the specific appearance of each type of bone is determined by the quantity and orientation of collagen fibers. For example, the appearance of lamellar bone is due to the presence of layers of parallel collagen bundles. This association between the microstructure of bone and the ultrastructure of collagen fibrils implies that the collagen may regulate osteoblasts in determining the microstructure of bone.[49] The lamellated pattern is also a result of the method by which bone is laid down by osteoblasts. They usually form a sheet of cells clinging to a previously formed bony surface and produce multiple thin layers of matrix that subsequently mineralize (Fig. 13–5).

Collagen accounts for about 90 percent of the organic matrix of bone. The collagen is largely genetic type I, the same as is found in tendon, with variations only in the number of amino acids rather than in the specific types of amino acids present. The synthesis of collagen has been described earlier in this chapter. The remaining 10 percent of the matrix is made up of proteoglycans, phosphoproteins, and other matrix proteins. At maturity, up to 80 percent of the weight of cortical bone is mineral. The mineral is almost exclusively calcium phosphate with minor components of carbonate, sodium, magnesium, and some other trace elements.[50] The calcium and phosphate join in the form of an hydroxyapatite crystal.[51] The displacement of collagen fibers in a staggered arrangement leaves regularly spaced holes that may be sites for deposition of mineral in the process of bone formation. Some authors believe that the three-dimensional structure of the collagen fibrils catalyzes the deposition of mineral in bone.[52] However, it is not clear whether the collagen itself plays an active or a passive role in directing the deposition of mineral crystallites within and around it.[53]

Cells probably control mineralization in several ways. These include spatial and temporal controls as well as alterations in pH and in cell organelles such as mitochondria. En-

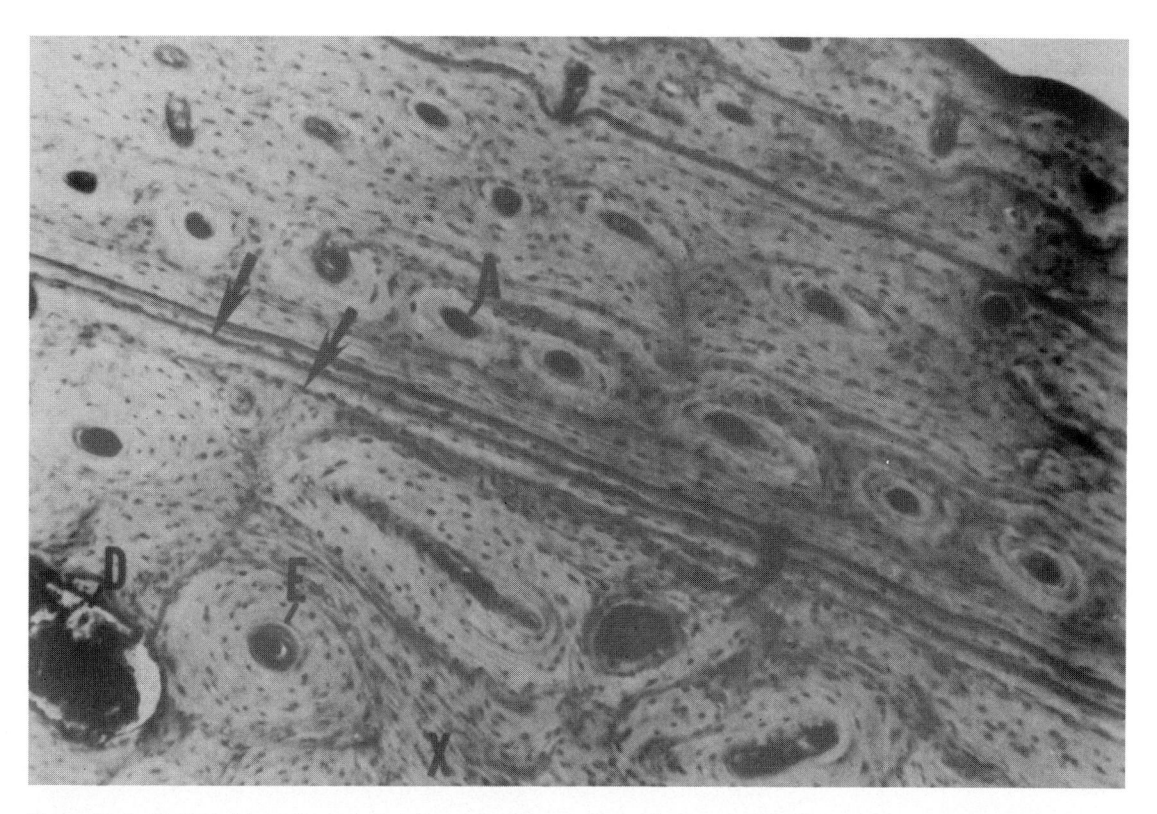

Figure 13–5 Periosteal bone formation. A layer of primary osteons (A), a reversal line (arrows) separates the younger periosteal zone from endosteal layers produced during an earlier growth stage. Resorption spaces (D), secondary osteons (E), and convoluted interstitial lamellae (X) can be identified. (From Enlow DH. Principles of bone remodeling. Springfield, IL: CC Thomas, 1963. Courtesy of Charles C. Thomas, Publisher.)

zymes such as alkaline phosphatase and pyrophosphatases may also play a role in mineralization. A loss of proteoglycans from the osteoid matrix may be involved in the initiation of mineralization. These substances may mask the site of crystal nucleation on the collagen fibril.[54] Alternatively, other matrix proteins such as phosphoproteins may positively influence the spatial growth of mineral crystallites. Extracellular matrix vesicles contain many of the membrane-bound enzymes needed for calcification and "may facilitate calcification (1) by concentrating ions, (2) providing a protective environment free of mineralization inhibitors, or (3) providing enzymes involved in matrix modification."[55] In other words, the process of mineralization of osteoid is an extracellular process, whereas matrix production is a cellular process. The precise mechanism by which all of these factors interact still contains some missing links, but the cells appear to be central to the process.[56]

Bone contains three types of cells: osteoblasts, osteocytes, and osteoclasts. *Osteoblasts* are rectangular, usually having their long axis perpendicular to the surface of bone. Typically they can be found in a single layer on a surface of actively forming bone. The osteoblast produces *osteoid*, which is a combination of collagen, glycosaminoglycans, and glycoproteins. Osteoid is often seen between the osteoblast cell membrane and the mineralized matrix of extant bone. The osteoblasts also provide storage sites for calcium and phosphorus. The principal organelle within the cell appears to be the *mitochondrion*, which serves as a calcium sink, releasing calcium under specific conditions. Low oxygen tension is associated with anaerobic glycolysis and the mitochondrial release of calcium.[41] Osteoblasts also contain a great deal of rough endoplasmic reticulum and Golgi apparatus. Enzymes, such as alkaline phosphatase distributed over the outer surface of the osteoblast cell membrane and ATPase produced by these cells, are responsible for controlling the flux of calcium and phosphate into and out of the matrix.

The *osteocyte* has a greater nuclear:cytoplasmic ratio and fewer organelles than the osteoblast. The osteocyte is essentially an osteoblast surrounded by mineralized matrix. Usually osteocytes are located concentrically around the lumen of an osteon, with extensive cell processes extending into canaliculi that radiate parallel to the radius of the osteon. These canaliculi communicate between adjacent osteocytes. Cells lie in and between lamellae and orient along them. Both osteoblasts and osteocytes can regulate calcium exchange more or less independently of surface resorption and accretion.[55] Bone mineral exchange with extracellular fluid takes place on the surfaces of haversian canals and lacunar and canalicular walls.

Osteoclasts, which resemble giant cells containing multiple nuclei, are phagocytic cells that resorb bone. Osteoclasts are thought to originate from mononuclear precursors derived either from bone marrow or from perivascular mesenchymal cells. They generally lie in cavities of bone resorption. Intracellularly, they contain very little rough endoplasmic reticulum, a moderate number of ribosomes, and well-developed mitochondria. When active, osteoclasts have a ruffled or brush border that is made up of extensive infoldings and projections of the cell membrane adjacent to the resorptive surface (Fig. 13–6). These infoldings increase the surface area with which the osteoclast can make

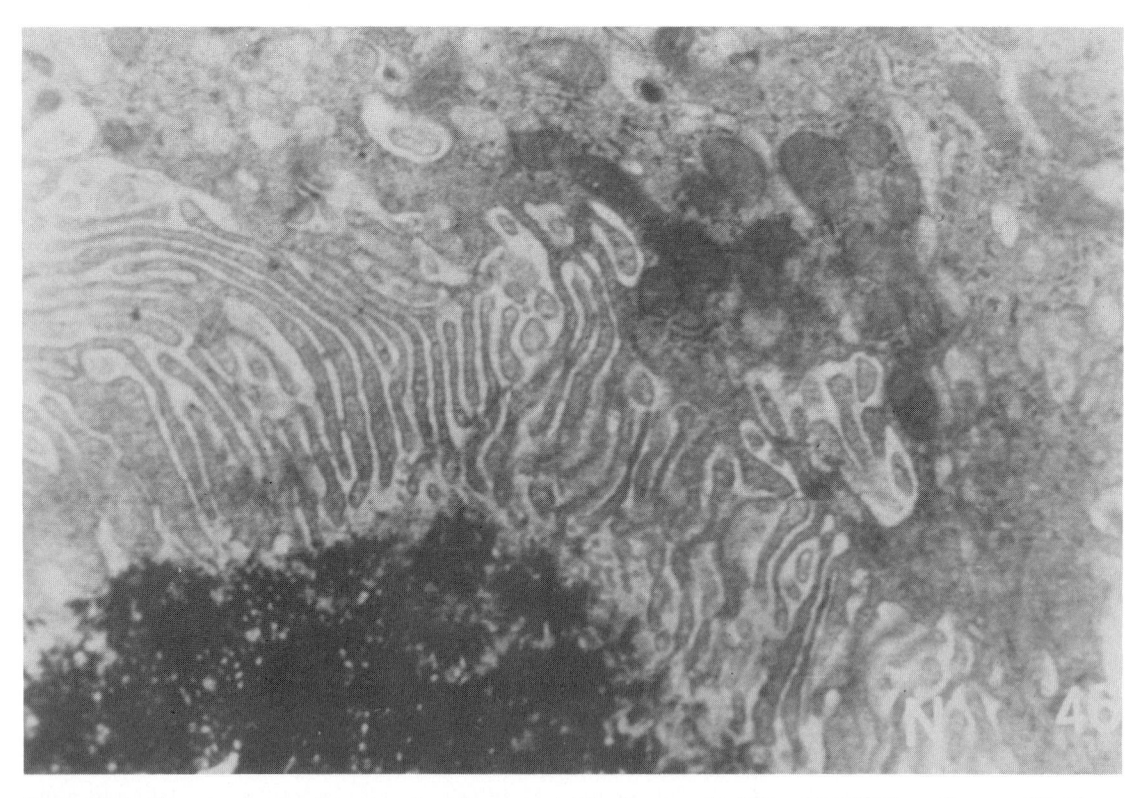

Figure 13–6 The osteoclast brush border. Crystalline material lies between the folds ×33,000. (From Cameron DA. The ultrastructure of bone. In: Bourne GH, ed. The biochemistry and physiology of bone. New York: Academic Press, 1972. Reprinted with permission.)

contact with the intact bone. They form channels that end in cytoplasmic vacuoles on the interior of the osteoclast. The ruffled border appears to come and go with initiation and cessation of osteoclast activity, and the size of the ruffled border is proportional to the degree of osteoclastic resorption activity. The clear space seen within the ruffled border is an acidic microenvironment in which resorption occurs. The osteoclast contains a proton pump (similar to that in the renal tubular cell), which transfers protons to keep the environment acidic so that acid phosphatase, collagenase, and other hydrolytic enzymes can digest bone into crystals and components of collagen and organic matrix. Proteases then degrade the matrix. Teitlebaum's work suggests that vitamin D and parathyroid hormone stimulate osteoblasts to secrete a substance that tells osteoclasts to resorb bone. This finding may explain the apparent tandem operation of osteoblasts and osteoclasts.[57] When this process is complete, the osteoclast loses contact with the bone surface and leaves behind a Howship's lacuna.[58] The stimulus for this resorption is not completely known but seems to be a combination of chemical and physical factors.

Biomechanics

The mechanical properties of bone are a function not only of its composition but also of its shape and structural relationships. Bone has tensile strength similar to cast iron. It also exhibits plastic behavior and deforms permanently when stressed beyond its elastic limit. Prior to failure, bone can absorb six times as much energy after it has yielded than it can during elastic deformation. When bone fails, energy is released. When a stress–strain curve is plotted, the stored energy is equal to the area under the curve (Fig. 13–7).

Three biomechanical zones have been identified: the *load zone*, in which bone responds in an elastic fashion; the *fatigue zone*, in which repetitive loading weakens the bone; and the *overload zone*, in which a single load produces plastic deformation.[59] In the elastic zone the deformation is proportional to the force applied, and fatigue failure does not occur. In the fatigue zone, progressive plastic deformation occurs, and prefailure slip lines appear in compressed cortex. Prefailure slip lines are caused by shear and rupture of collagen fibers in the lamellae, as well as disruption of the crystal lattices. The duration of the plastic phase varies as a function of age, with a greater degree of deformation prior to fracture occurring in children. Eventually a fatigue fracture develops, with the fracture localized in the middle of the area crossed by the slip lines. In the overload zone, deformation usually occurs obliquely at an angle of about 30 degrees to the long axis of the diaphysis.

A force acting on bone produces external as well as internal effects. The external effects result in movement of the bone about a joint whereas the internal effects include stress and strain in the bone (see Table 13–1). Stress perpendicular to the surface is known as *normal stress*, whereas stress parallel to the surface is known as *shear stress*. Strain can also take various forms. Toughness depends on strain as well as stress and describes the strain energy built up in a material as load is applied. Two materials with the same breaking strength may absorb markedly different amounts of energy.[47] Bone is viscoelastic, so its properties vary with the rate of loading. "A viscoelastic material combines the elastic properties of a spring, where maximum deformation is dependent upon the load, and the viscous properties of a . . . syringe, where the rate of flow is dependent on

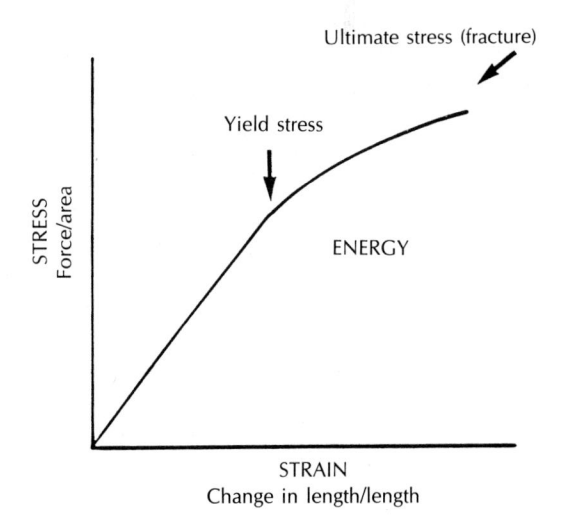

Figure 13–7 A stress–strain curve for bone.

load. The elastic element determines the maximum deformation possible for a given load, while the viscus element determines the time required to reach this limit."[48] The ultimate strength, i.e., the stress at the point of fracture, thus is directly related to the strain rate. The toughness is much greater at high than at low loading rates. Longitudinal strains of 2 to 4 percent may occur prior to fracture as a function of the rate of loading and the age of the patient.

Bone is also anisotropic; therefore, its physical properties vary with the direction of loading. In long bones, the greatest tensile strength is along the longitudinal axis. This is an efficient design for resisting loads placed on long bones. The resistance of bone to deformation is one of its most important physical properties. In tension, bone can elongate approximately 0.75 percent of its original length before permanent deformation occurs. Whereas the collagenous component of bone (one-third) is primarily responsible for resisting tensile stresses, the mineral component (two-thirds) is responsible for its resistance to compression. The greater the mineral content, the greater the stiffness and static strength of bone. The mechanical properties of bone (shape, strength, elasticity) may change as a function of hormonal, vascular, and physical stimuli.

Metabolism

Bone, although it appears relatively inert, is actually a metabolically active tissue that is continually remodeling. Bone remodeling is a surface phenomenon that occurs on periosteal and endosteal, haversian canal, and trabecular surfaces. The rate of remodeling in cortical bone ranges from 50 percent per year in the first 2 years of life to between 2 and 5 percent per year in the elderly. Trabecular bone remodeling rates may be five to 10 times higher. In normal bone there is a balance between bone formation and resorption, such that the mineralization of the bone remains relatively constant. How this balance is maintained is incompletely understood.

Frost has likened the process to the maintenance of an ice skating rink in which the surface area and the thickness of the ice are kept constant. He found that there was a constant relationship between the mass of organic matrix removed or made and the volume of this matrix. He described a basic multicellular unit (BMU) of action in bone remodeling found in both cortical and trabecular bone.[60] An initial stimulus causes mesenchymal cells to become osteoclasts and osteoblasts. The osteoclasts appear first and, by means of cutting cones, resorb approximately 0.05 cubic millimeters of bone (Fig. 13–8). The osteoclasts advance about 4 μ per hour, and during a 24-hour period they can resorb a cavity 100 to 300 μ in diameter. A capillary loop and osteoblasts are generally found a short distance behind the cutting cone. They produce new bone, which progressively fills the cavity formed by the cone. The bone matrix formed by osteoblasts calcifies after an 8- to 10-day interval. The osteoblasts remain as osteocytes, which are isolated in lacunae. It is the osteocyte that maintains the viability of mature bone tissue. The time it takes for the process to reverse from bone resorption to bone formation can be estimated by the distance between the osteoclasts and the osteoblasts on a longitudinal section through an osteon, and the new bone made by a remodeling unit can be identified by a cement (reversal) line that forms at the outer limit of bone resorption (see Fig.

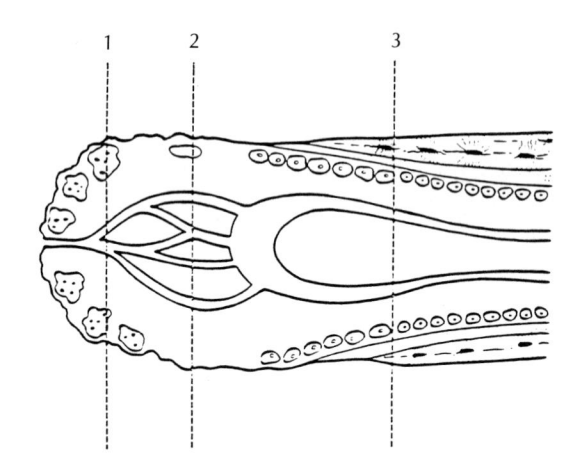

Figure 13–8 A longitudinal section through an active BMU. (*1*) The cutting cone (resorption front). (*2*) Interim phase between resorption and formation. (*3*) Active osteoblasts bordering a layer of unmineralized osteoid to fill the cavity formed by 1. (From Albright JA, Skinner SCW. Bone: structural organization and remodeling dynamics. In: Albright JA, Brand RA, eds. The scientific basis of orthopaedics. Norwalk, CT: Appleton and Lange, 1987. Reprinted with permission.)

13–5). Adjacent sections of bone do not communicate across cement lines.

Bone modeling and remodeling may be regulated systemically, locally, or in both ways. The systemic factors regulating bone modeling and remodeling include calcium-regulating hormones such as parathyroid hormone and vitamin D, systemic hormones such as insulin and thyroxin, and growth factors such as platelet-derived growth factor and somatomedin. Local factors include prostaglandins, cyclic nucleotides, bone-derived growth factor, and calcium and phosphate ions. The hypothesis that modeling and remodeling are regulated locally at the tissue level rather than by systemic hormones does not explain uncoupling of bone formation and resorption seen with age and various hormonal disorders such as Cushing's syndrome, osteomalacia, or osteoporosis.[61] The activation of bone metabolic units is partially under the control of parathyroid hormone, which appears to activate mesenchymal precursor cells to become osteoclasts. Parathyroid hormone also is capable of modulating cAMP levels in bone cells through the cell membrane. Growth hormone, thyroxine, and physical loading of the bone also have been found to activate precursor cells. Calcitonin, estrogen, and corticosteroids inhibit activation. Systemic growth factors, such as epidermal growth factor and fibroblast growth factor, stimulate cell replication in skeletal and nonskeletal tissues but inhibit differentiated function. Platelet-derived growth factor stimulates cell replication and protein synthesis by differentiated cells and makes fibroblasts competent to replicate. Insulin and somatomedin stimulate bone cell replication and differentiation.[62] New bone formation may be secondary to the activation of resting osteoblasts or to the proliferation and differentiation of preosteoblasts. Hormones can regulate the level of osteoblast replication and function. Osteoblasts in turn, may regulate mineralization. Vitamin D is required for the normal mineralization of osteoid. Osteoblasts synthesize osteocalcin when stimulated by 1,25 dihydroxy vitamin D. Osteocalcin is another bone-specific protein that is present in the extracellular matrix. Its function is unknown, but current concepts suggest it has a role in resorption.

Locally synthesized factors include an autologous bone-derived growth factor that stimulates bone collagen and DNA synthesis. Bone morphogenetic protein has been found to induce differentiation of perivascular mesenchymal cells into cartilage and bone.[63] It also stimulates DNA synthesis and replication in fibroblasts but not in postdifferentiated bone cells.[64] Transforming growth factor beta is present in a variety of cells and is known to induce fibroblast chemotaxis and differentiation to enhance collagen synthesis.[65,66] The collagen fraction in bone is associated with local osteoinductive activity.[67] Collagen and its fragments are mitogens and inducers of fibroblast chemotaxis.[68,69] Prostaglandins may be involved in the coupling of resorption and bone formation, because they are stimulators of both processes and can be produced by osteoblasts. Their action may be mediated by cyclic nucleotides. In chick tibae, compressive loads of physiologic magnitude changed the carbohydrate metabolism and the cell division in the specimen. Less cAMP was found in the epiphyses of bones exposed to load than in controls. Levels of cGMP went up or down depending on the cell observed. Load applied to isolated cells produced changes in their cyclic nucleotide content as well. Changes were cell specific and dependent on the matrix. The distortion of cell membranes produced by mechanical, electrical, or chemical perturbation may initiate remodeling by cyclic nucleotide messengers.[70]

In addition to factors already mentioned, biomechanical stresses and electrical stimulation are known to influence the rate of turnover of bone. The ability of bone to change its shape or mass as a function of applied mechanical stress was described in 1892 and is known as Wolff's law.[71] In essence, Wolff's law states "that a bone, when bent by a mechanical load, adapts by depositing new bone on the concave side and resorbing the bone on the convex side."[48] This is clearly seen during remodeling after a fracture. Bone adapts to stress by altering its shape, its inner structure, and the material distribution within the bone.[72] As mentioned above, applied muscular and gravitational forces generate stresses and strains within bone. The anisotropic nature of bone causes the strains to be variable in different parts of the bone in conformance with the varying microstructure. Clark and associates placed strain gauges and found that bone responded to both the size and the direction of strain imposed by locomotion.[73]

Muscle pull also affects osteonal remodeling.[74] During disuse, immobilization, or weightlessness, resorption predominates. This is associated with calcium loss and increased osteoclastic activity. In studies from the aerospace industry, weightlessness produced muscle loss and an average total loss of calcium per crew member of 25 g in an 84-day flight.[75] The loss of muscle can be retarded by exercise, but the type of exercise used thus far has had no effect on calcium loss. The adaptation of bone to changes in stress often neutralizes the change, so that the new configuration of bone is more capable of withstanding the stress applied. This resembles a closed-loop negative feedback system. As bone is resorbed, the stress increases until balance occurs but at a decreased bone mass. When stresses are greater than usual, bone formation predominates, thereby decreasing the stress until balance is restored. When stress is optimal, bone remodeling and resorption are balanced. In a study in pigs in which the ulna was removed unilaterally and strain gauges were placed on the radius, the compressive strains on the radius increased 2 to $2^1/_2$ times. The radius then remodeled; 3 months later, its cross-sectional area and the area enclosed by the radial periosteum were equal in value to that of the radius plus the ulna in the contralateral limb. At this point in time, the compressive strains measured in the limb containing only the radius were equal to those measured in both the radius and ulna in the contralateral limb.[76] It may be that the strains seen during plastic deformation are the major stimulus to bone hypertrophy, per Wolff's Law.

Frost described a minimum effective strain as that which evokes adaptive architectural bone modeling. Strains less than an average range of 0.0008 to 0.002 unit of bone surface strain evoke no response in bone modeling. According to this concept of minimum effective strain, "(1) a feedback mechanism exists in bone, (2) this feedback mechanism senses an effect of mechanical loads, (3) it converts that effect into some type of signal that controls the adaptive modeling, and (4) the mechanism operates in the negative feedback mode," thus eliminating the cause of the initial signal.[77] Using this concept of a minimum effective strain, Frost was able to predict lamellar bone architectural adaptations. For example, the typical bone adaptation to load is to increase trabeculae along lines of stress, thus actually reducing the risk of fracture under subsequent similar loads. Mechanically evoked remodeling is thought to occur faster in young and recently fractured bone, because it is a function of strain not stress, and strain is greater in more compliant bone, such as immature bone or incompletely mineralized callus.

Mechanically evoked remodeling can occur because of exercise, which is known to increase bone mass in normal individuals of any age. Anderson and co-workers found that exercise conserves both the collagen and the mineral components of bone.[78] Exercise appears to stimulate bone formation and calcium retention. Physical studies of bone have reported denser, stronger, and thicker bones following exercise. A number of studies have correlated bone marrow content and physical activity.[79,80] When the type of exercise is analyzed, it appears that mild exercise maintains bone but does not increase it. Short-term, high-resistance activities are necessary to increase bone mass and strength. Many authors have found consistently positive effects on the skeleton in athletes compared to control subjects, particularly when comparing the dominant limb to the nondominant limb.[81-84] Exercise is also beneficial in retarding mineral loss in the postmenopausal female.[85] However, the relationship between biophysical stress and hormones is complex. Most recently, it has become apparent that mineral loss can occur in a premenopausal woman who is exercising extensively, if the intensity of exercise is such that amenorrhea occurs.[86,87] Bone mineral loss due to amenorrhea in premenopausal women resembles the process that occurs in postmenopausal osteoporosis. The hormonal influence in this situation seems to be more potent than the influence of the physical stresses produced by the exercise.

What is still not clear is the physical or chemical nature of the transducer that converts biomechanical stress and strain into the biological signals that control the cells. This transducer is thought by some to be perturbations in the cell membrane that cause changes in intracellular prostaglandin E synthesis and production of cAMP and cGMP, which in turn initiate a number of cellular processes. Others feel the transducer is bioelectrical in nature. There are at least two types of electrical charges present in bone—piezoelectrical potentials and streaming potentials.[88] Piezoelectricity is caused by mechanical distortion of bonds in a crystalline solid. *Piezoelectrical potentials* arise from stress-induced formation of electrical dipoles in the material, from the stress-induced orientation of these dipoles, or from charge separation in materials whose structure lacks a center of symmetry. The piezoelectrical potentials are strain related or stress induced. Collagen is thought to account for the piezoelectrical properties found in dry bone. In wet bone the electrical properties may be due to *streaming potentials*, i.e., the voltage developed between two points in an electrolyte when it flows past a charged solid surface. Such potentials can arise in vascular channels and in the extravascular fluid spaces in bone as a result of pulsatile blood flow, muscle activity, and physiologic loading. Fluid spaces in bone have been identified between cells lining the bone surfaces and the calcified tissue, and perivascularly, i.e., in the space between the capillary wall and the bone cells; they have also been noted intravascularly, in haversian canals, and in the mineral crystal.[89,90] This fluid appears to move from the lacunae to the haversian canals by way of canaliculi. A third type of bioelectrical potential, whose origin is not clear, is dependent upon cell viability and metabolic effort. This electrical charge is negative in areas of active growth and positive in less active areas. It is not dependent on mechanical stress.[91] Pollack tries to combine the cellular and bioelectrical theories, offering the hypothesis that applied physical stresses generate electrical potentials which then cause a cellular response leading to remodeling.[91] The electrical potentials may stimulate the release of prostaglandins which, in turn, influence the level of cyclic nucleotides.

Brighton, as well as Bassett, Mitchell, and Gaston, have shown the effectiveness of electrical stimulation in fracture healing and have found that the tension side of bone and the compression side of bone have opposite electrical charges.[92,93] During bending, the concave (compression) side of bone develops a negative potential, whereas the convex (tension) side develops a positive potential. Percussive bone impact also generates minute measurable electrical fields. In experimental studies the positive charge associated with tension is capable of producing resorption. New bone formation is generally associated with the negative pole of a current passed through two electrodes in bone. This correlates with the fact that more bone is seen on the compression side than on the tensile side of bone. Justus and Luft found that hydroxyapatite crystals become increasingly soluble when tension is applied, and that they become less soluble, causing calcium salts to precipitate, when compression is applied.[94] The fact that physical activity produces electrical potentials in bone does not necessarily mean that there is a causative relationship with bone remodeling. Exercise also produces systemic and circulatory changes that may affect bone homeostasis.

In summary, control of osteoblast and osteoclast activity involves biochemical changes; however, it is not clear whether the stimulus to these changes occurs through physical, electrical, or chemical stimuli or combinations thereof. In order for adaptation to occur, intermittent deformation is necessary. Adaptation is a function of the number of loading cycles, the frequency of cycling, and the amount of strain, strain rate, and strain duration per cycle. One of the distinct characteristics of living bone is its ability to cycle indefinitely depending upon the frequency of loading. Because living bone is self-repairing, fracture occurs from overuse only when frequency of loading exceeds the remodeling necessary to prevent failure, i.e., remodeling is outpaced by fatigue. When mechanical stress increases at a subfracture level, one finds an increase in bone tissue.[95] Intermittent compression, a form of biological irritation that continually reactivates osteogenesis, causes hypertrophy. Bone remodeling activity is much greater in areas exposed to greater forces, producing newer, more strain-sensitive bone that enables bone to function better as a supporting structure. This strain-sensitive remodeling ensures that commonly encountered strains do not lead to fracture and that the body can compensate for slow changes in weight that might occur, such as during pregnancy.

Pathophysiology—Fracture

Bone is loaded in compression, tension, torsion, bending, shear, or combinations thereof. When excessive load is applied to bone, it fractures. Fractures tend to follow cement lines, which appear to be the weakest material in bone. Because bone is capable of energy storage, when loading speeds are low, energy can dissipate through the formation of a crack, and little or no displacement occurs. Bone and soft tissues remain relatively intact. At high loading speed, the greater energy stored cannot dissipate rapidly enough, and comminution and extensive soft tissue damage occur.[96] Hence, depending upon the rate of loading, the fracture site may be smooth (slow loading) or rough. The fracture pattern in a bone also reveals the direction and type of load applied to that bone. Pure tension, when applied at either end of a long bone, produces a fracture perpendicular to the long axis of the bone. When shear is involved, the fracture line is at 45 degrees to the direction of pull. An oblique fracture generally results from a combination of compression and shear loads. A torsional load produces a spiral fracture at 45 degrees to the longitudinal axis. With pure bending, the fracture often starts perpendicular to the long axis and then splits along two oblique planes. This pattern is thought to be due to a shear component on the concave side of the bone.

A stress fracture is not due to a single excessive load but rather to frequent repetitions of relatively low or normal loads. As such, stress fractures represent overuse injuries. Frequency of loading is critical in living bone and distinguishes it from various metals that also may fracture from fatigue after a finite number of load cycles have been applied. In living bone, the number of cycles leading to fatigue is not finite, in that the bone continues to adapt depending upon the frequency of loading. Stress fractures occur when the remodeling of bone is outpaced by the fatigue process. Stresses on the bone may be imposed by impact, muscle pull, or muscle fatigue.[97] Nordin and Frankel theorize that during continuous strenuous exercise, fatigued muscles are less capable of storing energy and neutralizing the stresses imposed on the bone.[96] Therefore, the bone may encounter abnormally high loads in this setting (Fig. 13–9). Muscle fatigue in the lower extremity may also change the gait pattern leading to abnormal loading, altered stress distributions, and subsequent stress fracture in the lower extremity bones. Thus, overuse can produce a clinical stress fracture directly caused by increased frequency of either impact-generated or muscle-generated loading cycles, or indirectly by altered mechanics or muscle fatigue, leading to abnormal loading cycles.

In a study in rabbits of tibial stress fractures produced by excessive jumping and running, vascular changes were the first pathologic change to occur in the development of a tibial stress fracture. Disturbances of circulation in the haversian systems with engorgement, vasodilatation, and hyaline thrombosis were observed initially. Cracks that initially appeared in the bone occurred at the cement lines of the haversian system. The convergence of several neighboring cracks produced the ultimate fracture line. Ischemia and anoxia may have been responsible for the subsequent acceleration of osteoclastic activity creating resorption cavities. Li and co-workers showed that early osteoclastic resorption of bone followed by osteoblastic new bone formation is part of the response to physical stress. It may be that during the initial phase of osteoclastic resorption, the bone is temporarily weakened. Continued activity at this time could produce an area of overload in the weakened bone and thereby, a stress fracture.[98]

The process of fracture healing is similar

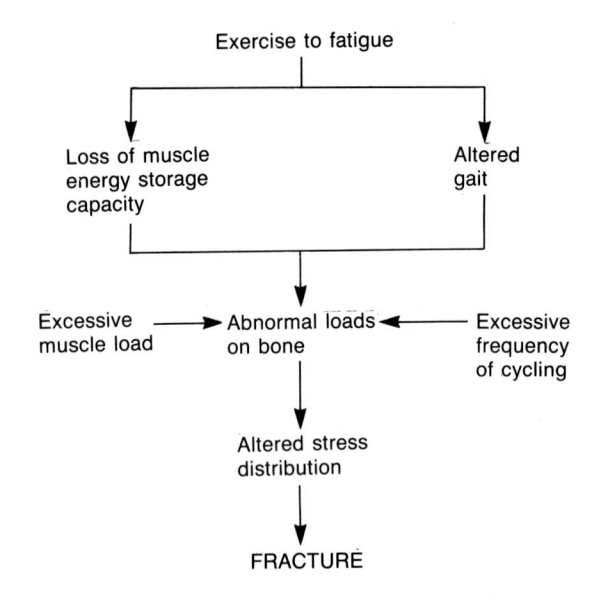

Figure 13–9 Factors leading to stress fracture.

in many ways to that of healing in other collagenous tissue, at least in its initial phases. Fracture healing initially requires an inflammatory phase, which is subsequently followed by repair and remodeling phases. The inflammatory process is identical to that seen in repair of other collagenous tissue, beginning with disruption of blood supply, hemorrhage, formation of clot, and influx of inflammatory cells. Damaged blood vessels and thrombus formation lead to bone death at the fractured bone ends. The osteocytes soon begin to degenerate, and within a few days empty lacunae may already be found 1 or 2 mm away from the fractured ends of the bone.[99]

As the reparative phase of fracture healing begins, usually within the first week following fracture, the phagocytic osteoclasts remove dead bone at the fracture surfaces.[100] This process can be seen radiographically as bone loss or apparent widening of the fracture line. Pluripotential mesenchymal cells in the periosteum and periosteal blood vessels proliferate in such a way that capillaries, fibroblasts, and cartilage cells predominate, and collagen and osteoid begin to be laid down to form callus (Fig. 13-10). Callus generally surrounds the ends of the fractured bone and is nature's way of providing internal fixation. The amount of callus produced is a function of both the mechanical and metabolic environments. When motion predominates, cartilage is formed and proceeds through an endochondral sequence to become bone. Direct bone repair occurs as well. When motion is limited as, for example, when internal fixation is used, little or no cartilage forms, and repair proceeds directly through woven bone to lamellar bone. Low oxygen tension is conducive to cartilage and bone production, whereas high oxygen tension and tensile stresses are associated with production of fibrous tissue leading to nonunion.[41] Despite the marked increase in vasculature at the fracture site, there is so much cell proliferation that the average bone or cartilage cell exists in relative hypoxia. Each type of cell present in the callus—fibroblast, chondroblast, and osteoblast—produces its metabolic products, e.g., type I and type II collagen, proteoglycans, and matrix proteins. Mineralization proceeds in cartilage and in new osteoid to bridge the fracture site with restoration of both periosteal and endosteal vasculature. As mineralization occurs, callus becomes visible on radiographs. Some authors have suggested that bioelectrical signals may activate cell replication, differentiation, and matrix production in callus.[101] In addition, the electrical potential seen on the surface of callus is strongly negative throughout healing.[102] This negative electrical potential encourages mineral deposition. Thus, fibrocartilaginous callus converts to woven bone. During remodeling, woven bone converts to lamellar bone. Although there is overlap between the remodeling and the repair phases of fracture healing, the end of the reparative phase is the point at which the fracture is structurally sound enough to allow normal function. Technically then remodeling begins.

Remodeling proceeds through the same process as does normal bone deposition and resorption, but at a greater rate.[103] Piezoelectrical messages are thought to aid in the remodeling process.[104] A fracture may be functionally healed early in the remodeling phase when the strength of the fractured bone equals its pre-fracture strength. Healing may not be apparent on radiographs, because mineralization of the callus surrounding the fracture line may proceed for months, and remodeling of bone to the point at which the medullary cavity is reestablished and the usual architecture is restored may take a year or more.

The phases of fracture healing may also be examined from a biochemical perspective. Hydroxyproline, RNA and DNA, calcium, magnesium, and phosphate increase progressively throughout fracture healing; the peak in mineral content occurs later than the peak in hydroxyproline and hexosamine content.[105]

Inductors of fracture healing may include the oxygen gradient, electrical potentials, and various growth factors previously discussed. The age and diet of the patient, as well as the presence or absence of normal amounts of growth hormone, thyroid hormone, parathyroid hormone, and corticosteroid, also affect fracture healing. NSAIDs that inhibit prostaglandin synthesis also may slow fracture healing by inhibiting the early inflammatory phase.[106,107]

A stress fracture may fail to heal because of the location of the fracture, inadequate immobilization, distraction, damage to the blood supply, or persistence of activity that causes the inflammatory process and resorption to continue at a rate exceeding that of repair, deposition, and remodeling. Just as in soft tissues,

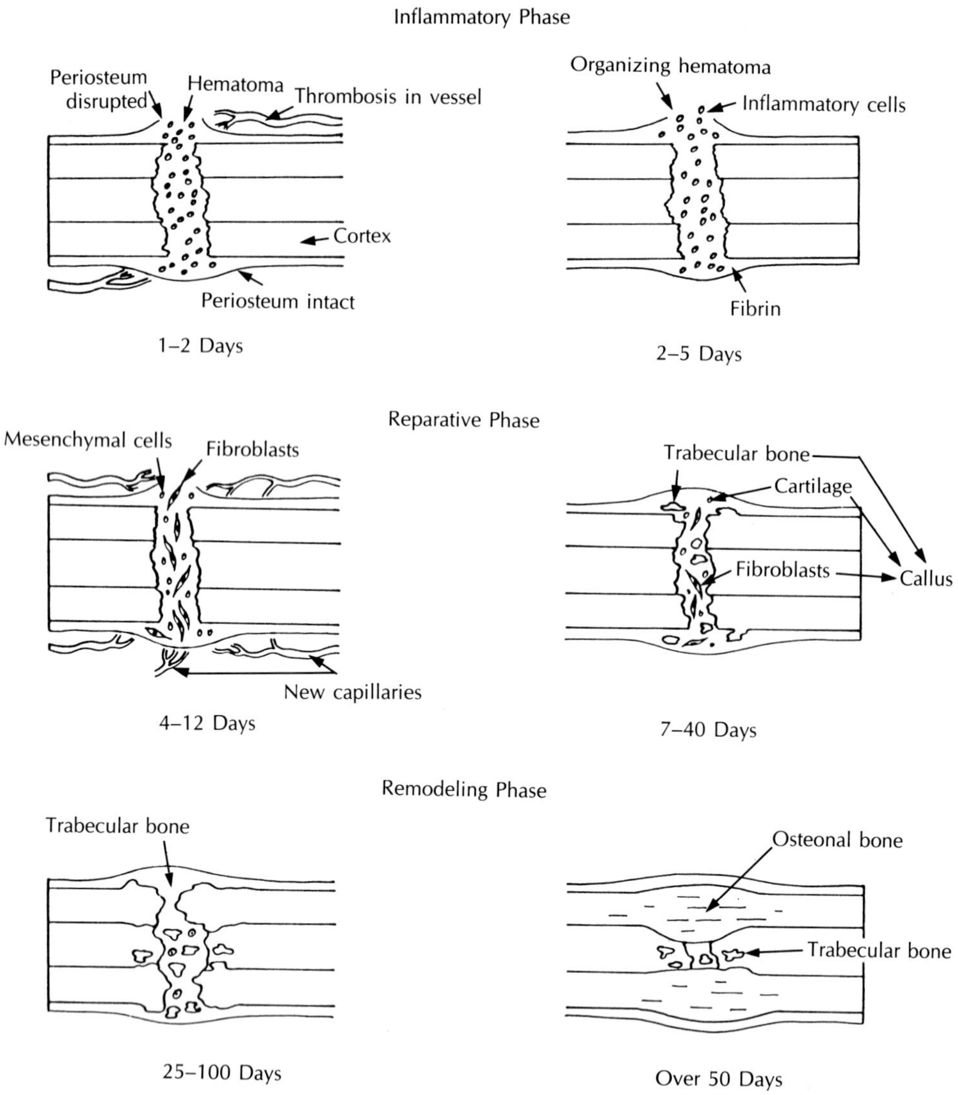

Figure 13-10 Schematic diagram of fracture healing sequence. (From Brand RA. Fracture healing. In: Albright JA, Brand RA, eds. The scientific basis of orthopaedics. New York: Appleton-Century-Crofts, 1979. Reprinted with permission.)

functional use of bone promotes healing. It is thought that early protected weight bearing following a fracture produces stress-generated potentials in the fracture callus that determine the orientation of collagen fibers, favoring mineralization and increasing the strength of the new bone.[41] The necessity for immobilization and the determination of the quantitative or qualitative type of loads necessary for fracture healing are yet to be determined, and they differ from one bone to the next.[108]

Clinical Correlation

Stress fractures were first described in the military and were known as march fractures. They occurred most commonly in the metatarsals when unconditioned recruits were subjected to strenuous activity. Subsequently, these fractures have been described in almost all of the lower extremity bones as well as in a number of upper extremity bones as a function of overuse. The clinical diagnosis of stress fracture is based on a history consistent with overuse and the physical finding of tenderness to palpation of a discrete area of bone. A stress fracture usually takes the form of a crack through the bone with no displacement. In many cases the crack is not visible on routine radiographs. As long as sufficient strength is present from new periosteal or endosteal bone, and movement at the fracture site is minimal, radiographically evident callus may not form. In other cases, the stress fracture can be recognized radiographically during the resorption phase between 7 and 10 days following fracture. Callus formation is most commonly seen in the metatarsals, and thickening of the cortex is seen in the tibia.

Bone scans (pictures taken of the involved limb following systemic injection of radioactive diphosphonate) are useful diagnostically when stress fractures are invisible on routine radiographs. "Positive" bone scans reflect the increased metabolic activity occurring during fracture healing. They often remain positive for up to a year after the time of stress fracture owing to continued remodeling at the fracture site.[103]

When treating a stress fracture, significant percussive load must be avoided, but other uses of the limb are helpful in providing the stresses necessary for growth of normal collagenous and skeletal tissue. For example, in a runner with a lower extremity stress fracture, running should be prohibited, but walking, swimming, rowing, and bicycling might be suggested as alternative means of remaining fit, using the limb, and avoiding further injurious forces.

MYOFASCIAL COMPARTMENTS

Normal Physiology

A myofascial compartment consists of a group of muscles, a major artery, and a nerve bounded by bone and relatively inelastic fascia. Because of the inelastic boundaries, any swelling that occurs within a compartment can lead to elevated intracompartmental pressure and ischemia of muscle and nerve. The swelling can be caused by trauma-induced hemorrhage, pooling of venous blood due to maintenance of the upright position, and drugs that produce fluid retention, such as birth control pills or danocrine. Elevated intracompartmental pressure also can arise from transient increases in skeletal muscle volume and from externally applied elastic wraps. During exercise, capillary pressure and capillary surface area within muscle increase, leading to greater transcapillary filtration of intravascular fluid and therefore greater skeletal muscle volume; "during prolonged exercise a muscle may retain so much extracellular fluid as to increase its weight by 20 percent. . . ."[109] The combination of the increased volume and the mechanical factors involved in muscle contraction produces an increase in the total intramuscular and intracompartmental pressure, the height of which is a function of the size and compliance of the surrounding fascia.

Pathophysiology

A compartmental syndrome begins when increased intracompartmental pressure produces local ischemia. Because intracompartmental tissue pressure is usually less than arterial blood pressure, distal arterial blood flow often remains intact. Similarly, because the digital capillary bed drains into extracompartmental veins, capillary circulation in the digits remains intact (Fig. 13–11). However, within the compartment, blood flow is determined by the local arteriovenous (AV) gradient and the local vas-

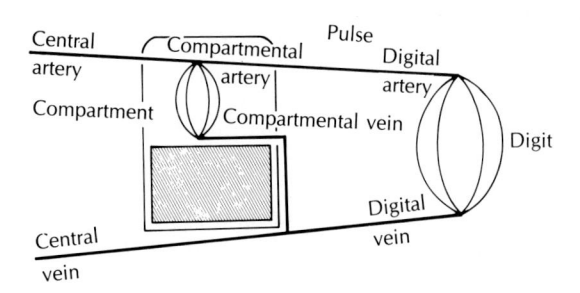

Figure 13–11 Comparison of local and distal effects of increased tissue pressure. (From Matsen FA III. Compartment syndromes. New York: Grune & Stratton, 1980. Reprinted with permission.)

cular resistance. As local tissue pressure increases, venous pressure increases, thereby lowering the AV gradient within the compartment. Any cause of lowered arterial pressure further compromises the local AV gradient and blood flow. As the AV gradient narrows, ischemia produces local vasodilatation so that the local vascular resistance decreases. Nevertheless, capillary circulation slows to the extent that it does not meet the metabolic demands of the muscle and nerve tissue. Rapidly metabolizing tissue may require more blood flow to maintain its viability than does resting muscle. Reneman and associates, in a study using rabbits, observed that when the applied pressure was 25 to 30 mm Hg less than mean arterial pressure, capillary blood flow ceased. Even with applied pressures as high as 60 mm Hg, no evidence of microvascular occlusion was found.[110]

The absolute intramuscular pressure that collapses blood vessels is determined by the geometric dimensions of interstitial spaces, the amount of fluid in the cells, and the physical characteristics of the surrounding tissues. In laboratory studies, the amount of external pressure required to elevate compartmental pressure ranges from 20 to 70 mm Hg. The variation in amount of pressure required to produce a compartmental syndrome and in pressure tolerance seen among individuals is related to duration of pressure, local arterial pressure, and metabolic demands of the tissue. Hargens and co-workers quantitated the decrement in nerve conduction velocity as a function of intracompartmental pressure in the canine leg anterolateral compartment. The time required to produce a conduction block was inversely proportional to the intracompartmental pressure.[111] Higher pressures required progressively less time to arrest nerve conduction.

Posttraumatic compartmental syndromes are acute and usually due to intracompartmental hemorrhage. In the athletic setting, compartmental syndrome is an intermittent yet chronic problem, i.e., one that comes and goes as a function of the degree of activity of the athlete; it has been called exertional compartmental syndrome and medial tibial syndrome.[109] The rapidity and degree of muscular swelling and the distensibility of the fascial wall determine whether the condition is acute (producing muscle necrosis) or chronic (producing pain during exercise).

Clinical Correlation

Wiley and associates described the clinical picture of exertional compartmental syndrome as the presence of crampy muscle pain precipitated by a fixed work load.[112] Because it takes a certain period of time for exercise-induced swelling to occur, pain related to ischemia in chronic compartmental syndrome does not occur upon initiation of exercise but rather at some point after beginning exercise. For a given individual, the time to onset of pain after initiation of exercise is often standard and may be related to the individual's circulatory status and venous competence. When exercise is stopped, allowing normal venous drainage, the arteriovenous gradient returns to normal and symptoms subside. This explains the usual course of chronic compartmental syndrome in athletes. Pain in the anterior or deep posterior tibial compartments, which began at a certain time after starting exercise, subsides within a few hours following cessation of exercise. Rarely is there associated numbness as is noted with acute compartmental syndromes, probably because resolution of the intracompartmental pressure occurs fairly rapidly after exercise stops. Clinically, muscle hernias are seen in 40 to 60 percent of patients with chronic compartmental syndromes.[113,114] Most frequently these hernias are in the anterolateral distal half of the leg. They represent a decompression of the compartment by a spontaneous opening in the tough fascial membrane.

In order to confirm the diagnosis of chronic compartmental syndrome, compartmental pressures must be measured before and immediately after exercise and after a recovery period of 10 to 20 minutes. Patients with chronic compartmental syndromes usually have high resting pressures and consistently require prolonged periods of time for compartmental pressures to return to preexercise levels.[115,116] In Qvarfordt's study of 108 athletic patients with leg pain, 14 percent were found to have exertional compartmental syndromes. Their resting pressures ranged from 18 to 28 mm Hg, with a mean of 22; the resting mean pressure of asymptomatic controls was 8 mm Hg (ranging from 2 to 23 mm Hg). After exercise, mean compartmental pressure in the symptomatic patients was 80 mm Hg, with a range from 48 to 135; in controls, the mean was 26 mm Hg (range from 8 to 60 mm Hg). In the controls, the return to resting pressure took approximately 1 minute. In the symptomatic patients, the return to resting pressures averaged 40 minutes, with a range from 10 to 120 minutes. Biopsy in these patients showed an increase in water content in the anterior tibial muscles. Blood flow, as measured with xenon-133, was found to be decreased, particularly after exercise. Qvarfordt and associates also found an increased level of lactic acid in the involved muscles. Following surgical compartmental release, blood flow after exercise increased, lactic acid decreased, but water content remained unchanged.[113] This evidence supports the theory that the increase in pressure found in muscular compartments of patients with exertional compartmental syndrome is caused by an increase in the interstitial fluid pressure (Fig. 13–12).[117]

The treatment of exertional compartmental syndrome can take the form of decreasing the exercise below the individual's ischemic threshold, stopping, when possible, any medication that is causing fluid retention, or surgically releasing the fascia of the involved compartments.[118,119] Because ischemia normally leads to vasodilatation, attempts at decreasing vascular resistance further by sympathectomy or vasodilator drugs have not proven useful in the treatment of compartmental syndromes. Similarly, diuretics have not proven effective, because they dehydrate the athlete without changing the intracompartmental fluid mechanics.

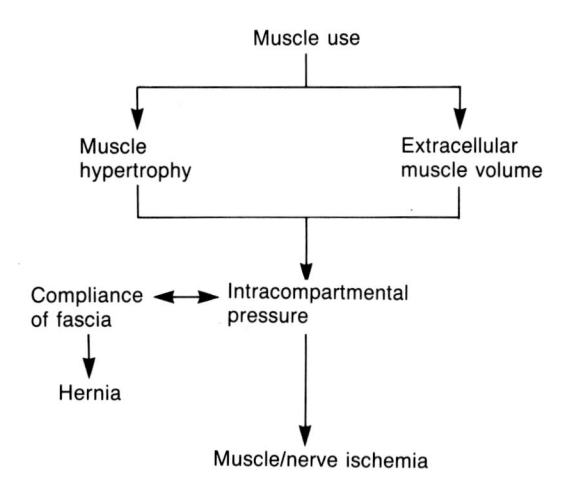

Figure 13–12 Factors leading to exertional compartmental syndrome

TREATMENT PRINCIPLES

Treatment of overuse injuries must include identification of exacerbating factors. Relative rest of the injured part is a critical early component of treatment. The active individual may not require total rest, but can decrease the frequency or duration of the involved activity or change components of that activity so as not to stress the injured area. In other cases the injured part may be taped, braced, or immobilized. The patient can be kept physically active either in the same activity in which he was injured or in a different activity, as long as the stresses to the injured part can be avoided.

If the training schedule is identified as a factor in the production of injury, it must be changed. The old adage of "taking one's time" applies here. From the discussion above, it should be apparent that if the musculoskeletal tissues are given the opportunity to remodel in response to stress, they will do so. One must consider the frequency, intensity, and duration of training. The duration and intensity of activity should not produce delayed onset muscle soreness or bone pain. A conservative training schedule might include a 10 percent increment in amount of activity each week. We generally suggest this in combination with a peak-and-valley type of training method so that the tissues are given a chance to adapt (Fig. 13–13). We also suggest to an athlete who wishes to train on a daily basis that the activities on alternate days emphasize use of different body parts, so that parts previously stressed can initiate an adaptive response before being subject to significant load again. A person should not necessarily be running daily but might alternate running with swimming, rowing, biking, or weight lifting.

Technique, as mentioned earlier in this chapter, is often critical in the production of overuse injuries, because poor technique produces inefficient use of musculature. Hence, any methods for improving technique are useful,

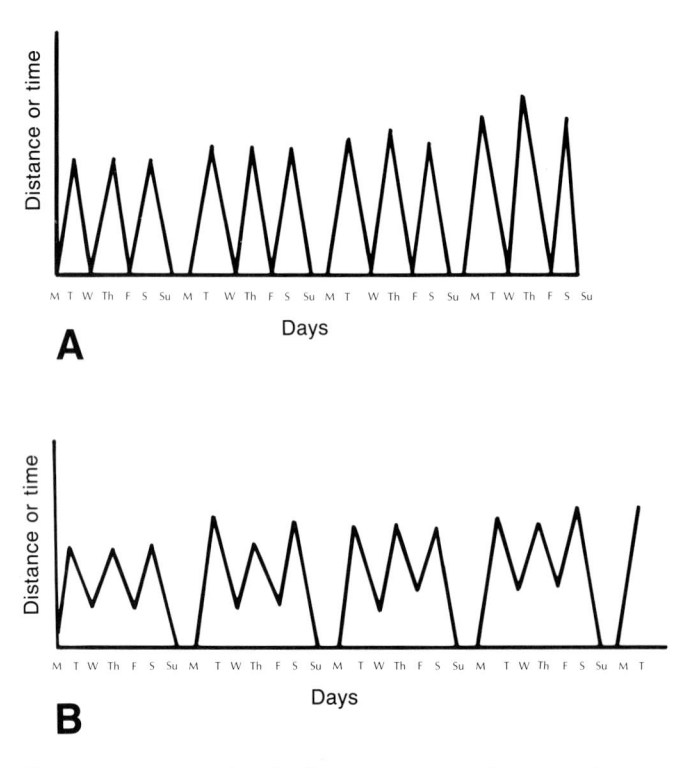

Figure 13–13 (A) Peak-and-valley training method utilizing the concepts of alternate-day activity and 10 percent increment in amount of activity per week. (B) Peak-and-valley training method utilizing daily training and a 10 percent increment in amount of activity per week.

including coaching and proprioceptive neuromuscular facilitation.[120]

When possible, alignment should be changed actively or passively. Increasing vastus medialis strength might actively alter patellar tracking and therefore patellofemoral alignment. Similarly, it may be possible to provide some active support for the arch by strengthening the posterior tibialis muscle and the digital flexors in the foot. Passive alignment changes can be produced with arch supports in the shoes, knee sleeves with lateral patellar pads, and various orthotic devices. Lateral shoe wedges may be useful for the patient with hindfoot varus, just as medial supports are useful for those patients with excessive midfoot pronation, cavus feet, and pes planus. True leg length discrepancies can be modified with heel lifts. Rarely is alignment changed surgically.

Patterns of wear in shoes often provide important clues, particularly to dynamic alterations in lower extremity alignment. Worn shoes also can contribute to overuse injury when they lack proper support or shock absorption. The latter can be improved using insoles made of Sorbothane or similar viscous rubberlike materials. Poorly fitted pointe shoes prevent accurate positioning and lead to posterior tibial and peroneal tendinitis in the ballet dancer. Equipment must be considered as a factor contributing to injury and should be adjusted accordingly.

Strengthening of limbs and trunk should be specific to the patient as well as to the sport. To avoid recurrent injury, the injured part needs to be strengthened to regain and perhaps exceed its preinjury strength. Certain injuries are more common in some sports than others, e.g., swimmer's shoulder, runner's knee, bowler's thumb, tennis elbow. For a patient who is going to engage in a throwing sport, for example, strengthening of the rotator cuff proves useful;

adductor strengthening in the thigh would be particularly useful for an avid horseback rider. Often one can identify areas of potential injury in a given patient as a function of the specific sport planned and that patient's anatomical structure. These areas should be strengthened or, in some cases, attempts should be made to make the associated joints more flexible.

Flexibility requirements also may be sport specific as well as patient specific. A patient who has particularly tight hamstring muscles or Achilles tendons is likely to benefit from flexibility exercises oriented specifically to these areas. Dance and gymnastics in particular demand a great amount of flexibility in the shoulders, hips, and ankles. Except in the case of the hypermobile individual, flexibility exercises should be encouraged for patients engaged in these types of activities. Because collagen is sensitive to temperature, flexibility exercises should be undertaken not as the warm-up but after the body is warm, in order to produce plastic deformation in the collagenous tissue, rather than elastic deformation. This should produce more permanent changes in flexibility. Patients who are already hyperflexible may need to refrain from additional flexibility exercises and work more on strengthening.[121,122]

Finally, aerobic conditioning is useful, because it decreases fatigue and increases capillarization of muscles, both of which make subsequent injury less likely.[123]

In summary, soft and bony tissues are markedly similar in their responses to normal stress, to overuse, and to injury. How these tissues respond to stress is not completely understood. It is widely assumed that all connective tissues contain cells that retain their embryonic potential for division and differentiation. The message to multiply and differentiate can be evoked by a variety of stimuli.[124] These stimuli may include a combination of electrical, physical, and biomechanical stresses that get translated biochemically at the level of the cell membrane by cyclic nucleotides to regulate the necessary reparative processes.

Overuse injuries occur when the normal physiologic response to stress is exceeded and remodeling cannot keep up with the frequency and duration of cyclical loading. In response to stress, both bone and soft tissues respond in accordance with Wolff's law.[71] Soft tissue responds by thickening and by increasing collagen content, glycosaminoglycans, weight, and volume. Bone responds by increasing the formation of trabeculae. The healing response in both soft and bony tissues requires an inflammatory phase initially, followed by repair and remodeling phases. Because inflammation is necessary for healing to occur, NSAIDs used too early in the treatment of overuse injuries may interfere with the repair process. In addition, if one continues to load the injured tissue, the tissue is likely not to proceed from the early inflammatory phase to the subsequent necessary phases of repair and remodeling. Treatment of overuse injuries must include a careful analysis and modification of contributing factors.

REFERENCES

1. Armstrong RB. Mechanisms of exercise-induced delayed onset muscle soreness. A brief review. Med Sci Sports Exerc 1984; 16:529–538.
2. Veis A, Sabsay B. The collagen of mineralized matrices. In: Peck WA, ed. Bone and mineral research. Amsterdam: Elsevier, 1987:1.
3. Curwin S, Stanish WD. Normal tendon. In: Tendinitis: its etiology and treatment. Lexington, MA: DC Heath, 1984:1–24.
4. Smart GW, Taunton JE, Clement DB. Achilles tendon disorders in runners—a review. Med Sci Sports Exerc 1980; 12:231–243.
5. Bistevins R, Awad EA. Structure and ultrastructure of mechanoreceptors at the human musculotendinous junction. Arch Phys Med Rehabil 1981; 62:74–82.
6. Gotte L, Mammi M, Pezzin G. Scanning electron microscope observation on elastin. Connect Tiss Res 1972; 1:61–67.
7. Nordin M, Frankel VH. Biomechanics of collagenous tissues. In: Basic biomechanics of the skeletal system. Philadelphia: Lea & Febiger, 1980:87–110.
8. Elliott DH. Structure and function of mammalian tendon. Biol Rev 1965; 40:392–421.
9. Walker LB, Harris EH, Benedict JV. Stress–strain relationships in human plantaris tendon: a preliminary study. Med Elect Biol Eng 1964; 2:31–38.
10. Wahrenberg H, Lindbeck L, Ekholm J. Dynamic load in the human knee during voluntary active impact to the lower leg. Scand J Rehabil Med 1978; 10:93–98.
11. Wahrenberg H, Lindbeck L, Ekholm J. Knee muscular movement, tendon tension, and EMG activity during a vigorous movement in man. Scand J Rehabil Med 1978A; 10:99–106.
12. Zernicke RF, Garhammer J, Jobe FW. Human patellar tendon rupture. J Bone Joint Surg 1977; 59A:179–183.
13. Curwin S, Stanish WD. Tendinitis. In: Tendinitis: its

etiology and treatment. Lexington, MA: DC Heath, 1984:25–44.
14. Barfred T. Experimental rupture of the Achilles tendon: comparison of different types of experimental rupture in rats. Acta Orthop Scand 1971; 42:528–543.
15. Newham DJ, Mills KR, Quigley BM, Edwards RHT. Pain and fatigue after concentric and eccentric muscle contractions. Clin Sci 1983; 64:55–62.
16. Rathbun J, Macnab I. The microvascular pattern of the rotator cuff. J Bone Joint Surg 1970; 52B:540–553.
17. Okuda Y, Gorski JP, An KN, Amadio PC. Biochemical, histological, and biomechanical analysis of canine tendon. J Orthop Res 1987; 5:60–68.
18. Soft tissue disorders. In: Simon SR, Riggins RS, Wirth CR, Fox ML, eds. Orthopaedic science. Park Ridge, IL: American Academy of Orthopedic Surgeons, 1986:72.
19. Landi AP, Altman FP, Pringle J, Landi A. Oxidative enzyme metabolism in rabbit intrasynovial flexor tendons. I. Changes in enzyme activities of the tenocytes with age. J Surg Res 1980; 29:276–280.
20. Lehmann JF, Masock AJ, Warren CG, et al. Effect of therapeutic temperatures on tendon extensibility. Arch Phys Med Rehabil 1970; 51:481–487.
21. Sapega AA, Quedenfeld TC, Moyer RA, Butler RA. Biophysical factors in range-of-motion exercise. Phys Sportsmed 1981; 9:57–65.
22. Woo SL-Y, Gomez MA, Woo Y-K, et al. Mechanical properties of tendons and ligaments: II. The relationships of immobilization and exercise on tissue remodeling. Biorheology 1982; 19:397–408.
23. Viidik A. Tensile strength properties of Achilles tendon systems in trained and untrained rabbits. Acta Orthop Scand 1969; 40:261–272.
24. Tipton CM, Matthes RD, Maynard JA, Carey RA. The influence of physical activity on ligaments and tendons. Med Sci Sports Exerc 1975; 7:165–175.
25. Woo SL-Y, Matthews JV, Akeson WH et al. Connective tissue response to immobility. Arthritis Rheum 1975; 18:257–264.
26. Vailas AC, Tipton CM, Matthes RD, Gart M. Physical activity and its influence on the repair process of medial collateral ligaments. Connect Tiss Res 1981; 9:25–31.
27. Weissmann G, Zurier RB, Hoffstein S. Leukotactic proteases and the immunologic release of lysosomal enzymes. Am J Pathol 1972; 68:539–564.
28. Janoff A. Human granulocyte elastase. Am J Pathol 1972; 68:579–592.
29. Taubman SB, Goldschmidt PR, Lepow IH. Effects of lysosomal enzymes from human leukocytes on human complement components. Fed Proc 1970; 29:434.
30. Weissman G, Dukor P, Zurier RB. Effect of cyclic AMP on release of lysosomal enzymes from phagocytes. Nature 1971; 231:131–135.
31. Bourne HR, Lichtenstein LM, Melmon KL, et al. Modulation of inflammation and immunity by cyclic AMP. Science 1974; 184:19–28.
32. DiSabatino CA. Inflammation. In: Albright JS, Brand RA, eds. The scientific basis of orthopaedics. New York: Appleton-Century-Crofts, 1979:415–436.
33. Ross R. The fibroblast and wound repair. Biol Rev 1968; 43:51–96.
34. Forrester JC, Zederfelt BH, Hayes TL, et al. Wolff's law in relation to the healing skin wound. J Trauma 1970; 10:770–779.
35. Akeson WH, Amiel D, LaViolette D. The connective tissue response to immobility: a study of the chondroitin-4 and 6 sulfate and dermatan sulfate changes in periarticular connective tissue of control and immobilized knees of dogs. Clin Orthop 1967; 51:183–197.
36. Gelberman RH, Manske PR, Akeson WH, et al. Flexor tendon repair. Orthop Res 1986; 4:119–128.
37. Weber ER. Nurtritional pathways for flexor tendons in the digital theca. In: Hunter JM, Schneider LH, Mackin EJ, eds. Tendon surgery in the hand. St Louis: CV Mosby, 1987:91.
38. Mason ML, Allen HS. The rate of healing of tendons. Ann Surg 1941; 223:424–459.
39. Woo SL-Y, Gelberman RH, Cobb NG, et al. The importance of controlled passive mobilization on flexor tendon healing. Acta Orthop Scand 1981; 52:615–622.
40. Gelberman RH, Goldberg VM, An K, Banes A. Tendon. In: Woo SL-Y, Buckwalter JA, eds. Injury and repair of the musculoskeletal soft tissues. Park Ridge, IL:American Academy of Orthopaedic Surgeons, 1988:1.
41. Brighton CT. Principles of fracture healing. In: Instructional course lectures. St. Louis: CV Mosby, 1984; 33:60–82.
42. Curwin S, Stanish WD. Exercise and the muscle-tendon unit. In: Tendinitis: its etiology and treatment. Lexington, MA: DC Heath, 1984:45.
43. Laughman RK, Youdas JW, Garrett TR, Chao EYS. Strength changes in the normal quadriceps femoris muscle as a result of electrical stimulation. Phys Ther 1983; 63:494–499.
44. Almekinders LC, Gilbert JA. Healing of experimental muscle strains and the effects of nonsteroidal anti-inflammatory medication. Am J Sports Med 1986; 14:303–308.
45. Kennedy JC, Baxter-Willis R. The effects of local steroid injections on tendons: a biochemical and microscopic correlative study. Am J Sports Med 1976; 4:11–18.
46. Halpern AA, Horowitz BG, Nagel DA. Tendon ruptures associated with corticosteroid therapy. West J Med 1977; 127:378–382.
47. Albright JA. Bone: physical properties. In: Albright JA, Brand RA, eds. The scientific basis of orthopaedics. Norwalk, CT: Appleton and Lange, 1987:213–240.
48. Albright JA. Bone: Physical properties. In: Albright JA, Brand RA, eds. The scientific basis of orthopaedics. New York: Appleton-Century-Crofts, 1979:135–183.
49. Ascenzi A, Bonucci E. Relationship between ultrastructure and "pin test" in osteons. Clin Orthop 1976; 121:275–294.
50. Skinner HC, Kempner E, Pak CY. Preparation of the mineral phase of bone using ethylene diamine extraction. Calcif Tissue Res 1972; 10:257–268.
51. Skinner HCW. Bone mineralization. In: Albright JA,

Brand RA, eds. The scientific basis of orthopaedics. Norwalk, CT: Appleton and Lange, 1987:199.
52. Katz EP, Li ST. Structure and function of bone collagen fibrils. J Mol Biol 1973; 80:1–15.
53. Wuthier RE. A review of the primary mechanism of endochondral calcification with special emphasis on the role of cells, mitochondria, and matrix vesicles. Clin Orthop 1982; 169:219–242.
54. Baylink D, Wergedal J, Thomson E. Loss of protein polysaccharides at sites where bone mineralization is initiated. J Histochem Cytochem 1972; 20:279–292.
55. Anatomy. In: Orthopaedic science. Park Ridge, IL: American Academy of Orthopaedic Surgeons, 1986:2–40.
56. Boskey AL. Current concepts of the physiology and biochemistry of calcification. Clin Orthop 1981; 157:225–258.
57. Teitlebaum SL. The cellular mechanisms of bone resorption. Presented at 55th annual meeting: American Academy of Orthopaedic Surgeons. Atlanta, GA: Feb 4, 1988.
58. Bonucci E. New knowledge on the origin, function, and fate of osteoclasts. Clin Orthop 1981; 158:252–269.
59. Chamay A, Tschantz P. Mechanical influences in bone remodeling. Experimental research on Wolff's law. J Biomech 1972; 5:173–180.
60. Frost HM. Tetracycline-based histological analysis of bone remodeling. Calc Tiss Res 1969; 3:211–237.
61. Risz LG, Kream BE. Regulation of bone formation. N Engl J Med 1983; 309:29–35.
62. Canalis E. Effect of growth factors on bone cell replication and differentiation. Clin Orthop 1985; 193:246–263.
63. Urist MR, Lietze A, Mizutani H, et al. A bovine low molecular weight bone morphogenetic protein (BMP) fraction. Clin Orthop 1982; 162:219–232.
64. Canalis E, Centrella M, Urist M. Effect of partially purified morphogenetic protein on DNA synthesis and cell replication in calvarial and fibroblast cultures. Clin Orthop 1985; 198:289–296.
65. Postlethwaite AE, Keski-Oja J, Moses HL, et al. Stimulation of the chemotactic migration of human fibroblasts by transforming growth factor beta. J Exp Med 1987; 165:251–256.
66. Sporn MB, Roberts AB, Wakefield LM, et al. Transforming growth factor beta: biological function and chemical structure. Science 1985; 223:532–534.
67. Sampath TK, Reddi AH. Distribution of bone inductive proteins in mineralized and demineralized extracellular matrix. Biochem Biophys Res Commun 1984; 119:949–954.
68. Rath NC, Reddi AH. Collagenous bone matrix is a local mitogen. Nature 1979; 278:855–857.
69. Postlethwaite AE, Seyer JM, Kang AH. Chemotactic attraction of human fibroblasts to type I, II, and III collagens and collagen-derived peptides. Proc Natl Acad Sci USA 1978; 75:871–875.
70. Rodan G, Bourret LA, Harvey A, Mensi T. Cyclic AMP and cyclic GMP: mediators of the mechanical effects on bone remodeling. Science 1975; 189:467–469.
71. Wolff J. Das Gesetz, der Transformation, der Knochen. Berlin: Hirschwold, 1892.
72. Kummer BFK. Biomechanics of bone: mechanical properties, functional structure, functional adaptation. In: Fung YC, Perrone N, Anliker M, eds. Biomechanics. Its foundations and objectives. Englewood Cliffs, NJ: Prentice-Hall, 1972:237.
73. Clark EA, Goodship AE, Lanyon LE. Locomotor bone strain as the stimulus for bone's mechanical adaptability. J Physiol 1975; 245:57P.
74. Johnson LC. The kinetics of skeletal remodeling. In: Structural organization of the skeleton. Birth defects original article series. New York: National Foundation, 1966:66.
75. Rambaut P, Johnson RS. Prolonged weightlessness and calcium loss in man. Acta Astron 1979; 29:1113–1122.
76. Goodship AE, Lanyon LE, McFie H. Functional adaptation of bone to increased stress. J Bone Joint Surg 1979; 61A:539–546.
77. Frost HM. A determinant of bone architecture. Clin Orthop 1983; 175:286–292.
78. Anderson JJ, Milin L, Crackel WC. Effect of exercise on mineral and organic turnover in swine. J Appl Physiol 1971; 30:810–813.
79. Frisancho AR, Montoye HJ, Frantz ME, et al. A comparison of morphological variables in adult males selected on the basis of physical activity. Med Sci Sports Exerc 1970; 2:209–212.
80. Skrobak-Kaczynski J, Andersen KL. Age dependent osteoporosis among men habituated to a high level of physical activity. Acta Morph Neerl Scand 1974; 12:283–292.
81. Eisenberg E, Gordon GS. Skeletal dynamics in man measured by nonradioactive strontium. J Clin Invest 1961; 40:1809–1825.
82. Dalen N, Olsson KE. Bone mineral content and physical activity. Acta Orthop Scand 1974; 45:170–174.
83. Nilsson BE, Westlin NE. Bone density in athletes. Clin Orthop 1971; 77:179–182.
84. Jones HH, Priest JD, Hayes WC, et al. Humeral hypertrophy in response to exercise. J Bone Joint Surg 1977; 59A:204–208.
85. Aloia JF, Cohn SH, Ostuni JA, et al. Prevention of involutional bone loss by exercise. Ann Intern Med 1978; 89:356–358.
86. Cann C, Martin MC, Genant HK, Jaffe RB. Decreased spinal mineral content in amenorrheic women. JAMA 1984; 251:626–629.
87. Drinkwater BL, Nilson K, Chesnut CH III et al. Bone mineral content of amenorrheic and eumenorrheic athletes. N Engl J Med 1984; 311:277–281.
88. Singh S, Saha S. Electrical properties of bone. Clin Orthop 1984; 186:249–271.
89. Chakkalakal DA, Johnson MW. Electrical properties of compact bone. Clin Orthop 1981; 161:133–145.
90. Hughes S, Davies R, Kahn R, Kelly P. Fluid space in bone. Clin Orthop 1978; 134:332–341.
91. Pollack SR. Bioelectrical properties of bone. Orthop Clin North Am 1984; 15:3–14.
92. Brighton CT. Current concepts review. The treatment of nonunions with electricity. J Bone Joint Surg 1981; 63A:847–851.
93. Bassett CA, Mitchell SN, Gaston SR. Pulsing electromagnetic field treatment in ununited fractures and failed arthrodeses. JAMA 1982; 247:623–628.
94. Justus R, Luft JH. A mechanochemical hypothesis for

association with marching), were not seen in children involved in recreational play. All this changed, of course, with the advent of intense sports training for children.[4]

Children, we now know, may actually be more vulnerable to overuse injury than adults because of the presence of an especially susceptible tissue, growth cartilage, and because of the growth process itself, which may induce muscle imbalances around joints and increase the risk of injury.[3] A third factor that appears to be assuming increased importance is the variability of coaching and training available to this group of young athletes, in particular the growing trend toward more intense training in children's sports programs. Some swimming programs now have 11-year-olds swimming 7,000 to 10,000 yards per day.

ANATOMY AND PATHOPHYSIOLOGY

The child's growing bone has a complex architecture, defined in part by the three sites of growth cartilage: at the ends of the long bones underlying the joint surface; at the growth plate or physis, which is responsible for the majority of skeletal growth; and at the sites of major muscle-tendon insertions, the traction apophyses (Fig. 14–1). Cartilage cells that blend into the hyaline cartilage at the joint surface differentiate, mature, and undergo endochondral ossification, resulting in growth in size and shape of the bone end. The end of the bone,

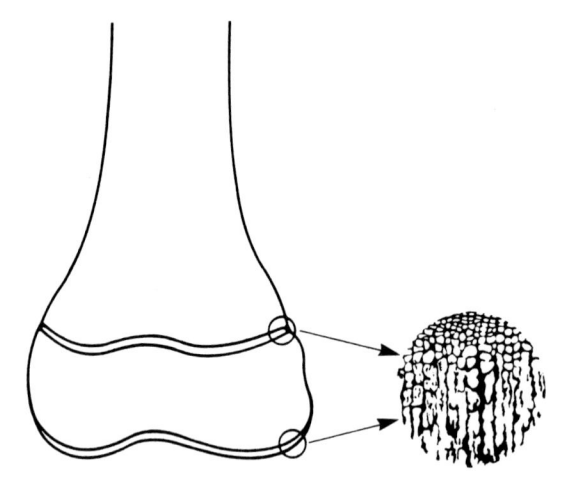

Figure 14–1 Growth cartilage is present at three sites in the child: the growth plate, or physis; the joint surface; and the apophyses, sites of major muscle-tendon insertions.

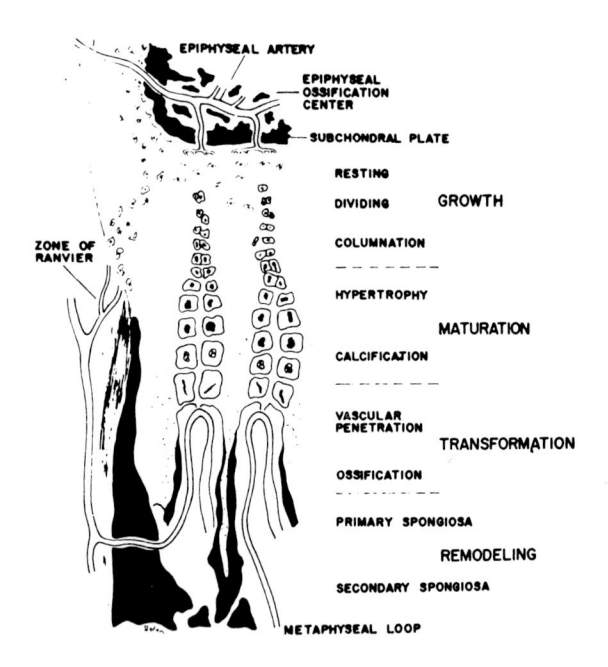

Figure 14–2 Microanatomy of the human growth plate. (From Ogden J. Postnatal development and growth of the musculoskeletal system. In: Albright JA, Brand RA, eds. The scientific basis of orthopaedics. East Norwalk, CT: Appleton & Lange, 1987.)

or epiphysis, has as its base the physis or growth plate. This growth plate is responsible for longitudinal growth of the bones.

For purposes of discussion, the growth plate is often described in zones (Fig. 14–2). However, it should be realized that the zones are not totally discrete, that cells merge between zones, and that the basic underlying collagen framework is interspersed throughout.[5] In long bones, the physes progress from planar to undulating structures.[6] The zone closest to the epiphysis is the reserve zone. This zone is richly supplied by arterioles from the epiphyseal vessels. Cells may arise not only from the resting chondrocytes in this zone, but also from the perivascular regions and the zone of Ranvier (see below). The collagen in this zone is randomly distributed. Cells in this zone contain glycogen, appear to store lipids, and have abundant endoplasmic reticulum. The reserve zone also contains more hydroxyproline than any other zone in the plate, as well as aggregated proteoglycan.[7] In the adjacent proliferative zone, cellular division occurs. Division occurs in a direction corresponding to the long axis of the bone, creating columns of cells. The collagen in this zone becomes longitudinally oriented and lies between the columns of cells. The cells in the proliferative zone, as those in the reserve zone, also contain glycogen and rich endoplasmic reticulum. The matrix in this zone contains matrix vesicles, neutral glycoproteins, and proteoglycan aggregates. These two zones together are considered the region of growth.

The next region, that of maturation, consists of a zone of hypertrophy and a zone of calcification. In the hypertrophic zone, cartilage matrix is generated, and the chondrocytes swell and gradually lose their cytoplasmic organelles and glycogen. As the cells die, mitochondrial calcium is given up and may be involved in matrix calcification. When calcification occurs, diffusion of nutrients and oxygen to the hypertrophic chondrocyte is decreased, and anaerobic glycolysis with glycogen consumption occurs until all the glycogen is depleted. The calcification that then occurs does so within or upon matrix vesicles that are present in the longitudinal septa of the matrix. Degradation of proteoglycan aggregates also occurs in this region and is associated with mineral growth. It is postulated that the three-dimensional structure of the proteoglycans in the reserve and part of the hypertrophic zone may inhibit mineralization.[7] Vessels invade from terminal branches of the metaphyseal arteriolar loops, and the chondroid septa then transform into trabecular bone through the elaboration of osteoid matrix by osteoblasts. These osteoblasts may come from perivascular cells or from preexisting chondrocytes.[8] Subsequent remodeling occurs in the metaphysis, which is immediately adjacent to the diaphysis. The diaphysis, or shaft of the bone, connects the two ends. It consists of a cylinder of cortical bone and a central medullary canal. In the child, its endosteal and periosteal tissues also are active in forming, resorbing, and remodeling the cortical bone, and they contribute to growth in diaphyseal circumference and cortical thickness.

In addition to the structures mentioned above, at the periphery of the growth plate is an anatomic structure bordered on its exterior by fibrous periosteum and on its interior by the physeal and epiphyseal cartilage. This circumferential zone contains a fibrous component consisting of a wedge-shaped groove of cells (the groove of Ranvier) and a ring of fibrous tissue and bone demarcating the periphery of the physis (the ring of Lacroix).[9] Although they are part of the same structure, these two components have different functions. The groove of Ranvier supplies chondrocytes for circumferential growth, whereas the perichondrial ring mechanically limits and supports the growth plate, much like the bark on a tree. The ring of Lacroix is an extension of the metaphyseal cortex; together with the groove of Ranvier it acts as an anchor for the periosteum and the growth plate. In addition, osteoblast precursors may originate in this zone, as may cartilage progenitor cells contributing to circumferential growth by apposition.

In the carpal and tarsal bones more spherical physes are found. The process of ossification is similar to that in the physis at the ends of long bones. The spherical physis assumes the shape of its future bone by progressive centrifugal expansion modified by the morphology of the bone in which it is contained. Some of these small bones develop additional centers of ossification, for example the os trigonum of the talus or the accessory tarsal navicular bone.

Apophyses are traditionally thought of as bony protuberances, where a tendon inserts in bone whose growth plates are responsive to traction. They do not contribute to longitudinal growth. The differences among various types of growth plates lie in the overall height of the physis and the cellular density in each zone. In addition, in the apophyses, the zone of hypertrophy is replaced with a zone of fibrocartilage.[10] Ogden and Southwick studied the development of the apophysis on the anterior aspect of the tibia, the tibial tuberosity, and found that this physis showed structural adaptations to accommodate the large tensile stresses imposed by the quadriceps mechanism.[11] While the main proximal tibial physis expands distally toward the tuberosity, the apophyseal growth plate grows proximally and anteriorly. These two ossification centers remain separated by a zone of cartilage until close to skeletal maturity. Therefore this chondro-osseous region where the patellar tendon inserts is relatively weak and may be acutely or chronically traumatized to create the classic clinical and radiographic features of Osgood-Schlatter disease (Fig. 14–3). Other entities previously classed as osteochondroses—Sever's disease of the heel and Köhler's disease of the tarsal navicular—most probably result from

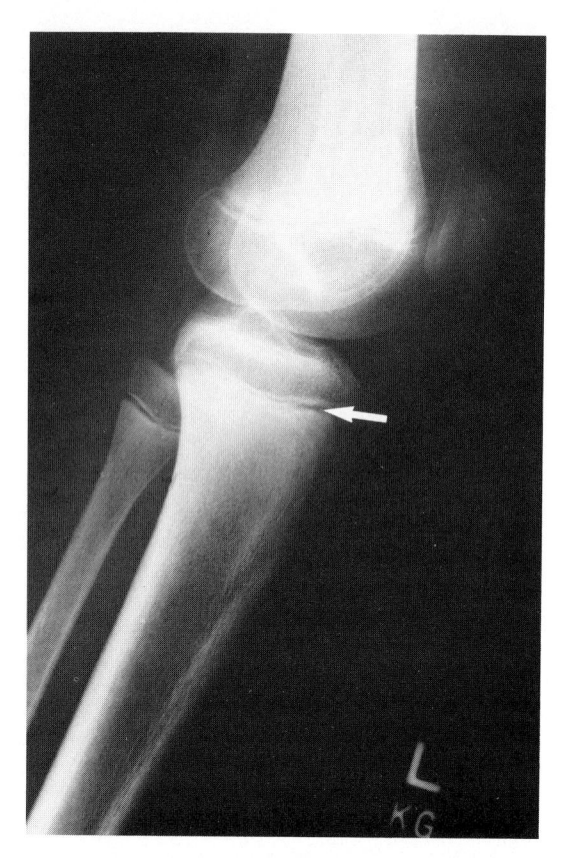

Figure 14-3 Osgood Schlatter apophysitis of the tibial tubercle is the result of repetitive microavulsions of the tendon insertion in the adolescent.

repetitive microtrauma to the apophyseal growth plate and are really stress fractures or vascular insults, not developmental disorders of cartilaginous growth. This group of disorders was named apophysites, the suffix "itis" used because of the inflammatory response that often accompanies these tiny avulsion injuries.[12] Other apophyses injured in the adolescent athlete include that of the lesser trochanter, the ischial tuberosity, and the iliac spine.[13,14]

The growth plate gets its blood supply from epiphyseal, metaphyseal, and perichondrial vessels. However, the central zone of the physis is relatively avascular. Once the small arteries cross the subchrondal plate, they become endarterioles. The variation in vascularity and therefore in oxygen tension in different regions of the growth plate is thought to play a role in cell differentiation.[15] When vasculature is compromised, as for example during fracture, the cells cannot undergo their usual growth and maturation processes, whereas the unaffected areas continue to grow. This may result in deformity, particularly if the injured area is near the periphery of the physis.[16] Because interruption of the metaphyseal blood supply does not directly affect the division and growth of the chondrocytes in the physis, injury in this region of the growth plate does not usually result in abnormal growth.

On the basis of this knowledge, Salter and Harris developed a classification of physeal injuries.[17] This classification has been extremely useful in predicting prognosis after physeal fracture. The fractures are classed from type I through type V, based on the site of fracture, the extent of involvement of adjacent epiphysis and metaphysis, the hypothesized mechanism of injury, and the potential for subsequent growth arrest, with type I being considered the most innocuous and type V the most likely to produce growth arrest (Fig. 14-4).

Ogden has recently expanded this classification to include types VI through IX. In a type VI fracture, there is injury to the peripheral margin of the growth plate including the groove of Ranvier. These injuries may result in localized marginal growth arrest with bone bridging and angular deformity. A type VII injury is an injury of the growth cartilage of the epiphyseal surface. A macrotrauma injury of this type would be properly described as an osteochondral fracture, whereas an injury of the repetitive microtrauma type would correspond to the older terminology of osteochondritis dissecans (Fig. 14-5). Type VIII injuries result in disruption of the metaphyseal growth and remodeling mechanisms, whereas type IX injuries affect the diaphyseal growth and remodeling mechanisms, including endosteal and periosteal bone turnover.[18] It was initially thought that the incidence of subsequent growth arrests following Salter I or II injuries was quite low, approximately 3 to 4 percent.[19] However, several studies have shown an unexpectedly high incidence of resulting disturbance, especially when these injuries involve the distal radial epiphysis or distal femoral physis.[20]

The controllers of growth include the genetic makeup of the individual, biomechanical influences that determine shape predominantly, and the periosteal sleeve, which acts as an anatomic restraint.[21] As mentioned above,

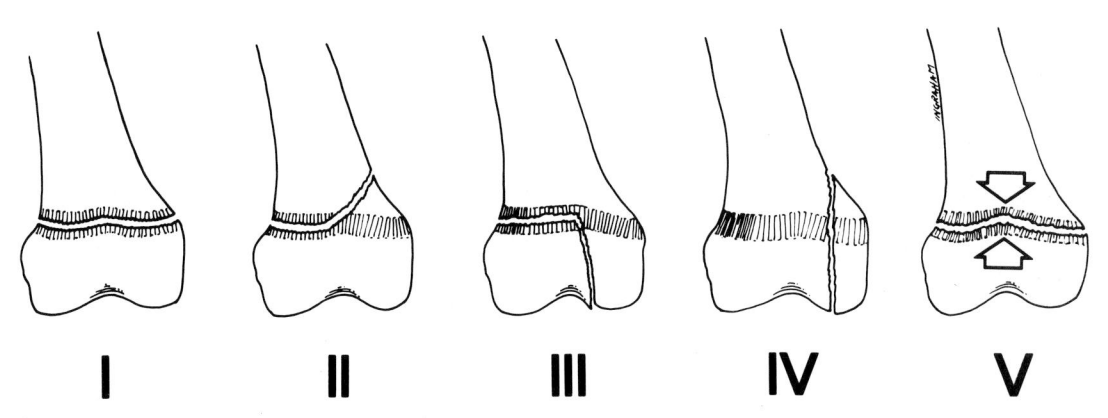

Figure 14–4 The Salter-Harris classification of physeal fracture.

the periosteum is anchored to the ends of long bones by the zone of Ranvier. However, it is only loosely attached to the metaphysis and diaphysis. When the intrinsic elasticity of this periosteal sleeve is disrupted, as in fracture, overgrowth of the bone, compared with the contralateral one, occurs.[18] Growth and the cessation of growth are also regulated by hormones including thyroxine, growth hormone, and the sex hormones. Thyroxine and growth hormone seem to act synergistically to stimulate growth. Although testosterone initially stimulates the physis during the growth spurt, eventually it, like estrogen, suppresses growth plate activity leading to ultimate closure of the physis.

Finally, while the bones are growing, the muscle-tendon units spanning the bones and joints may become sequentially tighter, particularly during growth spurts.[2,22,23] Ligaments and tendons generally insert into fibrous and fibrocartilaginous (periosteal) regions in bone. This attachment allows for relatively well-integrated growth of muscular and chondro-osseous structures. Late in skeletal maturation, collagen fibers develop that are continuous between the bone and the tendon or ligament (Sharpey's fibers). This explains why in adults, a given angular force may produce a disruption of a ligament, whereas in a child, the same force may produce a bony injury. When these growth processes are not synchronous, relative tightness of the soft-tissue structures, particularly those traversing joints, occurs. This can lead not only to apophyseal avulsions but also to less severe traction apophysitis such as Osgood-Schlatter disease.[10] Apophyseal avulsions (e.g., ischial tuberosity) are predominantly due to weakness in the apophyseal physis during adolescence, but loss of flexibility during the growth spurt also contributes. Therefore, a violent muscular contraction while the muscle (e.g.,

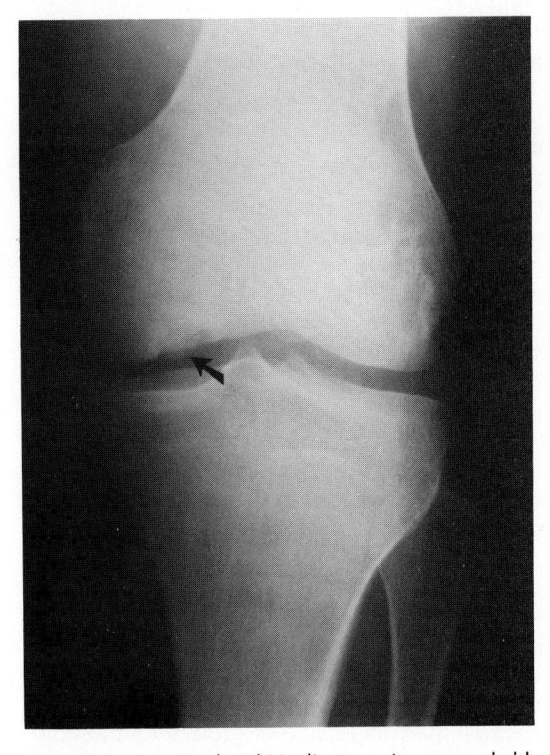

Figure 14–5 Osteochondritis dissecans is most probably a stress fracture of the epiphyseal surface, classed as a type VII injury in the Ogden classification.

semitendinous) is stretched will likely lead to an apophyseal avulsion in the adolescent and a muscle strain in the adult.[19] In addition, Beunen, Malina and colleagues, have found in boys that the adolescent spurt in muscle tissue and strength (with the exception of trunk muscles, which do not undergo a spurt) occurs after peak height velocity and is relatively coincident with peak weight velocity. Thus, muscle tissue apparently increases first in mass and then in strength during male adolescence.[24] In contrast, the most rapid gains in flexibility precede the peak height velocity. There may be more optimal strength–lever arm relationships at this time. In our own study of changes occurring around the knee at the time of the adolescent growth spurt, we demonstrated the development of patella alta in two of seven adolescent females paralleling their accelerated bone growth rate (Fig. 14–6).[25] This loss of flexibility increases the chance of injury both from a single impact such as a sudden forced elongation while jumping or hurdling and from repetitive strains as in running or throwing. During periods of rapid growth, intensity of training should be reduced and, in our opinion, specific, slow stretching exercises should be initiated in order to prevent injury.

Biomechanical studies have suggested that the growth plate and, in particular, the growing cartilage of the joint surface may be more susceptible to stress, especially shear stress, than mature adult articular cartilage.[26] Fatigue wear of articular cartilage results from microscopic damage within the load-bearing material. As in bone, this may occur from repeated applications of high loads over a relatively short period, or from low loads over an extended period.[27]

Clinical experience has demonstrated the susceptibility of the growth plate to injury from single impact trauma, particularly during growth spurts, and there is some evidence that repetitive microtrauma, as in running or jumping, may cause injury at the physis of the hip or knee.[1,28] Concern for the increased risk of growth plate injuries in organized sports for children has been the focus of much public and medical debate. However, there are no data supporting an increased incidence of growth cartilage injury in organized sports as compared with free play or recreational sports activities.

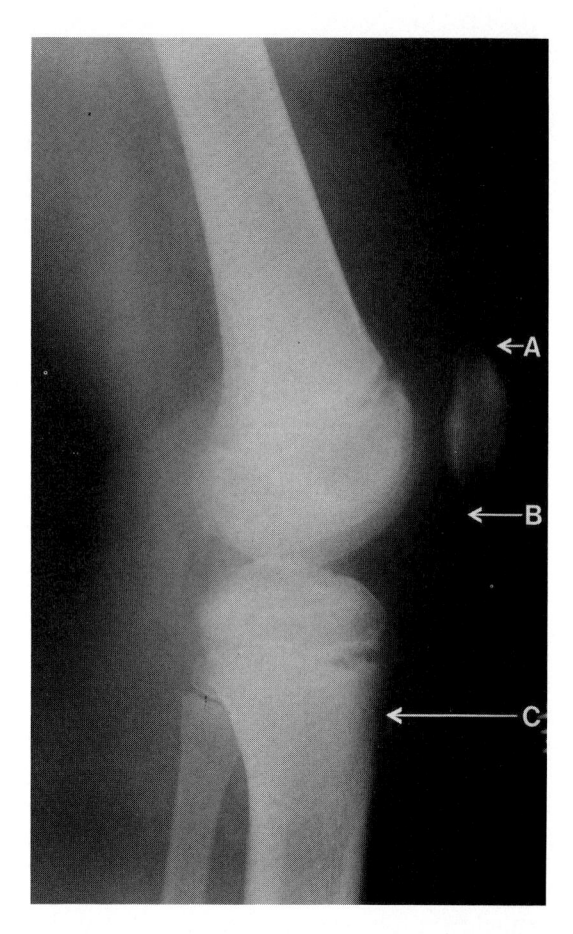

Figure 14–6 With a growth spurt, rapid elongation of the bones results in an increased tightness of the muscle-tendon units spanning the joints. At the knee, this may result in pain at the patella (A), patellar tendon (B), or tibial tubercle (C).

Injuries to the growing bone of the child can have a dramatic impact on subsequent growth of the extremity. The anatomic site of injury must be accurately determined. With macrotrauma fractures, the anatomic location of the fracture, especially if the fracture involves the physis; the degree of initial displacement of the fracture fragments; and the subsequent deformation resulting from the fracture may affect the ultimate growth and function of the extremity.

In the growing child, the stage of relative maturation may affect the location of tissue disruption and the pattern of injury. As an example, a fall on the outstretched hand in the prepubescent child, Tanner stage I or II, usually results in a fracture at the junction of the diaphysis and metaphysis of the radius and ulna distally. In the adolescent, a similar fall would result in a fracture through the distal radial physis and ulnar styloid. In the young adult, the usual result would be a fracture of the scaphoid bone.

A second way in which maturation stage affects patterns of injury can be seen when childhood knee injuries are studied. In the prepubescent child, the physis and its attachment site to adjacent hard bone, the zone of Ranvier, may be stronger than the ligamentous structures of the contiguous joints. Thus, a blow or twist to the knee of the 8- or 9-year-old may result not in a growth plate injury, but in ligamentous injury of the knee, including the cruciates or collateral ligaments. The high incidence of unsuspected ligamentous injuries of the knees in the prepubescent child has received increased attention in recent years.[29]

The same mechanism of injury in the rapidly growing adolescent may result in a growth plate injury. Morscher demonstrated in animal studies that tensile strength of the physis decreased during sexual maturation.[30] Propagation of a fracture through the physis usually occurs through the zone of hypertrophic cartilage cells (see Fig. 14–2). This may be because of a well-accepted mechanical principle, the stress riser. A stress riser is a weak area that is subject to stress caused by sudden changes in material properties. Between the hypertrophic zone and the zone of provisional calcification, the ratio of ground substance to cellular material in the physis changes radically, and the ground substance becomes calcified.[19] This region is therefore a weak zone. Fortunately, fractures through this zone leave the germinal cells unharmed, and growth can continue. Speer has suggested that because this zone is also the zone of least collagen fiber concentration, collagen fiber deficiency may play a role in predisposing this transitional zone to separation.[5] Although change in the structure and strength of this zone is thought to occur during adolescence, possibly because of the relative influences of growth versus sex hormones, the biomechanics and histology of injury at this site have not, as yet, been studied.

As mentioned above, bony injuries in the child can result from macrotrauma or microtrauma. It is well known that macrotrauma to the physis may result in angular deformity or cessation of growth.[31] The mechanisms of growth arrest following physeal injury are often complex in a given injury. Experimental studies have demonstrated that four different mechanisms may contribute to physeal arrest: injury to the epiphyseal blood supply of the plate, direct injury of the germinal cell layer of the plate, injury to the metaphyseal blood supply, or formation of a bony bridge across the plate at a site of major mechanical disruption. This bony bar may result in angular deformity or exert sufficient mechanical resistance to further growth that premature closure of the entire remaining physis may occur.

Approximately 15 percent of all fractures in children involve the physis.[18] Of these only a portion result in growth arrest or angular deformity, depending on the specific physis involved, the type of physeal injury, and the age of the child at the time of injury. Although the Salter-Harris classification was initially developed to describe macrotrauma to the physis, repetitive microtrauma or overuse injuries to the growth cartilage are receiving increased attention, particularly in injuries of the child involved in intense athletic training. Repetitive microtrauma to the growth cartilage of the joint surface was once classified among the osteochondroses and was described as osteochondritis dissecans based on the anatomic appearance of the lesion. It is now hypothesized that this lesion is a stress fracture of the joint surface and should be classed as an Ogden type VII epiphyseal injury, because in the growing child articular cartilage acts as a load-bearing structure besides having a deeper zone that is the growth plate of the epiphysis.

Repetitive microtrauma or stress injury to the physis has only very recently been documented. However, it has been hypothesized for some years that repetitive impact to the lower extremities in such activities as distance running and, in particular, marathon training might cause microscopic injury to the physis with inhibition of subsequent growth in the child. In 1976 Kato and Ishiko presented an initial report suggesting that certain children in rural areas of Japan who were subjected to heavy work activities demonstrated decreased height owing to physeal microinjury.[32] More recently, Roy, Caine, and Singer described a high incidence of positive ulnar variance, a relative overgrowth of the distal ulna with respect to the radius, in young gymnasts with open physes.[33] The authors hypothesized that this disorder resulted from injury to the growth tissue of the distal radial epiphysis from repetitive microtrauma of landings and vaults (Fig. 14–7). Essentially, although the effects of normal biologic forces on the physis, epiphysis, and metaphysis are not well understood, as in adult bone, the response to mechanical forces is a function of the magnitude, duration, and direction of the force (see previous chapter) and may result in normal remodeling or in fracture or deformation.

OVERUSE INJURIES

Children with overuse injuries usually present with complaints of pain when a particular maneuver is performed, and there may be accompanying complaints of swelling or tenderness.

The history of pain onset and the circumstances in which the pain occurs may prove critical in making a proper diagnosis and in instituting proper treatment, because certain types of injuries are seen with greater frequency in certain sports. As an example, the young gymnast complaining of back pain should be suspected of having spondylolysis of the lower lumbar spine, a result of repetitive flexion and extension of the back in gymnastic maneuvers.[34,35] With this suspicion of spondylolysis based on the history of gymnastic preparation, sophisticated diagnostic techniques may then be used to confirm the diagnosis. It is essential to make the diagnosis early and to institute proper treatment in order to increase the chance of healing the stress fracture and to ensure return to painless competition. It would be an error, indeed, to attribute these complaints sim-

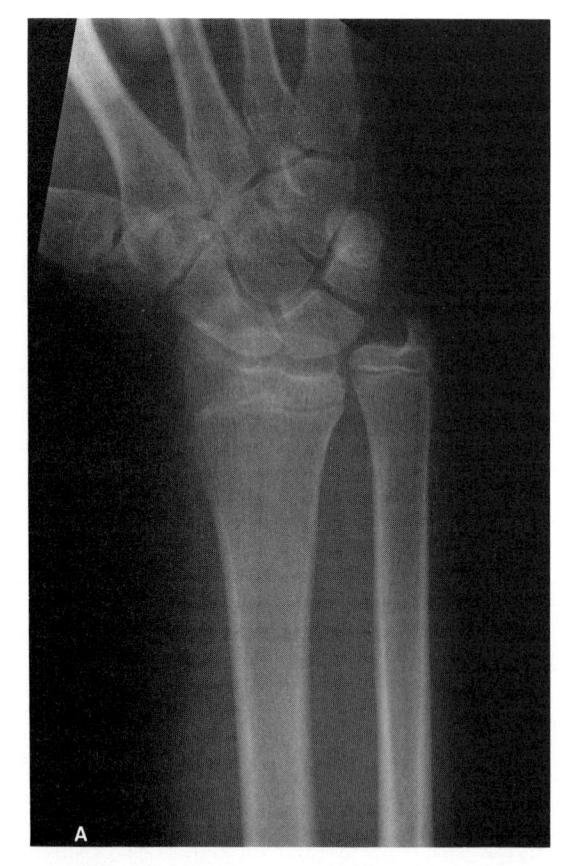

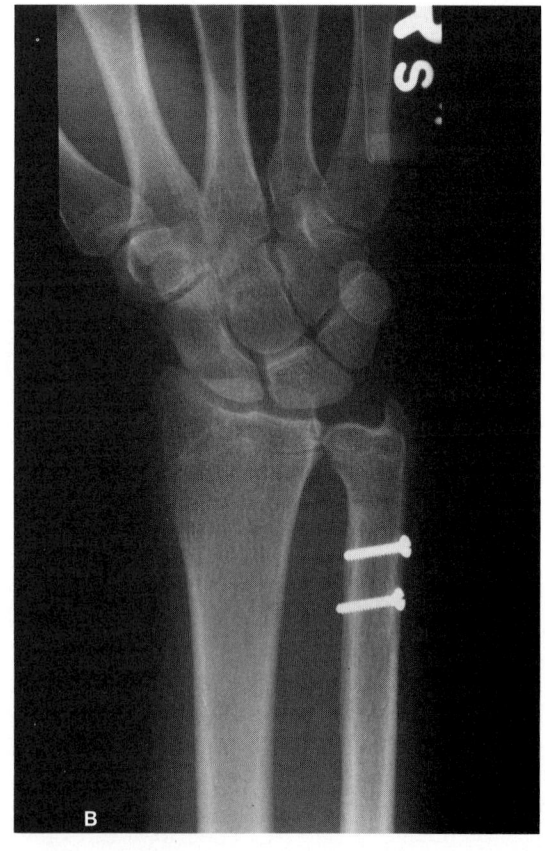

Figure 14–7(*A*) Injury from repetitive impact to the distal radial physeal plate, resulting in relative ulnar lengthening (positive ulnar variance). (*B*) Correction by ulnar shortening and distal ulnar epiphysiodesis.

ply to a back strain or "growing pains" and to encourage the child to continue in gymnastic participation without proper treatment.

Children's overuse injuries include bursitis, tendinitis, apophysitis, stress fractures of long bones, and, in certain cases, osteochondral injuries of the joint surface.[3,12] As noted above, there is growing evidence that "osteochondritis dissecans" of the elbow and knee also may be due to repetitive microtrauma, which results in fracture of the underlying bone and subsequent cartilage injury.[36-38] In addition, repetitive rotational stresses at the shoulder may cause microfracture through the growth plate of the proximal humerus—dubbed "Little League shoulder," but in effect a Salter I stress fracture—again the result of the repetitive microtrauma.[39-42]

If detected early and properly diagnosed, many of these overuse injuries require nothing more than a brief period of "relative rest" of 3 to 4 weeks. During this time, while the injured tissue heals, additional steps are taken to correct and reverse detected risk factors responsible for the injury.

Risk Factors in Overuse Injury

The physician dealing with the sports-injured child must have some knowledge of the sport or training program pursued by the child. This can be important in making the proper diagnosis initially, as well as in aiding in the management and, ultimately, the prevention of these injuries.

In dealing with overuse injuries in particular, I have found it useful to attempt to determine the factors contributing to the occurrence of a given overuse injury. Often, two or more factors may have actually contributed to the occurrence of injury. The most common "risk factors" encountered in sports injuries are summarized in Table 14-1 and were discussed in the previous chapter.

The first risk factor, training error, is seen with greatest frequency. This usually involves changes in the rate or intensity of training, or the use of inappropriate training.[43] We have learned from studies of running injuries and observations of running coaches that the rate, duration, or intensity of training usually should not be increased more than 10 percent per week.

As an example, a child running 20 minutes per day, five days per week, may safely run 22 minutes per day the following week. Similarly, a young swimmer doing 1,000 yards per day, may safely be advanced to 1,100 per day the following week. The ultimate limits of training depend on the sport or event being prepared for and on the capacity of the individual child. At present, we are dependent on such "clinical" observations by coaches and team physicians to give guidelines for changing the rate of intensity of training, because measurement of tissue "fitness" for repetitive impact loading is not yet available.

A recent observation by many coaches and sports scientists has been that many elite athletes have been overtrained, consequently increasing the chance of overuse injury without significantly enhancing performance. This risk is also of particular concern in children's sports. The adults responsible for coaching children's sports may often have no specific training in the physiology or psychology of the child. In certain instances, well-meaning volunteers may also be relatively ignorant of the sports that they are coaching and the specific skills required for these sports.[44] In such a circumstance, the untrained coach may encourage greater duration of training, paying little attention to training technique. Unfortunately, the coaching philosophy "more is better" may be particularly detrimental to the young athlete.

TABLE 14-1 Apparent Risk Factors in Overuse Injury

1. Training errors, including abrupt changes in intensity, duration, or frequency of training.
2. Errors in technique.
3. Anatomic malalignment of the lower extremities, including difference in leg lengths, abnormalities of rotation of the hips, position of the kneecaps, and bow legs, knock knees, or flat feet.
4. Musculotendinous imbalance of strength, flexibility, or bulk.
5. Footwear: improper fit, inadequate impact-absorbing material, excessive stiffness of the sole, and/or insufficient support of hindfoot.
6. Running surface: concrete pavement versus asphalt versus running track versus dirt or grass.
7. Associated disease state of the lower extremity, including arthritis, poor circulation, old fractures, or other injury.
8. Cultural deconditioning from decreased general exercise and activity.

The second risk factor, errors in technique, is also of particular concern in the child. The young overhand thrower in baseball or cricket has an increased risk of injury to the growing cartilage of the shoulder or elbow joint if he or she is pitching improperly.[38,39] The young dancer is at particular risk of injury to the cartilage of the patella if the plié is performed incorrectly, with too much forced turnout below the knee.[45] In such cases, proper treatment of the injury and prevention of recurrence is not a matter of drugs or surgery but of a change in the athlete's technique. The physician must be aware of this as a potential etiologic factor and be prepared to discuss corrective measures with patients, coaches, or parents.

The third risk factor, anatomic malalignment, is a matter of much debate and, on occasion, an invitation to error in assessing the etiology of the child's overuse injury. Common anatomic abnormalities include excessive femoral anteversion, genu varum, genu valgum, hyperextension, pes planus, and leg length discrepancies. In actuality, the body can adjust to a wide range of anatomic combinations and function without pain or injury, provided that changes in stress patterns are gradual.[46]

Unfortunately, a detected anatomic malalignment may be indicated as a major contributor to pain or injury simply because it is obvious, despite the fact that the injury was, in fact, due to poor training or muscle imbalance. As an example, a child who suddenly begins soccer training, is progressed too rapidly, and also has extremely tight calf muscles may complain of calf or heel pain. At the time of examination, the child may have flexible pes planus, and the leg pain may be attributed to this malalignment. The child may be incorrectly treated with arch supports or, worse, advised that sports are contraindicated for him or her, instead of having appropriate treatment, which would consist of a proper progression of training and corrective exercises.[47]

The fourth risk factor, muscle-tendon imbalance, can be an important contributor to sports injury in both acute injuries and overuse injuries. For example, there is some evidence that the risk of ankle sprain is increased by excessive tightness of the calf muscles.[48] As noted earlier, muscle-tendon-bone imbalance during the adolescent growth spurt may contribute to traction apophysitis and to apophyseal avulsions.

This increased risk of injury at the time of a growth spurt is well known to ballet teachers, who often decrease the intensity of training during the growth spurt in order to avoid injury. A careful assessment of the relative strength and flexibility of an individual child preparing to play sports or complaining of pain in association with sports is necessary, because imbalances are individual and joint specific.[49,50] A young gymnast may have strong thigh muscles but weak abdominal muscles. A young runner may have flexible calf muscles but dangerously tight hamstrings.

Another risk factor, which may be more important than we realize, is a generalized decrease in physical activity of the children and adolescents living in technologically advanced societies. Children who are driven to school, play computer games, watch television, and vie with increased loads of homework in today's competitive academic environment may be getting much less general exercise than is healthy, resulting in weaker tissues. Exposing these deconditioned tissues to short bursts of heavy training of a repetitive nature may be a further invitation to injury. Recent studies that describe a declining level of physical fitness of our youth and increased levels of adolescent obesity lend further support to this concern.[51]

SPECIFIC INJURIES

Knee Injuries

The knee is the most frequent site of injury in most childhood sports. Acute knee injuries in the child must be carefully assessed for the possibility of ligamentous injury, internal derangement, or extensor mechanism injury, as in the adult. The possibility of injury to the growth plates of the distal femur or proximal tibia must also be considered.[34] When a child complains of acute knee injury, it is useful to obtain a description of the injury. Was the injury the result of a direct blow to the knee, or the result of an indirect force transmission to the knee? Was the player's weight alone involved, or was he or she struck by another player?

Acute knee injuries include ligamentous

sprains, internal derangements, including tears of the menisci and loose bodies; injuries to the extensor mechanism, such as a dislocated patella; and contusions from direct blows. In addition, an epiphyseal fracture through the distal femoral or proximal tibial physis must always be considered, particularly during the final adolescent growth spurt (Fig. 14–8).

An accurate diagnosis is essential for proper injury management. The easy label of "sprained knee" must not be used for every knee injury, particularly in the young. A careful physical examination can determine the site of maximal tenderness, the range of motion of the knee, and the presence of abnormal motion, if it exists. A complete radiographic assessment may be necessary. In certain cases, when an internal derangement or injury of the cruciate ligaments is suspected, arthroscopy can be used to confirm the diagnosis and perform immediate and definitive treatment, such as partial resection or repair of meniscal tears.[29]

Overuse injuries of the knee are actually more common in the young athlete than are acute traumatic injuries. Overuse injuries usually involve the extensor mechanism, either at the site of insertion on the tibia (Osgood-Schlatter disease), the patellar tendon (tendinitis), or the patella itself (patellofemoral stress syndrome).[52,53] As with acute injuries, parapatellar pain must not simply be labeled "chondromalacia patella," because this specific pathologic diagnosis, which in actuality is rarely encountered in the child, indicates fibrillation of the patellar articular cartilage. Other overuse injuries around the knee that result in pain include osteochondritis dissecans of the joint surface and pain on either the medial or lateral aspects of the knee resulting from bursitis or tendinitis.[36,37]

As noted above, once it has been determined which tissues have been injured, it is essential to determine the risk factors associated with the occurrence of injury (e.g., training error, poor technique, shoewear) in order to assist with initial management and to prevent recurrence. As an example, a child complaining of pain at the tibial tubercle may be clinically diagnosed as having Osgood-Schlatter apophysitis. In the past, cast immobilization was frequently used for this condition. At present, we do not immobilize children with this condition; rather, we institute a program of "rela-

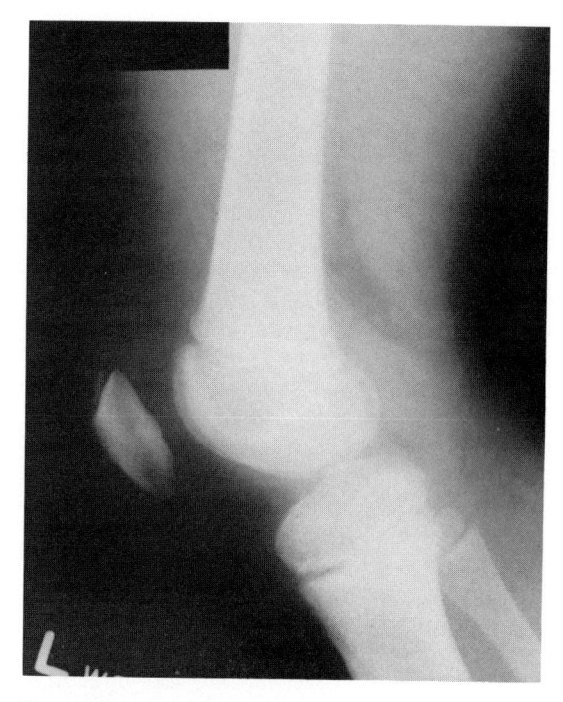

Figure 14–8 Avulsion of the patella in a young basketball player, following a jump.

tive rest," substituting biking for running and stopping jumping and kicking activities. We may also suggest better impact-absorbing shoes or a softer playing surface. Most important, this overuse injury is associated with a relative tightness and weakness of the quadriceps muscle, with secondary repetitive microavulsions at the tibial tubercle. It is therefore important to institute progressive exercises to restore both the strength and the flexibility of the lower extremity, particularly of the quadriceps muscle.[54]

Elbow Injuries

An acutely painful, swollen elbow in a child must be considered an emergency, because injuries around the elbow can result in permanent disability or even loss of the extremity. These injuries range from a simple sprain to a completely displaced supracondylar fracture of the distal humerus with progressive neurovascular compromise of the forearm and hand.[55]

Initial management includes determination of the distal neurovascular status, including radial pulse, capillary refill, and sensory and motor activity of the ulnar, radial, and median nerves. Immobilization in a position of relative comfort should be the next step. This position is often not that of flexion to a 90-degree angle in a sling. In fact, this position may increase the potential for swelling and further neurovascular compromise. If possible, ice should be applied immediately, as well as a gentle compression dressing. A splint made of a folded newspaper, Ace bandages, and bags of crushed ice may be ideal.

High-quality radiographs, often with multiple views, are essential for diagnosis and subsequent management. It is important to include the joints at both ends of the injured extremity; e.g., with elbow injuries, this means shoulder and wrist. The incidence of ipsilateral fractures of the forearm with elbow injuries is often higher than is realized.[56]

In addition to supracondylar fractures, a variety of different macrotrauma fractures may occur about the elbow that are less emergent in nature but that often require careful assessment and reduction. Acute avulsion of the medial epicondyle in the young thrower may occur. Usually preceded by a period of elbow pain, suggesting a combination of microtrauma and macrotrauma, these are generally best treated by open reduction.

"Little League" elbow, a general label applied to the overuse injuries sustained by some young pitchers, can include osteochondritis of the capitellum, with or without associated loose bodies in the joint; injury and premature closure of the proximal radial epiphysis; overgrowth of the radial head; and irritation or frank avulsion of the medial epicondyle (Fig. 14–9). The mechanism of injury appears to be the repetitive valgus strain applied to the elbow by throwing, with compression laterally and traction medially.[57] We would hypothesize a second mechanism of injury, based upon our own clinical observation that most of the children with capitellar injury have an associated tightness of the anterior elbow structures. When the involved elbow is forced into extension at the end of delivery, this imparts a shear stress to the capitellum from the edge of the radial head. This mechanism may be particularly important in younger throwers.

If detected early, relative rest and exercises to improve the strength of the entire arm, as well as attention to throwing technique to minimize the valgus strain at the elbow, can stop the process. A child with a history of repetitive throwing who presents with pain around the elbow with associated swelling and complete loss of motion must be examined very closely using anteroposterior, lateral, and oblique radiographs of the elbow, as well as possibly an elbow arthrogram, to determine injury.

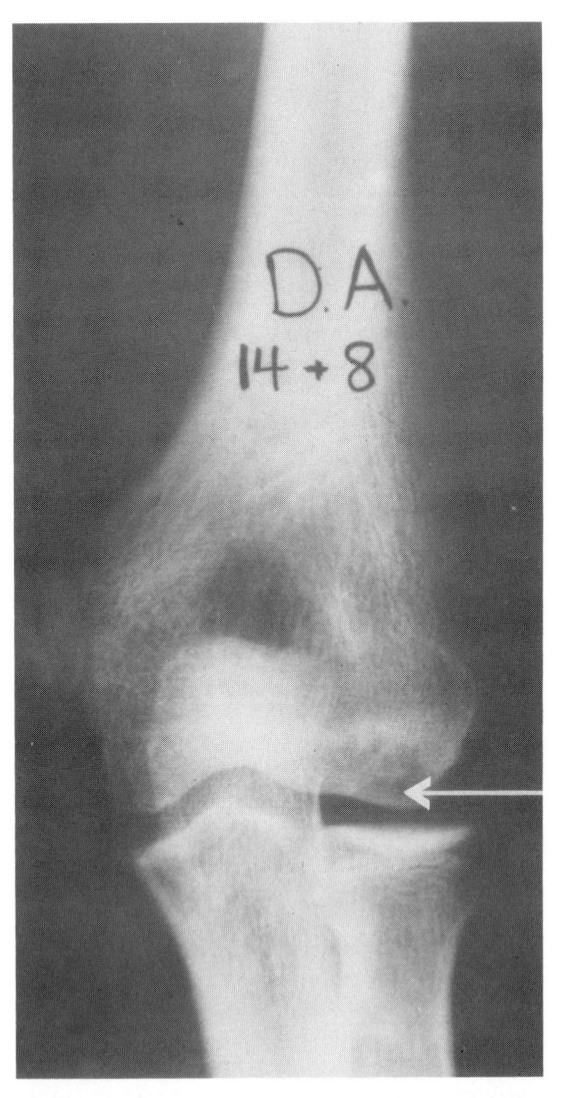

Figure 14–9 The repetitive microtrauma of overhand throwing in the child may result in osteochondral injury of the capitellum and the formation of loose bodies in the joint.

Spine Injuries

Especially during the growth spurt, there appears to be a tendency to develop lordosis of the lumbar spine. This is because of the enhanced growth anteriorly in the vertebral bodies and the relative tightness of the lumbodorsal fascia. I have observed, associated with excessive lumbar lordosis, a relative flexion contracture at the hips, tight hamstrings, and, because normal forward excursion of the lumbar spine is limited, a tendency to develop forward bending at the thoracolumbar junction or in the thoracic spine itself. If, at the time this posture is developing, repetitive sports training is done that requires repetitive flexion, extension, or rotation of the spine, a characteristic pattern of injuries may develop.

Research on lumbar spine mechanics has suggested that increased lumbar lordosis increases the tendency both to posterior element failure at the pars interarticularis and to disk failure.[58]

This theoretical concern appears to be consistent with clinical observations. The overuse back problems seen in the young athlete generally fall into one of three categories: stress fracture of the pars interarticularis (spondylolysis), hyperlordotic mechanical low back pain, or disk herniation, all of which appear to be helped to a greater or lesser extent by an antilordotic program of exercises and, sometimes, bracing.[59]

At the thoracolumbar junction, back pain can develop that is associated with radiographic deformation of some or more vertebral bodies anteriorly. Although the etiology of this atypical Scheuermann's disease is still being debated, the mode of onset, the frequent association with repetitive sports activity, and the physical findings suggest that this is a repetitive microtrauma compression fracture of the vertebral bodies anteriorly.[60] With early recognition and, usually, bracing, rapid healing and bony reconstitution can be seen.

INJURY PREVENTION

Both the rate of occurrence and the relative severity of many children's sports injuries may be decreased by proper preparticipation assessment, advice, and rehabilitation after injury. To be effective, this advice must be based both upon a working knowledge of the sports involved and their potential for injury, and upon a careful assessment of the pediatric sports candidate.[49,50] This includes weighing individual fitness, or lack thereof, against the demands of the sport. In certain instances, the child may not be sufficiently fit to participate safely in the sport in question. Recommendations, in such instances, may include a prescription of strengthening, stretching, or aerobic exercises to correct the deficiency. In certain instances, special protective equipment might be required. In some cases, the child may not, under any circumstances, be able to participate safely in the sport in question.

In such instances, the physician and physical educator must be prepared to suggest alternative sports or fitness activities. This becomes particularly important when dealing with the handicapped child or the child with other medical conditions such as hypertension or diabetes, where sports participation and exercise can have profound benefits for both the physical and psychological health of the child.[61-64]

Rehabilitation after childhood or adolescent injury has received little emphasis or attention, except in the case of severe injuries, such as those involving limb loss or neurologic involvement. This laissez faire attitude may delay any child's recovery and return to full function, but it can be especially dangerous when applied to the sports-injured child. The child who is active in sports desires a safe and effective return to full athletic participation, with complete restoration of strength, muscle bulk, and flexibility. Studies have shown that incomplete rehabilitation increases the risk of reinjury in young athletes.[54,65,66]

As noted above, the most important environmental factor in the occurrence of youth sports injuries is the quality of adult coaching and supervision. Parents should be counseled to assess the qualifications and coaching techniques of their children's coaches and sports teachers.

REFERENCES

1. Micheli LJ. Pediatric and adolescent sports medicine. Boston: Little, Brown, 1984.
2. Jackson DW, Jarrett H, Bailey D, et al. Injury prediction in the young athlete: a preliminary report. Am J Sports Med 1978; 6:6–16.

3. Micheli LJ. Overuse injuries in children's sports; the growth factor. Orthop Clin North Am 1983; 14:337–360.
4. Micheli LJ, Santopietro FJ, Gerbino PG, Crowe P. Etiologic assessment of the overuse stress fractures in athletes. Nova Scot Bull 1980; 59:43–47.
5. Speer DP. Collagenous architecture of the growth plate and perichondrial ossification groove. J Bone Joint Surg (Am) 1982; 64:399–407.
6. Speer DP, Pitt MJ. Peripheral and central contours of the growth plate. Trans Orthop Res Soc 1982; 7:53.
7. Anatomy. In: Orthopaedic science. Park Ridge, IL: American Academy of Orthopaedic Surgeons, 1986: 1.
8. Robles-Marin D, Smith-Agreda V, Marti-Faus M, et al. Histochemical and enzymatic changes in the chondrocytes next to the vascular invasion during endochondral ossification. In: Arlet J, Ficat RP, Hungerford DS, eds. Bone circulation. Baltimore: Williams & Wilkins, 1984.
9. Lacroix P. The organization of bones. Philadelphia: Blakiston, 1951.
10. Ogden J. Postnatal development and growth of the musculoskeletal system. In: Albright JA, Brand RA, eds. The scientific basis of orthopaedics. East Norwalk, CT: Appleton & Lange, 1987.
11. Ogden JA, Southwick WD. Osgood Schlatter's disease and tibial tuberosity development. Clin Orthop 1976; 116:180–189.
12. Micheli LJ. The traction Apophysitises. Clin Sports Med 1987; 6:389–404.
13. Metzmaker JN, Pappas AM. Avulsion fractures of the pelvis. Am J Sports Med 1985; 13:349–358.
14. Waters PM, Millis MB. Hip and pelvic injuries in the young athlete. Clin Sports Med 1988; 7:513–526.
15. Mooar PA, Brighton CT, Wisneski RJ, Pollack SR. Stimulation of in-vivo epiphyseal plate growth by a time varying electric field. Trans Orthop Res Soc 1982; 7:56.
16. Ogden J. Hip development and vascularity. Relationship to chondro-osseous trauma in the growing child. In: The hip. Proceedings of the hip society. St. Louis: CV Mosby, 1981.
17. Salter RB, Harris WR. Injuries involving the epiphyseal plate. J Bone Joint Surg (Am) 1963; 45:587–622.
18. Ogden JA. Skeletal injury in the child. Philadelphia: Lea & Febiger, 1982.
19. Singer K. Injuries and disorders of the epiphyses in young athletes. In: Broekhoff J, Ellis MJ, Tripps DG, eds. Sport for children and youths. Champaign IL: Human Kinetics Publishers, 1984; 141.
20. Peterson CA, Peterson HA. Analysis of the incidence of injuries to the epiphyseal growth plate. J Trauma 1972; 12:275–281.
21. Eyre-Brook AL. The periosteum: its function reassessed. Clin Orthop 1984; 189:300–307.
22. Guerewitsch AD, O'Neill M. Flexibility of healthy children. Arch Phys Ther 1944; 25:216–221.
23. Malina RN. Adolescent changes in size, build, composition, and performance. Hum Biol 1974; 46:117–131.
24. Beunen G, Malina RM, Van't Hof MA, et al. Adolescent growth and motor performance: a longitudinal study of Belgian boys. Champaign, IL: Human Kinetics Publishers, 1988.
25. Micheli LJ, Slater JA, Woods E, Gerbino PG. Patella alta and the adolescent growth spurt. Clin Orthop 1986; 213:159–162.
26. Bright RW, Burstein AH, Elmore SM. Epiphyseal plate cartilage—a biomechanical and histological analysis of failure modes. J Bone Joint Surg (Am) 1974; 56:668–703.
27. Mow V, Rosenwasser M. Articular cartilage: biomechanics. In: Woo SL-Y, Buckwalter JA, eds. Injury and repair of the musculoskeletal soft tissues. Park Ridge, IL: American Academy of Orthopaedic Surgeons, 1988: 427.
28. Murray RO, Duncan C. Athletic activity in adolescence as an etiological factor in degenerative hip disease. J Bone Joint Surg (Br) 1971; 53:406–419.
29. Mayer PJ, Micheli LJ. Avulsion of the femoral attachment of the posterior cruciate ligament in an eleven-year-old boy. J Bone Joint Surg (Am) 1979; 61:431–432.
30. Morscher E. Strength and morphology of growth cartilage under hormonal influence of puberty. Animal experiments and clinical study on the eitology of local growth disorders during puberty. Reconstr Surg Traumatol 1968; 10:3–104.
31. Harris WR, Hobson KW. Histological changes in experimentally displaced upper femoral epiphysis in rabbits. J Bone Joint Surg (Br) 1956; 38:914–921.
32. Kato S, Ishiko T. Obstructed growth of children's bones due to excessive labor in remote corners. In: Proceedings of International Congress of Sports Sciences. Tokyo: Japanese Union of Sports Sciences, 1976.
33. Roy S, Caine D, Singer KM. Stress changes of the distal radial epiphysis in young gymnasts. Am J Sports Med 1985; 13:301–308.
34. Jackson DW, Wiltse LL, Cirincione RJ. Spondylolisthesis in the female athlete. Clin Orthop 1976; 117:68–73.
35. Micheli LJ. Back injuries in gymnastics. Clin Sports Med 1985; 4:85–93.
36. Conway FM. Osteochondritis dissecans: description of the stages of the condition and its probable traumatic etiology. Am J Surg 1937; 38:691–699.
37. Green WT, Banks HH. Osteochondritis dissecans in children. J Bone Joint Surg (Am) 1953; 35:26–44.
38. McManama GB, Micheli LJ, Berry MV, Sohn RS. The surgical treatment of osteochondritis of the capitellum. Am J Sports Med 1985; 13:11–21.
39. Cahill BR, Tullos HS, Fain RH. Little league shoulder. J Sports Med 1973; 2:150–153.
40. Jackson DW. Chronic rotator cuff impingement in the throwing athlete. Am J Sports Med 1971; 4:231–240.
41. Larson RL. Epiphyseal injuries in adolescent athletes. Orthop Clin North Am 1973; 4:839–851.
42. Richardson AB, Jobe FW, Collins RH. The shoulder in competitive swimming. Am J Sports Med 1980; 8:159–163.
43. Pollock ML, Cureton TK, Greninger L. Effects of frequency of training on work capacity, cardiovascular function, and body composition of adult men. Med Sci Sports 1969; 1:70–74.
44. Gross RH. Training programs for volunteer coaches: more time, more money. Phys Sportsmed 1982; 10(11):183–185.
45. Walaszek A. Physical therapy rehabilitation of dance

46. Gross RH. Leg length discrepancy: how much is too much? J Orthop 1978; 1:307–310.
47. Subotnick SL. Orthotic foot control and the overuse syndrome. Phys Sportsmed 1975; 3:75–79.
48. Santopietro FJ, Micheli LJ, Gerbino PG. Anatomic malalignment associated with chronic inversion ankle sprains: a preliminary study. In Rinaldi RR, Sabia ML Jr, eds. Sports medicine '79. New York: Futura Publishing, 1979:209.
49. Goldberg B, Saraniti A, Witman P. Preparticipation sports assessment—an objective evaluation. Pediatrics 1980; 66:736–745.
50. Micheli LJ, Stone KR. The presports physical: only the first step. J Musculoskeletal Med 1984; 1(6):56–60.
51. Gortmaker SL, Dietz WM Jr, Wehler CA. Increasing pediatric obesity in the United States. Am J Dis Child 1987; 141:535–540.
52. Ficat RP, Hungerford DS. Disorders of the patello-femoral joint. Baltimore, William & Wilkins, 1977.
53. Micheli LJ. Lower extremity injuries: overuse injuries in the recreational adult athlete. In: Cantu RC, ed. The exercising adult. Lexington, MA: Collamore Press, 1982.
54. Micheli LJ. Special considerations in children's rehabilitation programs. In: Hunter LY, Funk FJ, eds. Rehabilitation of the injured knee. St. Louis: CV Mosby, 1984: 406.
55. Skolnick MD, Hall JE, Micheli LJ. Supracondylar fractures of the humerus in children. Orthop Trans 1979; 3:287.
56. Stanitski CL, Micheli LJ. Simultaneous ispilateral fractures of the arm and forearm in children. Clin Orthop 1980; 153:205–209.
57. Tullos HS, King JW. Lesions of the pitching arm in adolescents. JAMA 1972; 220:264–271.
58. Kraus H. Effect of lordosis on the stress in the lumbar spine. Clin Orthop 1976; 117:56–58.
59. Micheli LJ, Hall JE, Miller ME. Use of the Boston brace for back injuries in athletes. Am J Sports Med 1980; 8:351–356.
60. Hensinger RN. Back and vertebral changes simulating Scheuermann's disease. Orthop Trans 1982 6:1.
61. Fitch KD, Godfrey S. Asthma and athletic performance. JAMA 1976; 236:152.
62. Leon AL, Fitzwiler DD, Costill DL. Diabetes and exercise. Phys Sportsmed 1979; 7:49–61.
63. Lieberman E. Essential hypertension in children and youth; a pediatric perspective. J Pediatrics 1974; 85:1–11.
64. Micheli LJ. Rehabilitation: expanding the definition. In: Bernhardt DB, ed. Physical and occupational therapy in pediatrics—recreation for the disabled child. New York: Haworth Press, 1984:3.
65. Nicholas JA. Risk factors, sports medicine, and the orthopedic system: an overview. J Sports Med 1976; 3:243–259.
66. Gleim GW, Nicholas JA, Webb JW. Isokinetic evaluation following leg injuries. Phys Sportsmed 1978; 6:74–81.

Chapter 15
Principles of Rehabilitating Sports Injuries

GLEN A. HALVORSON

FIRST AID PHASE: DECREASING THE ACUTE RESPONSE TO INJURY

Cellular Response to Injury

Acute soft tissue injury results in a cascade of vascular, cellular, and chemical events that lead to bleeding, inflammation, swelling, and pain with subsequent loss of motion, joint stiffness, and impaired motor function. Cellular injury results in the release of such chemical mediators as histamine, bradykinin, and prostaglandins that encourage increased cellular permeability and vasodilatation of capillaries. Intracapillary volume and pressure cause extravasation of fluid into the interstitial tissues (transudate) followed by a cellular response (exudate) that results in soft tissue swelling. The amount of swelling is proportional to the extent of injury, the changes in vascular permeability, and the influence of chemical mediators. Swelling causes tissue hypoxia, which enhances cellular damage both directly and indirectly by increasing release of chemical mediators. This further increases capillary permeability and vasodilatation with increased swelling, increased cellular debris, and a prolonged cellular response to injury. The end result is delayed tissue repair and healing. Therefore, control of swelling is critical to reducing recovery time from acute athletic injury.

Connective tissue is made up of specialized tissue cells and collagen. The healing response depends on both soft tissue cellular regeneration and collagen formation. Different tissues repair at different rates according to the degree of cellular versus collagen response in each tissue. Fibroblasts produce collagen in areas in which primary cellular tissue fails to recover. Increased collagen response leads to scar formation and shortening of the healing soft tissues. The amount of scar versus primary tissue repair depends upon the type of cell and type of injury. The duration of recovery is also affected by the amount of tissue swelling and the extent of the inflammatory response, which may last as long as 2 weeks.

Pain Response to Injury

Pain perception is modulated by complex neurocircuits using neurotransmitters. Pain relief can be achieved either by inhibition of pain-stimulating pathways or by facilitation of pain-inhibiting pathways.[1] Nociceptors are free nerve endings that transmit pain impulses in response to such stimuli as heat, cold, pressure, deformation, and chemical changes in soft tissues. Pain is perpetuated following soft tissue injury by the inflammatory response and also by involuntary contraction of skeletal muscle in response to pain. Persistent muscle spasm with increased relative ischemia in the area of injury facilitates chemical mediator-induced nociceptor activity. Chemical mediators of the inflammatory response are known to decrease the threshold of nociceptors to other stimuli such as heat or mechanical deformation.[2] This sets up a positive feedback loop of reflex muscle spasm (pain–spasm–pain cycle). Inhibition of voluntary muscular function secondary to pain results in decreased range of motion, muscle atrophy, and a loss of strength and endurance in muscles of the affected extremity. Control of pain is necessary in acute and chronic injury to avoid the adverse effects of immobility and to restore normal neuromuscular function.

Response to Immobility

Immobility adds to the complications of acute cellular injury by encouraging fibrous contractures of joints, atrophy of muscle, and impaired cardiopulmonary efficiency.[3,4] Studies have extensively documented soft tissue changes in response to inactivity. There is a change in structure and orientation of collagen in joint capsules and ligaments after 2 weeks of immobilization.[5] Noyes reported a 40 percent decrease in ability of monkey anterior cruciate ligament to resist failure after 8 weeks of immobilization. Approximately 12 months were required to restore normal function to the injured monkey ligament.[6] Enneking and Horowitz described progressive contracture of joint capsule and pericapsular structures caused by immobilization.[7] Rapid cartilage degeneration and infiltration of fibrofatty connective tissue were observed. In addition to weakening of extracapsular structures and cartilage degeneration, the joint itself becomes stiff and there is decreased lubrication. Salter and co-workers reported a marked improvement in rate of articular cartilage healing in rabbit joints when continuous passive motion was used compared with either intermittent active range of motion or immobilization after injury.[8] Early range of motion is advocated as soon as possible to minimize the effects of immobility and avoid longer periods of recovery.

Muscle Atrophy

Muscle atrophy occurs rapidly after injury and is due to cellular response to injury, pain, and immobility. Decreases of 25 to 30 percent in quadriceps strength have been seen after 2 weeks of knee immobilization.[9] Similar decreases in strength were also measured in the hamstring and gastrocnemius soleus muscles following knee injury.[9,10] Deficits in quadriceps strength up to 50 percent have been observed 4 weeks after knee surgery.[10,11] Some studies show that weakness in an affected joint can occur secondary to inflammation or joint effusion.[12,13]

As mentioned above, muscle weakness occurs even without immobilization when there is persistent pain. Eriksson demonstrated a significant decrease in degree of quadriceps atrophy after knee surgery when epidural anesthesia was used for control of pain.[14] Decreased neuronal input secondary to pain inhibition (and inactivity) results in cellular changes that promote muscle atrophy.[15] There is a decrease in protein and a change in enzyme content of injured or inactive muscle.[16,17] Immobilized muscle usually shortens and decreased electrical activity can be measured.[17] Changes in neuromuscular excitation after immobilization include impaired contractile properties of muscle including decreased contraction time and decreased tetanus: twitch ratio.[18] Jokl and Konstadt noted that atrophy is more rapid when the muscle is immobilized in a shortened position.[19] Booth found predominantly type I muscle atrophy after immobilization.[17] These studies support the concept that early range of motion and relief of pain facilitate recovery by limiting the extent of atrophy and weakness following injury.[20,21] Significant impairment of motor function associated with atrophy is likely to occur whenever there is inactivity, immobility, pain, swelling, or joint effusion.

First Aid

Proper treatment in the first 24 to 72 hours can have a significant impact on the extent of soft tissue injury. It is important to be aggressive in the first aid treatment of acute injuries. It has been well documented in clinical and laboratory studies that greater immobilization and swelling lead to weaker muscles, stiffer ligaments and joints, and progressive soft tissue contracture.[22-28] The more extensive the changes, the longer it takes to control pain and restore normal function. The goals of first aid are to minimize this acute reaction to injury so that the rehabilitation phase can begin as soon as possible.

The first aid phase of treatment is typically represented by the pneumonic RICE: rest, ice, compression, and elevation of the injured body part.[29] The duration of first aid treatment depends on the type and severity of injury. Less severe injuries with less bleeding and swelling respond more quickly to ice, compression, and elevation than more severe injuries. Minor injuries may require only 24 hours of ICE. Most of the bleeding in the acute inflammatory response can be resolved within 1 to 3 days of injury.

Rest or Immobilization

Rest, immobility, or protected joint range of motion decrease the amount of bleeding and protect the injured area from further mechanical trauma in the acute phase of cellular injury. Rest is required when there is an active inflammatory response but is encouraged only to control the acute reaction. Early mobilization is advocated to avoid the adverse long-term consequences of stiffness and soft tissue contracture.

Ice

The application of cold decreases the acute reaction to injury by decreasing swelling, bleeding, pain, inflammation, and muscle spasm.[30] Cold slows cellular metabolism and impairs the inflammatory response.[31] Decreased bleeding and decreased swelling are probably secondary to vasoconstriction in response to cold.[32] Pain is decreased by a direct effect of cold on pain receptors and nerve fiber transmission and by a secondary decrease in swelling and inflammation. Muscle spasm is inhibited by reflex response to skin cooling and by direct cooling of muscle tissue.[33] Direct effect on muscle includes decreased muscle spindle sensitivity to stretch and impaired large diameter nerve fiber conduction of afferent sensory input from the myotatic stretch reflex. Decreased nociception results in secondary relief of muscle spasm. Sensory stimulation of the skin by the application of cold may also inhibit pain sensory input through neuronal blockade (gate theory).[34]

Compression

Compression decreases swelling by inhibiting the flow of cellular exudate into the interstitium and by increasing dispersion of excessive interstitial fluid.[35] Too much interstitial fluid leads to hypoxic cellular death, increased inflammation, and increased pain. Excessive swelling can also mechanically separate tissue layers and delay or prevent primary tissue repair. Combined compression and cold therapy appear to be more effective than either compression or ice alone for control of acute swelling. Clinical studies demonstrate a much faster return to sports participation when ice and compression are combined in the acute phase of treatment.[36] Compression is commonly achieved with an elastic wrap. Pads shaped from surgical felt conform to areas around bony prominences for more effective local compression. Pneumatic compression devices provide more aggressive and controlled compression of distal extremities.

Elevation

Elevation of the injured part above heart level decreases the amount of bleeding secondary to controlled vascular flow and increases efficiency of venous and lymphatic drainage from the injured area. Venous and lymphatic flow can be further increased during elevation by active muscle contraction, intermittent pneumatic or static compression, and high-voltage electrical stimulation.[37]

Heat

Heat is generally *not* recommended in the first aid phase of treatment. Heat facilitates bleeding and swelling through vasodilatation and may increase the acute inflammatory response to injury. The application of superficial heat in the first 24 to 72 hours after acute athletic injury is not advocated by most authors, although it has been observed that the application of superficial heat in acute strains of underlying deep muscle may facilitate reflex relaxation of painful muscle spasm. In selected athletes, reflex relaxation of acute muscle spasm using heat may be more effective than cold therapy.

Despite firm guidelines suggesting that heat is completely contraindicated in the acute phase of athletic injury and the common practice of not using cold after the acute phase, there may be advantages to such heat therapy based on the athlete's response to a given modality. Pegg and others have, for example, found cryotherapy to facilitate active range of motion of arthritic joints in which perception of decreased joint stiffness was experienced by patients.[30,38-41] This is in contrast to the traditional opinion that cold increases stiffness in rheumatoid joints. Likewise, the injured athlete may find it easier to move a joint actively following cold application rather than heat application, or vice versa. The choice of heat or cold for inhibition of muscle spasm or pain control may be different depending upon the type of patient and how comfortable the specialist is with one method or another of facilitating pain-free range of motion and increased voluntary effort during muscle rehabilitation. It is apparent from the above discussion that proper treatment involves daily evaluation of progress and daily change in the treatment protocol.

After control of the acute response to injury, modalities and exercise are used to promote soft tissue repair, restore pain-free range of motion, and prepare the athlete for neuromuscular rehabilitation. Modality selection needs to incorporate indications, contraindications, and consideration of persistent pain. Pain inhibition may deter progress from the first aid to the modality phase of treatment.

MODALITY PHASE: PROMOTING SOFT TISSUE HEALING

Modalities are used to promote soft tissue healing and bridge the gap between acute first aid and rehabilitation. Treatment goals include decreasing or eliminating pain, preventing further inflammatory changes, reducing joint stiffness, encouraging normal range of motion, softening scar tissue, and increasing blood flow to areas of injury for restoration of normal neuromuscular function. In this sense, modalities are regarded as a physiologic tool because of their direct and indirect effects on soft tissue. Modalities are also a psychological tool helping to achieve goals of improved function when there is impaired voluntary effort because of pain or restricted range of motion.

Both art and science are involved in the application of modalities. It is important to know the physiologic effects produced by a given modality (e.g., selective heating of capsule or tendon with ultrasound), but it is also important to acquire judgment through experience in modality selection (e.g., patient tolerance with respect to heat or cold). These decisions are contingent on the type of injury, the personality and motivation of the injured athlete, and the experience of the health care professional. At times the personal relationship between health care professional and athlete may be more important than the scientific basis for use of a specific modality. This is not an excuse for lack of understanding of the precise physiologic effect of the modality being applied, but it does take into consideration such variables as emotional status, motivation, and the placebo effect.

Therapeutic Cold (Cryotherapy)

Therapeutic cold is perhaps the most important modality, with broad application to many areas of rehabilitation of athletic injuries. Studies have shown ice to be more effective than heat in raising pain thresholds of joints or extremities prior to and during treatment.[42] Cold also results in a longer pain-relieving effect.[33] This is a critical concept in cryotherapy, in which sufficient time may be required to achieve goals of improved flexibility or strength after a modality such as ice is used to reduce pain and muscle spasm. Cooling agents may include ice pack, ice bath, cold towel, ice massage, vapocoolant spray (fluorimethane, ethylchloride), chemicals or gels. Consideration should be given to type, duration, and frequency of application for each specific injury and individual athlete.

The effect of ice on swelling, bleeding, inflammation, pain, and muscle spasm has been reviewed. Ice is probably the most effective, safe, inexpensive, and readily available form of cold therapy.[43] Ice applied to the extremity produces immediate skin cooling, a slight delay in cooling of subcutaneous tissue, and a much more delayed cooling response in underlying muscle.[44,45] Decreases in muscle temperature depend on the amount of subcutaneous insulation, effective vascular response to skin cooling, limb circumference, and duration of application. Significant cooling of muscle in thin athletes with less than 1 cm of fat occurs within 10 minutes. A maximum depth of efficient cooling is approximately 2 cm into muscle. Athletes with more than 2 cm of fat require about 20 to 30 minutes to achieve significant cooling approximately 1 cm into superficial muscle. After removal of ice, there is immediate warming of the skin but a delayed return of muscle temperature to normal. Forty to 60 minutes may be required to achieve normal muscle temperature after 10 to 30 minutes of ice application to the skin.[30]

To achieve a therapeutic response to cold, it is necessary to understand the variability in response proportional to body type. The bigger the athlete, the longer the duration of ice application must be. The deeper the extent of suspected injury, the longer is the duration of ice application. The greater the amount of pain or muscle spasm, the more frequent is ice application. One cannot use a single cookbook formula for treating every athlete. Several methods of cryotherapy are discussed below.

Ice Pack, Ice Towel, Ice Bath

The ice pack, ice towel, and ice bath are typical methods of applying ice in the acute phase of injury. This more static form of ice application is also useful during the rehabilitation phase for relief of pain and swelling associated with exercise. Ice is routinely applied after rehabilitation exercise. Examples include an ice pack to the knee after quadriceps strengthening, an ice towel to the hamstring after stretching or to the shoulder after rotator cuff isokinetic exercise, and an ice bath for the foot and ankle after running or biking when there is residual ligament soreness, joint aching, or mild swelling. Duration of application is usually 20 to 30 minutes. Direct ice application to the skin works best, with little danger of frostbite, in contrast to the risk from direct application of chemical preparations.[43] Wet towels are more effective than dry ones, which decrease the cooling effect secondary to increased insulation.

Ice Massage

The application of ice with slow circular strokes for 5 to 10 minutes provokes a characteristic clinical response of cold, burning, aching, and numbness. This is an effective method of relieving pain and inflammation from superficial conditions such as tendonitis, bursitis, or soft tissue contusion.[46] Longer durations (10 to 20 minutes) produce a cooling response in superficial muscle and can be effective in the treatment of acute and chronic muscle strain.[47-49] A reflex vasodilatation of underlying tissue has been observed 20 to 30 minutes after completion of ice massage and is thought to play a part in improved healing times seen with regular use of this modality.[32] Ice massage is commonly a part of home treatment programs and is often combined with strength and flexibility exercise. For example, tennis elbow treatment protocols may include heat, followed by stretching of forearm muscles, followed by ice massage to the epicondyle. During progression to strengthening exercises, continued use of ice massage before and after exercise may facilitate improved voluntary muscle contraction. Treatment two or three times daily with ice massage appears to be a useful adjunct to other superficial modality treatments for a variety of common injuries such as rotator cuff tendonitis, tennis elbow, patellar tendonitis, superficial muscle strain, plantar fasciitis, and persistent muscle spasm following painful injury.[50]

Cryostretch

Cold therapy facilitates stretching after muscle or joint injury by decreasing pain and muscle spasm so that passive and active range of motion are possible. Where painful muscle spasm is present, increased muscle spindle input to the central nervous system exaggerates muscle response to stretch.[51] Cold dampens this excessive response to stretch by decreasing the activity of muscle spindles and by decreasing the rate of nerve fiber transmission of pain input. The combination of ice massage and proprioceptive neuromuscular facilitation (PNF) techniques for muscle stretching has been extremely effective in improving flexibility.[52-54] Ice massage is applied to the affected muscle for 10 to 20 minutes. Passive range of motion to a sticking point at which motion cannot proceed secondary to pain or contracture is guided by pain and voluntary resistance to movement. An isometric contraction (hold) is maintained for 5 seconds, followed by a pause and then passive range of motion to pain tolerance. This cycle of hold, relax, stretch is repeated. Many protocols have been described in the literature with excellent results achieved from 5 to 30 seconds of stretching, depending upon patient response to passive range of motion.[52,53,55]

Stretching may also be facilitated by simultaneous application of vapocoolant spray (fluorimethane) to the skin over a tight muscle. "Stretch is the action, spray is the distraction" refers to the counterirritant principle by which the vapocoolant spray is thought to cause a burst of cutaneous afferent impulses to the spinal cord (closing the gate), which decreases sensory pain input from the slower conducting C fibers reacting to painful muscle stretch.[56-58]

Cryokinetics

Cold therapy prior to strengthening exercise may improve voluntary effort by eliminating pain inhibition. Just as more effective stretching is possible when local soft tissue pain is reduced, ice massage to the elbow or patellar tendon prior to strengthening allows more effective strengthening of the respective forearm or quadriceps muscles.[46,55] Care must be taken not to mask pain and to increase injury. It is wise to progress slowly, with passive or active range of motion well within pain tolerance limits. Progress should be evaluated daily to increase or decrease the intensity of effort based on clinical response. The goal of cryokinetics is normal pain-free range of motion.

Contraindications to cold therapy include cold urticaria, cold allergy, Raynaud's disease, cryoglobulinemia, and paroxysmal cold hemoglobinuria. Cold urticaria is a hypersensitivity reaction presumably mediated by histamine with initial erythema, itching, flushing, and swelling that may progress to systemic shock. Gastrointestinal (GI) disturbances may be present as well. In Raynaud's disease there is an acute vascular response with distal ischemic changes secondary to vasoconstriction. Nerve palsy has also been described secondary to prolonged ice application over superficial nerves.[59]

Cryotherapy has been advocated for treatment of a variety of athletic injuries in which there is significant pain, tenderness, inflammation, swelling, stiffness, or impaired motor function. Some health care practitioners advocate almost exclusive use of cryotherapy as opposed to therapeutic heat or other modalities.[31,53] A common mistake repeated through the literature is the standard use of heat 3 days after acute injury. The athlete starts out with first aid management of ice, compression, elevation, and is then subjected to a sudden heat application with active or passive range of motion, which may result in increased swelling and pain. The more appropriate choice might be 3 days of ice followed by cryotherapy. Further cold application to produce pain relief and facilitate increased range of motion may avoid the progression of swelling. This is certainly not a golden rule, because many athletes tolerate cold poorly, and heat can be quite helpful in the early phase of rehabilitation after the acute bleeding and swelling have stopped. A common treatment for chronic muscle strain includes heat application, followed by stretching and strengthening, followed by ice massage. For patellar tendonitis with quadriceps inflexibility, moist heat to the quadriceps is followed by passive range of motion of the knee and ice massage to the patellar tendon. This is repeated several times daily as necessary to provide pain relief and to achieve goals of normal quadriceps flexibility. When the tendonitis has resolved, quadriceps strengthening exercise is added after heat and stretch. Ice massage may continue, depending on the individual patient response. Alternating heat and cold may allow the athlete to choose the modality subjectively felt to be the most helpful in relieving pain and improving range of motion.[60]

Therapeutic Heat

Therapeutic responses to heat include increased collagen extensibility, increased blood flow, decreased pain, decreased muscle spasm, and decreased joint stiffness.[30] Heat is helpful in a subacute phase to resolve local posttraumatic swelling by improving vascular and lymphatic flow. Soft tissue repair can also be stimulated by changes in tissue temperature, changes in cellular metabolism, and reflex responses to superficial heating of the skin. Range of motion of joint, ligament, tendon, and muscle can be facilitated through application of heat, which increases extensibility of collagen and reduces muscle spasm.[61,62] Muscle spasm is reduced by direct effect of heat on primary and secondary muscle spindle afferents and an indirect reflex inhibition in which decreased gamma activity inhibits the excitability of the muscle spindle.[63] Heat also acts as a counterirritant to reduce pain (gate theory), as mentioned above.[30] A secondary decrease in pain may also result from reflex relaxation of muscle spasm in response to local heat.

Common forms of heat used in sports injury rehabilitation include hot packs, whirlpool, and ultrasound. Therapeutic response to local heat depends on the intensity and duration of treatment. Modality selection is based on selective heating principles, including temperature distribution, heating pattern for a given modality, conductivity of specific injured tissue, and technique of application. Concepts of vigorous versus mild heating and deep versus superficial heating need to be understood when selecting a specific modality.[30]

Moist Heat

Moist heat is the most readily available form of application of superficial heat for both supervised therapy and home programs. Moist heat is frequently used for relief of pain and facilitation of stretching and strengthening programs. In the supervised setting, hydrocollator packs are used, providing superficial heat by conduction. Silica gel and cotton hold water heated in a tank at 160 to 176° F. The amount of heat conduction depends on the thickness of protective toweling, which controls the amount of heat transfer. After hot pack application there is a rapid rise in skin temperature, followed by equilibrium as vascular reflexes cause a cooling response in subcutaneous tissues. Muscles are protected by an insulating subcutaneous fat layer, and the vasodilatation response in skin results in constant cooling with less dramatic temperature changes in deeper soft tissues. Maximum skin temperature elevation occurs approximately 8 to 10 minutes after application of a hydrocollator pack. Reapplication of a new hydrocollator pack does not significantly increase maximum skin temperature but may slightly increase the depth of heat penetration and change the temperature of underlying muscle. Equilibrium is achieved at approximately 15 to 20 minutes, with a maximum temperature change of approximately 2° C at 1 cm depth in underlying muscle and 1° C at 2 cm in underlying muscle.[30] In summary, hot packs replaced every 8 to 10 minutes maintain a maximum therapeutic heating response, which occurs at approximately 8 to 10 minutes in skin and 15 to 20 minutes in superficial muscle layers. Only minimal temperature changes can be achieved in deeper muscle tissues because of subcutaneous insulation and vascular cooling responses. Application of moist heat beyond 20 minutes does not change tissue temperature levels but may be beneficial in generating muscle relaxation secondary to peripheral reflex mechanisms. Most treatment protocols, therefore, suggest 20 to 30 minutes' duration for moist heat. Hot packs need to be reheated or replaced every 8 to 10 minutes. Moist towels heated in hot water or a microwave oven provide easy application of moist heat at home. Home treatment towels retain heat less effectively than hydrocollator packs and should be reheated approximately every 5 minutes to maintain a maximum elevation of tissue temperature.

Whirlpool

Whirlpools or immersion baths produce temperature changes through convection. A safe transfer of heat can be accomplished in a warm whirlpool of 100 to 105° F. Highest temperature changes occur in the skin; core temperature changes depend on the amount of tissue immersed in the whirlpool. With near total immersion of the athlete, it is possible to provoke potentially dangerous rises in core temperature with application beyond 20 to 30 minutes. This type of treatment is primarily for relaxation and facilitation of range of motion exercises, because deep heating of joint, tendon, or ligament is not physiologically achieved through convection.

Contrast Baths

Contrast therapy is an effective method of combining heat, cold, and exercise modalities for treating joint stiffness or residual swelling and for facilitating early range of motion of peripheral joints.[64] Alternating cycles of hot and cold water produce a pumping type of vascular response that decreases soft tissue swelling. The affected area is immersed first in a warm bath (100 to 110° F) for 4 minutes and then in a cold bath of half ice and half water (55 to 60° F) for 1 minute. These contrast baths are alternated for an entire treatment cycle of approximately 20 minutes. Range of motion exercises are done during the warm phase, and the extremity is rested in cold water to control pain and swelling. Most protocols suggest ending contrast therapy with cold. This may be followed by strengthening exercise. It is important not to start contrast therapy too soon after acute injury and risk increased bleeding or inflammation during the warm phase.

Ultrasound

Ultrasound is a popular deep heating modality that is frequently cited for instances of overuse or abuse. The heating effect of ultrasound depends on conversion of absorbed acoustic vibrations at tissue interfaces where there are changes in acoustic impedance.[65] The pattern of relative heating for ultrasound has been extensively studied.[30,66,67] Comparison of fat, muscle, and bone indicate that the highest temperature changes occur at the interface between bone and soft tissue. Uniform tissues do not absorb enough ultrasound to provide an effective heating response. Therefore, ultrasound does not selectively heat normal muscle tissue. It does heat scar tissue that develops following muscle contusion or strain, and it generates a heating response at myofascial interfaces. Ultrasound is most effective for dense collagen tissues such as ligaments, joint capsules, and tendons.[30]

Technique of ultrasound application is important.[68] Maximum response at the interface of soft tissue and bone makes ultrasound potentially harmful if proper techniques are not observed. A field of treatment should be less than 5 inches square in order to ensure heating that is uniform and adequate to a given area. Overlapping circular or longitudinal strokes are encouraged to achieve this effect without causing excessive concentration of sound waves in a small area. Multiple fields need to be treated if the area is too large or if there is a bony configuration that would interfere with total joint heating from one area of application. For example, the shoulder and hip require approximately 5 to 10 minutes for each of three fields (anterior, middle, and posterior) to get adequate circumferential heating of the joint capsule.

Indications for ultrasound include desired heating of joint capsule, tendon, ligament, and fibrous scar. Ultrasound combined with active and passive range of motion can be more effective than moist heat in the treatment of soft tissue contractures. Ultrasound enhances the therapeutic effect of joint and soft tissue injection.[69] Ultrasound combined with topical anesthetic and hydrocortisone cream (phonophoresis) is effective in the treatment of superficial inflammatory conditions including lateral epicondylitis, patellar tendonitis, shin splints, and bursitis.[70-74] Ultrasound has been used for resolution of hematoma and other soft tissue swelling after contusion. Ultrasound is contraindicated in the presence of acute bleeding or suspected heterotopic ossification.

Selective Injection Technique

Several techniques of selective injection therapy have been advocated in the literature for relief of pain and muscle spasm in acute soft tissue injury. Krecji and Koch described a technique of intradermal infiltration of procaine used by European physicians.[75] Tender sites over the injured muscle were located by palpation or by changes in skin impedance measured by an electrical instrument (e.g., punctoscope). The authors noted a marked decrease in subjective pain and spasm following injection which correlated with an objective increase in blood flow to underlying muscle (as measured by rheoplethysmography) and a more rapid return to athletic participation. These intradermal sites are not to be confused with tenderness on deeper palpation of muscle tissue for tender nodules or bands, referred to as trigger points. Intramuscular injection of dilute (0.5 percent) procaine into muscle trigger points following acute or chronic muscle strain results in a significant immediate improvement in range of motion.[76-78] I have observed quicker return to full sports participation with no adverse ill effects on muscle function, in more than 50 college athletes following injection of trigger points in injured muscles, especially hamstrings.

Motor point blocks with phenol have been used extensively for relief of spasticity induced by chronic lesions of the upper motor neuron (e.g., cerebral palsy).[79] Injection of motor points with phenol is contraindicated in athletic injury, but the technique of locating motor points followed by injection of local anesthetic has been successfully used to reduce severe muscle spasm. Motor points (myoneural junctions) are localized grossly with surface electrical stimulation and then more precisely with special Teflon-coated needles.[80] Local anesthetic is injected until the electrically stimulated motor response is abated. Local anesthetic applied to a myoneural junction reduces alpha motor neuron input and thereby produces temporary relief of severe spasm unresponsive to more conservative means.

Zoltan described joint aspiration and Xylocaine infiltration of the joint and tender ligaments combined with early mobilization following ankle sprain.[81] Statistical comparison of nearly 100 patients showed a significantly faster recovery time in the group treated with injection therapy and RICE compared to a control group treated with RICE only.

Selective injection therapy in acute soft tissue injury is regarded as more aggressive management than many health care professionals would advocate. Corticosteroid injections are contraindicated in tendon injuries, not recommended for muscle strains, useful in bursitis and joint synovitis unresponsive to other modalities, and helpful in reducing the inflammatory response to traumatic joint effusion.[82] The health care professional is encouraged to read the literature carefully to determine the relative merits of injection therapy (see chap. 13). Additional skill is mandatory to achieve an appropriate therapeutic response with minimal risk of further injury to the athlete.

Mobilization

Early range of motion therapy has been advocated throughout the literature for the treatment of acute and chronic athletic injuries.[83-87] Early range of motion promotes healing of tendons and ligaments, limits formation of joint contractures, and decreases the amount of muscle atrophy seen after injury or surgery. Range of motion exercise, whether active, passive, or assisted, should be pain free. Amazingly, despite impressive clinical support for early mobilization, there are health care practitioners who still inappropriately and excessively splint knees, cast ankles, restrict activity, and never recommend a progressive program of properly prescribed and supervised therapeutic exercise.

Electrotherapy

Electrical stimulation modalities most commonly used when treating athletic injuries are transcutaneous electrical nerve stimulation (TENS) for pain relief, high-voltage electrical stimulation (HVES) for pain and swelling, galvanic current, and electrical muscle stimulation (EMS). TENS has been most successfully used for the relief of pain associated with acute injury or surgery.[34,88,89] Benefits of TENS after arthroscopic knee surgery include decreased use of narcotic medication, increased early ambulation, quicker return to normal range of motion, and decreased duration of hospitalization.[90,91] TENS facilitates early range of motion that otherwise is inhibited by pain in conditions such as mild sprains of the knee and ankle, shoulder dislocation, lumbar strain, acromioclavicular separation, and stress fracture.[92] TENS is very helpful for pain relief in conditions in which active or passive range of motion is not contraindicated but is limited by pain, including hip pointer, lateral epicondylitis, Osgood-

Schlatter disease, or mild contusion.[93] Care must be taken to avoid complete analgesia when excessive activity could result in increased soft tissue injury.

Traditional TENS utilizes high-frequency, low-intensity pulse current and a comfortable sensory threshold. Electrodes can be placed over areas of pain, peripheral nerves, trigger points, or acupuncture sites.[94,95] Treatment may be continuous in the postoperative phase or intermittent for 5 to 30 minutes per treatment to facilitate range of motion. Pain relief depends on stimulation of large myelinated A fibers that increase presynaptic inhibition at the spinal cord level and interfere with pain input from slowly conducting unmyelinated C fibers (gate theory).

Stimulation parameters vary widely in the literature in pulse width, pulse rate, and intensity. As a general rule, lower intensity stimulation with frequencies in the 50 to 100 pulses per second (PPS) range provide sensory threshold stimulation without a motor response.

Acupuncturelike TENS has also been prescribed (e.g., neuroprobe).[96] High-intensity, low-frequency (10 PPS) modulated current is thought to stimulate endogenous opiates (enkephalins, endorphins), which bind to neurotransmission sites in the central nervous system to alter pain perception and peripheral nerve responses.[34,97-99] This type of TENS is usually more painful and depends on a knowledge of acupuncture sites for effective results.[100] Duration of treatment is shorter and may be effective in combination with traditional TENS or in lieu of traditional TENS when exercise is inhibited by persistent pain.[91,101] Acupuncture sites on the affected extremity are treated prior to mobilization and exercise. Fox and Melzack described significant relief in 50 to 75 percent of patients with chronic pain treated with either TENS or acupuncturelike TENS.[34,102]

HVES has been prescribed to obtain pain relief, increased joint range of motion, decreased muscle spasm, and decreased swelling in joints and soft tissue. A variety of current forms including alternating current, direct current, interferential and microamperage alternating current have been advocated.[90,93,103-110] The "body electric" responds to electrical stimulus by changes in polarity as a flow of current is generated in tissue. These changes in the electromagnetic field reduce pain by the presumed mechanisms of the gate theory and the endogenous opiate system, and they also facilitate healing by presumed changes in vascular and lymphatic flow. There are also changes in the bioelectrical field in an area of treatment that result in ion exchange and have an impact on cellular response to injury. Although precise mechanisms of cellular response to electrical stimulation may not be completely understood, clinical observations show an impressive response to electrical stimulation, including progressive or rapid decreases in joint swelling with only a few daily sessions of 20 minutes' duration. HVES to motor threshold can be an effective adjunct to ice massage for the relief of acute muscle spasm in smaller muscle groups. Continuous stimulation at approximately 100 PPS decreases the force of muscle contraction (presumably secondary to fatigue) in 20 to 30 minutes.

Direct galvanic current for the introduction of ionized molecules into subcutaneous tissue (iontophoresis) has also been described as an effective modality for treating superficial inflammatory conditions including tendonitis.[111-113] Comparative studies with ultrasonic phonophoresis favor phonophoresis as more effective in the introduction of ionized molecules into the subcutaneous tissues and as having a shorter treatment duration and better patient tolerance, because the degree of electrical stimulation required for iontophoresis may be clinically uncomfortable for the patient.

Electrical muscle stimulation (EMS) is used to retard atrophy during immobilization and to provide neuromuscular reeducation when voluntary contraction is inadequate secondary to marked atrophy or pain inhibition.[114-116] Studies of the postoperative use of EMS to stimulate the quadriceps have documented decreased muscle atrophy, increased succinic dehydrogenase (SDH), decreased myofibrillar ATPase, earlier range of motion, decreased pain, and earlier return to activity.[9,16,117] Studies also show that, although the biochemical response in muscle to electrical stimulation is similar to the response to isometric exercise, EMS and isometrics combined are more effective than isometric exercise alone to retard the atrophic effects of prolonged immobilization.[118-120]

Clinical observations of EMS support a significant decrease in the time required to make the transition from modalities to rehabilitation to return to play. For example, daily EMS to the quadriceps may aid patients with symptoms of patellofemoral arthralgia or chondromalacia, in whom quadriceps atrophy or pain inhibition is present.[121-123] The strength of the electrically induced contraction is proportional to the intensity and pulse duration of the stimulus.[109] EMS stimulates large motor units near the surface in a synchronous continuous contraction with rapid fatigue.[124] Voluntary muscle contraction results in stimulation of small, slow twitch fibers first, and a subsequent gradual synchronous full muscle contraction.

Common errors leading to treatment failure include the following:

1. Use of a battery operated EMS unit that is not capable of intensive enough current for tetany of large muscle groups.
2. Use of an HVES unit with shorter duration pulse capabilities, which requires too intense a current to achieve tetany in larger muscle groups. The stimulation is then too painful to be tolerated on a repetitive basis by the patient.
3. Inappropriate use of an appropriate muscle stimulator, so that stimulation is either inadequate (electrode placement) or too painful (pulse parameters) to achieve full muscle contraction or to allow the athlete to learn how to increase voluntary effort.
4. Failure to instruct the athlete to contract the stimulated muscle voluntarily as it is stimulated, to achieve maximal contraction of both fast and slow twitch fibers.[125]

Although EMS effectively strengthens muscles weakened by immobilization, surgery, or pain, studies do not consistently document any significant advantage of electrical muscle stimulation over progressive resistance exercise for strengthening of normal muscle.[126-129]

Rehabilitation Phase: Restoring Normal Neuromuscular Function

The rehabilitation phase is designed to restore normal neuromuscular function, including strength and endurance, cardiovascular fitness, coordination, proprioception, and sport-specific skills. As mentioned earlier, muscle atrophy occurs quickly following injury, owing in part to persistent pain or joint effusion with or without immobilization.[9,10,130] Mueller estimated strength losses from 1 to 5 percent per day during cast immobilization of the elbow.[131] Strength deficits may not always be clinically apparent, as indicated by studies of manual muscle testing that demonstrate unreliability until as much as a 50 percent strength deficit has occurred.[10] Muscle atrophy may not be visually apparent. Computed tomography (CT) studies of the thigh reveal as much as a 10 percent loss of muscle bulk (especially in the vastus medialis) with no change in thigh circumference.[132] Loss of strength and flexibility often occurs throughout the affected extremity but may go unnoticed because of a primary focus on the local site of injury.[10]

Comprehensive rehabilitation programs should, therefore, include proper flexibility and strengthening exercise for all muscles of the affected extremity. An overemphasis on strengthening exercises may overlook persistent dysfunction secondary to inflexibility, e.g., when mild muscle strains respond more slowly than expected to rehabilitation exercise. It is common to see dramatic improvement in patellofemoral arthralgia when unilateral tightness of the quadriceps muscle is recognized and an aggressive stretching program is started before emphasizing strength and endurance exercise. Runners with distal lower extremity complaints often remain symptomatic, because weakness of the hip abductors or tightness of the iliotibial band is ignored during treatment protocols for inflammatory overuse conditions of the distal extremity.

Flexibility

Flexibility can be defined in simplest terms as normal joint and soft tissue range of motion in response to active or passive stretch. Stretching is advocated throughout the sports medicine and sports training literature to decrease risk of injury, increase musculoskeletal performance, and decrease muscle soreness associated with exercise.[10,52,133-137]

Range of motion in response to passive and

active stretch is affected by tensile properties of connective tissue and neurophysiologic responses to lengthening of muscle and tendon.[138] Soft tissue structures are made up of collagen fibers with viscoelastic properties. The viscous properties of collagen allow plastic deformation after stretching that is dependent on the intensity, rate, and duration of stretch at a given tissue temperature.

Low stretching forces at longer durations during a 1 to 2° C elevation of tissue temperature result in more permanent elongation of connective tissue.[139,140] This is analogous to gradual stretching of a coiled spring, which does not return to the prestretch resting state. Tissue temperature elevation is necessary for plastic deformation to occur.[141] Increased range of motion may also be more permanent if stretching is continued until soft tissue cools after application of heat or during the cooling down period after exercise.[140] Higher intensity, rapid stretching of the cold limb affects the elastic more than the viscous properties and results in only temporary elongation of soft tissue. This is analogous to the rubber band that is stretched out and then returns to its previous resting length when stretch is removed. The viscoelastic responses of connective tissue to stretch are verified by the clinical difference in flexibility with slow static versus ballistic stretching.[142] Prolonged stretching of 15 to 60 seconds at lower intensities overcomes the elastic resistance and results in more plastic deformation. Rapid stretching of the elastic component only produces temporary elongation of soft tissue and also increases the risk of injury by potentially exceeding the tensile threshold of soft tissue.

Soft tissue responses to stretching may be altered by injury or immobilization. Collagen fibers change in orientation and tensile strength because of injury and repair. Shortening or weakening of collagen fibers, scar formation, adhesions, and fibrous contractions may affect range of motion in tendons, ligaments, joint capsule, aponeurosis, fascial sheaths, and supportive structures of muscle. All or any of these structures may limit the range of motion and may require specific attention during a stretching program. An understanding of the primary and secondary structures limiting normal range of motion is important if selective heating is to be used as a therapeutic modality, because increased temperature is probably the single most important factor in increasing permanent changes in range of motion after injury. This is in contrast to clinical studies that advocate cryotherapy and stretching as more effective than heat and stretching.[51] Cryotherapy may be appropriate when pain limits stretching but may increase the risk of soft tissue injury, because cold does not encourage viscous or plastic deformation of connective tissue.

Neurophysiologic responses to stretching can be summarized in the stretch reflex. Muscle spindle fibers and Golgi tendon organs of the agonist muscle tendon complex respond to stretch by feedback communications between peripheral muscles, spinal cord, and the central nervous system to modulate muscle tone in response to position or movement. Stretching of muscle spindles activates efferent impulses that stimulate a central response through the alpha motor neuron to increase muscle contraction in response to stretching. Stretching longer than 6 seconds' duration activates Golgi tendon organ afferent impulses in the tendon of the agonist muscle. This stimulates a spinal cord-mediated reflex relaxation of the antagonist muscle by the gamma motor neuron. These balanced neurologic responses are sensitive to rate and intensity of stretching, gravitational position, and voluntary or pain-induced reflex contraction of the involved agonist and antagonist muscles. Rapid or ballistic stretching enhances muscle spindle activity to cause increased agonist muscle contraction, which inhibits stretching of that agonist muscle. Slow sustained stretching overcomes the inhibitory component of the muscle spindle response and also allows more effective reflex relaxation of the antagonist muscle.[142]

Isometric contraction of the antagonist muscle causes reflex relaxation of the stretched agonist muscle by the reciprocal Golgi tendon organ response of the antagonist muscle. Manipulation of the stretch reflex for increased stretch of the agonist muscle has been referred to as proprioceptive neuromuscular facilitation (PNF).[143] Many studies recommend PNF as the most effective means of achieving increased flexibility and increased strength.[52,142,144]

Several different techniques have been described, of which contract–relax or hold–relax is probably the most popular.[145] The agonist muscle is isometrically or isotonically contracted for 5 to 10 seconds, followed by a brief period of relaxation and then passive stretch for 5 to 10 seconds. A second passive stretch is executed after a second brief contraction and relaxation period. The entire sequence is repeated for several minutes for each muscle. A variation of this technique is slow-reversal-hold. The agonist muscle is contracted, relaxed, and then stretched, with isometric contraction of the antagonist occurring during stretching of the agonist. This is followed by a brief period of relaxation and a second stretching of the agonist muscle. The entire sequence is repeated for several minutes.[146] The first method has been referred to as "autogenic" inhibition, and the second method, as "reciprocal" inhibition.[147]

Relaxation of certain muscles can be facilitated by eliminating antigravity reflexes during stretching activity. Sitting down may allow more effective stretching of the hamstring muscles than standing, which activates muscle spindles and increases tone. PNF patterns often rely on positional changes to eliminate as much reflex muscle tone as possible and to facilitate the desired movement.[148]

Recommendations for effective stretching include adequate warm-up before stretching, slow sustained stretching of 15 to 60 seconds to threshold of discomfort, and PNF techniques, when a knowledgeable partner is available to assist in passive range of motion.[145,146,149-151] Increased tissue temperature is achieved by direct application of selective heating modalities or by moderate aerobic activity until a light sweat is achieved. Slow stretching to the threshold of discomfort or to tightness effectively stretches the muscle without increasing inhibition secondary to overstretching which increases the pain response. General stretching is advocated after warm-up and before sports participation. Selective stretching based on specific sports activity is recommended after sports participation. Runners, for example, experience tightness of the primary extensors including erector spinae, hamstrings, and gastrocnemius soleus muscles, so they should stretch these structures after running, when the musculotendinous unit is warm and optimal plastic (permanent) deformation is achieved.

Range of motion is limited not just by tight muscles but also by ligaments, joint capsules, tendons, and myofascial elements of muscle. Connective tissue scar, fibrous adhesions, shortened muscles, stiff joints, or pain inhibition may require modality treatment to help restore normal range of motion. As mentioned above, heat enhances stretching of connective tissue. The choice of superficial or deep heating methods depends on the structures involved in restriction of range of motion and on whether the goal is elevated soft tissue temperature or reflex inhibition of muscle spasm and pain. Although heat facilitates deformation of collagen tissue, pain inhibition may be more effectively overcome with cryotherapy. Advocates of cryostretching need to weigh the relative risks of stretching cold tissue versus the need to overcome active resistance to stretch secondary to a low pain threshold.[51]

Sports injury studies reveal inconsistent correlations between improved flexibility, improved sports performance, and decreased risk of injury.[10,136,152] However, clinical observations suggest an increased frequency of reinjury when an injured muscle remains inflexible following a strain, and a definite improvement in symptoms when normal range of motion is restored prior to beginning a strengthening program.[135,137,153] Quantitative computerized muscle testing has been helpful in providing objective evidence to support increased strength and endurance responses in muscles that have been tested before and after good flexibility programs.[9] Subtle limitations of normal movement may be a significant contributor to impaired muscle function. For example, the standard evaluation of patellofemoral symptoms should always include assessment of knee flexion in the prone position to look for unilateral tightness of the rectus femoris, and assessment of hip motion in the sidelying position for restriction of hip extension and tightness of the iliotibial band. Inflexibility of these muscles is a frequent source of impaired progress during quadriceps rehabilitation. A tight heel cord may be a limiting factor in ankle rehabilitation.[154]

The goals of stretching are normal pain-free range of motion, decreased joint stiffness, decreased muscle soreness after exercise, and early mobilization to reduce swelling and to inhibit scar formation. Increased flexibility allows earlier and more aggressive muscle strengthening and, subsequently, earlier functional participation in sport-specific skills.

Strength

Strength and endurance exercises are cornerstones of athletic rehabilitation. Studies of athletic injury closely correlate strength with decreased risk of reinjury and improved athletic performance.[11,137,155–158] Responses to resistance exercise include increased muscle strength and endurance, increased thickness and strength of tendons and ligaments, faster recovery of tendons and ligaments from injury, increased joint stability, and increased metabolic efficiency.[124,159–162]

Experts disagree on the most efficient way to achieve improved muscle strength and endurance after injury.[163–166] They do agree that exercise must be of sufficient intensity, duration, and frequency to develop maximum tension and generate muscle fatigue.[124,167,168] This is commonly referred to as the *overload principle* and is the basis for most progressive resistance exercise programs.[169,170] Strength can be defined isometrically as the maximum force generated against immovable resistance; isotonically, as the heaviest weight lifted with a shortening (concentric) or lengthening (eccentric) contraction of muscle; or isokinetically, as the maximum torque generated against a limited angular velocity. *Endurance* can be defined as isometric strength over time; isotonic strength, as maximum repetitions for a given resistance; or isokinetic strength, as having a fatigue curve demonstrating limitations of torque at a specific angular velocity over time.

Regardless of definition, strength is directly proportional to cross-sectional area (size) of muscle, number of motor units recruited, and efficiency of motor unit recruitment (synchronization ratio).[171–173] Initial improvement in strength in response to exercise is thought to be secondary to increased neuromuscular facilitation, because rapid strength responses occur before muscle hypertrophy can be documented. Although synchronization ratios improve with exercise (weight lifters have significant increases in synchronization ratios), many other factors appear to be involved, such as rate and type of contraction and type of muscle fibers involved in the contraction.[174] It is possible, for example, to have visible atrophy in the presence of normal muscle strength.[175] This suggests factors other than muscle hypertrophy in the development of maximum muscle strength.[176,177] Concentric or positive contractions develop greater tension at slower rates, and eccentric or negative contractions develop greater tension at faster rates. Studies indicate that work efficiency is significantly increased with eccentric rather than concentric contractions.[178–180] Prestretch of the muscle facilitates the stretch reflex and increases the amount of tension generated in a given muscle. (This is the basis of structural design in such equipment as Nautilus, which attempts to stretch a given muscle prior to concentric contraction) (Fig. 15–1). The time required to reach peak motor unit recruitment varies with types of muscles and individuals.[181–184] The type of muscle fiber recruited also varies with speed and duration of exercise.[185–187] There is a difference between fast twitch and slow twitch fibers in response to exercise and sport-specific skills. This serves as the basis for the recommendation that weight training be velocity specific, depending on the desired athletic skill.[188] Both slow and fast twitch fibers change in chemical composition and levels of metabolic activity in response to disuse or increased exercise.[114,124,189] Slow twitch (type 1) fibers appear to atrophy more quickly where there is immobilization.

Studies of the biochemical, physiologic, and neuromuscular parameters of muscle function have resulted in a variety of recommended approaches to muscle rehabilitation.[24,168,172,190–194] It is unclear, for example,

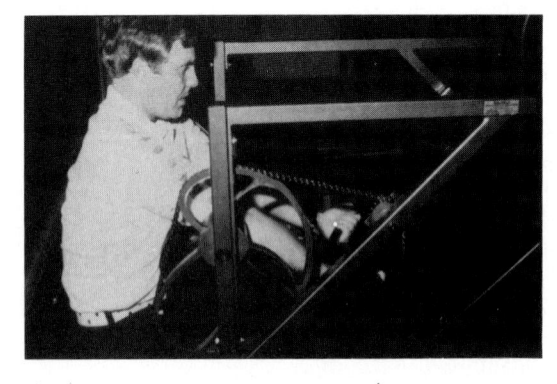

Figure 15–1 Exercise to regain strength.

whether fatigue is primarily a metabolic response to exercise with impaired function, secondary to decreased substrates for energy production, or whether it is primarily neuronal with impaired excitation or activation of the neuromuscular unit. Laboratory and clinical investigations suggest that, despite our incomplete understanding, some generalized conclusions and recommendations can be made.

Isometric Exercise

Isometric exercise decreases the amount of atrophy after acute injury and appears to facilitate a quicker transition to dynamic exercise. Whether this results from a direct effect on the metabolic status of the muscle or is secondary to neuronal mechanisms such as decreased pain inhibition is not entirely clear. Improved strength from isometric exercise appears to be limited to the joint angle used during the exercise and does not correlate with increased functional performance.[195] Isometric exercise is started in the acute phase when joint range of motion is painful, contraindicated, or impossible secondary to immobilization. Isometric exercises are begun as soon as the injured athlete is able to tolerate voluntary contraction. When significant isometric effort is tolerated at multiple joint angles, dynamic exercises are begun. In contrast to strength gained from isometric exercise, strength gained from dynamic exercise correlates more with improved functional performance.

Isokinetic Exercise

The traditional progression from isometric to isotonic exercise has changed with the development of isokinetic exercise equipment.[196] The popularity of isokinetic exercise can be attributed to its ability to accommodate resistance at variable speeds.[197] A fixed rate of speed of the resistance lever arm adjusts to patient effort. Resistance (torque) is directly proportional to effort and is objectively measurable on a hydraulic dynamometer (e.g., Cybex). This permits controlled exercise protocols at variable speeds up to approximately 300 degrees per second, during which risk of injury from overload with excessive weight is less likely than during isotonic exercise. The equipment accommodates the variable strengths of athletes; it allows decreased effort through painful arcs of joint motion and maximal concentric effort throughout the pain-free range of joint motion. Isokinetic exercise on the Cybex permits only concentric contractions, which generate less muscle tension and less delayed muscle soreness than eccentric contraction.[198–202] This allows safe early rehabilitation at a level tolerated by the individual patient.[175] It also allows exercise at higher speeds that may correlate more closely with improved sport performance.

Isokinetic equipment has expanded the knowledge of muscle response to rehabilitation by providing objective measurements of performance, including peak torque, peak torque recruitment time, and fatigue and strength ratios of agonist and antagonist muscles.[203–205]

Hydraulic Exercise

Hydraulic exercise equipment (e.g., Hydrafitness) provides a variation on the theme of isokinetic exercise. This equipment operates on hydraulic cylinders that allow variable speed and provide accommodating resistance proportional to patient effort. Muscle does not physiologically shorten at a constant rate throughout the range of motion, so there is some argument to support this type of equipment as being more physiologic. Practical advantages include accommodating concentric resistance and the ability to maintain a training heart rate on equipment that is safe, durable, and relatively inexpensive.

Isotonic Exercise

Isotonic exercise also results in greater strength gains than isometric exercise. Some studies indicate that similar gains in strength may be seen with isotonic and isokinetic exercise.[194,206] These similarities may be predominantly in endurance and power, for sport-specific activities in which higher speeds of training are more beneficial. Training for power lifting requires large eccentric loads that cannot be obtained on isokinetic equipment.[207]

During isotonic exercise, a fixed resistance is moved at a variable rate through both concentric and eccentric range of motion. Eccentric training may be disadvantageous during early phases of rehabilitation, when muscle soreness can interfere with progress secondary to pain inhibition. During later phases of rehabilitation, when isokinetic exercise is well tolerated through the full range of motion, isotonic exercise becomes desirable for many reasons: availability of equipment (e.g., Nautilus, Universal, free weights), adaptability of exercise programs (e.g., home programs with hand weights, surgical tubing, variability of movement patterns), and the fact that the most rapid gains of muscle bulk are seen in strengthening programs that utilize eccentric contractions. Disadvantages of isotonic equipment include increased muscle soreness and increased risk of strain compared with isokinetic equipment. The competitive nature of "lifting weights" and the frequent tendency for the athlete to progress beyond his level may result in increased injury.

A comprehensive rehabilitation program may take advantage of all three forms of exercise for strength and endurance. Programs need to be custom fit to each patient. The following discussion uses patellofemoral arthralgia as an example of how functional progressions are utilized in the rehabilitation program. The goal is to achieve increased strength and endurance without increasing pain or dysfunction.

Isometric Phase. When joint range of motion is painful, isometric contractions of the quadriceps muscle are used initially to minimize the adverse effects of atrophy during immobilization. Eight seconds of maximal isometric contraction is alternated with 2 seconds of relaxation. This sequence is repeated for intervals of 3 to 5 minutes until the quadriceps is fatigued. This exercise is followed immediately by straight leg raises, three sets of 10 to 20 repetitions with 1-mintue rest periods between sets. Straight leg raises are performed with the knee in full extension as tolerated, from 0 to 45 degrees of hip flexion. Subsequently, isometric contractions of the quadriceps muscle are performed with the knee in 30, 60, and 90 degrees of flexion.

The entire isometric protocol is preceded by moist heat for 10 minutes, is followed by ice massage for 5 to 10 minutes, and is repeated twice daily. If there is significant pain inhibition or poor voluntary effort during isometric quadriceps contraction, a program of electrical muscle stimulation is prescribed. The initial protocol uses the same interval of 8 seconds on, 2 seconds off, with a short delay from onset to maximal electrical stimulation (ramp time) for "neuromuscular reeducation." Some patients do not tolerate high-intensity electrical stimulation or fatigue too easily with this protocol.[208] A longer duration stimulus (e.g., 20 seconds) at lower intensity with a longer rest interval (e.g., 20 to 60 seconds) may be required initially. The parameters of intensity, duration, frequency, and interval rest period are changed on a progressive basis as the patient accommodates to electrical stimulation during each treatment session and becomes more accustomed to this modality in follow-up sessions. Electrical muscle stimulation appears to be an effective means of overcoming pain inhibition or weakness associated with patellofemoral complaints in patients with significant pain or extreme muscle atrophy. Better results are seen with daily treatment.[121]

Isokinetic Phase. Transition to dynamic exercise is made as soon as isometric contractions are tolerated at 0, 30, 60, and 90 degrees of flexion. The patient must also be able to tolerate resisted range of motion without increased pain. This may include limited-range isotonic exercise (terminal knee extensions) or full range of motion with isokinetic or hydraulic exercise. In patients having patellofemoral arthralgia, isotonic exercise at slower speeds is limited by the amount of weight tolerated through the painful arc. Isokinetic exercise or hydraulic exercise permits full effort through a pain-free range of motion, with an accommodating decrease in effort through the arc of pain. Isokinetic accommodating resistance thus allows more efficient strengthening when there is a significantly painful arc. Accommodating concentric exercise is also favored initially in an effort to avoid increased muscle soreness from eccentric exercise or from excessive isotonic overload. During early rehabilitation of patellofemoral arthralgia, the athlete continues a home program of isometric quadriceps sets and starts on a full range of motion isokinetic resistance program. Quadriceps resistance exercise may still be limited, to exclude approximately 30 to 60 degrees of knee flexion at the point of maximal patellofemoral compression while encouraging full isokinetic resistance throughout hamstring powered knee flexion. Higher speeds are used to avoid increased patellofemoral compression.

Isotonic Phase. Increased tolerance of isokinetic resistance exercise through a full range of motion is followed by an isotonic progressive resistance program that starts with light weights and higher repetitions until it is clear that the patient is able to tolerate the eccentric load on the patellofemoral joint. Range of motion is initially restricted as noted above and is increased as tolerated. Rate of progress depends on the individual patient. Once efforts are pain free with minimal delayed muscle soreness and no increase in patellofemoral symptoms, a more aggressive strengthening program can be pursued. It should be noted that some patients may never be able to tolerate significant resistance through a specific arc of motion.

Isotonic exercise programs are most effective when resistance is increased at frequent intervals. This may require modifications of the traditional DeLorme method of three sets of 10 repetitions at 50 percent, 75 percent, and 100 percent of a 10-repetition maximum. Resistance is increased 5 to 10 percent on a weekly basis. The DeLorme method has the disadvantage of arbitrary adjustments in resistance that may not accommodate to potentially rapid strength changes in the early phases of rehabilitation. The goal of maximum muscle tension and fatigue is not as effectively achieved as with daily adjustable progressive resistance exercise (DAPRE), which provides daily changes in resistance to accommodate more rapid gains in strength.[193,209]

Practical conclusions for strength and endurance rehabilitation exercise include the following:

1. Stretching for increased flexibility should be performed before and after strengthening. Muscle strength is impaired when muscle is shortened after injury. Stretching after strengthening also decreases muscle soreness.
2. Functional progressions are guided by range of motion, pain, swelling, and type of injury. Therapeutic exercise may be passive, assisted, active, or resistive, with care taken to avoid increased pain or increased joint swelling in the early phases of rehabilitation, because pain and swelling interfere with function and correlate with decreased muscle strength.[130,210]
3. Dynamic exercise should be preceded by static exercise to protect against injury from inappropriate sudden stress on healing tissue. Isometric muscle contractions can be facilitated with electrical muscle stimulation in the presence of significant pain, weakness, or immobility.[118]
4. When tolerated, exercise must be progressive (overload principle) and must stimulate a maximum tension response to increase muscle strength efficiently. Intensity of exercise requires five to seven maximum repetitions, with a rest interval of 1 minute or less. Three to five sets are usually performed every other day or three times weekly. Isokinetic studies suggest that effort must be greater than 50 percent of maximum voluntary contraction to recruit fast twitch fibers effectively.[211]
5. Eccentric exercise is avoided early when pain inhibition or patient confidence is a factor. Patients are sometimes unable to distinguish soreness of exercise from pain because of the original soft tissue injury.
6. Adequate warm-up to raise body core temperature and improve metabolic efficiency is necessary before starting even a modest strengthening program. Stationary bicycle, treadmill, upper extremity ergometer, and stair climbing equipment can be effectively incorporated into a strengthening program.
7. It is good to work the muscle at variable speeds and at functional tasks. Studies show comparable strength gains when isokinetic and isotonic exercises are used, but improved functional performance levels following isokinetic exercise, presumably secondary to the higher speeds of training. Smith and Melton noted significant improvement in vertical jump, standing broad jump, and 40-yard dash in isokinetically trained subjects versus those trained isotonically.[206] The advantage of using free weights is the ability to mimic sport-specific movements involving cocontracting stabilizers while concentrating on specific agonist–antagonist muscle groups.
8. All muscles of the affected extremity should be strengthened. Clinical studies clearly show losses of strength and endurance in muscles

distant from a given site of injury.[69] Nicholas and co-workers specifically noted significant hip weakness following ankle and foot injuries, quadriceps weakness associated with knee ligament injuries, and quadriceps and hamstrings and hip flexor weakness in patients having patellofemoral pain problems.[10] The contralateral extremity should also be strengthened. Studies demonstrate a cross-over effect in which strengthening of the unaffected extremity results in improved strength response (without hypertrophy) in the affected extremity.[174,212-214]

Proprioception

The goal of neuromuscular rehabilitation is restoration of maximal physical function. Traditional rehabilitative exercise programs place an emphasis on strength, endurance, and flexibility. Recent clinical studies indicate that optimization of physical skill levels also requires an understanding of neuromuscular control mechanisms such as proprioception, coordination reflexes, and methods of improving the power, agility, and speed components of sport-specific skills.[52,144,215,216]

Sensory awareness of body position and movement is referred to as *kinesthesia*. Kinetic sensations arise from sensory receptors in muscle, ligament, tendon, and joint to provide an awareness of very fine movements. For example, it is normal to appreciate 1 to 2 degrees of motion at the interphalangeal joint. Impulses arising from muscle and tendon spindles provide input on direction, force, and range of motion. This input is finely tuned to provide instant awareness of position of body parts in space, and it serves as a complex feedback loop to increase reflex response during physical movements that require rapid changes in position or weight bearing. Coordination involves complex communication among the cerebellum, basal ganglia, the premotor cortex, and visual stimuli. Proprioceptive sensations tested clinically include motion, position, vibration, and pressure. When injury results in inflammation, swelling, pain, and immobility, there is an apparent decrease in neuromuscular efficiency. Reflexes are slowed, and body awareness is impaired. Specific exercises that require balance, weight shift, stimulation of antigravity reflexes, and coordination between agonist and antagonist muscle contractions appear to facilitate proprioceptive feedback mechanisms.[191,215,217] These, in turn, increase coordination and reflex response and improve functional sports performance.

Plyometrics

Plyometrics is a popular term used to describe exercises that emphasize explosive muscle contractions to increase strength, speed, and power. Recent studies of sports performance suggest this type of exercise, which incorporates speed, strength, quick reflexes, and coordination skills, improves performance more effectively than traditional progressive resistance exercises that focus primarily on strength, endurance, and flexibility.

Plyometrics is based on physiologic principles of the myotatic stretch reflex and the elastic component of skeletal muscle tissue.[191] Rapid lengthening (eccentric) contractions of muscle are thought to facilitate more rapid and powerful concentric or shortening contractions, by activation of sensory fibers in the muscle spindle.[191,215] These afferent fibers respond to lengthening of muscle fibers by sending a barrage of impulses to the central nervous system, which, in turn, activates increased efferent input to the contracting muscle fibers to increase the speed and force of shortening contraction. As mentioned above, there is a complex balance of muscle spindle fibers, Golgi tendon organs, and efferent gamma and alpha motor neurons that controls muscle tension, rate, and intensity of contraction. The rate of passive or active muscle stretch directly affects the type of muscle response. A sustained stretch in which interfusal fibers are stretched slowly results in an accommodation of muscle tone to the stretch stimulus. As the rate of stretch increases, the rate of afferent input to the central nervous system also increases. With the first application of intense stimulus, there is a more rapid and intense efferent alpha motor neuron response. This results in a rapid intense shortening contraction of muscle. With repetition, the interval between eccentric contraction and concentric response appears to shorten. Rapid stretch also stores elastic energy in muscle and tendon, which facilitates a more rapid and explosive concentric contraction than can be explained solely on a neuromuscular basis.

Repetitive movements increase the speed of response to change in direction and are used in training on the assumption that a decrease in the interval between eccentric and concentric contractions increases speed and power. Exercises that incorporate antigravity reflex movements such as stepping, jumping, hopping, bounding, and leaping are thought to improve jumping and running ability by decreasing the interval between bending and straightening while jumping and between forward and back while running. These movements require complex coordinated control of agonist–antagonist movements during changes in direction. There is a generalized emphasis on hip flexion with knee flexion, knee extension with hip extension, and cocontraction of dynamic stabilizers of the trunk, hip, knee and ankle (e.g., adductors and abductors of the hip).

Plyometric exercises are beneficial for training as well as rehabilitation. Explosive power demands in sports that require a rapid change in direction include the cocking phase of the baseball pitch or tennis serve, basketball rebounding, the volleyball spike, the baseball swing, the soccer kick, coming out of stance for a football lineman, and the golf swing. Six weeks of plyometric jumping exercise combined with weight training increased average vertical jump by 3 to 4 inches in college basketball players at the University of Arizona (information from personal communication).

Cardiopulmonary Fitness

Athletic rehabilitation would be incomplete without a discussion of aerobic and anaerobic fitness.[218] Cardiopulmonary responses to inactivity include decreased cardiac output (increased resting heart rate, decreased stroke volume), decreased vital capacity, and decreased oxygen consumption capacity. These decrements result in less total work capability for the athlete despite participation in a progressive resistance exercise program for muscle strength and endurance. Whenever possible, aerobic exercise is included early in the phases of rehabilitation to minimize the effects of inactivity on cardiovascular and cardiopulmonary function.

An aerobic program is based on the principles of intensity, duration, frequency, and mode of exercise. Intensity of exercise can be monitored by direct measurement of training heart rate, according to recommended guidelines of the American College of Sports Medicine. A minimum intensity for aerobic fitness should be above 50 percent of maximum oxygen consumption rate, which correlates with at least 60 percent of maximum heart rate. For healthy athletes, duration of exercise at 60 to 80 percent of maximum heart rate should be at least 30 minutes daily to maintain an adequate aerobic level during rehabilitation. Interval training at higher levels of intensity above 90 percent of maximum heart rate may be included as tolerated during the rehabilitation phase, in order to provoke an anaerobic training response. Frequency of exercise for the competitive athlete is different from that for the recreational athlete, who may have different fitness goals. Competitive athletes usually participate in aerobic training on a daily basis, with less frequent rest intervals than the noncompetitive athlete. Deconditioned or less fit athletes may need 24 to 48 hours of rest between periods of longer-duration aerobic exercise. These athletes may respond more appropriately to 3 to 4 aerobic sessions a week. Competitive athletes and more physically fit athletes may be able to tolerate daily exercise with infrequent rest intervals of 1 or 2 days weekly or biweekly.

Mode of exercise depends on sport-specific requirements and type of injury. The athlete with a lower extremity injury is asked to perform aerobic exercise on an upper extremity ergometer. The athlete with an upper extremity injury may be able to continue lower extremity exercise such as treadmill, StairMaster, stationary bicycle, or walking, while waiting for the upper extremity injury to heal.

Circuit weight training is a less efficient means of achieving aerobic fitness. Studies indicate approximately 5 percent improvement in oxygen consumption rates with circuit weight training, compared to 15 to 25 percent improvement with continuous aerobic exercise such as running, walking, swimming, or biking.[219,220] A modest improvement in aerobic fitness with circuit weight training justifies the inclusion of this mode of exercise for specific athletes who desire generalized musculoskeletal conditioning as part of their training program. A typical prescription is 30 minutes of circuit weight training combining upper and lower extremity exercises at 50 percent of maximum repetition ability for 10 to 15 repetitions with 15 to 30 seconds of rest between sets. The number of sets per circuit may vary from one set to a maximum of three sets, depending on the time interval. Circuit training can be added to a conditioning program from one to three times weekly.

RETURN TO ATHLETIC PARTICIPATION

Criteria for Return to Play

It is critical to the success of athletic injury rehabilitation to have objective criteria for returning to full participation in sports. These return-to-play criteria may include objective measurements of flexibility and strength.[221] Return-to-play criteria are best incorporated into a program of progressive rehabilitation.[222] Each phase of treatment is designed to accommodate anticipated performance capabilities of the injured athlete. The goal is increased function, but each phase also provides an objective means of evaluating improvement. It is much easier to evaluate strength, endurance, and flexibility than it is to evaluate proprioception, reflex time, coordination, and agility. Thus, an incomplete course of rehabilitation may result if the athlete is not observed in the performance of sport-specific skills. For example, the football player can be observed on the practice field during agility and coordination drills before a final recommendation for return to play is made.

A positive correlation exists between normal neuromuscular function and decreased risk of reinjury. Examples include reducing recurrent shoulder dislocation with rotator cuff strengthening, decreasing symptomatic tennis elbow with forearm strengthening, decreasing shoulder pain in swimmers by using rotator cuff strengthening, decreasing joint injuries with correction of muscular weakness or imbalance, and decreasing recurrent ankle injury after strengthening either ankle evertors or dorsiflexors.[11,223-226] Studies of the efficacy of flexibility exercises show decreased low back pain in female rowers after lumbar stretching programs, decreased recurrence of ankle sprains after heel cord stretching, and decreased muscle strain after adequate strengthening prior to activity.[146,154,227]

Studies also document decreased risk of new injury with adequate conditioning or "prehabilitation" programs prior to sports participation.[228] Ekstrand and associates claimed a 75 percent decrease in injury rate in senior division male soccer players in Sweden when a comprehensive conditioning, rehabilitation, and injury prevention program was conducted under the supervision of physicians and therapists for a 6-month period.[157] This program included preseason conditioning, early recognition and treatment of musculoskeletal injury, prophylactic ankle taping, education in prevention of injury, and objective criteria for return to play after injury. Preseason conditioning programs for high school football players have resulted in a significant decrease in the number and severity of knee injuries.[156]

Principles of Prevention

Rehabilitation of the injured athlete is not complete until consideration is given to preventing future injury.[229,230] Prevention may require analysis of biomechanical factors and use of orthotic appliances, braces, taping or other devices, and special equipment.[231,232] It is important to look at the alterations in biomechanics caused by these devices from two perspectives—a beneficial one, and a detrimental one in which potential impairment of performance or increased risk of new injury occurs despite the intended protective purpose of such appliances.

Studies of ankle taping indicate a significant decrease in risk of new injury or reinjury without any significant impairment in function.[154,233,234] Orthotic arch supports alone often decrease overuse injuries associated with excessive subtalar joint pronation in runners.[235] Low-dye strapping is effective in the treatment of pronation and plantar fascial strain.[236] Patellar braces may significantly relieve anterior knee pain and objectively increase isokinetic strength measurements of quadriceps function in symptomatic patellofemoral arthralgia.[237] Recurrent patellar tendonitis may be prevented with the use of an infrapatellar strap.[238]

Braces for prevention of knee injury in football players may actually impair function and increase risk of injury.[239-243] Neoprene sleeves have been anecdotally described as being more effective (and more comfortable) than specialized braces for ACL instability in recreational athletes with symptomatic knee effusions from such sports as tennis, basketball, softball, or skiing. Some studies have found no measurable improvement in static knee joint stability with elaborate or bulky braces.[240] These findings have led to the assumption that braces may trigger increased dynamic stability through proprioceptive mechanisms, because there is an observed subjective improvement in function seen with soft supports such as elastic bands and Neoprene sleeves that is not significantly different from that seen when sturdier braces are used.

In summary, the goals of athletic injury rehabilitation are restoration of maximum physical function and sport-specific skills in the minimum amount of time. Proper treatment implies early recognition of injury and aggressive intervention to control soft tissue and neuromuscular responses to injury. A coordinated effort by physician, therapist or trainer, and athlete is required to progress efficiently through the phases of first aid, use of modalities, neuromuscular rehabilitation, and attainment of physical performance skills. Specific criteria for return to play provide an objective measure of function and decrease the risk of recurrent injury. The committed health care provider should communicate these principles to the athlete.

REFERENCES

1. Yaksh TL, Hammon DL. Peripheral and central substrates involved in the rostrad transmission of nociceptive information. Pain 1982; 13:1-85.
2. Edmeads J. The physiology of pain: a review. Prog Neuropsychopharmacol Biol Psychiatry 1983; 7:413-419.
3. Thaxter TH, Mann RA, Anderson CE. Degeneration of immobilized knee joints in rats. J Bone Joint Surg (Am) 1965; 47:567-585.
4. Herbison GJ, Jaweed MM, Ditunno JF. Muscle fiber atrophy after cast immobilization in the rat. Arch Phys Med Rehabil 1978; 59:301-305.
5. Noyes FR. Functional properties of knee ligaments and alterations induced by immobilization. Clin Orthop 1977; 123:210-242.
6. Noyes FR, DeLucas MS, Tovik PJ. Biomechanics of anterior cruciate ligament failure: an analysis of strain rate sensitivity and mechanisms of failure in primates. J Bone Joint Surg (Am) 1974; 56:236-253.
7. Enneking WF, Horowitz M. The intra-articular effects of immobilization on the human knee. J Bone Joint Surg (Am) 1972; 54:973-985.
8. Salter RB, Simmons DF, Malcom BW, et al. The biological effects of continuous passive motion on the healing of full thickness defects in articular cartilage. J Bone Joint Surg (Am) 1980; 62:1232-1251.
9. Morrissey MC, Brewster CE, Shields CL, Brown M. The effects of electrical stimulation on the quadriceps during postoperative knee immobilization. Am J Sports Med 1985; 13:40-45.
10. Nicholas JA, Strizak AM, Veras G. A study in thigh muscle weakness in different pathological states of the lower extremity. Am J Sports Med 1976; 4:6.
11. Grace TG. Muscle imbalance and extremity injury: a perplexing relationship. Sports Med 1985; 2:77-82.
12. Herbison GJ, Jaweed MM, Ditunno JF. Muscle atrophy in rats following denervation, casting, inflammation, and tenotomy. Arch Phys Med Rehabil 1979; 60:401-404.
13. Spencer JD, Hayes KC, Alexander IJ. Knee joint effusion and quadriceps reflex inhibition in man. Arch Phys Med Rehabil 1984; 65:171-177.
14. Eriksson E. Rehabilitation of muscle function after sport injury. Int J Sports Med 1981; 1:1-6.
15. Witzmann FA, Kim DH, Fitts RH. Recovery time course in contractile function of fast and slow skeletal muscle after hindlimb immobilization. J Appl Physiol 1982; 52(3):677-682.
16. Stanish WD, Galiant GA, Bonen A, Belcastro AN. The effects of immobilization and electrical stimulation on muscle glycogen and myofibrillar ATPase. Can J Appl Sport Sci 1982; 7(4):267-271.
17. Booth FW. Effect of limb immobilization on skeletal muscle. J Appl Physiol Respirat Environ Exerc Physiol 1982; 52:113-118.
18. Fischbach GD, Robbins N. Changes in contractile properties of disused soleus muscles. J Physiol 1969; 320:201-205.
19. Jokl P, Konstadt S. The effect of limb immobilization on muscle function and protein composition. Clin Orthop 1983; 174:222-229.
20. Appell HJ. Skeletal muscle atrophy during immobilization. Int J Sports Med 1986; 7:1-5.
21. Woo SLY, Matthews JV, Akeson WH, et al. Connective tissue response to immobility. Arthritis Rheum 1975; 18(3):275-281.
22. Akeson WH, Woo SLY, Amiel D, et al. The connective tissue response to immobility: biochemical changes in periarticular connective tissue of the immobilized rat knee. Clin Orthop 1983; 93:356-362.
23. Casey KL. Pain: a current view of neural mechanisms. Am Sci 1973; 61:194-200.

24. Lesmes GR, Costill DL, Coyle EF, Fink WJ. Muscle strength and power changes during maximal isokinetic training. Med Sci Sports Exerc 1978; 10(4):266–269.
25. Goldin B, Block WD, Pearson JR. Wound healing of tendon—I. Physical, mechanical and metabolic changes. J Biomech 1980; 13:241–256.
26. Hocutt JE, Jaffe R, Rylander R, Beebe JK. Cryotherapy in ankle sprains. Am J Sports Med 1982; 10:316–319.
27. Kolb P, Denegar C. Traumatic edema and lymphatic system. Athletic Training 1983; 18:339–341.
28. Kalenak A, Medlar CE, Fleagle SB, Hochberg WJ. Athletic injuries: heat vs. cold. Trauma 1977; 2(5): 131–134.
29. Knight KL. ICE for immediate care of injuries. Phys Sportsmed 1982; 10:2.
30. Lehmann JF, ed. Therapeutic heat and cold. Rehabilitation medicine library. 3rd ed. Baltimore: Williams & Wilkins, 1982.
31. Barnes L. Cryotherapy—putting injury on ice. Phys Sportsmed 1979; 7(6):130–136.
32. Clarke RSJ, Hellon RF, Lind AR. Vascular reactions of the human forearm to cold. Clin Sci 1958; 17:165–179.
33. Benson TB, Copp EP. The effects of therapeutic forms of heat and ice on the pain threshold of the normal shoulder. Rheumatol Rehabil 1974; 13:101–104.
34. Melzack R. Prolonged relief of pain by brief intense transcutaneous somatic stimulation. Pain 1975; 1:357–373.
35. Wilkerson GB. External compression for controlling traumatic edema. Phys Sportsmed 1985; 13:97–106.
36. Basur RL, Shepard E, Mouzas GL. A cooling method in the treatment of ankle sprains. Practitioner 1976; 216:708–711.
37. Wilkerson GB. Inflammation in connective tissue: etiology and management. Athletic Training 1985; 21:298–301.
38. Pegg S, Littler T, Littler E. A. trial of ice therapy and exercise in chronic arthritis. Physiotherapy 1969; 55:51–56.
39. Kern H, Fessl L, Trnavsky G, Hertz H. Changes in joint temperature due to ice application: basis for practical application. Wien Klin Wochenschr 1984; 96:832–837.
40. Kowal MA. Review of physiological effects of cryotherapy. J Orthop Sports Phys Ther 1983; 66–73.
41. Olson JE, Stravino VD. A review of cryotherapy. Phys Ther 1972; 52(8):840–853.
42. McMaster WC. Cryotherapy. Phys Sportsmed 1982; 10(11):112–119.
43. McMaster WC, Liddle S, Waugh TR. Laboratory evaluation of various cold therapy modalities. Am J Sports Med 1978; 6(5):291–294.
44. Hartviksen K. Ice therapy in spasticity. Acta Neurol Scand (Suppl. 3) 1962; 38:79–84.
45. Johnson DJ, Moore S, Moore J, Oliver RA. Effect of cold submersion on intramuscular temperature of the gastrocnemius muscle. Phys Ther 1979; 59(10):1238–1242.
46. Grant AE. Massage with ice (cryokinetics) in the treatment of painful conditions of the musculoskeletal system. Arch Phys Med Rehabil 1984; 65:233–238.
47. Waylonis GW. The physiologic effects of ice massage. Arch Phys Med Rehabil 1967; 48:37–42.
48. Lowdon BJ, Moore RJ. Temperature changes in muscle during cold therapy and following a sustained contraction. Aust J Sports Med 1977; 11:9–12.
49. Lowdon BJ, Moore RJ. Determinants and nature of intramuscular temperature changes during cold therapy. Am J Phys Med 1975; 54(4):223–233.
50. Yackzan L, Adams C, Francis KT. The effects of ice massage on delayed muscle soreness. Am J Sports Med 1984; 12(2):159–165.
51. Prentice WE. An electromyographic analysis of the effectiveness of heat or cold and stretching for inducing relaxation in injured muscle. J Orthop Sports Phys Ther 1982; 3:133–140.
52. Prentice WE, Kooima EF. The use of proprioceptive neuromuscular facilitation techniques in the rehabilitation of sport related injury. Athletic Training 1986; 21:26–31.
53. Knight KL. Cryostretch for muscle spasm. Phys Sportsmed 1980; 8:4.
54. Cornelius W, Jackson A. The effects of cryotherapy and PNF on hip extensor flexibility. Athletic Training 1984; 19:183–184.
55. Hayden CA. Cryokinetics in an early treatment program. J Am Phys Ther Assoc 1964; 44:990–993.
56. Nielsen AJ. Spray and stretch for myofascial pain. Phys Ther 1978; 58(5):567–569.
57. Sealy DG. Practical considerations in flexibility exercises for knee and lower extremity injuries. In: Hunter LY, Funk FJ Jr. eds. Rehabilitation of the injured knee. St. Louis: CV Mosby, 1984:319.
58. Kraus H. The use of surface anesthesia in the treatment of painful motion. JAMA 1941; 116(23):2582–2583.
59. Drez D, Faust DC, Evans JP. Cryotherapy and nerve palsy. Am J Sports Med 1981; 9(4):256–257.
60. Downey JA. Physiological effects of heat and cold. Phys Ther 1964; 44(8):713–717.
61. Warren CG, Lehmann JF, Koblanski JN. Elongation of rat tail tendon: effect of load and temperature. Arch Phys Med Rehabil 1971; 52(10):465–474.
62. Warren CG, Lehmann JR, Koblanski JN. Heat and stretch procedures: an evaluation using rat tail tendon. Arch Phys Med Rehabil 1976; 5:122–126.
63. Lehman JF, Masock A, Warren CG, Koblanski JN. Effect of therapeutic temperatures on tendon extensibility. Arch Phys Med Rehabil 1970; 51(8):481–487.
64. Cooper DL, Fair J. Contrast baths and pressure treatment for ankle sprains. Phys Sportsmed 1979; 7(4):143.
65. Hansen TI, Kristensen JH. Effect of massage, shortwave diathermy and ultrasound upon 133Xe disappearance rate from muscle and subcutaneous tissue in the human calf. Scand J Rehabil Med 1973; 5:179–182.
66. Lehmann JF, Stonebridge JB, deLateur BJ, et al. Temperatures in human thighs after hot pack treatment followed by ultrasound. Arch Phys Med Rehabil 1978; 59:472–475.
67. Lehmann JF, deLateur BJ, Silverman DR. Selective heating effects of ultrasound on human beings. Arch Phys Med Rehabil 1966; 47(6):331–339.

68. Houglum PA. Clinical use of ultrasound. Phys Sportsmed 1982; 10:5.
69. Newman M, Kill M, Frampton G. The effects of ultrasound alone and combined with hydrocortisone injections by needle or hydrospray. Am J Phys Med 1958; 37:206-209.
70. Novak FJ. Experimental transmission of lidocaine through intact skin by ultrasound. Arch Phys Med Rehabil 1964; 45:231-232.
71. Griffin JE, Touchstone JC, Liu ACY. Ultrasonic movement of cortisol into pig tissue. Am J Phys Med 1965; 44(1):20-25.
72. Antich TJ. Phonophoresis: the principles of the ultrasound driving force and efficacy in treatment of common orthopaedic diagnoses. J Orthop Sports Phys Ther 1982; 4(2):99-102.
73. Kleinhart JA, Wood F. Phonophoresis with one percent versus ten percent hydrocortisone. Phys Ther 1975; 55:1320-1324.
74. Quillin W. Ultrasonic phonophoresis. Phys Sportsmed 1982; 10:211.
75. Krejci V, Koch P. Muscle and tendon injuries in athletes. Chicago: Year Book Medical Publishers, 1979.
76. Cooper AL. Trigger point injection: its place in physical medicine. Arch Phys Med Rehabil 1961; 42:704-709.
77. Travell J, Simons D. Myofascial pain and dysfunction: the trigger point manual. Baltimore: Williams & Wilkins, 1983.
78. Peppard A, Riegler HF. Trigger point therapy for myofascial pain. Phys Sportsmed 1981; 9(6):161-164.
79. Awad EA. Phenol block for control of hip flexor and adductor spasticity. Arch Phys Med Rehabil 1972; 53:554-557.
80. Felsenthal G. Nerve blocks in the lower extremities. Anatomic considerations. Arch Phys Med Rehabil 1974; 55:504-507.
81. Zoltan JD. Treatment of ankle sprains with joint aspiration, Xylocaine infiltration, and early mobilization. J Trauma 1977; 17(2):93-96.
82. Kapetanos G. The effect of local corticosteroids on the healing and biochemical properties of the partially injured tendon. Clin Orthop 1982; 163:170-179.
83. Gelberman RH, Woo SLY, Lothringer K, et al. Effects of intermittent passive mobilization on healing canine flexor tendons. J Hand Surg 1982; 7:170-175.
84. Gelberman RH, Menon J, Gonsalves M, et al. Effects of mobilization on the vascularization of healing flexor tendons in dogs. Clin Orthop 1980; 153:283-289.
85. Appell HJ. Morphology of immobilized skeletal muscle and the effects of a pre- and postimmobilization training program. Int J Sports Med 1986; 7:6-12.
86. Rasch PH, Maniscalco R, Pierson WR, Logan GA. Effect of exercise, immobilization, and intermittent stretching on strength of knee ligaments of albino rats. J Appl Physiol 1960; 15(2):289-290.
87. Tipton CM, Matthes RD, Maynard JA, Carey RA. The influence of physical activity on ligaments and tendons. Med Sci Sports 1975; 7(3):165-176.
88. Cooperman AM, Hall B, Mikalacki K, et al. Use of transcutaneous electrical stimulation in the control of postoperative pain. Am J Surg 1977; 133:185-187.
89. Rosenberg M, Curtis L, Bourdke DL. Transcutaneous electrical nerve stimulation for the relief of postoperative pain. Pain 1978; 5:129-133.
90. Smith MJ. Electrical stimulation for relief of musculoskeletal pain. Phys Sportsmed 1983; 11(5):47-55.
91. Smith MJ, Hutchins RC, Hehenberger D. Transcutaneous neural stimulation use in postoperative knee rehabilitation. Am J Sports Med 1983; 11(2):75-82.
92. Jensen JE, Etheridge GL, Hazelrigg G. Effectiveness of transcutaneous electrical neural stimulation in the treatment of pain. Sports Med 1986; 3:79-88.
93. Roeser WM, Weeks LW, Venis R, Strickland G. The use of transcutaneous nerve stimulation for pain control in athletic medicine. A preliminary report. Am J Sports Med 1976; 4(5):210-213.
94. Dlin RA, Benmair J, Hanne N. Pain relief in sports injuries application of TENS to acupuncture points. Int J Sports Med 1980:203-206.
95. Wolf SL, Gersh MR, Rao VR. Examination of electrode placements and stimulating parameters in treating chronic pain with conventional transcutaneous electrical nerve stimulation (TENS). Pain 1981; 11:37-47.
96. Paris DL, Baynes F, Gucker B. Effects of the neuroprobe in the treatment of second degree ankle inversion sprains. Phys Ther 1983; 63:35-40.
97. Solomon RA, Viernstein MC, Long DM. Reduction of postoperative pain and narcotic use by transcutaneous electrical nerve stimulation. Surgery 1980; 87:142-146.
98. Basbaum AI, Fields HL. Endogenous pain control mechanisms: review and hypothesis. Ann Neurol 1978; 4:451-462.
99. Basbaum AI, Fields HL. Endogenous pain control systems: brainstem spinal pathways and endorphin circuitry. Ann Rev Neurosurg 1984; 7:309-338.
100. Melzack R, Stillwell DM, Fox EJ. Trigger points and acupuncture points for pain: correlations and implications. Pain 1977; 3:3-23.
101. Peppard A, Ruegker G. Ankle reconditioning with TNS. Phys Sportsmed 1980; 8(6):105-106.
102. Fox EJ, Melzack R. Comparison of transcutaneous electrical stimulation and acupuncture in the treatment of chronic pain. In: Bonica JJ, et al, eds. Advances in pain research and therapy. New York: Raven Press, 1976:797.
103. Cheng N, Van Hoof H, Bockx E, et al. The effects of electric currents on ATP generation, protein synthesis, and membrane transport in rat skin. Clin Orthop 1982; 171:264-271.
104. Assimacopoulos D. Wound healing promotion by the use of negative electric current. Am Surg 1968; 34:423-431.
105. Ray CD. Electrical stimulation: new methods for therapy and rehabilitation. Scand J Rehabil Med 1978; 10:65-74.
106. Ross CR, Segal D. High voltage galvanic stimulation—an aid to postoperative healing. Current Podiatry 1981; 30(5):19.
107. Schultz P. TNS—the new current in sportsmedicine. Phys Sportsmed 1979; 7(4):116-121.
108. Brown S. Ankle edema and galvanic muscle stimulation. Phys Sportsmed 1981; 9(11):137.
109. Jacobs SR, Jaweed MM, Herbison GJ, Stilwell GK. Electrical stimulation of muscle. Therapeutic electric-

ity and ultraviolet radiation. Vol. 4. Physical Medicine Library. New Haven, CT: Elizabeth Licht, 1971.
110. Gersh MR, Wolf SL. Applications of transcutaneous electrical nerve stimulation in the management of patients with pain. Phys Ther 1985; 65(3):314–323.
111. Bertolucci LE. Introduction to anti-inflammatory drugs by iontophoresis: double blind study. J Orthop Sports Phys Ther 1982; 3:103–108.
112. Glass JM, Stephen RL, Jacobson SC. The quantity and distribution of radiolabeled dexamethasone delivered to tissue by iontophoresis. Int J Dermatol 1980; 19:519–525.
113. Harris PR. Iontophoresis: clinical research in musculoskeletal inflammatory conditions. J Orthop Sports Phys Ther 1982; 3:109–112.
114. Gould N, Donnermeyer D, Pope M, Ashikaga T. Transcutaneous muscle stimulation as a method to retard disuse atrophy. Clin Orthop Rel Res 1982; 164:215–220.
115. Gould N, Donnermeyer D, Gammon GG, et al. Transcutaneous muscle stimulation to retard disuse atrophy after open meniscectomy. Clin Orthop Rel Res 1983; 178:190–197.
116. Knight KL. Electrical muscle stimulation during immobilization. Phys Sportsmed 1980; 8:2.
117. Eriksson E, Haggmark T. Comparison of isometric muscle training and electrical stimulation of supplementing isometric muscle training in the recovery after major knee ligament surgery: a preliminary report. Am J Sports Med 1979; 7:169–171.
118. Selkowitz DM. Improvement in isometric strength of the quadriceps femoris muscle after training with electrical stimulation. Phys Ther 1985; 65(2):186–196.
119. Godfrey CM, Jayawardena H, Quance TA, Welsh P. Comparison of electrostimulation and isometric exercise in strengthening the quadriceps muscle. Physiother Can 1979; 31:5.
120. Mohr T, Carlson B, Sulentic C, Landry R. Comparison of isometric exercise and high voltage galvanic stimulation on quadriceps femoris muscle strength. Phys Ther 1985; 65(5):606–612.
121. Johnson DH, Thurston P, Ashcroft PJ. The Russian technique of faradism in the treatment of chondromalacia patellae. Physiother Can 1977; 29:5.
122. Currier DP, Lehman J, Lightfoot P. Electrical stimulation in exercise of the quadriceps femoris muscle. Phys Ther 1979; 59(12):1508–1512.
123. Laughman RK, Youdas JW, Garrett TR, Chao EYS. Strength changes in the normal quadriceps femoris muscle as a result of electrical stimulation. Phys Ther 1983; 63:494–499.
124. Gibson H, Edwards RHT. Muscular exercise and fatigue. Sports Med 1985; 2:120–132.
125. Owens J, Malone T. Treatment parameters of high frequency electrical stimulation as established on the Electro-Stim 180. J Orthop Sports Phys Ther 1983; 4:162–168.
126. Halbach JW, Straus D. Comparison of electro-myostimulation to isokinetic training in increasing power of the knee extensor mechanism. J Orthop Sports Phys Ther 1980; 1:20–24.
127. Boutelle D, Smith B, Malone T. A strength study utilizing the Electro-Stim 180. J Orthop Sports Phys Ther 1985; 6:50–53.

128. Currier DP, Mann R. Muscular strength development by electrical stimulation in healthy individuals. Phys Ther 1986; 63(6):915–921.
129. Kramer JF, Mendryk SW. Electrical stimulation as a strength improvement technique: a review. J Orthop Sports Phys Ther 1982; 3:91–98.
130. De Andrade JR, Grant C, Dixon ASJ. Joint distention and reflex muscle inhibition in the knee. J Bone Joint Surg (Am) 1965; 47:313–322.
131. Mueller EA. Influence of training and of inactivity on muscle strength. Arch Phys Med Rehabil 1970; 51(8):449–462.
132. Haggmark T, Jansson E, Svane B. Cross-sectional area of the thigh muscle in man measured by computed tomography. Scand J Clin Lab Invest 1978; 38:355–360.
133. Ekstrand J, Gillquist J. The frequency of muscle tightness and injuries in soccer players. Am J Sports Med 1982; 10(2):75–78.
134. Moretz JA, Walters R, Smith L. Flexibility as a predictor of knee injuries of college football players. Phys Sportsmed 1982; 10(7):93–97.
135. Beaulieu JE. Developing a stretching program. Phys Sportsmed 1981; 9(11):59–69.
136. Greipp JF. Swimmer's shoulder: the influence of flexibility and weight training. Phys Sportsmed 1985; 13:92–105.
137. Agre JC. Hamstring injuries, proposed aetiological factors, prevention, and treatment. Sports Med 1985; 2:21–33.
138. Hubley CL, Kozey JW, Stanish WD. The effects of static stretching exercises and stationary cycling on range of motion at the hip joint. J Orthop Sports Phys Ther 1984; 5:104–109.
139. Kottke FJ, Pauley KL, Ptak RA. The rationale for prolonged stretching for correction of shortening of connective tissue. Arch Phys Med Rehabil 1966; 47:345–352.
140. Sapega AA, Quendefeld TC, Moyer RA, Butler RA. Biophysical factors in range of motion exercise. Phys Sportsmed 1981; 9(12):57–65.
141. Henricson A, Fredriksson K, Persson I, et al. The effect of heat and stretching on the range of hip motion. J Orthop Sports Phys Ther 1984; 5:110–115.
142. Sady SP, Wortman M, Blanke D. Flexibility training: ballistic, static, or proprioceptive neuromuscular facilitation? Arch Phys Med Rehabil 1982; 63:261–263.
143. Wilkerson GB. Developing flexibility by overcoming the stretch reflex. Phys Sportsmed 1981; 9(9):189–192.
144. Nelson AG, Chambers RS, McGown CM, Penrose KW. Proprioceptive neuromuscular facilitation vs. weight training for enhancement of muscular strength and athletic performance. J Orthop Sports Phys Ther 1986; 7:250–253.
145. Moeller M, Ekstrand J, Oberg B, Gillquist J. Duration of stretching effect on range of motion in lower extremities. Arch Phys Med Rehabil 1985; 66:171–173.
146. Shellock FG, Prentice WE. Warming up and stretching for improved physical performance and prevention of sports related injuries. Sports Med 1985; 2:267–278.
147. Surburg PR. Neuromuscular facilitation techniques in

148. Knolt M, Voss DE. Proprioceptive neuromuscular facilitation. New York: Harper & Row, 1968.
149. Wiktorsson-Moller M, Oberg B, Ekstrand J, Gillquist J. Effects of warming up, massage and stretching on range of motion and muscle strength in the lower extremity. Am J Sports Med 1983; 11(4):249–251.
150. Williford HN, East JB, Smith FH, Barry LA. Evaluation of warm-up for improvement in flexibility. Am J Sports Med 1986; 14:316–319.
151. Prentice WE. Comparison of static stretching and PNF stretching for improving hip joint flexibility. Athletic Training 1983; 18:56–59.
152. Wallin D, Ekholm B, Grahn R, Nordenborg T. Improvement of muscle flexibility. Am J Sports Med 1985; 13(4):263–268.
153. Burkett LN. Causative factors in hamstring strains. Med Sci Sports 1970; 2(1):39–42.
154. McCluskey GM, Blackburn TA, Lewis T. Prevention of ankle sprains. Am J Sports Med 1976; 4(4):151–157.
155. Abbott HG, Kress JB. Preconditioning in the prevention of knee injuries. Arch Phys Med Rehabil 1969; 50(6):326–333.
156. Cahill BR, Griffith EH. Effect of preseason conditioning on the incidence and severity of high school football knee injuries. Am J Sports Med 1978; 6:180–184.
157. Ekstrand J, Gillquist J, Liljedahl S. Prevention of soccer injuries. Am J Sports Med 1983; 11(3):116–120.
158. Christensen CS, Wiseman DC. Strength, the common variable in hamstring strain. Athletic Training 1971; 7(2):36.
159. Tipton CM, James SL, Mergner W, Tcheng TK. Influence of exercise on strength of medial collateral knee ligaments of dogs. Am J Physiol 1970; 218(3):894–902.
160. Edwards RH. New techniques for studying human muscle function, metabolism, and fatigue. Muscle Nerve 1984; 7:599–609.
161. Goldberg A, Etlinger J, Goldspink D, et al. Mechanism of work-induced hypertrophy of skeletal muscle. Med Sci Sports Exerc 1975; 7:185–198.
162. Gonyea WJ. Physiology of exercise-induced muscle hyperplasia and hypertrophy. Sportsmed Digest 1984; 6:2.
163. Weltman A, Stamford B. Strength training: free weight vs. machines. Phys Sportsmed 1982; 10(11):197.
164. Hickson RC. Interference of strength development by simultaneously training for strength and endurance. Eur J Appl Physiol 1980; 45:255–263.
165. LeVeau BF, Rogers C. Selective training of the vastus medialis muscle using EMG biofeedback. Phys Ther 1980; 60:1410–1415.
166. Pavone E, Moffat M. Isometric torque of the quadriceps femoris after concentric, eccentric, and isometric training. Arch Phys Med Rehabil 1985; 66:168–170.
167. Withers RT. Effect of varied weight training loads on the strength of university freshman. Res Quart 1970; 41(1):110–114.
168. O'Shea JP. Effects of selected weight training programs on the development of strength and muscle hypertrophy. Res Quart 1966; 37(1):94–103.
169. deLateur BJ, Lehmann JF, Forydce WE. A test of the DeLorme axiom. Arch Phys Med Rehabil 1968; 49(5):245–248.
170. DeLorme TL, Watkins AL. Technics of progressive resistance exercise. Arch Phys Med 1948; 29:263–273.
171. Guth L. An overview of motor unit structure and function. Arch Phys Med Rehabil 1983; 64:408–411.
172. Edstrom L, Grimby L. Effect of exercise on the motor unit. Muscle Nerve 1986; 9:104–126.
173. Gonyea WJ, Sale D. Physiology of weight lifting exercise. Arch Phys Med Rehabil 1982; 63:235–237.
174. Milner-Brown HS, Stein RB, Lee RG. Synchronization of human motor units: possible roles of exercise and supraspinal reflexes. Electroencephalogr Clin Neurophysiol 1975; 38:245–254.
175. Sherman WM, Pearson DR, Plyley MJ, et al. Isokinetic rehabilitation after surgery. Am J Sports Med 1982; 10(3):155–161.
176. Milner-Brown HS, Stein RB, Yemm R. The orderly recruitment of human motor units during voluntary isometric contractions. J Physiol 1973; 231:359–370.
177. Person RS, Kudina LI. Discharge frequency and discharge pattern of human motor units during voluntary contraction of muscle. Electroencephalogr Clin Neurophysiol 1972; 32:471–483.
178. Komi PV, Buskirk ER. Effect of eccentric and concentric muscle conditioning on tension and electrical activity of human muscle. Ergonomics 1972; 15(4):417–434.
179. Johnson BL, Adamcyzk JW, Tenn DO, Stromme SB. A comparison of concentric and eccentric muscle training. Med Sci Sports Exerc 1976; 8(1):35–38.
180. Newham DJ, McPhail G, Mills KR, Edwards RHT. Ultrastructural changes after concentric and eccentric contractions of human muscle. J Neurol Sci 1983; 61:109–122.
181. Herbison GJ, Jaweed MM, Ditunno JF. Muscle fiber types. Arch Phys Med Rehabil 1982; 63:227–230.
182. Brooke MH, Kaiser KK. Muscle fiber types: how many and what kind? Arch Neurol 1970; 23:369–379.
183. Marino M, Glein GW. Muscle strength and fiber typing. Clin Sports Med 1984; 3(1):85–100.
184. Sjostrom M, Angquist KA, Bylund AC, et al. Morphometric analysis of human muscle fiber types. Muscle Nerve 1982; 5:538–553.
185. Gollnick PD, Armstrong RB, Saubert CW, et al. Enzyme activity and fiber composition in skeletal muscle of untrained and trained men. J Appl Physiol 1972; 33(3):312–319.
186. Gollnick PD. Relationship of strength and endurance with skeletal muscle structure and metabolic potential. Int J Sports Med 1982; 3(Suppl 1):26–32.
187. Gollnick PD, Matoba H. The muscle fiber composition of skeletal muscle as a predictor of athletic success. Am J Sports Med 1984; 12(3):212–217.
188. Osternig LR. Isokinetic dynamometry: implications for muscle testing and rehabilitation. Exerc Sci Rev 1986; 14:45–80.
189. Holloszy JO. Muscle metabolism during exercise. Arch Phys Med Rehabil 1982; 63:231–234.
190. Bigland-Ritchie B, Woods JJ. Changes in muscle contractile properties and neural control during human

muscular fatigue. Muscle Nerve 1984; 7:691–699.
191. Bosco C, Komi PV. Potential of the mechanical behavior of human skeletal muscle through prestretching. Acta Physiol Scand 1979; 106:467–572.
192. Delisa JA, deLateur BJ. Therapeutic exercise: types and indications. Am Fam Physician 1983; 28(4):227–233.
193. Knight KL. Knee rehabilitation by the daily adjustable progressive resistive exercise technique. Am J Sports Med 1979; 7(6):336–337.
194. Sanders MT. A comparison of two methods of training on the development of muscular strength and endurance. J Orthop Sports Phys Ther 1981; 1:210–213.
195. Abdenour TE. Patellofemoral rehabilitation. Phys Sportsmed 1983; 11(2):207.
196. Thistle HG, Hislop JH, Moffroid M, Lowman EW. Isokinetic contraction: a new concept of resistive exercise. Arch Phys Med Rehabil 1967; 48:279–282.
197. Osternig LR. Optimal isokinetic loads and velocities producing muscular power in human subjects. Arch Phys Med Rehabil 1975; 56:152–155.
198. Fiden J, Sjostrom M, Ekblom B. Myofibrillar damage following intense eccentric exercise in man. Int J Sports Med 1983; 4:170–176.
199. Talag TS. Residual muscular soreness as influenced by concentric, eccentric, and static contractions. Res Quart 1973; 44:458–469.
200. Abraham WM. Exercise-induced muscle soreness. Phys Sportsmed 1979; 7(10):57–60.
201. Tiidus PM, Ianuzzo CD. Effects of intensity and duration of muscular exercise on delayed soreness and serum enzyme activities. Med Sci Sports Exerc 1983; 15(6):61–465.
202. Francis KT. Delayed muscle soreness: a review. J Orthop Sports Phys Ther 1983; 4:10–13.
203. Coyle EF, Feiring DC, Rotkis TC, et al. Specificity of power improvements through slow and fast isokinetic training. J Appl Physiol 1981; 51:1437–1442.
204. Grimby G. Isokinetic training. Int J Sports Med 1982; 3:61–64.
205. Watkins MP, Harris BA. Evaluation of isokinetic muscle performance. Clin Sports Med 1983; 2(1):37–53.
206. Smith MJ, Melton P. Isokinetic vs. isotonic variable resistance training. Am J Sports Med 1981; 9(4):275–279.
207. Stamford B. The difference between strength and power. Phys Sportsmed 1985; 13(7):155.
208. Parker MG, Berhold M, Brown R, et al. Fatigue response in human quadriceps femoris muscle during high frequency electrical stimulation. J Orthop Sports Phys Ther 1986; 7:145–153.
209. Knight KL. Quadriceps strengthening with the DAPRE technique: case studies with neurological implications. Med Sci Sports Exerc 1985; 17:646–650.
210. Kennedy JC, Alexander IJ, Hayes KC. Nerve supply of the human knee and its functional importance. Am J Sports Med 1982; 10:329–335.
211. Grimby G, Gustafsson E, Peterson L, et al. Quadriceps function and training after knee ligament surgery. Med Sci Sports Exerc 1980; 12:70–75.
212. Kniffki KD, Mense S, Schmidt FJ. Responses to group IV afferent units from skeletal muscle to stretch, contraction, and chemical stimulation. Exp Brain Res 1978; 31:511–522.
213. Grimby L, Hannerz J. Recruitment order of motor units in voluntary contractions: changes induced by proprioceptive afferent activity. J Neurol Neurosurg Psychiatry 1968; 31:565–573.
214. Gollnick PD, Armstrong RB, Saltin B, et al. Effect of training on enzyme activity and fiber composition of human skeletal muscle. J Appl Physiol 1973; 34(1):107–111.
215. Chu DA. Plyometric exercise. NSCA Journal 1984; 56–62.
216. Matteson JH. Cybernetic technology and high performance athletic training. NSCA Journal 1984; 6:3.
217. Bosco C, Ito A, Komi PV, et al. Neuromuscular function and mechanical efficiency of human leg extensory muscles during jumping exercises. Acta Physiol Scand 1982; 114:543–550.
218. Kraus H. Evaluation of muscular and cardiovascular fitness. Prev Med 1972; 1:178–184.
219. Hempel LS, Wells CL. Cardiorespiratory cost of the nautilus express circuit. Phys Sportsmed 1985; 13(4):82–97.
220. Gettman LR, Pollock ML. Circuit weight training: a critical review of its physiological benefits. Phys Sportsmed 1981; 9(1):44–59.
221. Stafford MG, Grana WA. Hamstring/quadriceps ratios in college football players: a high-velocity evaluation. Am J Sports Med 1984; 12:209–211.
222. Kegerreis S, Malone T, McCarroll J. Functional progressions; an aid to athletic rehabilitation. Phys Sportsmed 1984; 12(12):67–71.
223. Aronen JG, Regan K. Decreasing the incidence of recurrence of first time anterior shoulder dislocations with rehabilitation. Am J Sports Med 1984; 12:283–291.
224. Nirschl R. Tennis elbow. Orthop Clin North Am 1973; 1:787–800.
225. Fleck SJ, Falkel JE. Value of resistance training for the reduction of sports injuries. Sports Med 1986; 3:61–68.
226. Fiore RD, Leard JS. A functional approach in the rehabilitation of the ankle and rearfoot. Athletic Training 1980; 15:231–235.
227. Howell DW. Musculoskeletal profile and incidence of musculoskeletal injuries in lightweight women rowers. Am J Sports Med 1984; 12(4):278–282.
228. Heiser TM, Weber J, Sullivan G, et al. Prophylaxis and management of hamstring muscle injuries in intercollegiate football players. Am J Sports Med 1984; 12(5):368–370.
229. Glick JM. Muscle strains: prevention and treatment. Phys Sports Med 1980; 8(11):73–77.
230. Glick JM, Gordon RB, Nishimoto D. The prevention and treatment of ankle injuries. Sports Med 1976; 4(4):136–147.
231. Komi PV. Biomechanics and neuromuscular performance. Med Sci Sports Exerc 1984; 16(1):26–28.
232. Subotnick SI. The biomechanics of running: implications for the prevention of foot injuries. Sports Med 1985; 2:144–153.
233. Garrick JG, Requa RK. Role of external support in the prevention of ankle sprains. Med Sci Sports 1973; 5(3):200–203.
234. Garrick JG. The frequency of injury, mechanism of injury, and epidemiology of ankle sprains. Am J Sports Med 1977; 5(6):241–242.
235. James SL, Bates BT, Osternig LR. Injuries to runners.

Am J Sports Med 1978; 6:40–50.
236. Newell SG. Conservative treatment of plantar fascial strain. Phys Sports Med 1977; 5:68–73.
237. Lysholm J, Nordin M, Ekstrand J, Gillquist J. The effect of a patellar brace on performance in knee extension strength tests in patients with patellar pain. Am J Sports Med 1984; 12:110–112.
238. Levine J, Splain S. Use of the infrapatellar strap in the treatment of patellofemoral pain. Oakdale: Department of Orthopedic Surgery, The Oakdale Hospital Medical Center, 1979: 179.
239. Teitz CC, Hermanson BK, Kronmal RA, Diehr PH. Evaluation of the use of braces to prevent injury to the knee in collegiate football players. J Bone Joint Surg (AM) 1987; 69A:2–8.
240. Hewson GF, Mendini RA, Wang JB. Prophylactic knee bracing in college football. Am J Sports Med 1986; 14:262–266.
241. Paulos LE, Drawbert JP, France P, Rosenberg TD. Lateral knee braces in football: do they prevent injury? Phys Sportsmed 1986; 14:119–125.
242. Prentice WE, Toriscelli T. The effects of lateral knee stabilizing braces on running speed and agility. Athletic Training 1986; 21:112–113.
243. Grace TG, Skipper BJ, Newberry JC, et al. Prophylactic knee braces and injury to the lower extremity. J Bone Joint Surg (Am) 1988; 70:422–427.

Section IV
Psychological Components

Chapter 16
Competitive Stress and Young Athletes

FRANK L. SMOLL
RONALD E. SMITH

Sports place demands on the physiologic, behavioral, and psychological resources of the participants. Athletes are required to test the limits of their abilities in competition with themselves and others. Thus, like many aspects of modern life, the sport setting is one that is capable of generating high levels of stress. From youth leagues to the professional ranks, participants are forced to cope with the pressures inherent in striving for victory. For some individuals, athletic activities are an exhilarating challenge; for others, they prove to be threatening and aversive. Athletes at all competitive levels must learn to cope with the demands and pressures of competition if they are to enjoy and succeed at sports. It is an unfortunate fact that some who choose not to participate in sports or who eventually drop out do so because of fear of failure and anxiety. In this chapter we focus on stress in the young athlete.

Organized youth sports in the United States actually go back to the early 1900s. The first programs were instituted in public schools when it was recognized that physical activity was an important part of education. Over time, sponsorship and control of some sports have shifted to a host of local and national youth agencies.[1] These programs have flourished, and today more children are playing than ever before. Estimates of young people (ages 6 to 18 years) in the United States indicate that approximately 20 million of the 45 million youngsters in this age range participate in nonschool sports.[2]

As organized sports for children have become more highly structured and as adults have often shaped them to reflect a victory-oriented professional sport model, a vigorous debate has arisen over the desirability of such programs for developing children. Critics have frequently charged that extreme performance pressures are sometimes being placed on children before the youngsters are developmentally prepared to cope with them.[3-9] In fact, the results of a brief questionnaire administered to sport psychologists and to nonschool youth sport coaches and administrators indicated that learning more about competitive stress and helping children cope with stress were top priorities.[10] Pediatricians and sports medicine practitioners have become increasingly concerned with the psychological as well as the physical impact of sports participation on children. There also is increased recognition that, because of their contact with child athletes and parents and the consulting roles they occupy in many youth sports programs, physicians are in a position to influence positively the physical and psychological welfare of young athletes.[11]

It is our opinion that, given appropriate adult guidance, the youth sport setting can be one that fosters the psychological growth of the child. Moreover, physicians can play an important role in helping coaches, parents, and sport administrators to facilitate this process. This chapter begins with an analysis of the dynamics of competitive anxiety within a conceptual model of the stress process. Next, we address the consequences of stress among young athletes. We then discuss the question of whether sports are too stressful for youngsters. Finally, we present several promising intervention strategies designed to reduce stress in youth sports. In Chapter 17, we focus on psychological intervention at the level of the individual athlete and describe treatment techniques that might be used to reduce stress in athletes of all ages and at all levels of competition.

DYNAMICS OF ATHLETIC STRESS

People typically use the word *stress* in two different but related ways. First, we use the term to refer to situations that tax the physical or psychological capabilities of the individual.[12] For example, running a race against a superior opponent may be referred to as a *stressor*. The focus here is on the balance between the demands of the situation and the personal and social resources the person has to cope with these demands. Situations are likely to be labeled as stressful when their demands test or exceed the resources of a person. The second use of the word *stress* relates to the individual's response to the situation. Used in this manner, it refers to a person's cognitive, emotional, and behavioral responses to situational demands. For example, "I have a meeting with my lawyer about the malpractice suit, and I feel nervous and uptight about it." Clearly, these two uses of the word *stress* are not synonymous, because people may vary considerably in how "stressful" they find the same situation to be.

A conceptual model showing the dynamics of stress is presented in Figure 16–1.[13] The model emphasizes relationships among cognitions, physiologic responses, and behavior and has four major elements: the situation, the athlete's cognitive appraisal of various aspects of the situation, physiologic arousal responses, and behavioral attempts to cope with the situation. Each of these components is, in turn, influenced by personality and motivational variables.

Situational Component

The situational component involves interactions between environmental demands and personal or environmental resources. Whenever a young athlete encounters a demand, resources are mobilized to meet it. When demands or resources are relatively balanced, stress is minimal. When demands slightly exceed resources, the situation is likely to be viewed as challenging. But when a significant imbalance occurs because of increased demands or a decrease in resources for meeting them, then the situation is likely to be regarded as stressful.

Ordinarily we think of emotional responses as being stimulated by an *external* situation. In the youth sport setting, many exter-

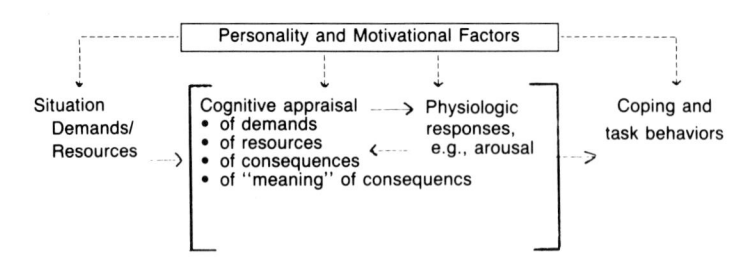

Figure 16–1 A conceptual model of stress showing hypothesized relationships among situational, cognitive, physiologic, and behavioral components. Motivational and personality variables are assumed to affect and interact with each of the components.

nal demands may be stressful, including abusive behaviors of coaches, a critical group of teammates, facing a strong opponent in an important contest, closeness of the score, and so on. Other situational demands have an *internal* cause, resulting from personality or motivational factors. Internal demands include desired goals, personal performance standards relating to values or commitments, or even unconscious motives or conflicts. In this regard, memories of past situations and anticipation of future consequences may interact with the current external situation to affect its psychological meaning and its effect on the young athlete.

In analyzing the numerous demands that are considered important by young athletes, Passer incorporated Martens' model of the competition process.[14,15] Accordingly, the fundamental demands of sports are the same as those in all competitive activities: first, some type of performance must occur, that is, an ability or attribute must be demonstrated; second, this performance must be compared with some standard, such as the performance of others or the person's past performance; and third, at least one person must be present, other than the performer, who can evaluate the comparison process. The significance of these demands to young athletes is clear. First, sports involve the demonstration of athletic ability, which is a highly valued attribute among children and adolescents. Second, the opportunity for comparison of athletic ability with that of peers is important, because it is a major means by which children acquire information about their physical competence. In this regard, social comparison takes on increasing significance during the elementary school years—a time when many children compete in organized sports. Third, children in youth sports are extensively evaluated by adults and peers. This social evaluation is readily transmitted by numerous verbal and nonverbal cues (e.g., praise and criticism, facial expressions, designation as a starter or a substitute). Social evaluation is important not only because it conveys substantial amounts of information to children about their ability, but also because it provides a direct means for obtaining adult social approval. Obviously, the youth sport setting involves many demands other than those concerning the demonstration, comparison, and evaluation of athletic ability. However, the demands of athletic competition to demonstrate physical skill, to compare this skill to that of peers, and to obtain evaluation from others are very important to youth sport participants.

Variables of personality and motivation play an important role in determining which of the complex environmental demands are most salient or demanding. For example, needs for competence, mastery, affiliation, or power each can cause the athlete to focus on and respond to particular aspects of the sport environment. Similarly, different types of resources (e.g., physical skills, social skills, or social support within the environment) may differ in their relative importance to individual athletes. Therefore, in any analysis of situational stress, it is important to take into account the specific demands, resources, and imbalances that are of concern to the individual athlete.

Typically, we think of stress as occurring when demands greatly exceed resources, producing a condition of "overload." However, psychological stress can also result when resources greatly exceed demands, or when the person is not challenged to use his or her resources. Feelings of boredom, stagnation, and "staleness" are common responses to this state of affairs. It is likely that a condition of "underload" may also take a toll on a young athlete. Thus, both overtaxing and undertaxing situations have been hypothesized to be predisposing factors for athletic burnout.[16]

Cognitive Component

Athletes generally view their emotions as being triggered directly by situational demands. However, in most instances, situations exert their effects on emotions through the intervening influence of thought.[17,18] Through their own thought processes, people create the psychological reality to which they respond. Thus, the second component of the stress model, cognitive appraisal, plays a central role in understanding stress, because the intensity of emotional responses is a function of what people tell themselves about situations, their meaning, and about their ability to cope with the demands of the situation.

As specified in the model, the active process of cognitive appraisal includes perception of four elements. People appraise not only the demands of the situation but also the nature and adequacy of the resources they have to cope with them. Such appraisal may or may not be accurate. For example, a young athlete low in self-confidence may perceive a greater discrepancy between demands and resources than is actually the case. Conversely, a self-assured athlete may perceive a smaller discrepancy than actually exists. It is the perception of balance and imbalance rather than the actual state of affairs that in the end determines how stressed a young athlete becomes. Here again, individual differences in such factors as self-efficacy and competitive trait anxiety can play a vital role.[19]

In addition to mental evaluation of demands and resources, people appraise the possible consequences of failure to meet the demands. If a perceived imbalance between demands and resources threatens harm or loss of desired goals, the situation is likely to be perceived as stressful.[12] Here again, the appraisal process may or may not be accurate. Thus, an athlete who exaggerates or "catastrophizes" about the consequences of failing to deal successfully with demands may experience needless stress. Distortions may occur about how negative the consequences will be as well as about how likely they are to occur. For example, one highly stressed athlete believed that any mistake on her part would certainly lead to demotion to the second team, despite assurances from her coach to the contrary. This distortion was clearly at the level of subjective probability of occurrence of a dreaded consequence.

The final aspect of the appraisal process is the personal meaning attributed to the consequences. These meanings derive from the athlete's personal beliefs, self-concept, and conditions of self-worth. Ellis has described in detail the central role of irrational assumptions and beliefs in psychological stress.[20] It is clear that athletes who believe that their basic self-worth is defined by their athletic success attribute different meanings to athletic outcomes than do athletes whose self-worth is more securely and realistically anchored. For the former, winning can become literally a life-or-death situation; in contrast, the athlete who can divorce self-worth from success can attribute a less urgent personal meaning to success and failure. Many young athletes appear to be victimized by irrational beliefs about the meaning and importance of success and approval of others, and such beliefs predispose them to inappropriate or excessive stress reactions.

Physiologic Component

The third component of the model, physiologic responses, is reciprocally related to appraisal processes. Despite the recent debate on whether cognition is a necessary condition for emotional arousal, we assume that whether and to what extent athletes respond with emotional arousal is largely dependent on cognitive mediational responses.[21,22] When appraisal indicates the threat of harm or danger, physiologic arousal occurs as part of the mobilization of resources to deal with the situation. Arousal, in turn, provides feedback about the intensity of the emotion being experienced, thereby contributing to the ongoing process of appraisal and reappraisal.[23,24] Thus, a young athlete who becomes aware of an increasing level of arousal may see the situation as threatening; this appraisal may, in turn, generate even more emotional arousal. Conversely, a young athlete who experiences low arousal in a potentially stressful situation is likely to appraise the situation as less threatening or as one with which he or she can cope successfully.

Behavioral Component

The fourth component of the model consists of output behaviors by which the athlete attempts to cope with the situation. These include task-oriented, social, and other classes of coping behaviors. Here the athlete is not directly affected by the demands of the situation; instead, instrumental behaviors are mediated by cognitive appraisal processes and by the nature and intensity of the physiologic responses that may occur. The adequacy or success of these coping behaviors affects the balance between demands and resources, as well as the ongoing appraisal process. Thus, each of the components of the model relates to the others, and changes in one component can ultimately affect all of the others.

CONSEQUENCES OF ATHLETIC STRESS

A substantial amount of research has been devoted to examining the determinants of anxiety experienced by child athletes prior to, during, and following competitive events. Passer's review of literature indicates that a variety of situational and intrapersonal factors influence precompetition stress.[14] These include the type of sport (individual or team), the importance of the contest, the passage of time as competition approaches, expectations about the quality of personal and team performance, perceived parental pressure to compete, self-esteem, and competitive trait anxiety. Stress during competition is affected by trailing or leading the opponent, the importance of the game and the particular situation within the game, the specific activity or role being performed, and competitive trait anxiety. Postcompetition stress is influenced by winning or losing and, regardless of outcome, is related to children's perceptions of how much fun they had. Some young athletes develop effective ways of coping with potential sources of stress. Others, who are not so fortunate, are prone to suffer adverse psychological, behavioral, and health-related effects (Fig. 16–2).

Effects on Participation, Enjoyment, and Withdrawal from Sports

Youngsters are affected by competitive stress in many different ways. Because of anticipated stresses, some children actually avoid playing sports. In one study, Orlick and Botterill reported that 75 percent of a sample of 8- and 9-year-old sport nonparticipants indicated that they would like to compete but were fearful of performing poorly or of failing to make a team.[25] In a more recent study of 10- to 17-year-olds, Pierce found that 26 percent of agency-sponsored sport participants, 26 percent of sport dropouts, and 32 percent of nonparticipants reported that various worries bothered them so much that they might not play in the future.[26]

In addition to influencing the decision about entering a sport program, competitive stress can detract from children's enjoyment of sports.

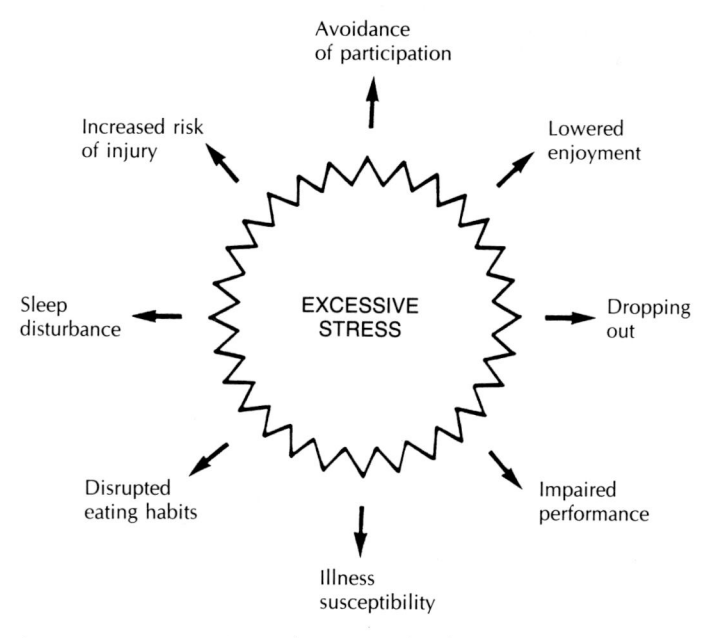

Figure 16–2 Negative effects of excessive stress in youth sports.

Youngsters who play for relatively punitive or critical coaches, who perceive more pressure and negative responses from their parents, who feel that their parents and coaches are less satisfied with their overall sport performance, and who view themselves as having less skill express less enjoyment from their participation and like their sport less.[27-29] Furthermore, young athletes who feel that winning is the most important aspect of sports (and who therefore may place themselves under added competitive stress) derive less enjoyment from their participation and are more apt to drop out.[25,30,31]

Whether stress causes young athletes to withdraw from competition is another important issue. Pooley found that 33 percent of 10- to 15-year-old youth soccer dropouts attributed quitting to an overemphasis on competition and negative coaching behaviors (e.g., frequent criticism of players, pushing them too hard).[32] Similarly, a study of 10- to 18-year-old former swimmers by Gould and co-workers revealed that over half of the youngsters rated "did not like the pressure" as either a very important (16 percent) or somewhat important (36 percent) reason for dropping out, and many rated "did not like the coach" as a very important (20 percent) or somewhat important (24 percent) factor.[33] In a study of more than 1,000 swimmers grouped by age and level of competition, McPherson and colleagues found that too much pressure, conflict with coaches, and insufficient success were among the reasons swimmers reported for why their teammates dropped out of competition.[34] Finally, in a recent study of 8- to 17-year-old wrestlers, a theoretically based comparison of dropouts' versus participants' won–lost records, performance expectations, attributions, and sport values led Burton and Martens to conclude that youngsters appeared to drop out when their perceived ability was threatened by consistent failure.[35] Existing evidence thus suggests that competitive stress contributes significantly to the dropout rate in youth sports.

Effects on Performance

It is widely recognized that stress can have adverse effects on motor skill and athletic performance. In empiric investigations of the stress–performance relationship, sport psychologists have assessed anxiety prior to or during competition and related it to actual measures of performance. For example, Klavora obtained pregame state anxiety scores for 145 male high school basketball players and related the measures to coaches' evaluations of the individual player's performance.[36] The results indicated that approximately 10 percent of the time the players were overexcited, and during this time their ability to achieve normal capacity was inhibited. Although results of other studies are less consistent than one might expect, it is generally held that stress causes performance impairment in young athletes.[37,38]

Another approach to assessing the stress–performance relationship involves having youngsters report how they feel their performance typically is affected by stress. Pierce found that 31 percent of a sample of youth sport participants and 50 percent of sport dropouts reported that various worries prevented them from playing up to their capabilities.[26] On the other hand, 39 percent of a sample of elite wrestlers and 50 percent of junior elite runners reported that anxiety and nervousness helped their performance.[39,40] Thus, although results are equivocal, it appears that some young athletes feel anxiety usually hurts their performance.

Health-Related Effects

A growing body of research literature is demonstrating positive, though modest, relationships between high levels of stress and the onset of a variety of medical and psychological dysfunction in children.[41-44] The unfortunate effects of severe competitive pressures are all too frequently seen in young athletes who develop stress-related dermatologic and gastrointestinal problems.[11,45] In addition, some data exist about the degree to which involvement in sports disrupts youngsters' eating and sleeping patterns. Skubic's survey of Little and Middle League baseball players revealed that 11 percent of the respondents experienced diminished appetite after losing a game, and 60 percent reported occasional or frequent sleep disturbance the night before or after competition.[46] A remarkably similar figure was obtained for a sample of junior elite wrestlers; 58 percent reported having "some" to "a lot" of difficulty sleeping the night before a match because of competitive anxiety.[39]

The most definitive data on sleep disruption are provided by the State of Michigan Youth Sports Study.[47] This comprehensive survey included a statewide sample of 1,118 male and female youth sport participants. Twenty-one percent of the children indicated that there were times when they did not receive enough sleep because of their involvement in sports. Of the athletes experiencing sleep loss, 46 percent rated worrying about performance as a contributing factor, and 25 percent indicated that being upset after losing was a cause. However, it should be noted that other sources of sleep disruption were not directly related to competitive stress. Moreover, youngsters' sleep was disrupted somewhat less by sports involvement than by other achievement-oriented recreational activities (e.g., music, drama, clubs).

The widely recognized contribution of life stress to the development of physical illness and psychological distress has stimulated research on the possible role of stress in athletic injuries. Several studies have examined whether athletes who experience a high degree of "life stress" are at greater risk for athletic injury. May and associates assessed life events, depression, and general well-being (health concerns, energy, life satisfaction, cheerfulness, tension, and emotional control) in 73 members of the U.S. Alpine Ski Team.[48] These psychological factors were compared with subsequent surveys of general health, illness, and athletic performance. Higher scores on the life-change scales were clearly related to greater duration of ear, nose, and throat (ENT) problems, headaches, musculoskeletal leg injuries, and sleep problems. On the other hand, positive well-being was associated with a shorter duration of ENT problems, headaches, digestive problems, sleep disturbances, and neurologic conditions. Overall, the psychological scales predicted (at statistically significant levels) seven of the top 10 health and injury problems of the alpine skiers.

Additional evidence derives from research on football injuries. Studies of college football players have shown injury rates of 68 to 73 percent in athletes who had recently experienced major life changes, compared to rates of 30 to 39 percent in athletes who had not experienced such events.[49,50] In another study of college football players, Passer and Seese obtained partial support for a relationship between injury and "object loss" (a subgroup of negative life events involving the actual or threatened loss of a close personal relationship).[51] In the sole study of younger athletes, Coddington and Troxell found no relationship between overall life stress and injury rates among high school football players.[52] However, athletes who suffered the actual loss of a parent were five times more likely to be injured than teammates who had experienced no object loss. It thus appears that life change, particularly negative events, may be a predisposing factor in youth sport injuries. This important issue warrants further empiric attention.

ARE YOUTH SPORTS TOO STRESSFUL?

The question of how stressful youth sports are for children has stimulated interest among researchers and practitioners alike. In approaching this topic, investigators have employed either physiologic arousal or self-report measures to assess young athletes' stress. Hanson used telemetry to monitor the heart rate of 10 male Little League baseball players.[53] Recordings were taken when the player was at bat, standing on base after a hit, sitting in the dugout after making an out, standing in the field, and sitting at rest before and after the game. The most striking finding was the magnitude of response shown when players came to bat. When at bat, players' heart rates escalated dramatically to an average of 166 beats per minute (bpm), 56 bpm above their mean pregame resting rate of 110 bpm. In fact, no other game situation caused arousal increases that even closely approximated the levels experienced when batting. Substantial variation was found within and among players. The highest heart rate recorded while at bat was 204 bpm; the lowest was 145 bpm. Interestingly, after the game most players reported that they did not feel particularly nervous while batting. Based on players' physiologic responses, Hanson concluded that the stress of being at bat was high, but short-lived.

In another study with 60 Little League players, Lowe and McGrath assessed pulse and respiration rates before batting, under conditions in which the consequences of performance varied in importance.[37] The two variables examined were the critical nature of the game and the critical nature of the situation. The importance of the game involved the ranking of the two teams within the league, the difference in their won-lost percentages, and the number of games left in the season. The importance of the situation included variables such as the inning and number of outs in the inning, the score, and the number and location of the base runners. The findings indicated higher autonomic arousal levels under conditions of increased importance, with importance of the game having a greater effect than importance of the situation.

These two field studies provide evidence that autonomic arousal increases as personal performance becomes accentuated and as the importance of the performance increases. Yet, arousal can be caused by many things besides stress, such as simple excitement or elation. Therefore, on the basis of physiologic data alone, it cannot be conclusively determined that the boys were manifesting aversive emotional reactions. It is likely that the arousal increases reflected stress reactions for some players and more positive emotional states for others.

Several studies have relied on self-report measures of state anxiety that require subjects to rate how tense, anxious, or worried they are at a particular moment. Scanlan and Passer obtained state anxiety measures from 11- and 12-year-old boys 30 minutes before and immediately after soccer matches.[54] For the majority of these young athletes, only slightly higher anxiety levels were reported than in preseason baseline measures. However, some children showed a preseason to pregame increase of as much as 20 points, and boys on losing teams showed higher points of postcompetition anxiety than those on winning teams. Similar results were obtained in Scanlan and Passer's follow-up research with 10- to 12-year-old girl soccer players.[55]

A landmark study by Simon and Martens assessed how stressful sports are compared with other evaluative activities in which children participate.[56] A self-report state anxiety inventory was administered to 468 9- to 14-year-old boys within 10 minutes before they competed in one of seven nonschool sports. The scores were compared with the anxiety experienced by 281 other boys just prior to their participation in four activities: interclass physical education softball games, academic tests, band group competitions, and music solo competitions. Of the various sports studied, individual sports evoked more anxiety than team sports. None of the sports elicited as much anxiety as band solos, and wrestling was the only sport that was significantly more anxiety arousing than school classroom tests (Fig. 16-3). However, like Scanlan and Passer, Simon and Martens reported that a minority of the young athletes experienced extremely high levels of anxiety before competing.[54,55]

Additional evidence about stress in youth sports versus other activities is provided by Skubic, who assessed the galvanic skin response (GSR) of 9- to 15-year-old boys during Little League baseball games and physical education (PE) class softball games.[57] For both activities, GSR measures were obtained immediately before, immediately after, and 1½ hours after competition. No significant differences occurred at any age level between players' precompetition GSR scores in league games and PE class softball. Few significant differences were found when league versus PE comparisons were made immediately after and 1½ hours after competition; when differences occurred, it was often softball competition that elicited greater arousal. Thus, Skubic's data are consistent with those of Simon and Martens in suggesting that the degree of children's emotional reaction to youth sport competition is similar to that experienced when participating in other achievement or competitive activities.

The studies described herein provide important information about the stress experienced by young athletes, but they do not determine whether competitive stress is excessive. In this regard, Martens noted that there are no absolute standards by which to judge how great a physiologic response or anxiety test score must be to indicate that a child is too psychologically stressed.[58] Passer's analysis reveals other salient considerations.[14] Specifically, children who experience the same operational level of stress (e.g., heart rate or anxiety score) may differ not only in how aversive they perceive that stress to be but also in their behavioral re-

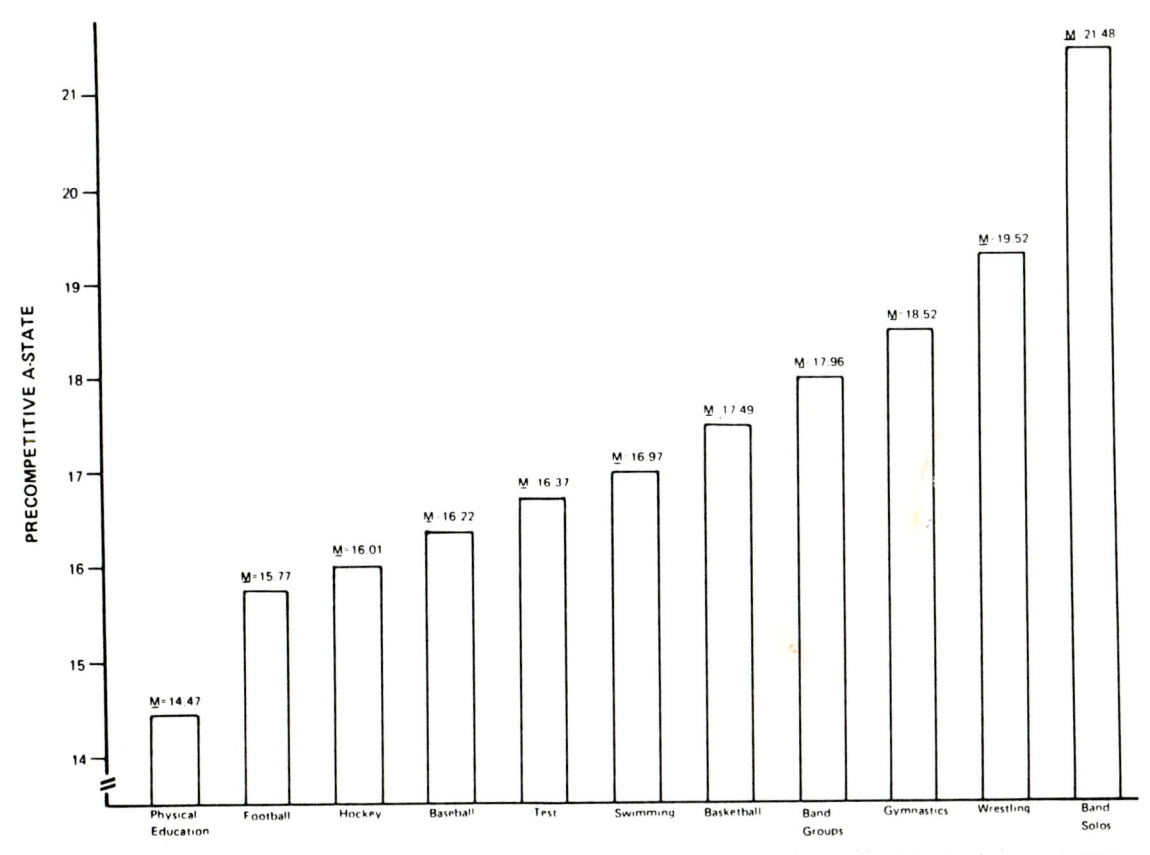

Figure 16-3 Children's precompetition state anxiety in 11 sport and nonsport evaluative activities (scale range is 10 to 30). (From Simon JA, Martens R. J Sport Psychol 1979; 1:160–169. Reprinted with permission.)

sponses. Furthermore, when evaluating the consequences of stress, we might ask how many children must drop out, endure sleep loss, or undergo performance impairment in order for youth sports to be declared too stressful, or, for an individual child, how chronic or severe must untoward stress effects be in order to constitute a "problem." We might also ask if children encounter too much stress in other evaluative activities. Obviously, the issue is quite complicated!

Although there is no simple answer to the question of whether youth sports are too stressful, research results indicate that, for most children, sport participation is not exceedingly stressful, especially in comparison with other activities involving performance evaluation. In other words, the amount of stress in youth sports does not appear to be as widespread or as intense as critics have claimed. Several authorities have thus suggested that the problem of competitive stress has been overemphasized.[58,59] However, it is evident that the sport setting can produce high levels of stress for a minority of youngsters. Such children undoubtedly find competition to be extremely threatening and, as emphasized earlier, the anxiety that they experience can have harmful psychological, behavioral, and health-related effects. Consequently, high priority should be given to developing and implementing intervention strategies designed to minimize sources of undue stress in youth sports.

APPROACHES TO STRESS REDUCTION

The practical as well as conceptual attractiveness of the stress model is that it has clear implications for stress reduction in youth sports.

We now consider how intervention might be directed at each of the four elements of the model: behavioral, physiologic, cognitive, and situational.

Behavioral Component

At the behavioral level, it is intuitively obvious, as well as theoretically consistent, that increasing the young athlete's physical prowess can make athletic demands easier to confront.[30] It follows that training to improve sport skills should be one way to reduce competitive stress, because youngsters' anxiety reactions are derived in part from perceived deficits in ability. Specifically, feelings of insecurity and heightened anxiety might arise because of perceived lack of skill to cope with a situation. Support for this assumption is provided by research indicating that all-star athletes had significantly lower competitive trait anxiety scores than playing substitutes.[60] However, other research is equivocal about whether athletes with high competitive trait anxiety experience competitive stress because of a lack of athletic ability.[39,61–63] For some youngsters, increasing their level of skill may serve to reduce the perceived imbalance between athletic demands and resources, but for others skill improvement may not be sufficient to reduce anxiety. For the latter, assistance in changing excessively high performance standards or distorted fears of the consequences of possible failure may be required.

Cognitive and Physiologic Components

Given that the amount of stress experienced by the young athlete is a joint function of the intensity of environmental stressors and the way the individual appraises and copes with them, it follows that active assistance in developing coping skills can increase youngsters' ability to deal effectively with athletic stress. Reduction of stress at the cognitive and physiologic levels is the focus of stress management programs that seek to teach specific physiologic and cognitive coping skills.

Training programs in stress management behaviors have promising applications with child athletes for several reasons. First, it is highly desirable to acquire adaptive coping responses prior to the turbulent years of adolescence. Second, unlike many adults, children have not generally developed maladaptive coping strategies that are deeply ingrained and therefore difficult to change. Third, the athletic arena requires child athletes to cope with stress-evoking situations on a regular and fairly predictable basis, thereby providing many opportunities to practice and strengthen coping skills in situations that are unlikely to exceed the children's adaptive ability. Finally, developing a range of highly generalizable coping skills should enhance children's ability to handle stress not only in athletics, but also in other aspects of their lives. In Chapter 17, we consider psychological intervention at the level of the individual athlete and describe several treatment approaches for providing young athletes with various stress-coping skills.

Situational Component

The most practical and economical approach to solving stress-related problems involves using measures at the situational level to alter dramatically their capacity to generate stress. The organization and administration of a sport program can be the focus of environmental change aimed at eliminating potential sources of stress. In this regard, it is well known that children vary greatly in physical and psychological maturation. Diverse programs should therefore be offered to allow for varied levels of athletic skill and degrees of competitive intensity. Youngsters can then select the level at which they prefer to play. Physicians, in consultation with parents and coaches, can help counsel athletes about the sports for which they are best suited.

Other methods of matching children to the appropriate level of competition can serve to combat stress associated with the inequity of competition and the risk of injury. Some youth leagues use homogeneous grouping procedures so that children compete against others of their own ability and size. Three examples of homogeneous grouping procedures are keeping the age range as narrow as possible (i.e., leagues for 9- to 10-year-olds and 11- to 12-year-olds, rather than 9- to 12-year-olds); using measures of height and weight in conjunction with chronologic age for grouping purposes; and using sports skills tests to group children.[64]

Organizational modification might also involve attempts to minimize situational demands that many youngsters find stressful. For example, to eliminate the stress-related emphasis on winning, some programs do not keep game scores, league standings, or individual performance statistics.

A more direct approach to change at the situational level involves modification of the sport itself. The purpose here is to decrease performance demands on growing children, thereby maximizing their chances of success and enjoyment. For example, Potter identified four categories in which sports are modified in the Eugene (Oregon) sports program: equipment, dimensions of the playing area, length of the contest, and rules.[65] Examples of equipment changes include reduced ball size and lowered hoops in basketball and nets in volleyball. Besides reducing the overall dimensions of the playing area, appropriate scaling modifications are applied to restraining lines for particular skills, such as serving in volleyball and shooting free throws in basketball. The length of the contest for all sports is shortened until at least the middle school grades. Finally, specific rule changes are implemented to reduce demands on players. Examples include no press defense in basketball, no fumble recovery in football (i.e., ball is dead), and no stealing in baseball and softball.

The kinds of modifications just described are highly desirable improvements. However, given that youth sport administrators and parents are often reluctant to implement change, it is important that reasonable proposals for adaptation be supported with factual information.[66] In this regard, the physician's input on a sports advisory council or management board can promote adoption of worthy policies and practices.

To this point, we have considered approaches to reducing situational sources of stress by changes in certain features of the sport itself. Two groups of adults, coaches and parents, occupy pivotal roles in youth sports and thus have potential for strongly influencing the stress process. In the final sections of this chapter, we describe how coaches and parents can be instructed to reduce the contributions they make to stress in youth sports.

WORKING WITH COACHES TO REDUCE STRESS

Obviously coaches occupy a central and critical role in the athletic setting. The nature of the relationship between athlete and coach is widely acknowledged as a primary determinant of the ways in which children are ultimately affected by their participation in organized athletic programs, and this influence extends to all levels of athletic competition.[58,59,67] The manner in which coaches structure the athletic situation, the priorities they establish explicitly and implicitly, and the ways in which they relate to their players can markedly influence how athletes appraise the situation and the amount of stress they experience.

Among the most important of environmental resources is the social support that coaches provide for young athletes. Substantial empiric evidence indicates that social support acts as an important buffer against stressors, and that low social support or a loss of support constitutes a significant stressor in its own right.[68,69] In this regard, the interpersonal climate that coaches create can vary considerably in the amount of social support that is available to serve as a potential buffer against the stresses of athletic competition. It follows, then, that one possible intervention approach is to assist coaches in creating a less stressful and more supportive team atmosphere.

The vast majority of athletes have their first sport experiences in programs staffed by volunteer coaches. Although many of these coaches are fairly well versed in the technical aspects of the sport, they rarely have had any formal training in creating a positive psychological environment for young athletes. Moreover, through the mass media, these coaches are frequently exposed to college or professional coaches who model aggressive behaviors and a "winning is everything" philosophy that is highly inappropriate in a recreational and skill development context. However, the vast majority of youth coaches are committed to providing a positive experience for their athletes, and our experience has shown that coaches are responsive to educational workshops that provide them with information and behavioral guidelines.[28,70] One such program, known as Coach Effectiveness Training (CET), is an effective and economical intervention that provides instruction for coaches in creating a more positive interpersonal environment for athletes.

Regardless of its nature, an intervention program is most likely to be successful if it has an empiric foundation. Accordingly, CET was developed in a 7-year research project carried out at the University of Washington. In the first phase of the project, research was done to establish empiric relationships between specific coaching behaviors and athletes' attitudes toward their coach, their teammates, the sport, and themselves. This research was guided by an information-processing model of coach–athlete relationships in which the impact of coaching behaviors is affected by the athlete's perceptions, evaluations, and recall of the behaviors.[71] Thus, if we wish to understand how coaching behaviors affect athletes' reactions, we need to take into account the mediating processes that occur in the athlete. From a methodologic perspective, we need to measure the actual coaching behaviors, the athletes' perception and recall of these behaviors, and the resulting evaluative reactions of the athletes.

To measure coaching behaviors, a behavioral assessment system was developed to permit direct observation and recording of coaches' behavior.[72] The Coaching Behavior Assessment System (CBAS) comprises 12 behavioral categories that are divided into two major classes: reactive (elicited) and spontaneous (emitted) behaviors. The reactive behaviors are responses to either desirable performance or effort (reinforcement, nonreinforcement), mistakes and errors (mistake-contingent encouragement, mistake-contingent technical instruction, punishment, punitive technical instruction, ignoring mistakes), or athletes' misbehaviors (keeping control). The spontaneous class includes general technical instruction, general encouragement, organization, and general communication. The CBAS was developed on the basis of extensive naturalistic observation of coaches, and it provides a direct means of assessing behaviors relating to social support, such as reinforcement, encouragement, and technical instruction, as well as nonsupportive behaviors, such as punishment.

Following development of the CBAS, a study was conducted to establish relationships between coaches' behaviors and the attitudes and reactions they ultimately evoke in athletes. Fifty-one male Little League baseball coaches were observed during a total of 202 complete games. A behavioral profile was established for each coach based on an average of 1,122 of his behaviors. After the season, a total of 542 players were interviewed and administered attitude and personality measures in their homes. Among the most important scales were measures of the degree of enjoyment experienced by players during the season, their liking for the coach and their teammates, their recall and perception of the coach's behaviors, and their levels of general and athletic self-esteem. These outcome measures were related to observed and player-perceived coaching behaviors, and the obtained relationships were used as the foundation for a set of behavioral guidelines that are the core of CET.[28]

The coaching guidelines are based primarily on social influence techniques that involve principles of positive control rather than aversive control, and a conception of success or "winning" as giving maximum effort.[73,74] An important goal of the guidelines is to increase the level of social support within the team and to increase the desire of athletes to learn and to give maximum effort while reducing fear of failure. The importance of reinforcement, encouragement, and sound technical instruction is emphasized, and aversive control procedures based on punishment and criticism are discouraged because they help foster fear of failure. If coaches demand of their athletes only that they give maximum effort, and if they reinforce effort rather than just outcome, athletes can learn to set similar standards for themselves. Athletes have complete control over effort and only partial control over outcome, and it is well established that lack of perceived control is an important aspect of stress responses.[75] As far as winning is concerned, CET emphasizes that if athletes are well trained, give maximum effort, and have positive achievement motivation rather than performance-disrupting fear of failure, winning will take care of itself within the limits of their ability. Moreover, athletes are more likely to develop their athletic potential in a supportive and enjoyable sport environment than in a stressful and nonsupportive one.

In the second phase of our project, we developed, implemented, and evaluated the CET intervention program. Thirty-one Little League baseball coaches were randomly assigned to an experimental (training) group or to a no-treatment control group. The two groups were matched as closely as possible on the behavioral and player attitude measures obtained the preceding year. The experimental group was given a preseason training program of approximately 3 hours' duration. The behavioral guidelines were presented both verbally and in written materials given to the coaches. The didactic presentation was supplemented by a modeling component in which the trainers demonstrated how to apply the principles effectively. In addition, coaches were given copies of their behavioral profiles, and specific self-monitoring procedures were introduced to increase their self-awareness of their behavior patterns, because the data from the first phase of the project indicated a striking lack of self-awareness on the part of most coaches.

The effects of the CET program were assessed by essentially repeating the phase 1 procedures. Coaches in both groups were observed four times during the course of the season by trained observers who were blind to the experimental procedure, and behavioral profiles were again generated for each coach. At the end of the season, 325 players who had played for the coaches were interviewed to obtain player outcome measures.

The results of the program evaluation were very encouraging. On both behavioral and player perception measures, the trained coaches differed from the controls in a manner consistent with the behavioral guidelines. They gave more reinforcement in response to good effort and performance and responded to mistakes with more encouragement and technical instruction and with fewer punitive responses. These behavioral differences were reflected in their players' attitudes as well, despite the fact that the average won–lost percentages of the two groups of coaches did not differ. Trained coaches were better liked and rated as better teachers, and players on their teams liked one another more and enjoyed their sport experience more. These results seemingly reflect the more socially supportive environment created by the trained coaches. Moreover, children who played for the trained coaches exhibited a significant increase in self-esteem as compared with scores obtained a year earlier, whereas those who played for the untrained coaches showed no significant change. Finally, children who were low in self-esteem exhibited the strongest differences in evaluative responses toward the trained, as opposed to the untrained, coaches. This was also encouraging, because it is the low-esteem athlete who is most in need of a positive athletic experience. Such children seemed to respond very positively to supportive coaches, and they exhibited an increase in their feelings of self-worth.[76]

It thus appears that coaches can be trained to relate more effectively to young athletes, to create a more supportive athletic environment, and to enhance athletes' self-esteem, all of which ultimately serves to decrease athletic stress. Adaptations of the original CET program have been offered to coaches at all competitive levels, including professional sports.

CONSULTING WITH PARENTS

Although coaches have the most direct contact with children within the sport environment, parents also play an important role. The literature on sport socialization confirms that parents are instrumental in determining children's sport involvement.[77,78] Moreover, the negative impact that parents can have on young athletes is all too obvious. Some parents assume an extremely active role in their children's sport involvement, and in some instances, their influence constitutes an important source of stress (see Passer and Scanlan).[19,79] Consider, for example, the following experience recounted by a youth coach:[80]

> One night last season my team lost a close game. I sat the whole team on the bench and congratulated them for trying, for acting like gentlemen. I said I couldn't have been prouder of them if they had won. Most of all, I said, it is as important to be a good loser as a gracious winner. As I talked I could see their spir-

its lifting. I felt they had learned more than just how to play baseball that night.

But as I mingled with the parents in the stands afterwards, I was shocked to hear what they were saying to the boys. The invariable theme was, "Well, what happened to *you* tonight?" One father pulled out a note pad and went over his son's mistakes play by play. Another father dressed down his son for striking out twice. In five minutes the parents had undermined every principle I had set forth.

Because of the harmful consequences caused by overzealous and unknowing adults, some youth leagues have banned parents from attending games in order to reduce the stress placed on young athletes and officials.[58] We view this as an unfortunate example of situational change, because parents can strongly and positively affect the quality of their children's sport experience. More desirable and constructive efforts are reflected in an increasing number of publications concerning parent responsibilities toward youth sport participation.[81-83] With specific reference to stress, *Parents' Complete Guide to Youth Sports* attempts to guide and educate parents about the nature and consequences of athletic stress.[45] This volume provides information on how parents might teach their children stress management relaxation skills, as well as how to prevent the development of fear of failure.

By establishing contact with parents, physicians may serve an important educational function. A key to reducing parent-induced stress in youth sports is to impress upon parents that such programs are for *children* and that children are not miniature adults. Parents need to acknowledge the right of each child to develop his or her potential as an athlete in an atmosphere that emphasizes participation, personal growth, and fun.

The conception of success or "winning" as giving maximum effort is as relevant to parents as it is to coaches. Indeed, it may be more important for parents to grasp its implications, because they can apply it in many areas of the child's life besides athletics. Likewise, the basic principles contained in the "positive approach" to coaching apply equally to parents. By encouraging youngsters to do as well as they are currently able, by reinforcing effort as well as outcome, and by avoiding use of criticism and punishment, parents might foster the development of positive motivation to achieve and help prevent fear of failure.

Acknowledgment

Preparation of this chapter was facilitated by grant 86-1066-86 from the William T. Grant Foundation.

REFERENCES

1. Berryman JW. From the cradle to the playing field: America's emphasis on highly organized competitive sports for preadolescent boys. J Sport History 1975; 2:112–131.
2. Martens R. Youth sport in the USA. In: Weiss MR, Gould D, eds. Sport for children and youths. Champaign, IL: Human Kinetics, 1986:27.
3. Brower JJ. The professionalization of organized youth sport: social psychological impacts and outcomes. Ann Am Acad Polit Soc Sci 1979; 445:39–46.
4. Michener JA. The jungle world of juvenile sports. Reader's Digest 1975; Dec: 109–112.
5. Ogilvie B. The child athlete: psychological implications of participation in sport. Ann Am Acad Polit Soc Sci 1979; 445:47–58.
6. Roberts R. Strike out little league. Newsweek 1975; July 21: 11.
7. Sayre BM. The need to ban competitive sports involving preadolescent children. Pediatrics 1975; 55:564.
8. Shah DK, Morris H. Peewee football. Newsweek 1978; Dec 4: 129, 131.
9. Underwood J. Taking the fun out of a game. Sports Illustrated 1975; Nov 17: 86–98.
10. Gould D. Sport psychology in the 1980s: status, direction, and challenge in youth sports research. J Sport Psychol 1982; 4:203–218.
11. Smith NJ, ed. Sports medicine for children and youth. Columbus, OH: Ross Laboratories, 1979.
12. Lazarus RS, Folkman S. Stress, appraisal, and coping. New York: Springer, 1984.
13. Smith RE. A component analysis of athletic stress. In: Weiss MR, Gould D, eds. Sport for children and youths. Champaign, IL: Human Kinetics, 1986:107.
14. Passer MW. Determinants and consequences of children's competitive stress. In: Smoll FL, Magill RA, Ash MJ, eds. Children in sport. 3rd ed. Champaign, IL: Human Kinetics, 1988:203.
15. Martens R. Social psychology and physical activity. New York: Harper & Row, 1975.
16. Smith RE. Toward a cognitive-affective model of athletic burnout. J Sport Psychol 1986; 8:36–50.
17. Lazarus RS. Thoughts on the relation between emotion and cognition. Am Psychol 1982; 37:1019–1024.
18. Smith CA, Ellsworth PC. Patterns of cognitive appraisal in emotion. J Pers Soc Psychol 1985; 48:813–838.
19. Passer MW. Competitive trait anxiety in children and adolescents: mediating cognitions, developmental an-

tecedents, and consequences. In: Silva JM, Weinberg RS, eds. Psychological foundations of sport and exercise. Champaign, IL: Human Kinetics, 1984:130.
20. Ellis A. Reason and emotion in psychotherapy. New York: Lyle Stuart, 1962.
21. Lazarus RS. On the primacy of cognition. Am Psychol 1984; 39:124–129.
22. Zajonc RB. On the primacy of affect. Am Psychol 1984; 39:117–123.
23. Lazarus RS. Psychological stress and the coping process. New York: McGraw-Hill, 1966.
24. Schachter S. The interaction of cognitive and physiological determinants of emotional states. In: Spielberger CD, ed. Anxiety and behavior. New York: Academic Press, 1966:193.
25. Orlick TD, Botterill C. Every kid can win. Chicago: Nelson-Hall, 1975.
26. Pierce WJ. Psychological perspectives of youth sport participants and nonparticipants. Unpublished doctoral dissertation. Blacksburg, VA: Virginia Polytechnic Institute and State University, 1980.
27. Scanlan TK, Lewthwaite R. Social psychological aspects of competition for male youth sport participants: IV. Predictors of enjoyment. J Sport Psychol 1986; 8:25–35.
28. Smith RE, Smoll FL, Curtis B. Coaching behaviors in little league baseball. In: Smoll FL, Smith RE, eds. Psychological perspectives in youth sports. Washington, DC: Hemisphere, 1978:173.
29. Wankel LM, Kreisel PSJ. Factors underlying enjoyment of youth sports: sport and age group comparisons. J Sport Psychol 1985; 7:51–64.
30. Roberts GC. The perception of stress: a potential source and its development. In: Weiss MR, Gould D, eds. Sport for children and youths. Champaign, IL: Human Kinetics, 1986:119.
31. Robinson TT, Carron AV. Personal and situational factors associated with dropping out versus maintaining participation in competitive sport. J Sport Psychol 1982; 4:364–378.
32. Pooley JC. Dropouts. Coaching Review 1980; 3:36–38.
33. Gould D, Feltz D, Horn T, Weiss M. Reasons for discontinuing involvement in competitive youth swimming. J Sport Behav 1982; 5:155–165.
34. McPherson B, Marteniuk R, Tihanyi J, Clark W. The social system of age group swimmers: the perception of swimmers, parents, and coaches. Can J Appl Sport Sci 1980; 4:142–145.
35. Burton D, Martens R. Pinned by their own goals: an exploratory investigation into why kids drop out of wrestling. J Sport Psychol 1986; 8:183–195.
36. Klavora P. An attempt to derive inverted-U curves based on the relationship between anxiety and athletic performance. In: Landers DL, Christina RW, eds. Psychology of motor behavior and sport—1977. Champaign, IL: Human Kinetics, 1978:369.
37. Lowe R, McGrath JE. Stress, arousal, and performance: some findings calling for a new theory. Report No. AF 1161–67. Washington, DC: Air Force Office of Strategic Research, 1971.
38. Scanlan TK, Lewthwaite R. Social psychological aspects of competition for male youth sport participants: I. Predictors of competitive stress. J Sport Psychol 1984; 6:208–226.
39. Gould D, Horn T, Spreeman J. Competitive anxiety in junior elite wrestlers. J Sport Psychol 1983; 5:58–71.
40. Feltz DL, Albrecht RR. Psychological implications of competitive running. In: Weiss MR, Gould D, eds. Sport for children and youths. Champaign, IL: Human Kinetics, 1986:225.
41. Coddington RD. The significance of life events as etiologic factors in disease of children: 2. A study of a normal population. J Psychosom Res 1972; 16:205–213.
42. Dohrenwend BS, Dohrenwend BP. Life stress and illness: formulation of the issues. In: Dohrenwend BS, Dohrenwend BP, eds. Stressful life events and their contexts. New York: Prodist, 1981:1.
43. Rabkin JG, Struening EL. Life events, stress, and illness. Science 1976; 194:1013–1020.
44. Rahe RH, Arthur RJ. Life changes and illness studies: past history and future directions. J Human Stress 1978; 4:3–15.
45. Smith RE, Smoll FL, Smith NJ. Parents' complete guide to youth sports. Reston, VA: American Alliance for Health, Physical Education, Recreation, and Dance, 1988.
46. Skubic E. Studies of little league and middle league baseball. Res Quart 1956; 27:97–110.
47. State of Michigan. Joint legislative study on youth sports programs: phase II. Agency sponsored sports. East Lansing, MI: Author, 1978.
48. May JR, Veach TL, Reed MW, Griffey MS. A psychological study of health, injury, and performance in athletes on the US Alpine Ski Team. Phys Sportsmed 1985; 13:111–115.
49. Bramwell ST, Masuda M, Wagner NN, Holmes TH. Psychosocial factors in athletic injuries: development and application of the Social and Athletic Readjustment Rating Scale (SARRS). J Human Stress 1975; 1:6–20.
50. Cryan PD, Alles WF. The relationship between stress and college football injuries. J Sports Med 1983; 23:52–58.
51. Passer MW, Seese MD. Life stress and athletic injury: examination of positive versus negative events and three moderator variables. J Human Stress 1983; 9:11–16.
52. Coddington RD, Troxell JR. The effect of emotional factors on football injury rates: a pilot study. J Human Stress 1980; 6:3–5.
53. Hanson DL. Cardiac response to participation in little league baseball competition as determined by telemetry. Res Quart 1967; 38:384–388.
54. Scanlan TK, Passer MW. Factors related to competitive stress among male youth sports participants. Med Sci Sports 1978; 10:103–108.
55. Scanlan TK, Passer MW. Sources of competitive stress in young female athletes. J Sport Psychol 1979; 1:151–159.
56. Simon JA, Martens R. Children's anxiety in sport and nonsport evaluative activities. J Sport Psychol 1979; 1:160–169.
57. Skubic E. Emotional responses of boys to little league and middle league competitive baseball. Res Quart 1955; 26:342–352.

58. Martens R. Joy and sadness in children's sports. Champaign, IL: Human Kinetics, 1978.
59. Seefeldt V, Gould D. Physical and psychological effects of athletic competition on children and youth. Report No. SP 015398. Washington, DC: ERIC Clearinghouse on Teacher Education, 1980.
60. Smith T. Competitive trait anxiety in youth sport: differences according to age, sex, race, and playing status. Percept Mot Skills 1983; 57:1235–1238.
61. Magill RA, Ash MJ. Academic psychosocial, and motor characteristics of participants and nonparticipants in children's sport. Res Quart 1979; 50:230–240.
62. Passer MW. Fear of failure, fear of evaluation, perceived competence, and self-esteem in competitive-trait-anxious children. J Sport Psychol 1983; 5:172–188.
63. Passer MW, Scanlan TK. A sociometric analysis of popularity and leadership status among players on youth soccer teams. Paper presented at the meeting of the North American Society for the Psychology of Sport and Physical Activity, Boulder, CO, May, 1980.
64. Martens R, Seefeldt V. Guidelines for children's sports. Washington, DC: American Alliance for Health, Physical Education, Recreation, and Dance, 1979.
65. Potter M. Game modifications for youth sport: a practitioner's view. In: Weiss MR, Gould D, eds. Sport for children and youths. Champaign, IL: Human Kinetics, 1986:205.
66. Haywood KM. Modification in youth sport: a rationale and some examples in youth basketball. In: Weiss MR, Gould D, eds. Sport for children and youths. Champaign, IL: Human Kinetics, 1986:179.
67. Smith RE, Smoll FL, Hunt E, et al. Psychology and the bad news bears. In: Roberts GC, Newell KM, eds. Psychology of motor behavior and sport—1978. Champaign, IL: Human Kinetics, 1979:109.
68. Heller K, Swindle RW. Social networks, perceived social support, and coping with stress. In: Felner RD, Jason LA, Moritsugu JN, Farber SS, eds. Preventive psychology: theory, research, and practice. Elmsford, NY: Pergamon, 1983:87.
69. Sarason IG, Sarason BR, eds. Social support: theory, research and applications. Boston: Nijhoff, 1985.
70. Martens R, Gould D. Why do adults volunteer to coach children's sports? In: Roberts GC, Newell KM, eds. Psychology of motor behavior and sport—1978. Champaign, IL: Human Kinetics, 1979:79.
71. Smoll FL, Smith RE, Curtis B, Hunt E. Toward a mediational model of coach–player relationships. Res Quart 1978; 49:528–541.
72. Smith RE, Smoll FL, Hunt E. A system for the behavioral assessment of athletic coaches. Res Quart 1977; 48:401–407.
73. Smoll FL, Smith RE. Improving relationship skills in youth sport coaches. East Lansing, MI: Michigan Institute for the Study of Youth Sports, 1979.
74. Smoll FL, Smith RE. Developing a health philosophy of winning in youth sports. In: Seefeldt V, Smoll FL, Smith RE, Gould D, eds. A winning philosophy for youth sports programs. East Lansing, MI: Michigan Institute for the Study of Youth Sports, 1981:17.
75. Folkman S. Personal control and stress and coping processes: a theoretical analysis. J Pers Soc Psychol 1984; 46:839–852.
76. Smith RE, Smoll FL, Curtis B. Coach effectiveness training: a cognitive-behavioral approach to enhancing relationship skills in youth sport coaches. J Sport Psychol 1979; 1:59–75.
77. Lewko JH, Greendorfer SL. Family influences in sport socialization of children and adolescents. In: Smoll FL, Magill RA, Ash MJ, eds. Children in sport. 3rd ed. Champaign, IL: Human Kinetics, 1988:287.
78. McPherson BD, Brown BA. The structure, processes, and consequences of sport for children. In: Smoll FL, Magill RA, Ash MJ, eds. Children in sport. 3rd ed. Champaign, IL: Human Kinetics, 1988:265.
79. Scanlan TK. Competitive stress in children. In: Weiss MR, Gould D, eds. Sport for children and youths. Champaign, IL: Human Kinetics, 1986:113.
80. McNeil DR. A coach speaks his mind: little leagues aren't big leagues. Reader's Digest 1961; June: 141.
81. Ferrell J, Glashagel J, Johnson M. A family approach to youth sports. La Grange, IL: Youth Sports Press, 1978.
82. Martens R. Parent guide to kids wrestling. Champaign, IL: Human Kinetics, 1980.
83. Vandeweghe E. Growing with sport: a parents' guide to the child athlete. Englewood Cliffs, NJ: Prentice-Hall 1979.

Chapter 17
The Psychology of "Mental Toughness": Theoretical Models and Training Approaches to Anxiety Reduction in Athletes

RONALD E. SMITH
FRANK L. SMOLL

The competitive sport environment is a setting that provides challenges, opportunities, and potential threats to physical and psychological well-being, and it is capable of eliciting a wide range of motivational and emotional states, including anxiety. It can produce high levels of anxiety in all age and competitive levels, from youth leagues to the professional ranks. The negative consequences of athletic stress on youth sport participants are summarized in Chapter 16.

Performance pressures increase in intensity at elite levels of competition. Smith has collected survey data on the frequency and intensity of anxiety reactions experienced before, during, and after games from more than 200 athletes on major college football teams.[1] Over 40 percent of the respondents indicated that they frequently experienced high levels of anxiety that they felt interfered with their performance. The potentially disruptive effects of heightened anxiety on the performance of college athletes have been objectively demonstrated in data reported by Weinberg and Genuchi.[2] They found that collegiate golfers who were high in competitive anxiety performed significantly more poorly during tournament rounds than did low-anxiety players of comparable ability as defined by scores during practice rounds.

There is also evidence that the stress produced by life changes that require readjustment (e.g., academic, athletic, and personal relationship concerns and disruptions) is related to an increased susceptibility to sport-related injuries, particularly when the athlete's coping resources are low.[3-6] We have recently completed a study revealing that college football players who are high in sport-related anxiety are significantly more likely to be injured during the course of the season than those with little anxiety.

Because of the potentially negative effects that anxiety can have on athletes' performance, physical health, and psychological well-being, much interest in reducing maladaptively high levels of anxiety has been expressed in the recent sport psychology literature. In the survey study of anxiety reactions in college football players cited above, fully 80 percent of those who indicated that they experienced high anxiety indicated interest in receiving stress management training.[1] Moreover, one of the most highly prized characteristics within the sport community, "mental toughness," is generally regarded as involving the ability to deal with stress and adversity in such a way that performance does not suffer (or even peaks) under conditions that place high physical and psychological demands on the competitor. It is therefore not surprising that anxiety reduction and control strategies are prominently discussed in recent books on psychological skills training for athletes.[7-9] From a scientific perspective, considerable interest exists in theoretical analyses of sport anxiety and the implications of various conceptual models for the development of effective anxiety reduction approaches.

This chapter describes the most important of the current conceptual models and the anxiety reduction approaches they have inspired, illustrating how they might be employed to reduce maladaptive anxiety responses in athletes. Because there is as yet no substantive body of research on the use of some of these techniques with athletes, we selectively review outcome studies of anxiety reduction performed with other client populations, as well as animal and human research bearing on the processes that appear to mediate anxiety reduction.

Four models of anxiety reduction have been particularly influential in recent psychological research on anxiety and anxiety reduction. Two models derived from the psychology of learning, the *extinction model* and the *counterconditioning model,* conceive of anxiety as a conditioned emotional response. Based on these models, two techniques employed to reduce anxiety, flooding and systematic desensitization, have been developed. A third model of anxiety reduction, known as the *cognitive mediational model,* addresses the thought processes that underlie anxiety and is aimed at modifying affect-eliciting cognitions. A fourth and increasingly influential model of anxiety reduction is the *coping skills model,* which underlies several approaches (e.g., anxiety management training, stress inoculation training, and cognitive-affective stress management training) that are designed to increase the individual's own control of anxiety responses.

EXTINCTION MODEL

Theoretical models derived from the psychology of learning conceptualize anxiety as a conditioned emotional response. Anxiety responses are elicited by formerly neutral stimuli through a process of classical conditioning. By virtue of being paired with aversive or painful stimuli (unconditioned stimuli or UCS), the formerly neutral stimuli become conditioned stimuli (CS) capable of eliciting a conditioned anxiety response. For example, after a professional baseball player was struck in the face by a pitched ball and suffered painful fractures and an eye injury, he found that going to bat elicited intense anxiety. Presumably this occurred because of the pairing of these stimuli, which had previously evoked no anxiety, with the primary aversive pain stimuli.

In many instances, people develop anxiety responses to particular situations when there is no history of their undergoing aversive classical conditioning themselves. It is possible for anxiety responses to develop through *vicarious classical conditioning,* in which the CS–UCS pairing is observed to occur to someone else.[10] For example, a gymnast began to experience intense anxiety that prevented him from attempting a difficult dismount after seeing one of his teammates fracture his back attempting a similar routine.

Once a conditioned anxiety response is established through direct or vicarious classical conditioning, it is capable of motivating and reinforcing avoidance responses. Because anxiety is an aversive state, people (and animals) are motivated to reduce, escape, or avoid it. When successful avoidance responses occur, the resulting reduction in anxiety constitutes a negative reinforcement that strengthens the avoidance responses.[11] This is one reason why the tendency to avoid anxiety-arousing stimuli often appears to become stronger over time, even though no further CS–UCS pairings occur.

Extinction is the process whereby classically conditioned responses are eliminated by repeatedly presenting the CS in the absence of the UCS. In Pavlov's classic studies of conditioning of salivary responses in dogs, the conditioned salivary response was extinguished by presenting the CS (i.e., the bell) repeatedly in the absence of food.[12] According to the extinction model, then, one way to reduce a conditioned anxiety response is to expose the individual to the anxiety-arousing stimuli in the absence of the primary aversive stimuli with which they were originally paired. This process occurs naturally in some people who are able to face up to their fears and remain in an anxiety-arousing situation until their anxiety is overcome. However, avoidance responses often prevent the natural process of extinction by removing the individual from the CS before extinction can occur. In animal studies, a technique of forced exposure to the CS while preventing the avoidance response from occurring (e.g., by restraining the animal) has been successfully employed in extinguishing anxiety responses.[13,14] The human therapeutic counterpart to this forced exposure procedure is known as flooding.

Flooding

Flooding refers to the general technique of exposing the individual to anxiety-provoking stimuli while preventing avoidance responses.[15] Clinically, the technique usually involves the use of imagined scenes, although *in vivo* exposure to the actual feared stimuli or situations can also be used, either alone or as an adjunct to the imaginal exposure. It is assumed that prolonged exposure to the anxiety-arousing stimuli in the absence of an aversive UCS extinguishes the anxiety. Thus, the client is "flooded" with the CS and the anxiety they elicit until the anxiety no longer occurs.

Because flooding is an aversive form of treatment, the client's informed consent should always be obtained before beginning the treatment. This can be accomplished by carefully explaining to the client the concepts discussed above: anxiety as a conditioned response, the concept of extinction, and the nature of and rationale for the treatment that is to be used. The client should be told that he or she will probably experience intense anxiety for a period of time before it diminishes. The client's informed commitment to the treatment technique is likely to enhance his or her willingness and ability to experience the aversive scenes and the anxiety they elicit.

A careful assessment should be made of the kinds of situations that are distressing to the client and the specific aspects of the situations that trigger the anxiety. In conjunction with the assessment phase, clients may be given imagery training in which they are asked to experience events vividly with all their senses.

The most common sources of anxiety in athletes are fears of failure and resulting social disapproval or rejection.[1] To illustrate the use of flooding, let us consider how we might approach a highly anxious male basketball player who has a tendency to "choke" in pressure situations. After establishing through interview what the most fearful situations might be, we would ask the player to close his eyes and imagine himself in pressure game situations being paralyzed by fear, failing miserably in the clutch, and anticipating the disapproval and possible rejection of teammates, the coach, spectators, and significant others such as parents, relatives, and (former) friends. Each scene would be presented in detail (with the player frequently being asked to provide additional details to enhance involvement) and would involve as many sensory modalities as possible. For example, the player might be asked to imagine standing at the foul line waiting to shoot crucial free throws late in the game. He can see every aspect of the scene—the crowd, with all eyes focused on him, opponents smiling confidently at him, his teammates avoiding his eyes, his parents watching intently and looking very anxious. He can hear the crowd screaming and one of his opponents muttering, "No way. You're going to choke." Kinesthetic cues (e.g., the trembling of his knees, his pounding heart, the weight of the ball in his slippery, sweaty hands) and olfactory-gustatory stimuli, such as the smell of sweaty bodies and the taste of sweat as he licks his lips with his dry, cottonlike tongue, would also be presented. The scene would be embellished and continued, depicting his missing the free throws badly and losing the game for his team. He would experience the booing and cries of "Choker!" from the crowd and sense rejection by his teammates, the coach, and perhaps even his parents.

Such scenes would be expected to elicit intense anxiety, and they would be prolonged until a visible and reported diminution of anxiety were observed. The extinction model emphasizes the importance of continuing stimulus presentation until extinction occurs; stimulus presentations that are too short are probably ineffective and could even increase the fear response.[13,16,17] Flooding sessions typically last from 30 to 40 minutes; an additional 15 to 20 minutes is spent discussing the client's experiences during the flooding and giving the client an opportunity to regain a relaxed emotional state.

Implosive Therapy

Implosive therapy, developed by Thomas Stampfl and Donald Levis, is a flooding procedure that adds to the learning-based extinction model concepts derived from psychodynamic theories, such as psychoanalysis.[18] The most important of these is the *avoidance serial cue hierarchy,* derived from the client's reports of fear-producing stimuli and the clinician's hypotheses about underlying psychodynamic conflicts of which the client is unaware. These underlying anxiety-arousing cues are typically related to themes of aggression and hostility, oral and anal scenes, sexual concerns, bodily injury, loss of impulse control, punishment, rejection, or guilt.[18] The psychodynamic cues high in the avoidance serial cue hierarchy are strongly avoided and repressed because they are extremely anxiety arousing. Stampfl and Levis maintain that these are often the cues to which the anxiety was originally conditioned and that in such instances, the elimination of anxiety requires exposure to them as well as to the external or symptom-contingent cues that can be identified by the client.

The effectiveness of flooding and implosion for anxiety reduction in athletes cannot yet be appraised because there have been too few clinical reports and experimental outcome studies with this treatment population. However, experimental evidence with animals indicates that prevention of avoidance responses and forced exposure to conditioned anxiety cues can be effective in reducing fear and avoidance.[13,14] Evidence also indicates that flooding can be an effective anxiety-reduction technique with human subjects.[19-22] Flooding can be highly effective both with severe anxiety disorders, such as agoraphobia, which are highly resistant to other forms of treatment, and with clients who have derived little benefit from other therapeutic approaches.[23]

The psychodynamic variant of flooding, implosive therapy, is a somewhat controversial intervention technique. Many behavior therapists challenge its psychodynamic tenets, and there is, in fact, no experimental evidence that the introduction of psychodynamic scenes facilitates therapy.[24] However, this conclusion is tempered by clinical reports in which clients spontaneously recalled, during flooding, earlier psychodynamically toned experiences that seemed related to the development of their symptoms. These recollections and the reexperiencing of the anxiety connected with them was followed by rapid improvement.[25] Thus, it is possible that in some cases exposure to psychodynamic cues may facilitate treatment.

The experience of clinicians who have used flooding as an intervention technique suggests that it is more variable in its effectiveness from client to client than other techniques.[26] When it is effective, improvement is often rapid and dramatic, as in one case in which a severe school phobia was eliminated in only two sessions.[27] This pattern of greater variability but quicker improvement when effective has also been reported in an experimental outcome study.[28] Flooding has often proved to be highly effective after other anxiety-reduction methods have failed.[19,29] Because it is more aversive than other techniques for clients, many clinicians tend to use flooding or implosion only after other approaches have failed. As should be evident, considerable clinical skill and experience are required to utilize the technique effectively.

COUNTERCONDITIONING MODEL

An alternative to extinguishing a conditioned emotional response is to condition a response that is incompatible with anxiety to the anxiety-arousing cues. The general principle was stated by Joseph Wolpe, the chief proponent of the counterconditioning approach: "If a response antagonistic to anxiety can be made to occur in the presence of anxiety-evoking stimuli so that it is accompanied by a complete or partial suppression of the anxiety responses, the bond between these stimuli and the anxiety responses will be lessened."[30]

According to Wolpe, anxious people have learned through a process of classical conditioning to experience excessively high levels of sympathetic nervous system arousal in the presence of certain stimuli. The goal of treatment is to replace sympathetic activity with competing behaviors that have a predominance of parasympathetic innervation, a process Wolpe termed *reciprocal inhibition*.

Systematic Desensitization

Systematic desensitization, the treatment devised by Wolpe, is designed to permit the gradual counterconditioning of anxiety, using relaxation as the incompatible response. Theoretically, other incompatible responses (Wolpe suggests assertion, sexual activity, vigorous muscular activity, and eating as possibilities) could also be used, but not as easily or dependably. The process of systematic desensitization is carried out in such a way that the client should experience little if any anxiety, a feature that differentiates this approach from flooding.

The desensitization procedure requires a careful assessment of the situations that elicit anxiety and of the client's ability to relax and imagine scenes with appropriate levels of emotion. The client should not have many different phobias if this approach is to be used, because the treatment is directed at each fear separately.

The client is first trained in deep muscle relaxation, using a variant of Jacobson's progressive relaxation procedure.[31] Relaxation is learned through a process of tensing and voluntarily relaxing the major muscle groups of the body. At the same time that relaxation is being mastered, the clinician begins to construct a stimulus hierarchy of scenes related to the client's anxiety. The hierarchy typically consists of 10 to 15 scenes arranged in terms of the intensity of anxiety they elicit. Hierarchies may be constructed along one or more of a variety of gradients, including time (gradually approaching a highly feared event), distance, seriousness, and so forth. The hierarchy should be constructed carefully in collaboration with the client, so that the steps are gradual and roughly equivalent in the increments of anxiety they elicit.

The hierarchy of the anxious basketball player discussed earlier (arranged from most to least anxiety arousing) might include scenes like the following:

1. Preparing to shoot a free throw, with 1 second left in a championship game and your team trailing by one point (high-anxiety scene)
2. Sitting in the locker room before the game as your coach tells you how important this game is (moderately high-anxiety scene)
3. Walking toward the arena where the game will be played (moderate-anxiety scene)
4. Awakening in the morning and thinking of the game that evening (moderately low-anxiety scene)
5. Thinking about the fact that the game will be played in 2 days (low-anxiety scene)

A complete hierarchy would obviously have other scenes interspersed between those above. Note that these scenes are arranged along an intensity dimension and a time dimension.

When the client has mastered the relaxation skill and the hierarchy has been developed, treatment begins. The client is deeply relaxed and is asked to imagine for perhaps 3 seconds the lowest (least anxiety-arousing) scene in the hierarchy. If any anxiety is experienced, the client is instructed to signal the clinician, who terminates the scene immediately and reinstates relaxation. However, if the client is deeply relaxed, the relaxation should inhibit the low level of anxiety aroused by a well-chosen initial hierarchy item. If no anxiety is experienced, the scene is presented again for a slightly longer interval, perhaps 5 seconds. If it is again successful, the scene is presented for 10 seconds, then 15. Each time the client is able to imagine the scene without experiencing anxiety, it is assumed that some of the total anxiety is being deconditioned through reciprocal inhibition, and the anxiety reduction is assumed to generalize to the items higher in the hierarchy.

After the first item has been counterconditioned, the relaxation may well be sufficient to inhibit the reduced amount of anxiety now elicited by the second item. In this manner, the clinician proceeds up the hierarchy. If the client cannot make the transition from a mastered item to the next highest item, the clinician may intersperse a new item to bridge the gap. Wolpe emphasized that great care should be taken to prevent anxiety from occurring, because this could partially undo the deconditioning that has occurred. As in flooding, it is assumed that the reduction of anxiety in response to imagined stimuli generalizes to corresponding life situations.

Probably no behavior therapy technique has been as widely researched as systematic desensitization, and its efficacy as an anxiety-reduction technique is well established. More than 100 controlled studies have found desensitization to be superior to placebo or treatment component controls with a wide range of anxiety-based disorders.[32] The technique has proved very effective in the treatment of test anxiety, a form of performance anxiety analogous to that experienced by many athletes. Positive changes have been observed on self-report test anxiety measures as well as on performance measures such as grade point average.[26] Therefore, there is every reason to believe that the technique would be valuable for athletes, particularly if the anxiety problem is a relatively circumscribed one; this qualifier applies to flooding as well. Because the extinction and counterconditioning models both focus on deconditioning responses to specific classes of stimuli, we should not expect a great deal of generalization of treatment gains to other areas of anxiety. Indeed, little generalization has been demonstrated with either flooding or desensitization.[32,33] Thus, other approaches are to be preferred for people who have multiple phobias or diffuse anxiety. Desensitization could prove to be a long and arduous process of working on hierarchy after hierarchy in dealing with the innumerable sources of anxiety in the lives of such people.

The generalization of treatment effects is a significant issue when considering the concepts of treatment efficacy and efficiency. Eliminating anxiety responses to specific situations may be a very worthwhile goal in and of itself for many clients, and the issue of generalization of treatment gains to other areas of the individual's life may be a moot one. However, some treatment approaches provide for the development of generalizable coping skills that are relevant not only to the specific anxiety-arousing situations on which treatment is focused but also to problem situations that may confront the individual in other circumstances or in the future.

COGNITIVE MEDIATIONAL MODEL

The extinction and counterconditioning models are based on a concept of anxiety as a classically conditioned emotional response. Radical behaviorists such as Wolpe eschew the use of cognitive concepts in accounting for the development, maintenance, and reduction of anxiety responses.[34] Other theorists, such as Arnold, Beck, Ellis, and Lazarus, have given cognitive mediational processes a prominent role in their theories of emotion.[35-38] These theorists assume that in most instances, emotional arousal is mediated by thoughts, images, and other cognitions rather than elicited directly by environmental cues. From this perspective, then, a powerful means of reducing maladaptive emotional responses, including anxiety, is to modify the cognitions that often elicit and perpetuate emotionality.

According to Ellis, many maladaptive emotions are the result of certain irrational beliefs that are learned early in life and reinforced within our culture.[37] Irrational beliefs that are likely to generate anxiety include the following:

1. One must be thoroughly competent and adequate and must achieve in every way in order to be worthwhile.
2. It is a dire necessity to be loved or approved of by virtually every significant other person.
3. It is catastrophic when things are not the way we would like them to be.
4. Unhappiness and anxiety are externally caused, and we have no control over our feelings.
5. If something is threatening or dangerous, one must keep thinking that it might happen.

Jones has developed an Irrational Beliefs Test to measure individual differences in endorsement of 10 of Ellis' list of irrational beliefs.[39] Scores on specific belief scales have been shown to be related to daily mood ratings of anxiety, anger, and depression in young adults over a 6-month period.[40] In addition, Mahoney and Avener have reported similar beliefs in highly anxious elite athletes.[41]

Cognitive Restructuring

Intervention directed toward the modification of anxiety-eliciting cognitions typically involves four related stages.[42] The first step is to help the client recognize that his or her beliefs, assumptions, perceptions, or ideas (i.e., cognitions) mediate emotional arousal. These cognitions have typically become automatized; they are, after all, overlearned habitual ways of thinking and tend to occur without the client's awareness. Once the client accepts this tenet, the second step is for the clinician to help him or her identify some of the underlying ideas and recognize their irrational and self-defeating nature. In the third phase, the client is helped to attack the irrational ideas and replace them with cognitions that prevent or reduce maladaptive anxiety. Finally, the client is helped to practice and rehearse the new modes of thinking and to apply them to the relevant life situations.

As stated earlier, the most common irrational beliefs noted among highly anxious athletes are that one must be thoroughly competent to be worthwhile (a belief that leads to fear of failure) and that one must be loved and approved of by everyone who is a significant other (a belief that leads to fear of social disapproval). Although we are unaware of any clinical outcome studies on the effectiveness of cognitive restructuring to reduce anxiety in athletes, the techniques have proved effective in reducing a related form of performance anxiety, test anxiety, which is typically mediated by similar beliefs.[43]

Cognitive restructuring approaches are likely to be very useful in reducing anxiety in athletes, particularly those who are fairly insightful and psychologically minded. As cognitive theorists have argued, the type of intervention likely to have the greatest impact in preventing maladaptive emotional arousal from occurring would be directed at modifying the cognitive mediators of emotionality.[36-38] We should also expect that the modification of key irrational beliefs and self-statements would result in generalization across related anxiety-arousing situations.

COPING SKILLS MODEL

In the extinction and counterconditioning models, the client is viewed as the rather passive recipient of a deconditioning procedure carried out by the clinician. Basically, something is done *to* the client to undo past conditioning experiences. In the cognitive restructuring approach, in contrast, the client plays a far more active role and assumes more personal responsibility for developing and applying new modes of thinking about problem situations.

The past decade has seen an emphasis on the development of active coping skills to deal with stressful life events, as well as several influential reconceptualizations of conditioning-based techniques. For example, Goldfried suggested that systematic desensitization could be more appropriately viewed as a procedure for learning and practicing relaxation as an active coping skill for the self-control of anxiety.[33]

Suinn and Richardson have introduced an approach called anxiety management training, which was based on a similar conception of relaxation as an active coping skill.[44] In this treatment, subjects practiced using relaxation to reduce anxiety elicited by the clinician.

Stress Inoculation Training

Meichenbaum's stress inoculation training provides a comprehensive treatment package that incorporates both cognitive and physiologic coping skills.[45] Meichenbaum conceives of the stress inoculation package as a kind of smorgasbord of coping skills that clients can master and apply as needed to deal with stressful situations. The coping skills are muscle relaxation and adaptive self-statements, learned through cognitive restructuring and *self-instructional training*. The latter involves teaching clients to give themselves adaptive instructions in dealing with stressors. Specific sets of self-statements are developed for four stages of the process: preparing for a stressor (e.g., "Just think about what you can do about it. That's better than getting anxious."); confronting and handling a stressor ("Relax: You're in control . . . Just think about what you have to do, not about fear."); coping with the feeling of being overwhelmed ("When fear comes, just pause."); and reinforcing oneself for effective coping ("You did great!").

As its name suggests, the stress inoculation technique is aimed at allowing clients to practice using their coping skills to cope with low and manageable doses of anxiety. The rehearsal phase takes the form of asking clients to imagine anxiety-arousing situations and to imagine themselves using their coping skills in these situations. This is combined with graded exposure to real-life stressors that approximate those that are dealt with through mental rehearsal. The notion is that practicing their coping skills to manage low levels of anxiety helps to "inoculate" clients against higher levels of anxiety in actual life situations.

The stress inoculation procedure has been employed successfully in a wide range of client populations to reduce anxiety and anger, as well as to increase pain tolerance, and nearly 100 controlled studies attest to its effectiveness as an intervention approach.[45] It would appear to be highly applicable to athletes. The self-instructional training could conceivably contain self-statements relevant to skill and strategy, as well as instructions relating to concentration and attentional processes.

Cognitive-Affective Stress Management Training

A coping skills approach that differs in several important respects from the stress inoculation training is cognitive-affective stress management training.[1,46] Like Meichenbaum's approach, this program involves the acquisition and rehearsal of both cognitive and relaxation skills. The relaxation skills involve both somatic relaxation, learned through progressive muscle relaxation training, and cognitive relaxation, acquired through training in Benson's meditation technique.[47] Cognitive coping skills are acquired through cognitive restructuring to modify irrational ideas or through self-instructional training to develop more adaptive cognitive control of attention and behavior.

A major difference between the stress inoculation and cognitive-affective approaches lies in the methods used to rehearse the coping skills once they have been acquired and the rationale underlying the favored rehearsal technique. Rather than rehearsing under low levels of anxiety, as in the inoculation approach, a technique known as *induced affect* is employed to allow rehearsal of coping responses under high emotional arousal. The client is asked to imagine a stressful situation, then to focus on the feeling the scene elicits. Suggestions that the feelings are growing more intense, and verbal encouragement and reinforcement for signs of increased arousal, are used to shape a strong affective response.[48] When the client is highly aroused, he or she is instructed to "turn it off" with his or her coping responses. Initially, relaxation alone is used, then self-statements alone. Finally, the two classes of coping responses are combined into an "integrated coping response" that is tied into the breathing cycle. As the client inhales, he or she emits a stress-reducing or task-relevant self-statement.

Then, while slowly exhaling, the client gives the mental self-instruction to relax, thus inducing somatic relaxation.

In terms of rehearsal procedures, then, the cognitive-affective approach provides rehearsal of coping skills to reduce levels of affective arousal that are as high as or higher than those experienced in the actual situation. The level of affect intensity evoked during induced affect is likely to approximate that elicited by flooding, whereas the stress inoculation procedures tend to elicit much lower anxiety levels. The assumption is that learning to master high levels of arousal ensures that lower levels can also be controlled, whereas the converse is not necessarily the case. One interesting finding here is that text-anxious subjects who were administered the cognitive-affective program expressed greater posttreatment confidence in their ability to cope in test situations than did subjects who rehearsed their coping skills with the stress inoculation procedures.[49] However, both treatment approaches greatly reduced test anxiety scores. Controlled outcome studies with a variety of populations, including medical students, heavy social drinkers, and athletes indicate that the cognitive-affective approach to coping skills training is an effective one.[46] In one study with athletes it was found that, compared with an untrained control group with whom they were matched on baseline endurance measures, trained subjects exhibited enhanced endurance during a posttraining submaximal treadmill run as defined by heart rate and oxygen consumption.[50] This difference was attributed to the acquisition of coping skills that the trained subjects reported using to manage the discomfort experienced during the endurance task.

The training of Mr. B, a college football player, illustrates the use of the coping skills approach to enhance self-control of maladaptive anxiety. Mr. B, a quarterback at a major university, suffered from intense competitive anxiety that interfered severely with his performance. Judged by his coaches to have exceptional talent, Mr. B rarely lived up to expectations under game conditions. He reported that he began experiencing severe anxiety several days before games. He was unable to sleep and frequently vomited before games. Severe muscular tension and high arousal interfered with motor performance during games, and thoughts about failure intruded frequently during competition. He reported that cognitive interference caused a kind of "tunnel vision" that impaired his reading of defenses during passing plays, resulting in poor judgments about where to throw the ball. Consequently, many of his passes were intercepted. His growing self-doubt and expectations of "choking" during competition threatened his career. On the positive side, he was intelligent, psychologically minded, and highly motivated to overcome his emotional problem.

The training was presented to Mr. B as an educational program in self-control of emotion. It was explained that with time and practice, he could learn coping skills that many successful athletes employ to control anxiety and enhance performance. Practice was begun in progressive muscle relaxation, and Mr. B practiced his relaxation exercises faithfully several times a day. Like many athletes, he learned the relaxation skills quickly because of his good muscular control.

While relaxation training was proceeding, Mr. B was helped to monitor his thought processes during competition and to isolate the self-statements that elicited and accompanied his anxiety responses. These typically involved telling himself how awful it would be if he played poorly or made a mistake and that he was a worthless failure if he did not perform up to his potential. Cognitive restructuring was used to attack the irrational elements of his fear of failure and his perfectionistic demands, to show him how the ideas were self-defeating, and to substitute a set of self-statements designed to reduce or prevent his anxiety by focusing on effort rather than outcome. His most effective thought was, "I can do no more than give 100 percent." Self-instructional training was also used to develop task-relevant thoughts such as, "Concentrate on what you have to do and nothing else," and to create imagery related to his desired performance.

During the rehearsal phase of the training program, Mr. B was asked to imagine vivid anxiety-arousing scenes involving pregame and game situations. The induced affect procedure was used to generate levels of arousal that he reported to be as high as or higher than those experienced in the actual competitive situations. He practiced reducing the arousal with relaxation, then with his new self-statements, and finally with an integrated coping response involving a coping self-statement during the inhalation phase and the mental command to relax (accompanied by voluntary relaxation) during exhalation (e.g., "I can do no more than give my best . . . so . . . relax.").

Having learned his coping responses well and having practiced them to reduce high levels of anxiety during induced affect, Mr. B found that he could employ them very effectively within the actual competitive situations. He used his training in meditation to control pre-event tension. His performance improved dramatically.

The coping skills approach to anxiety reduction in athletes offers two potential advantages over the extinction and counterconditioning approaches. First, rather than being the passive recipient of a deconditioning procedure, the athlete assumes major responsibility for developing the coping skills needed to reduce anxiety and is more likely to attribute improvement to his or her efforts. This should enhance maintenance of treatment gains, because self-attributed changes appear to be better maintained than change attributed to external agents.[51] Psychotherapy research has also shown that the more a specific treatment approach increases self-efficacy (confidence in one's own ability to cope), the more behavioral improvement is shown.[52]

The second advantage of coping skills approaches over those based on conditioning models relates to the issue of generalization introduced earlier. As we noted, neither flooding nor traditional desensitization gains generalize readily to other areas of anxiety.[24,33] To the extent that treatment is geared to the development of general and flexible coping skills that can be applied to a variety of situations, we should expect greater treatment generalization. Evidence to support this prediction comes from findings that subjects treated for test anxiety, using a self-control variant of desensitization developed by Goldfried, also showed a reduction in untreated speech anxiety, whereas subjects treated with traditional desensitization showed no speech anxiety reduction.[53] Thus, as applied to athletes, we should expect the results of coping skills programs to be useful over a wider range of both athletic and nonathletic situations.

The scientific study of intervention techniques designed to reduce anxiety in athletes is still in its infancy. Still needed are controlled outcome studies with well-defined and competently administered treatment procedures; dependent variable measures to tap behavioral, physiologic, and self-report outcome indices; and appropriate control groups (including attention-placebo control conditions that are as credible as the treatment conditions). Clearly the problem of anxiety is sufficiently widespread among athletes to justify the application and assessment of current anxiety-reduction techniques and the development of more powerful and cost-effective ones in the future. On a more general level, concepts such as "mental toughness" are being operationally defined in terms of specific psychological skills such as the ability to control emotional arousal and to focus attention in a task-relevant fashion under conditions of intense competitive demands and adversity. The development of an educational technology to train athletes in these and other psychological skills is one of the most exciting current frontiers of sport psychology.

Acknowledgment

Preparation of this chapter was partially supported by Grant 86–1066–86 from the William T. Grant Foundation.

REFERENCES

1. Smith RE. A cognitive-affective approach to stress management training for athletes. In: Nadeau CH, Halliwell WR, Newell KM, Roberts GC, eds. Psychology of motor behavior and sport—1979. Champaign, IL: Human Kinetics, 1980:154.
2. Weinberg RS, Genuchi M. Relationship between competitive trait anxiety, state anxiety, and performance: a field study. J Sport Psychol 1980; 2:148–154.
3. Bramwell ST, Masuda M, Wagner NN, Holmes TH. Psychosocial factors in athletic injuries: development and application of the Social and Athletic Readjustment Rating Scale (SARRS). J Human Stress 1975; 1:6–20.
4. Coddington RD, Troxell JR. The effect of emotional

factors on football injury rates: a pilot study. J Human Stress 1980; 6:3–5.
5. Cryan PL, Alles WF. The relationship between stress and college football injuries. J Sports Med 1983; 23:52–58.
6. Williams JM, Toneymon P, Wadsworth WA. Relationship of life stress to injury in intercollegiate volleyball. J Human Stress 1986; 12:38–43.
7. Gauron EF. Mental training for peak performance. Lansing, NY: Sport Science Associates, 1984.
8. Harris DV, Harris BL. The athlete's guide to sports psychology: mental skills for physical people. New York: Leisure Press, 1984.
9. Williams JM, ed. Applied sport psychology: personal growth to peak performance. Palo Alto, CA: Mayfield, 1986.
10. Berger SM. Conditioning through vicarious instigation. Psychol Rev 1962; 69:450–466.
11. Rescorla RA, Solomon RL. Two-process learning theory: relationships between Pavlovian conditioning and instrumental learning. Psychol Rev 1967; 74:151–182.
12. Pavlov I. Conditioned reflexes. London: Clarenden Press, 1927.
13. Baum M. Extinction of avoidance responding through response prevention (flooding). Psychol Bull 1970; 74:276–284.
14. Mineka S. The role of fear in theories of avoidance learning, flooding, and extinction. Psychol Bull 1979; 86:985–1010.
15. Boulougouris JC, Marks IM. Implosion (flooding): a new treatment for phobias. Br Med J 1969; 2:721–723.
16. McCutcheon BA, Adams HE. The physiological basis of implosive therapy. Behav Res Ther 1975; 13:93–100.
17. Staub E. Duration of stimulus exposure as a determinant of the efficacy of flooding procedures in the elimination of fear. Behav Res Ther 1968; 6:131–132.
18. Stampfl TG, Levis DJ. Essentials of implosive therapy: a learning theory-based psychodynamic behavioral therapy. J Abnor Psychol 1967; 72:496–503.
19. Boulougouris JC, Marks IM, Marset P. Superiority of flooding (implosion) to desensitization for reducing pathological fear. Behav Res Ther 1971; 9:7–16.
20. Girodo M. Yoga meditation and flooding in the treatment of anxiety neurosis. J Behav Ther Exp Psychiatry 1974; 5:157–160.
21. Krawitz G. Flooding versus an equally credible placebo in the treatment of acrophobia. Unpublished master's thesis. Norfolk, VA: Old Dominion University, 1978.
22. Yule W, Sacks B, Hersov L. Successful flooding treatment of a noise phobia in an eleven-year old. J Behav Ther Exp Psychiatry 1974; 5:209–211.
23. Marks IM. Fears, phobias, and rituals. New York: Oxford University Press, 1987.
24. Morganstern KP. Implosive therapy and flooding procedures: a critical review. Psychol Bull 1973; 79:318–334.
25. Boulougouris JC, Bassiakos L. Prolonged flooding in cases with obsessive-compulsive neurosis. Behav Res Ther 1973; 11:227–231.
26. Smith RE, Nye SL. A comparison of implosive therapy and systematic desensitization in the treatment of test anxiety. J Consult Clin Psychol 1973; 41:37–42.
27. Smith RE, Sharpe TM. Treatment of a school phobia with implosive therapy. J Consult Clin Psychol 1970; 35:239–243.
28. Barrett C. Systematic desensitization therapy versus implosive therapy. J Abnorm Psychol 1969; 74:587–592.
29. Kandel HJ, Ayllon T, Rosenbaum MS. Flooding or systematic exposure in the treatment of extreme social withdrawal in children. J Behav Ther Exp Psychiatry 1977; 8:75–81.
30. Wolpe J. Psychotherapy by reciprocal inhibition. Stanford, CA: Stanford University Press, 1958.
31. Jacobson E. Progressive relaxation. Chicago: University of Chicago Press, 1938.
32. O'Leary KD, Wilson GT. Behavior therapy: application and outcome. Englewood Cliffs, NJ: Prentice-Hall, 1987.
33. Goldfried MR. Systematic desensitization as training in self-control. J Consult Clin Psychol 1971; 37:228–234.
34. Wolpe J. Cognition and causation in human behavior and its therapy. Am Psychol 1978; 33:437–446.
35. Arnold MB. Emotion and personality. New York: Columbia University Press, 1960.
36. Beck AT. Cognitive approaches to stress. In: Woolfolk R, Lehrer P, eds. Principles and practice of stress management. New York: Guilford Press, 1984:162.
37. Ellis A, Grieger R. Handbook of rational emotive therapy. New York: Springer, 1977.
38. Lazarus RS, Folkman S. Stress, appraisal, and coping. New York: Springer, 1984.
39. Jones RG. A factored measure of Ellis' irrational belief systems with personality and maladjustment correlated. Wichita, KS: Test Systems, Inc, 1968.
40. Rohsenow D, Smith RE. Irrational beliefs as predictors of negative affective states. Motivation and Emotion 1982; 6:299–314.
41. Mahoney MJ, Avener M. Psychology of the elite athlete: an exploratory study. Cognitive Ther Res 1978; 1:135–141.
42. Haaga DA, Davison GC. Cognitive change methods. In: Kanfer FH, Goldstein AP, eds. Helping people change: a textbook of methods. 3rd ed. New York: Pergamon, 1986:236.
43. Goldfried MR, Linehan MM, Smith JL. The reduction of test anxiety through cognitive restructuring. J Consult Clin Psychol 1978; 46:32–39.
44. Suinn RM, Richardson F. Anxiety management training: a nonspecific behavior therapy program for anxiety control. Behav Ther 1971; 2:498–510.
45. Meichenbaum D. Stress inoculation training. New York: Pergamon, 1985.
46. Smith RE. Athletic stress and burnout: conceptual models and intervention strategies. In: Hackfort D, Spielberger CD, eds. Anxiety in sport: an international perspective. New York: Hemisphere (in press).
47. Benson H. The relaxation response. New York: Morrow, 1975.
48. Smith RE, Ascough JC. Induced affect in stress management training. In: Burchfield S, ed. Stress: psychological and physiological interactions. New York: Hemisphere, 1985:150.

49. Smith RE, Nye SL. A comparison of induced affect and covert rehearsal in the acquisition of stress management coping skills. J Counsel Psychol (in press).
50. Ziegler SG, Klinzing J, Williamson K. The effects of two stress management training programs on cardiorespiratory efficiency. J Sport Psychol 1982; 4:280–289.
51. Davison GC, Valins S. Maintenance of self-attributed and drug-attributed behavior change. J Pers Soc Psychol 1969; 11:25–33.
52. Bandura A, Adams NE, Hardy AB, Howells GN. Tests of the generality of self-efficacy theory. Cognitive Ther Res 1980; 4:39–66.
53. Zemore R. Systematic desensitization as a method of teaching a general anxiety-reducing skill. J Consult Clin Psychol 1975; 43:157–161.

A

Aerobic power gains, 44
Age and muscle fiber, 208
Age-related changes
  arterial oxygenation, 34
  cardiac output, 32–33
  heart rate, 33
  heart volume, 33
  hemoglobin concentrations, 34
  stroke volume, 33
  venous oxygenation, 34
Amenorrhea
  acute hormonal response, 128
  chronic hormonal response, 129–130
  diet, 127–128
  etiology of athletic, 121–130
  fat hypothesis, 121–124
  hormonal alterations, 128–130
  hypothalamic maturity, 126
  intense training prior to menarche, 124–125
  late menarche, 124
  and LH pulse, 129
  multiple factors, 130
  prior menstrual irregularity, 125
  psychological stress, 126–127
  quantity of training, 125–126
  reversibility, 130
  treatment, 130–132
  athletic, proposed causes of, 122
  body fat and, 123
  and meat consumption, 127
  and mileage increases, 125, 126
  prevalence of secondary, 119
Amenorrheic athlete, therapeutic approach to, 132
Angular momentum
  transfer of, 288
  conservation of, 284
Anthropometric measurements of human body, 290
Anxiety reduction, 391–400
  cognitive mediational model, 396–397
  cognitive restructuring, 397
  cognitive-affective stress management training, 398–400
  coping skills model, 397–400
  counterconditioning model, 395–396
  extinction model, 392–395
  flooding, 393–394
  implosive therapy, 394–395
  stress inoculation training, 398
  systematic desensitization, 395–396
Apophysitis of tibial tubercle, 332
Ariel, Gideon B., 271–297

Arterial insufficiency and effects of physical training, 191
Articular cartilage collagen alignment, 262
Athletic stress
  approaches to stress reduction, 383–385
  behavioral component, 378–379
  cognitive component, 377–378
  consequences of, 379–383
  dynamics of, 376–379
  effects on participation, enjoyment and withdrawal, 379–380
  effects on performance, 380
  health-related effects, 380–381
  physiologic component, 378
  situational component, 376–377
  in youth sports, 381–383

B

Berning, Jacqueline R., 135–152
Biomechanics, 271–296
  kinematics and kinetics, 289–296
  mechanics, 279–289
Blood flow, regional
  brain, 39
  heart, 40
  lungs, 39–40
  muscle, 37–38
  skin, 38
  viscera, 38–39
BMU, longitudinal section through active, 314
Body heat capacity
  thermal stress related to, 80–81
Body heat production rate and measurement, 79–80
Body temperature(s)
  extremes, 78–79
  mean, 81–82
  normal, 77–78
  rhythms, 78
  in neutral thermal conditions, 79
  and oxygen consumption, 114
  regulation, 100
Body temperatures, effector activity, and thermal balance
  change in fitness level, 112–114
  cold stress, 107–108
  core temperatures in zone of vasomotor regulation, 106
  effect of clothing, 108
  effects of changed power output and fitness level, 112

environments inside and outside zone of vasomotor regulation, 103
exercise, 108
heat stress, 105
minimal core temperature change with ambient temperature, 110–112
neutral environment, 104
new equilibrium, 105–106
skin temperatures during exercise, 108–109
skin temperatures in zone of vasomotor regulation, 105
sweat rate control during exercise, 110–112
vasomotor regulation zone, borders of, 104–105
Bone
biomechanics, 313–314
clinical correlation, 320–321
function, 309
metabolism, 314–317
pathophysiology—fracture, 317–320
structure, 309–313
Bone growth, phases of, 138
Bone mass of female athletes, 149
Breathing
central command, 63–65
central command and peripheral feedback integration, 67
CO_2 flux receptors, 66–67
control of during exercise, 62, 64
during prolonged dynamic exercise, 62
and locomotor rhythms, 61–62
skeletal muscle mechanoreceptors and metaboreceptors, 65–66
Brengelmann, George L., 77–116

C

Calcium intake for females, 141
Capillaries in muscle fiber, 223
effects of altitude on, 224
Capitellum, osteochondral injury of, 340
Cardiac output in cool and hot, 38
Cardiac regulation
adaptation to exercise, 35–36
cardioactive drugs, 35
general considerations, 34–35
systemic blood pressure and cardiac work rate, 36–37
Cardiovascular aspects
carbon dioxide homeostasis, 28
circulation and homeostasis, 27–30
oxygen transport, 27–28
thermal homeostasis, 28–30
Cardiovascular oxygen transport
arterial oxygenation, 31
cardiac output, 30
cardiac volume, 31
Fick Equation, 30
heart rate, 30
hemoglobin concentration, 32
stroke volume, 30–31
venous oxygenation, 31–32
Cardiovascular responses to exercise, 34

Cartilage resiliency from keratan sulfate, 262
Changes due to conditioning, 226
Cigar making, speed and skill in, 258
Collagen
degeneration, 266
production of, 302
Competitive stress, 375–388
Computer performance analysis, 294
Coplanar link system, 291
Core temperature
convection distribution of heat, 82–83
effect of external energy sources, 84
heat loss from lungs, 83
uniformity in organ blood flow changes, 83–84
Core temperature measurement, advantages of sites, 90–92
Core temperature uniformity, 83
Core-shell thermal model of body
analysis of thermal balance, 88–89
body shell and clothing as insulators, 87
insulation and conductivity of shell and clothing, 87–88
Coronary blood flow, 41
Coronary heart disease
other risk factors, 52
risk assessments, 52–53
Coronary heart disease risk assessments
primary coronary risk factors, 51–52
Cybex isokinetic exerciser, 253

D

Daily injury report, 10
Data analysis and display, 6–8
de Lateur, Barbara J., 243–260
Diaphyseal cortex of long bone, 310
Digestive system
anabolic corticosteroids, effect of on liver, 162
biliary secretion during exercise, 160–161
effect of exercise on, 153–162
exercise and colon, 161–162
exercise and peptic ulcer, 157
gastric acid secretion, 156–157
gastric emptying, 154–156
gastroesophageal reflux, 154
gastrointestinal symptoms and disorders in exercise, 162
gastrointestinal tract blood flow during exercise, 157–159
pancreatic secretion during exercise, 160
salivary secretion, 154
small intestinal motility, transit and absorption during exercise, 159–160
Distal radial physeal plate, injury from repetitive impact to, 336

E

Electrical activity in static work, 256
Energy balance equation, 168

Energy expenditure, daily, 171
Energy expenditure, effects of exercise on, 170
Environmental stress
 cold, 41
 heat, 40–41
 high altitudes, 41–42
 underwater, 42
Enzyme activities in human skeletal muscle, 190
Enzyme changes during conditioning, 215
Exercise, types of aerobic, 43
 anaerobic, 43
 isometric, 42–43
 isotonic, 42
Exercise EEG tests, influence of disease prevalence on, 49
Exercise performance with and without rest, 257
Exercise stress tests, reasons for false readings on, 49
Exercise table, 249
Exercise test, indications for halting, 50
Exercise test results, submaximal, 47
Exercise testing, contraindications, 50
Exercise testing, functional
 cardiac output, 48–50
 echocardiography, 48
 general considerations, 45
 lactate (anaerobic) threshold, 47
 maximum oxygen intake, 45
 myocardial ischemia, 47–48
 practical procedures and interpretation, 50–51
 submaximal tests, 45–46
Exertional compartmental syndrome, factors leading to, 323
Eyeguard, 17

F

Feedback control levels, 278
Feedback control of muscular contraction, 274
Fiber types, occurrence of, 209
Flexor muscles and contraction velocity, 251
Football injuries per 100 athletes/season, 8
Forces, analysis of, 281
Fracture healing sequence, 320
Fracture risk, 136
Fulkerson, John P., 261–270

G

GABA antagonist, cardiovascular, locomotor and respiratory effects of, 65
GnRH, hormonal response to, 131
Gollnick, Philip D., 185–241
Growth cartilage, 330
Growth spurt, 334

H

Halvorson, Glenn A., 345–371
Headgear, 14

Heat transfer coefficient at various air velocities, 93
Hormonal profile, 129
Human growth plate, microanatomy of, 330
Human skeletal muscle substrate, 190
Hypoxia, effects of, 49
Hypoxia, response to, 70

I

IEMG and force of contractions, 245
Injuries per 1000 athletes, 7
Injury data analysis, 1979–1987, 13
Injury reporting
 data collection, 5–6
 recognition, 4–5
Interscholastic injury summary, girls' soccer, 12
Intracellular ion concentrations, 207
Isometric contraction, endurance of, 38

J

Joints
 articular cartilage and subchondral bone, 261–264
 ligament reconstruction, 266–267
 ligament structure and healing, 265–266
 meniscus, 264–265
 mobility and instability, 269
 pathologic joint function, 267–269
 structure and function of, 261–269

K

Kinetic energy of collision, 20

L

Length-tension diagram, 251
Leverage curves, 252
Levers, 286
Luteal phase and training mileage, 120

M

Martin, Bruce J., 153–166
Maximal flows, effects of training on, 69
Maximal isometric force of triceps, 255
Maximal tension, 255
Maximum exercise heart rate, decline of, 33
Mechanisms of injury
 area safety, 17–19
 coaching, 21–22
 environment, 19
 equipment, 8–17
 mass and speed, 19–20
 skill and personality, 20–21
Menisci and vascular supply, 265
Menstrual cycle, 118
 defining amenorrhea, 120–121
 physiology of, 117–118
 short luteal phase, 120
Menstrual dysfunction in female athlete, 117–132
Menstrual irregularities, 118–120

Micheli, Lyle J., 329–343
Monthly injury summary, 10
Motor unit types, 194
Muscle contraction, forces produced during, 303
Muscle electrolytes in healthy subjects, 195
Muscle fiber typing, 189
Muscle fibers, parallel arrangement of, 244
Muscle size and distribution, 197–199
Muscle strength
 adaptive response to enzymes, 245–247
 cam-varied load exercise, 248
 Cybex system, 253–254
 DeLorme technique, 248
 fatigue, effects of, 254–257
 Hellebrandt technique, 249–250
 hypertrophy, 243
 improvement of motor control, 243–245
 isokinetic exercise, 248
 isometric exercise, 247
 isotonic exercise, 247
 motor learning, 257–258
 Nautilus system, 250–253
 Oxford technique, 249
 response of muscle to exercise, 243–247
 response of neuromuscular apparatus to exercise, 258
 specificity versus transferability, 258–260
 types of exercise, 247–254
 typical exercise training programs, 248–254
 University of Washington technique, 250
Muscle strength and local endurance training, 243–260
Muscular contraction, effects of, 66
Muscular metabolism available, 256
Musculoskeletal injuries, pediatric and adolescent, 329–341
Myofascial compartments
 clinical correlation, 322–323
 normal physiology, 321
 pathophysiology, 321–322

N

Nautilus system, 248

O

Obesity
 and activity and energy expenditure, 168
 components of daily energy expenditure, 171–173
 effect of exercise on body weight and adiposity, 168–169
 effect of exercise on caloric intake, 170–171
 effect of exercise on components of daily energy expenditure, 173–174
 effect of exercise on dietary weight loss programs, 174–175
 energy expenditure, regulation of, 167–168
 glucose and insulin homeostasis, 175–176
 other beneficial metabolic effects of exercise, 175–177
 plasma lipid and lipoprotein concentrations, 176–177
 resting metabolic rate, 171
 thermic effect of exercise, 171–172
 thermic effect of feeding, 172–173
 and exercise and energy expenditure, 167–179
Osteochondritis dissecans, 332
Osteoclast brush border, 311
Osteoporosis
 age-related, 136–137
 athletic amenorrhea and bone density, 147–149
 and bioavailability of calcium, 142–145
 bone mass measurements, 135–136
 bone mineral metabolism, 137
 and calcium, 140–142
 and diet, 140–145
 and exercise, 145–149
 and fiber, 144–145
 hormonal factors, 137–140
 and phosphorus, 142–143
 risk factors for, 137
 and vitamin D, 144
 diet, and exercise, 135–150
Ovarian cycle, 117
Overuse injuries, 299–325
 apparent risk factors in, 337
 tendon, 300–309
 treatment principles, 323–325
Oxygen consumption, 48
Oxygen intake, maximum, 45–46

P

Patella, avulsion of, 339
Peak-and-valley training method, 324
Periodic acid-Schiff, intensity of, 203
Periosteal bone formation, 311
Physeal fracture, 333
Precompetition state anxiety, 383
Principles of rehabilitation, 345–365
Pulmonary blood flow, 39
Pulmonary resistance and induced contractions, 66
Quadriceps, fatigued and nonfatigued, 256
Quadriceps board, 250
Quadriceps boot, 248

R

Respiratory
 and locomotor rates in horses, 61
Respiratory adaptations to exercise
 biochemical and contractile properties of diaphragm, 69–70

static lung volumes and ventilation, 67–68
ventilatory responses to hypoxia and hypercapnia, 70–71
ventilatory strength and endurance, 68–69
Respiratory responses
 to dynamic (rhythmic) exercise, 60–61
 to static exercise, 59
Respiratory responses and adaptations to exercise, 59–76
Respiratory responses to prolonged exercise, 62
Rice, Stephen G., 3–23

S

Sanborn, Charlotte F., 117–134, 135–152
Schwartz, Robert S., 167–181
SDH
 activity in response to conditioning and deconditioning, 217
 changes in training procedures, 216
 studies, 228
Shephard, Roy J., 27–57
Skeletal muscle(s)
 adaptation, significance of, 223–228
 adaptive response, 204–220
 aerobic metabolism and adaptation, 225–228
 biochemical basis for differences in twitch properties, 186–188
 capillaries, 220–223
 capillary anatomy, 221
 capillary density, 221–222
 capillary growth and development, 221
 capillary muscle fiber types and oxidative metabolism, 221–222
 capillary regulation, 222–223
 capillary use and disuse, 222
 connective tissue, 220
 contractile properties, 186
 contractile properties and fiber conversion, 217–219
 enzyme activities, 194–195
 enzyme activities and adaptation, 225–228
 fatigue characteristics, 192
 fiber cross-sectional area, 207–210
 fibers per motor unit, 186
 glycogen content, 194
 glycogen stores, 212–213
 glycolytic enzymes, 213–214
 histochemical differentiation of muscle fibers, 188
 hypertrophy versus hyperplasia, 210–212
 ionic composition, 195–196
 metabolic capacity, 212
 metabolic characteristics, 192–195
 maximal contractile force, 190–192
 mechanical properties, 219
 mitochondrial enzymes, 214–217
 motor unit, 185–196
 motor-unit recruitment, 202–204
 muscle fiber composition, 196–201
 muscle size, 205–212
 muscular size and adaptation, 223–224
 muscular strength, 207
 phosphagen content, 193
 phosphagen stores, 212
 postnatal development of metabolic capacity, 212
 postnatal development of muscle, 205–207
 regulation, 219–220
 speed of contraction, 192
 substrate stores and adaptation, 224–225
 substrates, 192–193
 triglyceride content, 194–195
 triglyceride stores, 213
 ultrastructural basis for fiber typing, 188–190
 use and disuse, 207–210, 212
 physiology, 185–228
Skin and core temperature in control of effectors, 101
Skin temperature versus ambient temperature, 110
Slow-twitch fiber distribution, 200
Smith, Ronald E., 375–390, 391–402
Smoll, Frank L., 375–390, 391–402
Sports injuries
 epidemiology, 3–8
 epidemiology and mechanisms of, 3–22
Sports medicine
 cardiovascular aspects of, 27–53
Sports participation
 risk of, 4
ST fibers
 distribution of, 200
 occurrence of, 201
Static discharge frequency of cold and warm fibers, 98
Static and rhythmic contractions, effects of, 68
Strength gain
 by hypertrophy, 245
 neural factors versus hypertrophy, 246
 through progressive resistance exercise, 245
Stress
 conceptual model of, 376
 negative effects of excessive, 379
Stress fracture, factors leading to, 318
Stress reduction
 behavioral component, 384
 cognitive and physiologic components, 384
 consulting with parents, 387–388
 situational component, 384–385
 working with coaches for, 385–387
Stress-strain curve(s), 263
 for bone, 313
 for tendon, 303
Study design, 6
Succinate dehydrogenase activities, 70

Sweat rate and core temperature, equilibrium levels, 107
Sweat rate versus core and skin temperature, 111
Sweat rate versus core and skin temperature, effects of change, 113
Synchronization ratios, 246
Systolic blood pressure by age and work rate, 37

T

Teitz, Carol C., 299–328
Temperature regulation, 77–114
Temperatures and heat loss in zone of vasomotor regulation, 104
Temperatures in superficial tissues
  in active muscle, 86–87
  cold stress, 84–86
  heat stress, 86
  skin temperature and increased local heat dissipation, 87
Tendon
  biomechanics, 303–305
  clinical correlation, 307–309
  function, 300–301
  metabolism, 305
  pathophysiology, 306–307
  structure, 301–303
Terms, 304
  Thermal balance, control of
    body heat content versus core temperature, 102–103
    central integration, 97
    control scheme, 99
    core temperature deviations in thermoregulation, 99–100
    core temperature thermoreception, 97–99
    cutaneous thermoreception, 97
    effector systems, 96–97
    set point, 100–101
    set point adjustment, 101–102
    setting of set point, 102
    thermal input from core and skin, interaction between, 100
    zones of regulation, 103
Thermal balance versus environmental temperature, 109
Thermal interaction with environment
  convection, 92–93
  dehydration, 95
  evaporation, 93–95
  evaporative heat loss, interference with, 95
  hidromeiosis, 95
  inappropriate evaporative heat loss, 95–96
  inevitable water loss, 93–94
  radiation, 93
  sweating, 94–95
Thermal profiles, 85
Thermic effect of feeding, 172
Thermoreceptors, general properties of, 99
Tissue pressure, effects of increased, 321
Torque computation, 252
Torque curves, 252
  of quadriceps, 254
  for flexion and extension, 253
  for pronation and supination, 253
Training intensity and frequency of elderly, effects of, 44
Training regimens
  aerobic (endurance), 43–44
  muscular, 44
  and myocardial ischemia, 47–48
  specificity of, 44
Transport of gases to working muscles, 29

V

Ventilation increase, explanation for, 63
Ventilation and oxygen consumption, 60
Ventilatory fatigue and exercise, 71
Ventilatory and lactate (anaerobic) thresholds, 72–73
Ventilatory response to rhythmic exercise, 60
Ventilatory response to static exercise, 60
Ventilatory responses to incremental exercise, 72
Vitamin D in liver, 138

W

Wagner, Wiltz W., 135–152
Waldrop, Tony G., 59–76
Water and protein concentration from development of muscle, 206

Y

Yearly injury summary, 11